Ross and Wilson
Anatomy & Physiology
in Health and Illness
12th Edition

Anne Waugh BSc(Hons) MSc CertEd SRN RNT FHEA

Senior Teaching Fellow and Director of Academic Quality, School of Nursing, Midwifery and Social Care, Edinburgh Napier University, Edinburgh, UK

Allison Grant BSc PhD RGN

Lecturer, Division of Biological and Biomedical Sciences, Glasgow Caledonian University, Glasgow, UK

Illustrations by Graeme Chambers

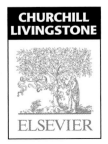

CHURCHILL LIVINGSTONE

ELSEVIER

Edinburgh   London   New York   Oxford   Philadelphia   St Louis   Sydney   Toronto   2014

CHURCHILL
LIVINGSTONE
ELSEVIER

© 2014 Elsevier Ltd. All rights reserved.

Twelfth Edition: 2014
Eleventh Edition: 2010
Tenth Edition: 2006
Ninth Edition: 2002
Eighth Edition: 2001
Seventh Edition: 1998

© 1997 Pearson Professional Limited

© 1990, 1987, 1981, 1973 Longman Group Limited

© 1968, 1966, 1963 E & S Livingstone Ltd.

ISBN 978-0-7020-5325-2
International ISBN 978-0-7020-5326-9
E-ISBN 978-0-7020-5321-4

British Library Cataloguing in Publication Data
A catalogue record for this book is available from the British Library

Library of Congress Cataloging in Publication Data
A catalog record for this book is available from the Library of Congress

Notices
Knowledge and best practice in this field are constantly changing. As new research and experience broaden our understanding, changes in research methods, professional practices, or medical treatment may become necessary.

Practitioners and researchers must always rely on their own experience and knowledge in evaluating and using any information, methods, compounds, or experiments described herein. In using such information or methods they should be mindful of their own safety and the safety of others, including parties for whom they have a professional responsibility.

With respect to any drug or pharmaceutical products identified, readers are advised to check the most current information provided (i) on procedures featured or (ii) by the manufacturer of each product to be administered, to verify the recommended dose or formula, the method and duration of administration, and contraindications. It is the responsibility of practitioners, relying on their own experience and knowledge of their patients, to make diagnoses, to determine dosages and the best treatment for each individual patient, and to take all appropriate safety precautions.

To the fullest extent of the law, neither the Publisher nor the authors, contributors, or editors, assume any liability for any injury and/or damage to persons or property as a matter of products liability, negligence or otherwise, or from any use or operation of any methods, products, instructions, or ideas contained in the material herein.

 ELSEVIER your source for books, journals and multimedia in the health sciences
www.elsevierhealth.com

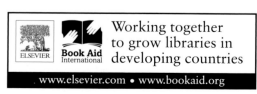

Working together to grow libraries in developing countries

www.elsevier.com • www.bookaid.org

The publisher's policy is to use paper manufactured from sustainable forests

Printed in China

Contents

ELSEVIER evolve

Register today

Additional online resources

To access your Student Resources, visit:

https://evolve.elsevier.com/Waugh/anatomy/

Register today and gain access to:

- **Body Spectrum Electronic Colouring Book** with illustrations you can colour in, to reinforce your learning in an enjoyable way.

- **Animations** to help you to learn in a fun, visual way.

- **Audio pronunciation guide** – you can hear the correct pronunciation of over 1,500 terms to check you have it right.

- **Self-assessment questions** in a variety of different styles give instant feedback to help you measure your knowledge and prepare for tests.

- **Case Studies,** with answers, help you understand real-life A&P scenarios.

- **Illustrations and photographs** bring your learning to life in a colourful way and can help with projects.

- **Weblinks** have been carefully selected to supplement each chapter of the book.

Preface

Ross and Wilson has been a core text for students of anatomy and physiology for over 50 years. This latest edition continues to be aimed at healthcare professionals including nurses, students of nursing, the allied health professions and complementary therapies, paramedics and ambulance technicians, many of whom have found previous editions invaluable. It retains the straightforward approach to the description of body systems and how they work. The anatomy and physiology of health is supplemented by new sections describing common age-related changes to structure and function, before considering the pathology and pathophysiology of some important disorders and diseases.

The human body is presented system by system. The reader must, however, remember that physiology is an integrated subject and that, although the systems are considered in separate chapters, all function cooperatively to maintain health. The first three chapters provide an overview of the body and describe its main structures.

The later chapters are organised into three further sections, reflecting those areas essential for normal body function: communication; intake of raw materials and elimination of waste; and protection and survival. Much of the material for this edition has been revised and rewritten. Many of the diagrams have been revised and, based on reader feedback, more new coloured electron micrographs and photographs have been included to provide detailed and enlightening views of many anatomical features.

This edition is accompanied by a companion website (https://evolve.elsevier.com/Waugh/anatomy/) with over 100 animations and an extensive range of online self-test activities that reflect the content of each chapter. The material in this textbook is also supported by the new 4th edition of the accompanying study guide, which gives students who prefer paper-based activities the opportunity to test their learning and improve their knowledge.

The features from the previous edition have been retained and revised, including learning outcomes, a list of common prefixes, suffixes and roots, and extensive in-text chapter cross-references. The comprehensive glossary has been extended. New sections outlining the implications of normal ageing on the structure and function of body systems have been prepared for this edition. Some biological values, extracted from the text, are presented as an appendix for easy reference. In some cases, slight variations in 'normals' may be found in other texts and used in clinical practice.

Anne Waugh
Allison Grant

Acknowledgements

Authors' Acknowledgements

The twelfth edition of this textbook would not have been possible without the efforts of many people. In preparing this edition, we have continued to build on the foundations established by Kathleen Wilson and we would like to acknowledge her immense contribution to the success of this title.

Thanks are due once again to Graeme Chambers for his patience in the preparation of the new and revised artwork.

We are indebted to the many readers of the eleventh edition for their feedback and constructive comments, many of which have influenced the current revision.

We are also grateful to the staff of Elsevier, particularly Mairi McCubbin, Sheila Black, Caroline Jones for their continuing support.

Thanks are also due to our families, Andy, Michael, Seona and Struan, for their continued patience, support and acceptance of lost evenings and weekends.

Publisher's Acknowledgements

The following figures are reproduced with kind permission.

Figures 1.1, 1.16, 3.15C, 3.19B, 6.6, 8.2, 10.12B, 12.5B, 13.6, 14.1, 14.5, 16.55, 18.18A Steve G Schmeissner/Science Photo Library

Figure 1.6 National Cancer Institute/Science Photo Library

Figure 1.19 Thierry Berrod, Mona Lisa Production/Science Photo Library

Figure 1.21 United Nations (2012) *Population Ageing and Development 2012,* wall chart. Department for Economic and Social Affairs, Population Division, New York.

Figure 3.2B Hermann Schillers, Prof. Dr H Oberleithner, University Hospital of Muenster/Science Photo Library

Figure 3.3 Bill Longcore/Science Photo Library

Figure 3.4 Science Photo Library

Figure 3.5 Dr Torsten Wittmann/Science Photo Library

Figure 3.6 Eye of Science/Science Photo Library

Figure 3.9 Dr Gopal Murti/Science Photo Library

Figures 3.14, 4.4A, 5.3, 12.21 Telser B, Young AG, Baldwin KM (2007) *Elsevier's integrated histology* Mosby: Edinburgh

Figure 3.17 Medimage/Science Photo Library

Figures 3.18B, 4.2, 5.46A, 16.68 Biophoto Associates/Science Photo Library

Figure 3.23B Professors PM Motta, PM Andrews, KR Porter & J Vial/Science Photo Library

Figure 3.24B R Bick, B Poindexter, UT Medical School/Science Photo Library

Figures 3.27, 7.10, 13.18 Young B, Lowe JS, Stevens A et al (2006) *Wheater's functional histology: a text and colour atlas* Edinburgh: Churchill Livingstone

Figure 3.41 Cross SS Ed. 2013 *Underwood's Pathology: a Clinical Approach* 6th edn, Churchill Livingstone: Edinburgh

Figure 4.3 Telser AG, Young JK, Baldwin KM (2007) *Elsevier's integrated histology* Mosby: Edinburgh; Young B, Lowe JS, Stevens A et al (2006) *Wheater's functional histology: a text and colour atlas* Edinburgh: Churchill Livingstone

Figure 4.4D Professors PM Motta & S Correr/Science Photo Library

Figures 4.15, 10.8A, 12.47 CNRI/Science Photo Library

Figures 4.16, 12.26B Eye of Science/Science Photo Library

Figure 5.11C Thomas Deerinck, NCMIR/Science Photo Library

Figure 5.13C Philippe Plailly/Science Photo Library

Figure 5.54 Zephyr/Science Photo Library

Figure 5.56A Alex Barte/Science Photo Library

Figure 5.56B David M Martin MD/Science Photo Library

Figure 7.4 CMEABG – UCBL1, ISM/Science Photo Library

Figures 7.11, 17.1 Standring S et al (2004) *Gray's anatomy: the anatomical basis of clinical practice* 39th edn Churchill Livingstone: Edinburgh

Figure 7.22 Penfield W, Rasmussen T (1950) The cerebral cortex of man. Macmillan, New York. © 1950 Macmillan Publishing Co., renewed 1978 Theodore Rasmussen.

Figure 7.37 Thibodeau GA, Patton KT (2007) *Anthony's Textbook of anatomy and Physiology* 18th edn Mosby: St Louis

Figure 8.27 Martini, Nath & Bartholomew 2012 *Fundamentals of Anatomy and Physiology* 9th edn Pearson (Fig. 17.13, p. 566)

Figures 8.11C, 8.12 Paul Parker/Science Photo Library

Figure 8.25 Sue Ford/Science Photo Library. Reproduced with permission.

Figures 8.26, 9.20, 10.27 Dr P Marazzi/Science Photo Library. Reproduced with permission

Figure 9.14 George Bernard/Science Photo Library

Figure 9.15 John Radcliffe Hospital/Science Photo Library

Figures 9.16, 9.17 Science Photo Library

Figure 10.19 Hossler, Custom Medical Stock Photo/Science Photo Library

Figure 10.29 Dr Tony Brain/Science Photo Library

Figure 11.3 Tony McConnell/Science Photo Library

Figure 13.5 Susumu Nishinaga/Science Photo Library

Figure 13.8 Christopher Riethmuller, Prof. Dr H Oberleithner, University Hospital of Muenster/Science Photo Library

Figure 14.3 Anatomical Travelogue/Science Photo Library

Figure 14.14 James Stevenson/Science Photo Library

Figure 15.1 Biology Media/Science Photo Library

Figure 16.4 Jean-Claude Révy, ISM/Science Photo Library

Figures 16.5B, 16.67 Prof. P Motta/Dept of Anatomy/University 'la Sapienza', Rome/Science Photo Library

Figure 16.7 Innerspace Imaging/Science Photo Library

Figure 16.57 Kent Wood/Science Photo Library

Figure 16.69 Alain Power and SYRED/Science Photo Library

Figure 18.8 Professors PM Motta & J Van Blerkom/Science Photo Library

Figure 18.8B Susumu Nishinaga/Science Photo Library

Common prefixes, suffixes and roots

Prefix/suffix/root	To do with	Examples in the text
a-/an-	lack of	anuria, agranulocyte, asystole, anaemia
ab-	away from	abduct
ad-	towards	adduct
-aemia	of the blood	anaemia, hypoxaemia, uraemia, hypovolaemia
angio-	vessel	angiotensin, haemangioma
ante-	before, in front of	anterior
anti-	against	antidiuretic, anticoagulant, antigen, antimicrobial
baro-	pressure	baroreceptor
-blast	germ, bud	reticuloblast, osteoblast
brady-	slow	bradycardia
broncho-	bronchus	bronchiole, bronchitis, bronchus
card-	heart	cardiac, myocardium, tachycardia
chole-	bile	cholecystokinin, cholecystitis, cholangitis
circum-	around	circumduction
cyto-/-cyte	cell	erythrocyte, cytosol, cytoplasm, cytotoxic
derm-	skin	dermatitis, dermatome, dermis
di-	two	disaccharide, diencephalon
dys-	difficult	dysuria, dyspnoea, dysmenorrhoea, dysplasia
-ema	swelling	oedema, emphysema, lymphoedema
endo-	inner	endocrine, endocytosis, endothelium
enter-	intestine	enterokinase, gastroenteritis
epi-	upon	epimysium, epicardium
erythro-	red	erythrocyte, erythropoietin, erythropoiesis
exo-	outside	exocytosis, exophthalmos
extra-	outside	extracellular, extrapyramidal
-fferent	carry	afferent, efferent
gast-	stomach	gastric, gastrin, gastritis, gastrointestinal
-gen-	origin/production	gene, genome, genetic, antigen, pathogen, allergen
-globin	protein	myoglobin, haemoglobin
haem-	blood	haemostasis, haemorrhage, haemolytic
hetero-	different	heterozygous
homo-	the same, steady	homozygous, homologous

COMMON PREFIXES, SUFFIXES AND ROOTS

Prefix/suffix/root	To do with	Examples in the text
-hydr-	water	dehydration, hydrostatic, hydrocephalus
hepat-	liver	hepatic, hepatitis, hepatomegaly, hepatocyte
hyper-	excess/above	hypertension, hypertrophy, hypercapnia
hypo-	below/under	hypoglycaemia, hypotension, hypovolaemia
intra-	within	intracellular, intracranial, intraocular
-ism	condition	hyperthyroidism, dwarfism, rheumatism
-itis	inflammation	appendicitis, hepatitis, cystitis, gastritis
lact-	milk	lactation, lactic, lacteal
lymph-	lymph tissue	lymphocyte, lymphatic, lymphoedema
lyso-/-lysis	breaking down	lysosome, glycolysis, lysozyme
-mega-	large	megaloblast, acromegaly, splenomegaly, hepatomegaly
micro-	small	microbe, microtubules, microvilli
myo-	muscle	myocardium, myoglobin, myopathy, myosin
neo-	new	neoplasm, gluconeogenesis, neonate
nephro-	kidney	nephron, nephrotic, nephroblastoma, nephrosis
neuro-	nerve	neurone, neuralgia, neuropathy
-oid	resembling	myeloid, sesamoid, sigmoid
olig-	small	oliguria
-ology	study of	cardiology, neurology, physiology
-oma	tumour	carcinoma, melanoma, fibroma
-ophth-	eye	xerophthalmia, ophthalmic, exophthalmos
-ory	referring to	secretory, sensory, auditory, gustatory
os-, osteo-	bone	osteocyte, osteoarthritis, osteoporosis
-path-	disease	pathogenesis, neuropathy, nephropathy
-penia	deficiency of	leukopenia, thrombocytopenia
phag(o)-	eating	phagocyte, phagocytic
-plasm	substance	cytoplasm, neoplasm
pneumo-	lung/air	pneumothorax, pneumonia, pneumotoxic
poly-	many	polypeptide, polyuria, polycythaemia
-rrhagia	excessive flow	menorrhagia
-rrhoea	discharge	dysmenorrhoea, diarrhoea, rhinorrhoea
sarco-	muscle	sarcomere, sarcoplasm
-scler	hard	arteriosclerosis, scleroderma
sub-	under	subphrenic, subarachnoid, sublingual
tachy-	excessively fast	tachycardia, tachypnoea
thrombo-	clot	thrombocyte, thrombosis, thrombin, thrombus
-tox-	poison	toxin, cytotoxic, hepatotoxic
tri-	three	tripeptide, trisaccharide, trigeminal
-uria	urine	anuria, polyuria, haematuria, nocturia, oliguria
vas, vaso-	vessel	vasoconstriction, vas deferens, vascular

Key

Orientation compasses are used beside many of the figures, with paired directional terms above and below and on each side of the compass.

A/P: anterior/posterior. This indicates that the figure has been drawn from above or below using a transverse section, and shows the relationship of the structures to the front/back of the body.
L/R: left/right.
e.g. Figure 16.20

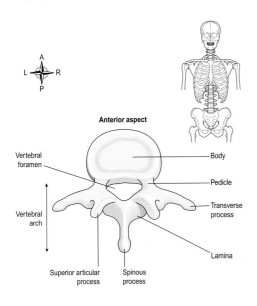

S/I: superior/inferior. This indicates that the figure has been drawn from the front, side or the back using either a sagittal or frontal section, and shows the relationship of the structures to the top/bottom of the body.
P/A: posterior/anterior.
e.g. Figure 7.42

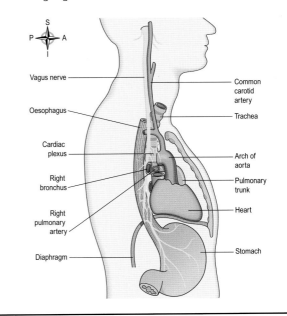

S/I: superior/inferior.
M/L: medial/lateral. This indicates that the figure has been drawn using a sagittal section, and shows the relationship of the structures to the midline of the body.
e.g. Figure 7.35 (posterior view)

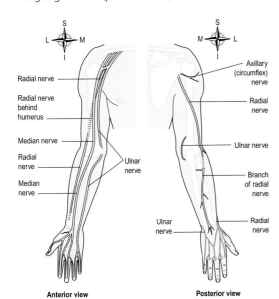

P/D: proximal/distal. This indicates the relationship of the structures to their point of attachment to the body.
L/M: Lateral/medial.
e.g. Figure 16.35

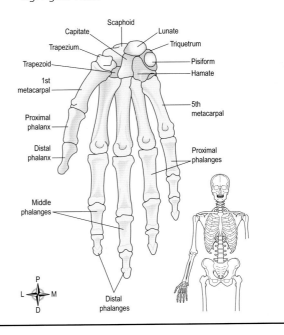

To help you locate bones of the skeleton, some artwork has either a skull or skeleton orientation icon beside it with the bone(s) under discussion clearly coloured.
e.g. Figures 16.17 and 16.39

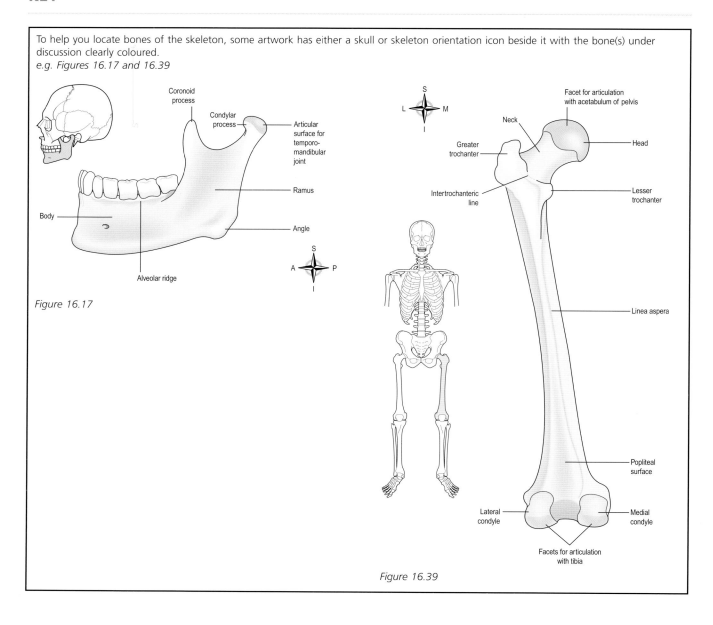

Figure 16.17

Figure 16.39

SECTION 1

The body and its constituents

Introduction to the human body

ANIMATIONS

The human body is rather like a highly technical and sophisticated machine. It operates as a single entity, but is made up of a number of systems that work interdependently. Each system is associated with a specific function that is normally essential for the well-being of the individual. Should one system fail, the consequences can extend to others, and may greatly reduce the ability of the body to function normally. Integrated working of the body systems ensures survival. The human body is therefore complex in both structure and function, and this book uses a systems approach to explain the fundamental structures and processes involved.

Anatomy is the study of the structure of the body and the physical relationships between its constituent parts. *Physiology* is the study of how the body systems work, and the ways in which their integrated activities maintain life and health of the individual. *Pathology* is the study of abnormalities and *pathophysiology* considers how they affect body functions, often causing illness.

Most body systems become less efficient with age. Physiological decline is a normal part of ageing and should not be confused with illness or disease although some conditions do become more common in older life. Maintaining a healthy lifestyle can not only slow the effects of ageing but also protect against illness in later life. The general impact of ageing is outlined in this chapter and the effects on body function are explored in more detail in later chapters.

The final section of this chapter provides a framework for studying diseases, an outline of mechanisms that cause disease and some common disease processes. Building on the normal anatomy and physiology, a systems approach is adopted to consider common illnesses at the end of the later chapters.

Levels of structural complexity

Learning outcome

After studying this section, you should be able to:

■ describe the levels of structural complexity within the body.

Within the body are different levels of structural organisation and complexity. The most fundamental of these is chemical. *Atoms* combine to form *molecules*, of which there is a vast range in the body. The structures, properties and functions of important biological molecules are considered in Chapter 2.

Cells are the smallest independent units of living matter and there are trillions of them within the body. They are too small to be seen with the naked eye, but when magnified using a microscope different types can be

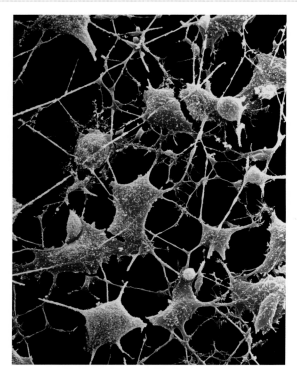

Figure 1.1 Coloured scanning electron micrograph of some nerve cells (neurones).

distinguished by their size, shape and the dyes they absorb when stained in the laboratory. Each cell type has become *specialised*, enabling it to carry out a particular function that contributes to body needs. Figure 1.1 shows some highly magnified nerve cells. The specialised function of nerve cells is to transmit electrical signals (nerve impulses); these are integrated and co-ordinated allowing the millions of nerve cells in the body to provide a rapid and sophisticated communication system. In complex organisms such as the human body, cells with similar structures and functions are found together, forming *tissues*. The structure and functions of cells and tissues are explored in Chapter 3.

Organs are made up of a number of different types of tissue and have evolved to carry out a specific function. Figure 1.2 shows that the stomach is lined by a layer of epithelial tissue and that its wall contains layers of smooth muscle tissue. Both tissues contribute to the functions of the stomach, but in different ways.

Systems consist of a number of organs and tissues that together contribute to one or more survival needs of the body. For example the stomach is one of several organs of the digestive system, which has its own specific function. The human body has several systems, which work interdependently carrying out specific functions. All are required for health. The structure and functions of the body systems are considered in later chapters. ▓ **1.1**

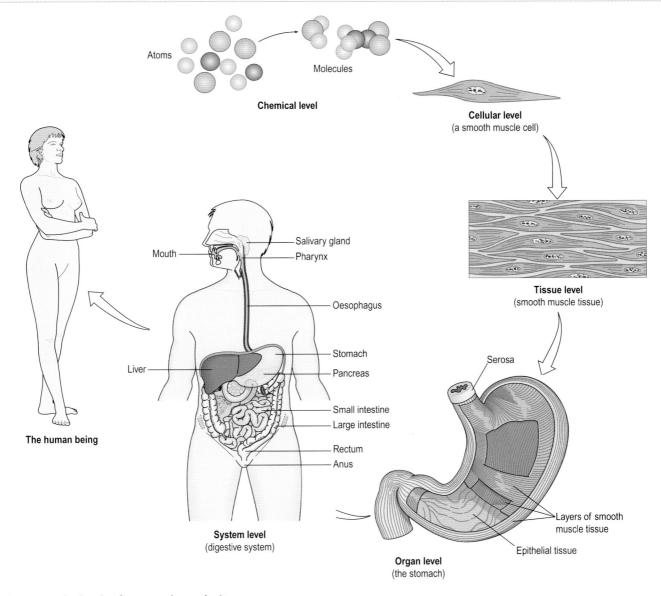

Figure 1.2 The levels of structural complexity.

The internal environment and homeostasis

Learning outcomes

After studying this section, you should be able to:

- define the terms internal environment and homeostasis

- compare and contrast negative and positive feedback control mechanisms

- outline the potential consequences of homeostatic imbalance.

The *external environment* surrounds the body and is the source of oxygen and nutrients required by all body cells. Waste products of cellular activity are eventually excreted into the external environment. The skin (Ch. 14) provides an effective barrier between the body tissues and the consistently changing, often hostile, external environment.

The *internal environment* is the water-based medium in which body cells exist. Cells are bathed in fluid called *interstitial* or *tissue fluid*. They absorb oxygen and nutrients from the surrounding interstitial fluid, which in turn has absorbed these substances from the circulating blood. Conversely, cellular wastes diffuse into the bloodstream via the interstitial fluid, and are carried in the blood to the appropriate excretory organ.

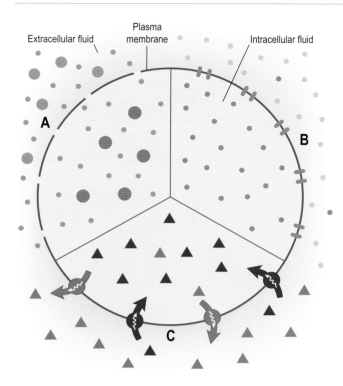

Extracellular fluid

Plasma membrane

Intracellular fluid

A

B

C

Figure 1.3 Role of cell membrane in regulating the composition of intracellular fluid. A. Particle size. **B.** Specific pores and channels. **C.** Pumps and carries.

Each cell is enclosed by its *plasma membrane*, which provides a selective barrier to substances entering or leaving. This property, called *selective permeability*, allows the cell (plasma) membrane (see p. 32) to control the entry or exit of many substances, thereby regulating the composition of its internal environment; several mechanisms are involved. Particle size is important as many small molecules, e.g. water, can pass freely across the membrane while large ones cannot and may therefore be confined to either the interstitial fluid or the intracellular fluid (Fig. 1.3A). Pores or specific channels in the plasma membrane admit certain substances but not others (Fig. 1.3B). The membrane is also studded with specialised pumps or carriers that import or export specific substances (Fig. 1.3C). Selective permeability ensures that the chemical composition of the fluid inside cells is different from the interstitial fluid that bathes them.

Homeostasis

The composition of the internal environment is tightly controlled, and this fairly constant state is called *homeostasis*. Literally, this term means 'unchanging', but in practice it describes a dynamic, ever-changing situation where a multitude of physiological mechanisms and measurements are kept within narrow limits. When this balance is threatened or lost, there is a serious risk to the

Box 1.1 Examples of physiological variables

Core temperature
Water and electrolyte concentrations
pH (acidity or alkalinity) of body fluids
Blood glucose levels
Blood and tissue oxygen and carbon dioxide levels
Blood pressure

well-being of the individual. Box 1.1 lists some important physiological variables maintained within narrow limits by homeostatic control mechanisms.

Control systems

Homeostasis is maintained by control systems that detect and respond to changes in the internal environment. A control system has three basic components: detector, control centre and effector. The *control centre* determines the limits within which the variable factor should be maintained. It receives an input from the *detector*, or sensor, and integrates the incoming information. When the incoming signal indicates that an adjustment is needed, the control centre responds and its output to the *effector* is changed. This is a dynamic process that allows constant readjustment of many physiological variables. Nearly all are controlled by *negative feedback* mechanisms. *Positive feedback* is much less common but important examples include control of uterine contractions during childbirth and blood clotting.

Negative feedback mechanisms (Fig. 1.4)
Negative feedback means that any movement of such a control system away from its normal set point is negated (reversed). If a variable rises, negative feedback brings it down again and if it falls, negative feedback brings it back up to its normal level. The response to a stimulus therefore reverses the effect of that stimulus, keeping the system in a steady state and maintaining homeostasis.

Control of body temperature is similar to the non-physiological example of a domestic central heating system. The thermostat (temperature detector) is sensitive to changes in room temperature (variable factor). The thermostat is connected to the boiler control unit (control centre), which controls the boiler (effector). The thermostat constantly compares the information from the detector with the preset temperature and, when necessary, adjustments are made to alter the room temperature. When the thermostat detects the room temperature is low, it switches the boiler on. The result is output of heat by the boiler, warming the room. When the preset temperature is reached, the system is reversed. The thermostat detects the higher room temperature and turns the

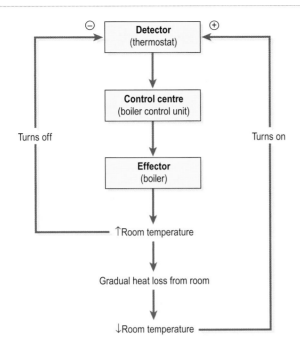

Figure 1.4 Example of a negative feedback mechanism: control of room temperature by a domestic boiler.

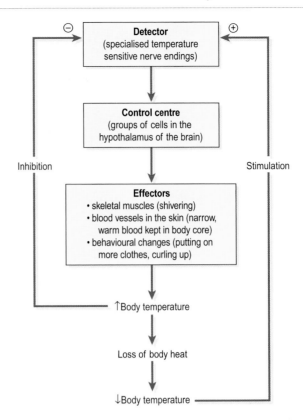

Figure 1.5 Example of a physiological negative feedback mechanism: control of body temperature.

boiler off. Heat production from the boiler stops and the room slowly cools as heat is lost. This series of events is a negative feedback mechanism that enables continuous self-regulation, or control, of a variable factor within a narrow range.

Body temperature is one example of a physiological variable controlled by negative feedback (Fig. 1.5). When body temperature falls below the preset level (close to 37°C), this is detected by specialised temperature sensitive nerve endings in the hypothalamus of the brain, where the body's temperature control centre is located. This centre then activates mechanisms that raise body temperature (effectors). These include:

- stimulation of skeletal muscles causing shivering
- narrowing of the blood vessels in the skin reducing the blood flow to, and heat loss from, the peripheries
- behavioural changes, e.g. we put on more clothes or curl up.

When body temperature rises within the normal range again, the temperature sensitive nerve endings are no longer stimulated, and their signals to the hypothalamus stop. Therefore, shivering stops and blood flow to the peripheries returns to normal.

Most of the homeostatic controls in the body use negative feedback mechanisms to prevent sudden and serious changes in the internal environment. Many more of these are explained in the following chapters.

Positive feedback mechanisms

There are only a few of these *cascade* or *amplifier* systems in the body. In positive feedback mechanisms, the stimulus progressively increases the response, so that as long as the stimulus is continued the response is progressively amplified. Examples include blood clotting and uterine contractions during labour.

During labour, contractions of the uterus are stimulated by the hormone *oxytocin*. These force the baby's head into the uterine cervix stimulating stretch receptors there. In response to this, more oxytocin is released, further strengthening the contractions and maintaining labour. After the baby is born the stimulus (stretching of the cervix) is no longer present so the release of oxytocin stops (see Fig. 9.5, p. 221).

Homeostatic imbalance

This arises when the fine control of a variable factor in the internal environment is inadequate and its level falls outside the normal range. If the control system cannot maintain homeostasis, an abnormal state develops that may threaten health, or even life itself. Many such situations, including effects of abnormalities of the physiological variables in Box 1.1, are explained in later chapters.

Survival needs of the body

By convention, body systems are described separately in the study of anatomy and physiology, but in reality they work interdependently. This section provides an introduction to body activities, linking them to survival needs (Table 1.1). The later chapters build on this framework, exploring human structure and functions in health and illness using a systems approach.

Communication

In this section, transport and communication are considered. Transport systems ensure that all body cells have access to the very many substances required to support them, as well as providing a means of excretion of wastes; this involves the blood and the cardiovascular and lymphatic systems.

All communication systems involve receiving, collating and responding to appropriate information. There are different systems for communicating with the internal and external environments. Internal communication involves mainly the nervous and endocrine systems; these are important in the maintenance of homeostasis and regulation of vital body functions. Communication with the external environment involves the special senses, and verbal and non-verbal activities, and all of these also depend on the nervous system.

Transport systems

Blood (Ch. 4)

The blood transports substances around the body through a large network of blood vessels. In adults the body contains 5 to 6 litres of blood. It consists of two parts – a fluid called *plasma* and *blood cells* suspended in the plasma.

Plasma. This is mainly water with a wide range of substances dissolved or suspended in it. These include:

- nutrients absorbed from the alimentary canal
- oxygen absorbed from the lungs
- chemical substances synthesised by body cells, e.g. hormones
- waste materials produced by all cells to be eliminated from the body by excretion.

Blood cells. There are three distinct groups, classified according to their functions (Fig. 1.6).

Table 1.1 Survival needs and related body activities

Survival need	Body activities
Communication	Transport systems: blood, cardiovascular system, lymphatic system Internal communication: nervous system, endocrine system External communication: special senses, verbal and non-verbal communication
Intake of raw materials and elimination of waste	Intake of oxygen Ingestion of nutrients (eating) Elimination of wastes: carbon dioxide, urine, faeces
Protection and survival	Protection against the external environment: skin Defence against microbial infection: resistance and immunity Body movement Survival of the species: reproduction and transmission of inherited characteristics

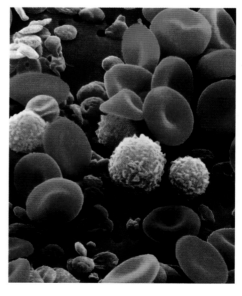

Figure 1.6 Coloured scanning electron micrograph of blood showing red blood cells, white blood cells (yellow) and platelets (pink).

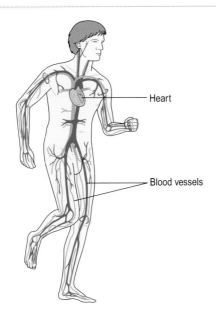

Figure 1.7 The circulatory system.

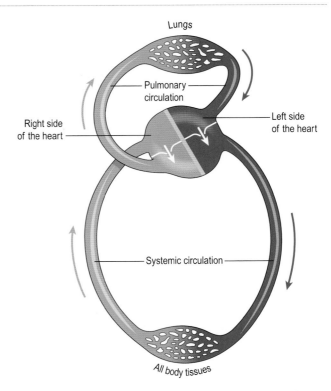

Figure 1.8 Circulation of the blood through the heart and the pulmonary and systemic circulations.

Erythrocytes (red blood cells) transport oxygen and, to a lesser extent, carbon dioxide between the lungs and all body cells.

Leukocytes (white blood cells) are mainly concerned with protection of the body against infection and foreign substances. There are several types of leukocytes, which carry out their protective functions in different ways. These cells are larger and less numerous than erythrocytes.

Platelets (thrombocytes) are tiny cell fragments that play an essential part in blood clotting.

Cardiovascular system (Ch. 5)
This consists of a network of blood vessels and the heart (Fig. 1.7). **1.2**

Blood vessels. There are three types:
- *arteries*, which carry blood away from the heart
- *veins*, which return blood to the heart
- *capillaries*, which link the arteries and veins.

Capillaries are tiny blood vessels with very thin walls consisting of only one layer of cells, which enables exchange of substances between the blood and body tissues, e.g. nutrients, oxygen and cellular waste products. Blood vessels form a network that transports blood to:
- the lungs (*pulmonary circulation*) where oxygen is absorbed from the air in the lungs and, at the same time, carbon dioxide is excreted from the blood into the air
- cells in all other parts of the body (*general* or *systemic circulation*) (Fig. 1.8).

Heart. The heart is a muscular sac with four chambers, which pumps blood round the body and maintains the blood pressure.

The heart muscle is not under conscious (voluntary) control. At rest, the heart contracts, or beats, between 65 and 75 times per minute. The rate is greatly increased when body oxygen requirements are increased, e.g. during exercise.

The rate at which the heart beats can be counted by taking the *pulse*. The pulse can be felt most easily where a superficial artery can be pressed gently against a bone, usually at the wrist.

Lymphatic system (Ch. 6)
The lymphatic system (Fig. 1.9) consists of a series of *lymph vessels*, which begin as blind-ended tubes in the interstitial spaces between the blood capillaries and tissue cells. Structurally they are similar to veins and blood capillaries but the pores in the walls of the lymph capillaries are larger than those of the blood capillaries. *Lymph* is tissue fluid that also contains material drained from tissue spaces, including plasma proteins and, sometimes, bacteria or cell debris. It is transported along lymph vessels and returned to the bloodstream near the heart.

There are collections of *lymph nodes* situated at various points along the length of the lymph vessels. Lymph is filtered as it passes through the lymph nodes, removing microbes and other materials.

The lymphatic system also provides the sites for formation and maturation of *lymphocytes*, the white blood cells involved in immunity (Ch. 15).

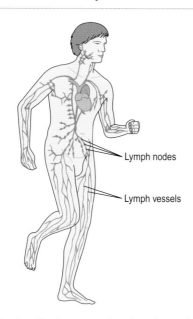

Figure 1.9 The lymphatic system: lymph nodes and vessels.

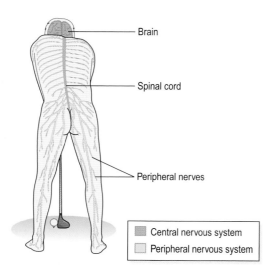

Figure 1.10 The nervous system.

Internal communication

This is carried out through the activities of the nervous and endocrine systems.

Nervous system (Ch. 7)

The nervous system is a rapid communication system. The main components are shown in Figure 1.10. The *central nervous system* consists of:

- the *brain*, situated inside the skull
- the *spinal cord*, which extends from the base of the skull to the lumbar region (lower back). It is protected from injury as it lies within the bones of the spinal column.

The *peripheral nervous system* is a network of nerve fibres, which are either:

- *sensory* or *afferent* nerves that transmit signals from the body to the brain, or
- *motor* or *efferent* nerves, which transmit signals from the brain to the effector organs, such as muscles and glands.

The *somatic* (*common*) *senses* are pain, touch, heat and cold, and these sensations arise following stimulation of specialised sensory receptors at nerve endings found throughout the skin.

Nerve endings within muscles and joints respond to changes in the position and orientation of the body, maintaining posture and balance. Yet other sensory receptors are activated by stimuli in internal organs and control vital body functions, e.g. heart rate, respiratory rate and blood pressure. Stimulation of any of these receptors sets up impulses that are conducted to the brain in sensory (afferent) nerves.

Communication along nerve fibres (cells) is by electrical impulses that are generated when nerve endings are stimulated. Nerve impulses (action potentials) travel at great speed, so responses are almost immediate, making rapid and fine adjustments to body functions possible.

Communication between nerve cells is also required, since more than one nerve is involved in the chain of events occurring between the initial stimulus and the reaction to it. Nerves communicate with each other by releasing a chemical (the *neurotransmitter*) into tiny gaps between them. The neurotransmitter quickly travels across the gap and either stimulates or inhibits the next nerve cell, thus ensuring the message is transmitted.

Sensory nerves transmit impulses from the body to appropriate parts of the brain, where the incoming information is analysed and collated. The brain responds by sending impulses along motor (efferent) nerves to the appropriate effector organ(s). In this way, many aspects of body function are continuously monitored and adjusted, usually by negative feedback control, and usually subconsciously, e.g. regulation of blood pressure.

Reflex actions are fast, involuntary, and usually protective motor responses to specific stimuli. They include:

- withdrawal of a finger from a very hot surface
- constriction of the pupil in response to bright light
- control of blood pressure.

Endocrine system (Ch. 9)

The endocrine system consists of a number of discrete glands situated in different parts of the body. They synthesise and secrete chemical messengers called *hormones* that circulate round the body in the blood. Hormones stimulate *target glands* or *tissues*, influencing metabolic and other cellular activities and regulating body growth and maturation. Endocrine glands detect and respond to levels of particular substances in the blood, including specific hormones. Changes in blood hormone levels are usually controlled by negative feedback mechanisms (see Figs 1.5 and 9.8). The endocrine system provides slower and more precise control of body functions than the nervous system.

In addition to the glands that have a primary endocrine function, it is now known that many other tissues also secrete hormones as a secondary function; some of these are explored further in Chapter 9.

Communication with the external environment

Special senses (Ch. 8)

Stimulation of specialized receptors in sensory organs or tissues gives rise to the sensations of sight, hearing, balance, smell and taste. Although these senses are usually considered to be separate and different from each other, one sense is rarely used alone (Fig. 1.11). For example, when the smell of smoke is perceived then other senses such as sight and sound are used to try and locate the source of a fire. Similarly, taste and smell are closely associated in the enjoyment, or otherwise, of food. The brain collates incoming information with information from the memory and initiates a response by setting up electrical impulses in motor (efferent) nerves to effector organs, muscles and glands. Such responses enable the individual to escape from a fire, or to subconsciously prepare the digestive system for eating.

Verbal communication

Sound is produced in the larynx when expired air coming from the lungs passes through and vibrates the *vocal cords* (see Fig. 10.8) during expiration. In humans, recognisable sounds produced by co-ordinated contraction of the muscles of the throat and cheeks, and movements of the tongue and lower jaw, is known as *speech*.

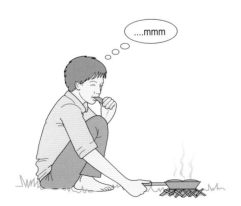

….mmm

Figure 1.11 Combined use of the special senses: vision, hearing, smell and taste.

Non-verbal communication

Posture and movements are often associated with non-verbal communication, e.g. nodding the head and shrugging the shoulders. The skeleton provides the bony framework of the body (Ch. 16), and movement takes place at joints between bones. Skeletal muscles move the skeleton and attach bones to one another, spanning one or more joints in between. They are stimulated by the part of the nervous system under voluntary (conscious) control. Some non-verbal communication, e.g. changes in facial expression, may not involve the movement of bones.

Intake of raw materials and elimination of waste

This section considers substances taken into and excreted from the body, which involves the respiratory, digestive and urinary systems. Oxygen, water and food are taken in, and carbon dioxide, urine and faeces are excreted.

Intake of oxygen

Oxygen gas makes up about 21% of atmospheric air. A continuous supply is essential for human life because it is needed for most chemical activities that take place in the body cells. Oxygen is necessary for the series of chemical reactions that result in the release of energy from nutrients.

The upper respiratory system carries air between the nose and the lungs during breathing (Ch. 10). Air passes through a system of passages consisting of the pharynx (throat, also part of the digestive tract), the larynx (voice box), the trachea, two bronchi (one bronchus to each lung) and a large number of bronchial passages (Fig. 1.12). These end in alveoli, millions of tiny air sacs in each lung. They are surrounded by a network of tiny capillaries and are the sites where vital gas exchange between the lungs and the blood takes place (Fig. 1.13). ▐ **1.3**

Nitrogen, which makes up about 80% of atmospheric air, is breathed in and out, but it cannot be used by the body in gaseous form. The nitrogen needed by the body is obtained by eating protein-containing foods, mainly meat and fish.

Ingestion of nutrients (eating)

Nutrition is considered in Chapter 11. A balanced diet is important for health and provides *nutrients*, substances that are absorbed, usually following digestion, and promote body function, including cell building, growth and repair. Nutrients include water, carbohydrates, proteins, fats, vitamins and mineral salts. They serve vital functions including:

- maintenance of water balance within the body
- provision of fuel for energy production, mainly carbohydrates and fats

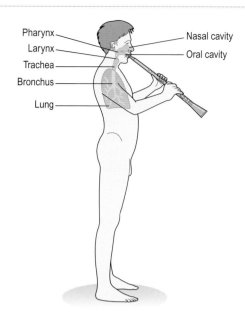

Figure 1.12 The respiratory system.

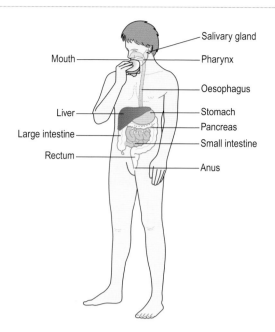

Figure 1.14 The digestive system.

- provision of the building blocks for synthesis of large and complex molecules, needed by the body.

Digestion

The digestive system evolved because food is chemically complex and seldom in a form that body cells can use. Its function is to break down, or digest, food so that it can be absorbed into the circulation and then used by body cells. The digestive system consists of the alimentary canal and accessory organs (Fig. 1.14).

Alimentary canal. This is essentially a tube that begins at the mouth and continues through the pharynx, oesophagus, stomach, small and large intestines, rectum and anus. ▉ **1.4**

Accessory organs. These are the *salivary glands, pancreas* and *liver* (Fig. 1.14), which lie outside the alimentary canal. The salivary glands and pancreas synthesise and release *digestive enzymes*, which are involved in the chemical breakdown of food while the liver secretes

bile; these substances enter the alimentary canal through connecting ducts.

Metabolism

This is the sum total of the chemical activity in the body. It consists of two groups of processes:

- *anabolism*, building or synthesising large and complex substances
- *catabolism*, breaking down substances to provide energy and raw materials for anabolism, and substances for excretion as waste.

The sources of energy are mainly dietary carbohydrates and fats. However, if these are in short supply, proteins are used.

Elimination of wastes

Carbon dioxide

This is a waste product of cellular metabolism. Because it dissolves in body fluids to make an acid solution, it must be excreted in appropriate amounts to maintain pH (acidity or alkalinity) within the normal range. The main route of carbon dioxide excretion is through the lungs during expiration.

Urine

This is formed by the kidneys, which are part of the urinary system (Ch. 13). The organs of the urinary system are shown in Figure 1.15. Urine consists of water and waste products mainly of protein breakdown, e.g. urea. Under the influence of hormones from the endocrine system, the kidneys regulate water balance. They also play a role in maintaining blood pH within the normal

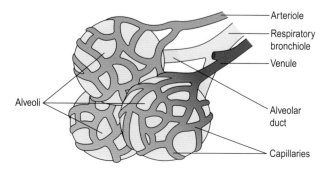

Figure 1.13 Alveoli: the site of gas exchange in the lungs.

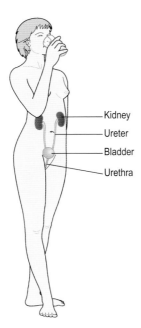

Figure 1.15 The urinary system.

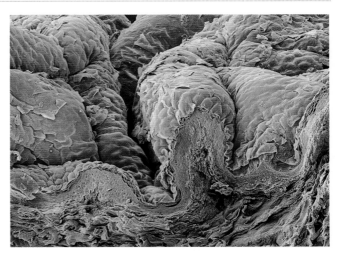

Figure 1.16 Coloured scanning electron micrograph of the skin.

range. The bladder stores urine until it is excreted during *micturition*. ⬛ **1.5**

Faeces

The waste materials from the digestive system are excreted as faeces during *defaecation*. They contain indigestible food residue that remains in the alimentary canal because it cannot be absorbed and large numbers of microbes.

Protection and survival

Body needs and related activities explored in this section are: protection against the external environment, defence against infection, movement and survival of the species.

Protection against the external environment

The skin (Fig. 1.16) forms a barrier against invasion by microbes, chemicals and dehydration (Ch. 14). It consists of two layers: the epidermis and the dermis.

The *epidermis* lies superficially and is composed of several layers of cells that grow towards the surface from its deepest layer. The skin surface consists of dead flattened cells that are constantly being rubbed off and replaced from below. The epidermis provides the barrier between the moist internal environment and the dry atmosphere of the external environment.

The *dermis* contains tiny sweat glands that have little canals or ducts, leading to the surface. Hairs grow from follicles in the dermis. The dermis is rich in sensory nerve endings sensitive to pain, temperature and touch. It is a vast organ that constantly provides the central nervous

system with sensory input from the body surfaces. The skin also plays an important role in the regulation of body temperature.

Defence against infection

The body has many means of self-protection from invaders, which confer resistance and/or immunity (Ch. 15). They are divided into two categories: specific and non-specific defence mechanisms.

Non-specific defence mechanisms

These are effective against any invaders. The skin protects most of the body surface. There are also other protective features at body surfaces, e.g. sticky *mucus* secreted by mucous membranes traps microbes and other foreign materials. Some body fluids contain *antimicrobial substances*, e.g. gastric juice contains hydrochloric acid, which kills most ingested microbes. Following successful invasion other non-specific processes that counteract potentially harmful consequences may take place, including the inflammatory response (Ch. 15).

Specific defence mechanisms

The body generates a specific (immune) response against any substance it identifies as foreign. Such substances are called *antigens* and include:

- pollen from flowers and plants
- bacteria and other microbes
- cancer cells or transplanted tissue cells.

Following exposure to an antigen, lifelong immunity against further invasion by the same antigen often develops. Over a lifetime, an individual gradually builds up immunity to millions of antigens. *Allergic reactions* are abnormally powerful immune responses to an antigen that usually poses no threat to the body, e.g. the effects of pollen in people with hay fever.

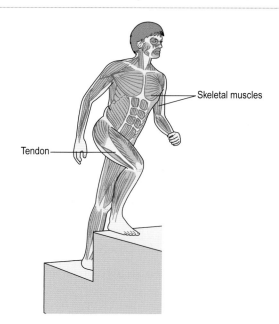

Figure 1.17 The skeletal muscles.

Movement

Movement of the whole body, or parts of it, is essential for many body activities, e.g. obtaining food, avoiding injury and reproduction.

Most body movement is under conscious (voluntary) control. Exceptions include protective movements that are carried out before the individual is aware of them, e.g. the reflex action of removing one's finger from a very hot surface.

The musculoskeletal system includes the *bones* of the skeleton, *skeletal muscles* and *joints*. The skeleton provides the rigid body framework and movement takes place at joints between two or more bones. Skeletal muscles (Fig. 1.17), under the control of the voluntary nervous system, maintain posture and balance, and move the skeleton. A brief description of the skeleton is given in Chapter 3, and a more detailed account of bones, muscles and joints is presented in Chapter 16.

Survival of the species

Survival of a species is essential to prevent its extinction. This requires the transmission of inherited characteristics to a new generation by reproduction.

Transmission of inherited characteristics

Individuals with the most advantageous genetic make-up are most likely to survive, reproduce and pass their genes on to the next generation. This is the basis of natural selection, i.e. 'survival of the fittest'. Chapter 17 explores the transmission of inherited characteristics.

Reproduction (Ch. 18)

Successful reproduction is essential in order to ensure the continuation of a species and its genetic characteristics

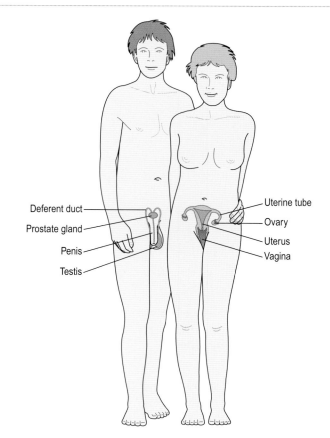

Figure 1.18 The reproductive systems: male and female.

from one generation to the next. Ova (eggs) are produced by two *ovaries* situated in the female pelvis (Fig. 1.18). During a female's reproductive years only one ovum usually is released at about monthly intervals and it travels towards the *uterus* in the *uterine tube*. In males, spermatozoa are produced in large numbers by the two *testes*, situated in the *scrotum*. From each testis, spermatozoa pass through the *deferent duct* (vas deferens) to the *urethra*. During sexual intercourse (coitus) the spermatozoa are deposited in the *vagina*.

They then swim upwards through the uterus and fertilise the ovum in the uterine tube. Fertilisation (Fig. 1.19) occurs when a female egg cell or *ovum* fuses with a male sperm cell or *spermatozoon*. The fertilised ovum (*zygote*) then passes into the uterus, embeds itself in the uterine wall and grows to maturity during pregnancy or *gestation*, in about 40 weeks.

When the ovum is not fertilised it is expelled from the uterus along with the uterine lining as bleeding, known as *menstruation*. In females, the *reproductive cycle* consists of phases associated with changes in hormone levels involving the endocrine system.

A cycle takes around 28 days and they take place continuously between *puberty* and the *menopause*, except during pregnancy. At *ovulation* (see Fig. 18.10, p. 457) an ovum is released from one of the ovaries mid-cycle. There

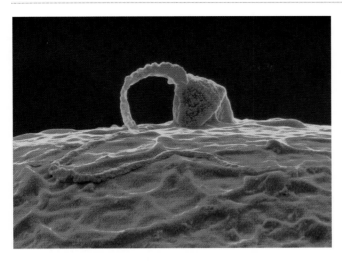

Figure 1.19 Coloured scanning electron micrograph showing fertilisation (spermatozoon: orange, ovum: blue).

is no such cycle in the male but hormones, similar to those of the female, are involved in the production and maturation of spermatozoa.

Introduction to ageing

Learning outcomes

After studying this section, you should be able to:

■ List the main features of ageing

■ Outline the implications of ageing human populations.

After birth many changes occur as the body grows and develops to maturity. The peak of mature physiological function is often relatively short lived, as age-related changes begin to impair performance; for example, kidney function begins to decline from about 30 years of age. At both extremes of the lifespan many aspects of body function are less efficient, for example temperature regulation is less effective in infants and older adults.

Maturity of most body organs occurs during puberty and maximal efficiency during early adulthood. Most organs are able to repair and replace their tissues, with the notable exceptions of the brain and myocardium (heart muscle). At maturity, many organs have considerable functional reserve, or 'spare capacity', which usually declines gradually thereafter. The functional reserve means that considerable loss of function must occur before physiological changes are evident. Alterations in body function during older life need careful assessment as ageing is generally associated with decreasing efficiency of body organs and/or increasing frailty. Although a predisposing factor for some conditions, the ageing process is not accompanied by any specific illnesses or diseases.

The process of ageing is poorly understood although it affects people in different ways. There is no single cause known although many theories have been proposed and there is enormous individual variation in the rate of ageing. The lifespan of an individual is influenced by many factors, some of which are hereditary (Ch. 17) and outwith individual control. Others not readily susceptible to individual influence include poverty, which is associated with poor health. However peoples' lifestyle choices may also strongly influence longevity, e.g. lack of exercise, cigarette smoking and alcohol misuse contribute to a shorter lifespan.

Several common age-associated changes that occur in particular organs and systems are well recognised and include greying hair and wrinkling of the skin. Further examples are shown in Figure 1.20 and these and others are highlighted together with their physiological and, sometimes, clinical consequences at the end of the physiology section in relevant chapters. Increasing age is a risk factor for some diseases, e.g. most cancers, coronary heart disease and dementia.

The World Health Organisation (WHO, 2012) predicts that the number of people aged 60 years and over globally will increase from 605 million to 2 billion between 2000 and 2050 (Fig. 1.21). The 20th century saw the proportion of older people increasing in high income countries. Over the next 40 years, this trend is predicted to follow in most areas of the world including low- and middle-income countries. Increasing life expectancy will impact on health care, and the role of prevention of and early interventions in ill-health will become increasingly important.

Physiological changes

Nervous system
- Motor control of precise movement diminishes
- Conduction rate of nerve impulses becomes slower

Special senses
- Ear – hair cells become damaged
- Eye – stiffening of the lens; cataracts (opacity of the lens)
- Taste and smell – diminished perception

Respiratory system
- Less mucus produced
- Stiffening of ribcage
- Decline in respiratory reflexes

Cardiovascular system
- Stiffening of blood vessel walls
- Reduction in cardiac function and efficiency

Endocrine system
- Pancreatic islet cells – decline in function of β-cells
- Adrenal cortex – oestrogen deficiency in post-menopausal women

Digestive system
- Loss of teeth
- Peristalsis reduced
- Decline in liver mass

Urinary system
- Fewer nephrons, lower glomerular filtration rate

Resistance and immunity
- Declines

Musculoskeletal system
- Thinning of bone
- Stiffening of cartilage and other connective tissue

Reproductive systems
- Female menopause

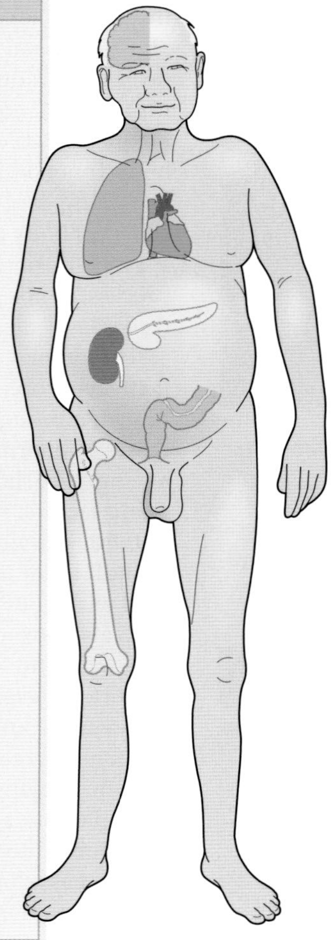

Common consequences

Nervous system
- Takes longer to carry out motor action, more prone to falls
- Poorer control of e.g. vasodilation, vasoconstriction and baroreceptor reflex

Special senses
- Hearing impairment
- Difficulty reading without glasses; good light needed for vision
- Food may taste bland, smells e.g. burning may go unnoticed

Respiratory system
- Increased risk of infections
- Reduced respiratory minute volume
- Less able to respond to changes in arterial blood gas levels

Cardiovascular system
- Increased blood pressure, increased risk of vessel rupture and haemorrhage
- Reduction in cardiac output and cardiac reserve

Endocrine system
- More prone to type 2 diabetes, especially if overweight

Digestive system
- Difficulty chewing
- Constipation
- Reduced liver metabolism with increased risk of e.g. drug toxicity

Urinary system
- Less able to regulate fluid balance
- More prone to effects of dehydration and overload

Resistance and immunity
- Increased risk of infection
- Longer healing times

Musculoskeletal system
- Increased risk of fractures
- Stiffening of joints
- Osteoporosis

Reproductive systems
- Cessation of female reproductive ability
- Reduced fertility in males

Figure 1.20 Effects of ageing on body systems.

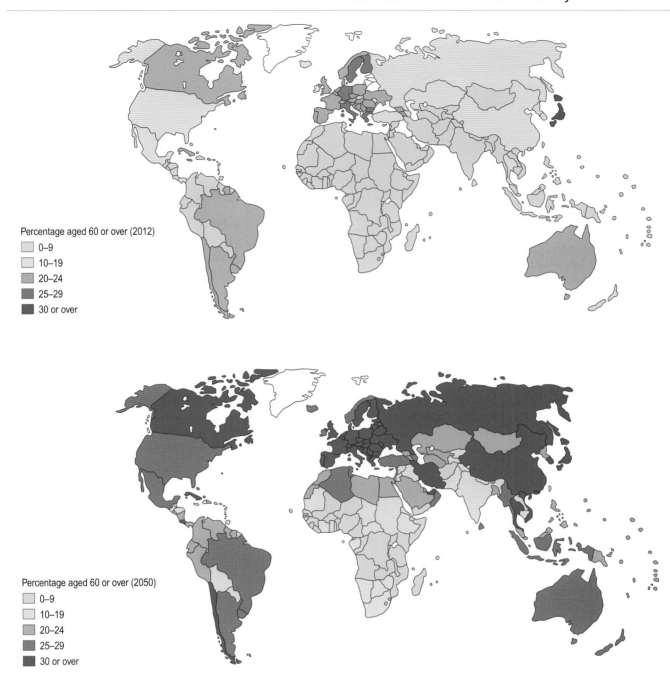

Figure 1.21 Global ageing trends.

Introduction to the study of illness

Learning outcomes

After studying this section, you should be able to:

■ list mechanisms that commonly cause disease

■ define the terms aetiology, pathogenesis and prognosis

■ name some common disease processes.

In order to understand the specific diseases described in later chapters, knowledge of the relevant anatomy and physiology is necessary, as well as familiarity with the pathological processes outlined below.

There are many different illnesses, disorders and diseases, which vary from minor, but often very troublesome conditions, to the very serious. The study of abnormalities can be made much easier when a systematic approach is adopted. In order to achieve this in later chapters where specific diseases are explained, the headings shown in Box 1.2 will be used as a guide. Causes (*aetiology*) are outlined first when there are clear links between them and the effects of the abnormality (*pathogenesis*).

Aetiology

Diseases are usually caused by one or more of a limited number of mechanisms that may include:

- genetic abnormalities, either inherited or acquired
- infection by micro-organisms, e.g. bacteria, viruses, microbes or parasites, e.g. worms
- chemicals
- ionising radiation
- physical trauma
- degeneration, e.g. excessive use or ageing.

In some diseases more than one of the aetiological factors listed above is involved, while in others, no specific cause has been identified and these may be described as *essential*, *idiopathic* or *spontaneous*. Although the precise cause

of a disease may not be known, *predisposing* (*risk*) *factors* are usually identifiable.

Pathogenesis

The main processes causing illness or disease are outlined below. Box 1.3 contains a glossary of disease-associated terminology.

Inflammation. (p. 377) – This is a tissue response to any kind of tissue damage such as trauma or infection. Inflammatory conditions are recognised by the suffix -itis, e.g. appendicitis.

Tumours. (p. 55) – These arise when abnormal cells escape body surveillance and proliferate. The rate of their production exceeds that of normal cell death causing a mass to develop. Tumours are recognised by the suffix -oma, e.g. carcinoma.

Abnormal immune mechanisms. (p. 385) – These are responses of the normally protective immune system that cause undesirable effects.

Thrombosis, embolism and infarction. (p. 119) – These are the effects and consequences of abnormal changes in the blood and/or blood vessel walls.

Degeneration. – This is often associated with normal ageing but may also arise prematurely when structures deteriorate causing impaired function.

Metabolic abnormalities. – These cause undesirable metabolic effects, e.g. diabetes mellitus, page 236.

Genetic abnormalities. – These may be either inherited (e.g. phenylketonuria, p. 446) or caused by environmental factors such as exposure to ionising radiation (p. 55).

Box 1.2 Suggested framework for understanding diseases

Aetiology: cause of the disease
Pathogenesis: the nature of the disease process and its effect on normal body functioning
Complications: other consequences which might arise if the disease progresses
Prognosis: the likely outcome

Box 1.3 Glossary of terminology associated with disease

Acute: a disease with sudden onset often requiring urgent treatment (compare with chronic)
Acquired: a disorder which develops any time after birth (compare with congenital)
Chronic: a long-standing disorder which cannot usually be cured (compare with acute)
Communicable: a disease that can be transmitted (spread) from one individual to another
Congenital: a disorder which one is born with (compare with acquired)
Iatrogenic: a condition that results from healthcare intervention
Sign: an abnormality seen or measured by people other than the patient
Symptom: an abnormality described by the patient
Syndrome: a collection of signs and symptoms which tend to occur together

Further reading

World Health Organization 2012 Good health adds life to years. Global brief for World Health Day 2012. WHO 2012, Geneva. Available online at http://whqlibdoc.who.int/hq/2012/WHO_DCO_WHD_2012.2_eng.pdf (p. 10) Accessed 3 September 2013

 For a range of self-assessment exercises on the topics in this chapter, visit Evolve online resources: https://evolve.elsevier.com/Waugh/anatomy/

Introduction to the chemistry of life

ANIMATIONS

Because living tissues are composed of chemical building blocks, the study of anatomy and physiology depends upon some understanding of biochemistry – the chemistry of life. This chapter introduces core concepts in chemistry that will underpin the remaining chapters in this book.

Atoms, molecules and compounds

Learning outcomes

After studying this section, you should be able to:

- define the following terms: atomic number, atomic weight, isotope, molecular weight, ion, electrolyte, pH, acid and alkali
- describe the structure of an atom
- discuss the types of bond that hold molecules together
- outline the concept of molar concentration
- explain the importance of buffers in the regulation of pH.

All matter in our universe is built of particles called *atoms*. An *element* contains only one type of atom, e.g. carbon, sulphur or hydrogen. Substances containing two or more types of atom combined are called *compounds*. For instance, water is a compound containing both hydrogen and oxygen atoms.

There are 92 naturally occurring elements, but the wide variety of compounds making up living tissues are composed almost entirely of only four: carbon, hydrogen, oxygen and nitrogen. Small amounts (about 4% of body weight) of others are present, including sodium, potassium, calcium and phosphorus.

Atomic structure

Atoms are mainly empty space, with a tiny central nucleus containing *protons* and *neutrons* surrounded by clouds of tiny orbiting *electrons* (Fig. 2.1). Neutrons carry no electrical charge, but protons are positively charged, and electrons are negatively charged. Because atoms contain equal numbers of protons and electrons, they carry no net charge.

These subatomic particles differ also in terms of their mass. Electrons are so small that their mass is negligible, but the bigger neutrons and protons carry one atomic mass unit each. The physical characteristics of electrons, protons and neutrons are summarised in Table 2.1.

Atomic number and atomic weight

What makes one element different from another is the number of protons in the nuclei of its atoms (Fig. 2.2). This

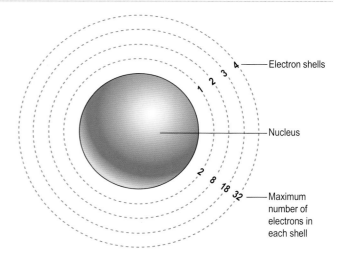

Figure 2.1 The atom, showing the nucleus and four electron shells.

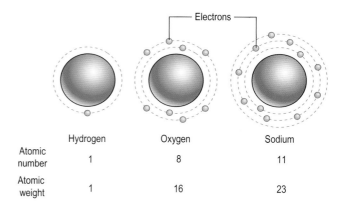

Figure 2.2 The atomic structures of the elements hydrogen, oxygen and sodium.

	Hydrogen	Oxygen	Sodium
Atomic number	1	8	11
Atomic weight	1	16	23

Table 2.1 Characteristics of subatomic particles

Particle	Mass	Electric charge
Proton	1 unit	1 positive
Neutron	1 unit	Neutral
Electron	Negligible	1 negative

is called the *atomic number* and each element has its own atomic number, unique to its atoms. For instance, hydrogen has only one proton per nucleus, oxygen has eight and sodium has 11. The atomic numbers of hydrogen, oxygen and sodium are therefore 1, 8 and 11, respectively. The *atomic weight* of an element is the sum of the protons and neutrons in the atomic nucleus.

The electrons are shown in Figure 2.1 as though they orbit in concentric rings round the nucleus. These shells represent the different energy levels of the atom's electrons, not their physical positions. The first energy level can hold only two electrons and is filled first. The second energy level can hold only eight electrons and is filled next. The third and subsequent energy levels hold increasing numbers of electrons, each containing more than the preceding level.

When the atom's outer electron shell does not contain a stable number of electrons, the atom is *reactive* and can donate, receive or share electrons with one or more other atoms to achieve stability. The great number of possible combinations of different types of atom yields the wide range of substances of which the world is built and on which biology is based. This is described more fully in the section discussing molecules and compounds.

Isotopes. These are atoms of an element in which there is a *different number of neutrons in the nucleus*. This does not affect the electrical activity of these atoms because neutrons carry no electrical charge, but it does affect their atomic weight. For example, there are three forms of the hydrogen atom. The most common form has one proton in the nucleus and one orbiting electron. Another form (*deuterium*) has one proton and one neutron in the nucleus. A third form (*tritium*) has one proton and two neutrons in the nucleus and one orbiting electron. Each is an *isotope* of hydrogen (Fig. 2.3).

Because the atomic weight of an element is actually an average atomic weight calculated using all its atoms, the true atomic weight of hydrogen is 1.008, although for most practical purposes it can be taken as 1.

Chlorine has an atomic weight of 35.5, because it contains two isotopes, one with an atomic weight of 35 (with 18 neutrons in the nucleus) and the other 37 (with 20 neutrons in the nucleus). Because the proportion of these two forms is not equal, the average atomic weight is 35.5.

Molecules and compounds

As mentioned earlier, the atoms of each element have a specific number of electrons around the nucleus. When the number of electrons in the outer shell of an element is either the maximum number (Fig. 2.1), or a stable proportion of this fraction, the element is described as *inert* or chemically unreactive, and it will not easily combine with other atoms. These elements are the inert gases – helium, neon, argon, krypton, xenon and radon.

Molecules consist of two or more atoms that are chemically combined. The atoms may be of the same element, e.g. a molecule of atmospheric oxygen (O_2) contains two oxygen atoms. Most substances, however, are compounds and contain two or more different elements, e.g. a water molecule (H_2O) contains two hydrogen atoms and an oxygen atom. ▓ **2.1**

Compounds containing carbon and hydrogen are classified as *organic*, and all others as *inorganic*. Living tissues are based on organic compounds, but the body requires inorganic compounds too.

Covalent and ionic bonds. The vast array of chemical processes on which life is based is completely dependent upon the way atoms come together, bind and break apart. For example, the humble water molecule is a crucial foundation of all life on Earth. If water was a less stable compound, and the atoms came apart easily, human biology could never have evolved. On the other hand, the body is dependent upon the breaking down of various molecules (e.g. sugars, fats) to release energy for cellular activities. When atoms are joined together, they form a chemical bond that is generally one of two types: *covalent* or *ionic*.

Covalent bonds are formed when atoms share their electrons with each other. Most molecules are held together with this type of bond; it forms a strong and stable link between its constituent atoms. A water molecule is built using covalent bonds. Hydrogen has one electron in its outer shell, but the optimum number for this shell is two. Oxygen has six electrons in its outer shell, but the optimum number for this shell is eight. Therefore, if one oxygen atom and two hydrogen atoms combine, each hydrogen atom will share its electron with the oxygen atom, giving the oxygen atom a total of eight outer electrons, making it stable. The oxygen atom shares one of its electrons with each of the two hydrogen atoms, so that each hydrogen atom has two electrons in its outer shell, and they too are stable (Fig. 2.4).

Ionic bonds are weaker than covalent bonds and are formed when electrons are transferred from one atom to another. For example, when sodium (Na) combines with chlorine (Cl) to form sodium chloride (NaCl), the only

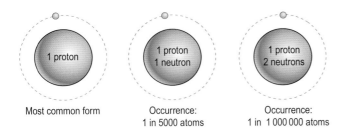

Most common form | Occurrence: 1 in 5000 atoms | Occurrence: 1 in 1 000 000 atoms

Figure 2.3 The isotopes of hydrogen.

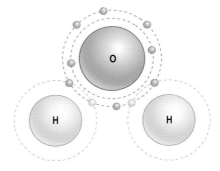

Figure 2.4 A water molecule, showing the covalent bonds between hydrogen (yellow) and oxygen (green).

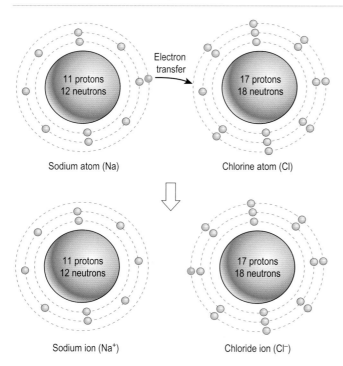

Figure 2.5 Formation of the ionic compound, sodium chloride.

Table 2.2 Examples of normal plasma levels

Substance	Molar concentrations	Equivalent concentration in other units
Chloride	97–106 mmol/L	97–106 mEq/L
Sodium	135–143 mmol/L	135–143 mEqL
Glucose	3.5–5.5 mmol/L	60–100 mg/100 mL
Iron	14–35 mmol/L	90–196 mg/100 mL

electron in the outer shell of the sodium atom is transferred to the outer shell of the chlorine atom (Fig. 2.5).

This leaves the sodium atom with eight electrons in its outer (second) shell, and therefore stable. The chlorine atom also has eight electrons in its outer shell, which, although not filling the shell, is a stable number. The sodium atom is now positively charged because it has given away a negatively charged electron, and the chloride ion is now negatively charged because it has accepted sodium's extra electron. The two atoms, therefore, stick together because they are carrying opposite, mutually attractive, charges.

When sodium chloride is dissolved in water the ionic bond breaks and the two atoms separate. The atoms are charged, because they have traded electrons, so are no longer called atoms, but *ions*. Sodium, with the positive charge, is a *cation*, written Na^+, and chloride, being negatively charged, is an *anion*, written Cl^-. By convention the number of electrical charges carried by an ion is indicated by the superscript plus or minus signs. 2.2

Electrolytes

An ionic compound, e.g. sodium chloride, dissolved in water is called an *electrolyte* because it conducts electricity. Electrolytes are important body constituents because they:

- conduct electricity, essential for muscle and nerve function
- exert osmotic pressure, keeping body fluids in their own compartments

- act as buffers (p. 24) to resist pH changes in body fluids.

Many biological compounds, e.g. carbohydrates, are not ionic, and therefore have no electrical properties when dissolved in water. Important electrolytes other than sodium and chloride include potassium (K^+), calcium (Ca^{2+}), bicarbonate (HCO_3^-) and phosphate (PO_4^{3-}).

Measurement of substances in body fluids

There is no single way of measuring and expressing the concentration of different substances in body fluids. Sometimes the unit used is based on weight in grams or fractions of a gram (see also pp. 479–80), e.g. milligrams, micrograms or nanograms. If the molecular weight of the substance is known, the concentration can be expressed as moles, millimoles or nanomoles per litre. A related measure is the *milliequivalent (mEq)* per litre.

Sometimes it is most convenient to measure the quantity of a substance in terms of its activity; insulin, for instance, is measured in *international units* (IU).

Table 2.2 gives examples of the normal plasma levels of some important substances, given in molar concentrations and alternative units.

Acids, bases and pH

pH is the measuring system used to express the concentration of hydrogen ions ($[H^+]$) in a fluid, which is an indicator of its acidity or alkalinity. Living cells are very sensitive to changes in $[H^+]$, and since the biochemical processes of life continually produce or consume hydrogen ions, sophisticated homeostatic mechanisms in the body constantly monitor and regulate pH.

An acid substance releases hydrogen ions when in solution. On the other hand, a basic (alkaline) substance accepts hydrogen ions, often with the release of hydroxyl (OH^-) ions. A salt releases other anions and cations when dissolved; sodium chloride is therefore a salt because in solution it releases sodium and chloride ions.

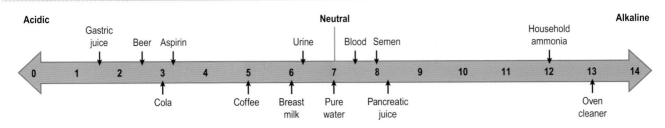

Figure 2.6 The pH scale.

The pH scale

The standard scale for measurement of hydrogen ion concentration in solution is the pH scale. The scale measures from 0 to 14, with 7, the midpoint, as neutral; this is the pH of pure water. Water is a neutral molecule, neither acid nor basic (alkaline), because when the molecule breaks up into its constituent ions, it releases one H^+ and one OH^-, which balance one another. With the notable exception of gastric juice, most body fluids are close to neutral, because they contain *buffers*, themselves weak acids and bases, to keep their pH within narrow ranges.

A pH reading below 7 indicates an *acid solution*, while readings above 7 indicate basic (alkaline) solutions. Figure 2.6 shows the pH of some common fluids (see also, p. 479). A change of one whole number on the pH scale indicates a 10-fold change in [H^+]. Therefore, a solution of pH 5 contains 10 times as many hydrogen ions as a solution of pH 6.

Not all acids ionise completely when dissolved in water. The hydrogen ion concentration is, therefore, a measure of the amount of *dissociated acid* (ionised acid) rather than of the total amount of acid present. Strong acids dissociate more extensively than weak acids, e.g. hydrochloric acid dissociates extensively into H^+ and Cl^-, while carbonic acid dissociates much less freely into H^+ and HCO_3^-.

Likewise, not all bases dissociate completely. Strong bases dissociate more fully, i.e. they release more OH^- than weaker ones.

pH values of body fluids

The pH of body fluids are generally maintained within relatively narrow limits.

The highly acid pH of the gastric juice is maintained by hydrochloric acid secreted by the parietal cells in the walls of the gastric glands. The low pH of the stomach fluids destroys microbes and toxins swallowed in food or drink. Saliva has a pH of between 5.4 and 7.5, which is the optimum value for the action of salivary amylase, the enzyme present in saliva which initiates the digestion of carbohydrates. Amylase is destroyed by gastric acid when it reaches the stomach.

Blood pH is kept between 7.35 and 7.45, and outwith this narrow range there is severe disruption of normal physiological and biochemical processes. Normal metabolic activity of body cells constantly produces acids and bases, which would tend to alter the pH of the tissue fluid and blood. Chemical *buffers*, which can reversibly bind hydrogen ions, are responsible for keeping body pH stable.

Buffers

Despite the constant cellular production of acids and bases, body pH is kept stable by systems of buffering chemicals in body fluids and tissues. These buffering mechanisms temporarily neutralise fluctuations in pH, but can function effectively only if there is some means by which excess acid or bases can be excreted from the body. The organs most active in this way are the *lungs* and the *kidneys*. The lungs are important regulators of blood pH because they excrete carbon dioxide (CO_2). CO_2 increases [H^+] in body fluids because it combines with water to form carbonic acid, which then dissociates into a bicarbonate ion and a hydrogen ion.

$$CO_2 + H_2O \leftrightarrow H_2CO_3 \leftrightarrow H^+ + HCO_3^-$$

carbon dioxide   water   carbonic acid   hydrogen ion   bicarbonate ion

The lungs, therefore, help to control blood pH by regulating levels of excreted CO_2. The brain detects rising [H^+] in the blood and stimulates breathing, causing increased CO_2 loss and a fall in [H^+]. Conversely, if blood pH becomes too basic, the brain can reduce the respiration rate to increase CO_2 levels and increase [H^+], decreasing pH towards normal (see Ch. 10).

The kidneys regulate blood pH by adjusting the excretion of hydrogen and bicarbonate ions as required. If pH falls, hydrogen ion excretion is increased and bicarbonate conserved; the reverse happens if pH rises. In addition, the kidneys generate bicarbonate ions as a by-product of amino acid breakdown in the renal tubules; this process also generates ammonium ions, which are rapidly excreted.

Other buffer systems include body proteins, which absorb excess H^+, and phosphate, which is particularly important in controlling intracellular pH. The buffer and excretory systems of the body together maintain the *acid–base balance* so that the pH range of body fluids remains within normal, but narrow, limits.

Acidosis and alkalosis

The buffer systems described above compensate for most pH fluctuations, but these reserves are limited and, in extreme cases, can become exhausted. When the pH falls below 7.35, and all the reserves of alkaline buffers are used up, the condition of *acidosis* exists. In the reverse situation, when the pH rises above 7.45, the increased alkali uses up all the acid reserve and the state of *alkalosis* exists.

Acidosis and alkalosis are both dangerous, particularly to the central nervous system and the cardiovascular system. In practice, acidotic conditions are commoner than alkalotic ones, because the body tends to produce more acid than alkali. Acidosis may follow respiratory problems, if the lungs are not excreting CO_2 as efficiently as normal, or if the body is producing excess acids (e.g. diabetic ketoacidosis, p. 237) or in kidney disease, if renal H^+ excretion is reduced. Alkalosis may be caused by loss of acidic substances through vomiting, diarrhoea, endocrine disorders or diuretic therapy, which stimulates increased renal excretion. Rarely, it may follow increased respiratory effort, such as in an acute anxiety attack where excessive amounts of CO_2 are lost through overbreathing (hyperventilation).

Important biological molecules

Learning outcomes

After studying this section, you should be able to:

■ describe in simple terms the chemical nature of sugars, proteins, lipids, nucleotides and enzymes

■ discuss the biological importance of each of these important groups of molecules.

Carbohydrates

Carbohydrates (sugars and starches) are composed of carbon, oxygen and hydrogen. The carbon atoms are normally arranged in a ring, with the oxygen and hydrogen atoms linked to them. The structures of glucose, fructose and sucrose are shown in Figure 2.7. When two sugar molecules combine to form a bigger sugar molecule, a water molecule is expelled and the bond formed is called a *glycosidic linkage*.

Glucose, the cells' preferred fuel molecule, is a *monosaccharide* (mono = one; saccharide = sugar). Monosaccharides can be linked together to form bigger sugars, ranging in size from two sugar units (*disaccharides*), e.g. sucrose (table sugar) (Fig. 2.7), to long chains containing many thousands of monosaccharides, such as starch. Such complex carbohydrates are called *polysaccharides*.

Glucose can be broken down in either the presence (*aerobically*) or the absence (*anaerobically*) of oxygen, but the process is much more efficient when O_2 is used. During this process, energy, water and carbon dioxide are released (pp. 315–6). To ensure a constant supply of glucose for cellular metabolism, blood glucose levels are tightly controlled. Functions of sugars include:

● providing a ready source of energy to fuel cell metabolism (p. 313)
● providing a form of energy storage, e.g. glycogen (p. 310)
● forming an integral part of the structure of DNA and RNA (pp. 438, 441)
● acting as receptors on the cell surface, allowing the cell to recognise other molecules and cells.

Amino acids and proteins

Amino acids always contain carbon, hydrogen, oxygen and nitrogen, and many in addition carry sulphur. In human biochemistry, 20 amino acids are used as the principal building blocks of protein, although there are others; for instance, there are some amino acids used only in certain proteins, and some are seen only in microbial products. The amino acids used in human protein synthesis have a basic common structure, including an amino group (NH_2), a carboxyl group (COOH) and a hydrogen atom. What makes one amino acid different from the next is a variable side chain. The basic structure and three common amino acids are shown in Figure 2.8. As in the formation of glycosidic linkages, when two amino acids join up the reaction expels a molecule of water and the resulting bond is called a *peptide bond*.

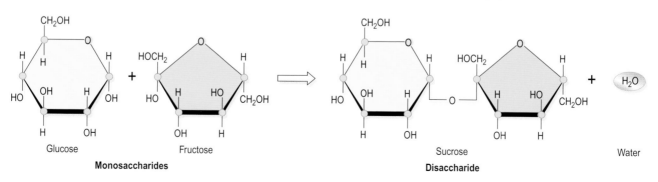

Figure 2.7 The combination of glucose and fructose to make sucrose.

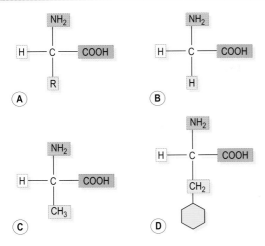

Figure 2.8 Amino acid structures. A. Common structure, R = variable side chain. **B.** Glycine, the simplest amino acid. **C.** Alanine. **D.** Phenylalanine.

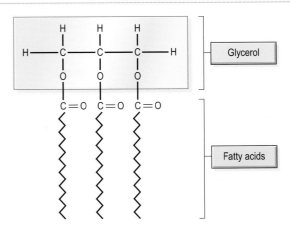

Figure 2.9 Structure of a fat (triglyceride) molecule.

Proteins are made from amino acids joined together, and are the main family of molecules from which the human body is built. Protein chains can vary in size from a few amino acids long to many thousands. They may exist as simple, single strands of protein, for instance some hormones, but more commonly are twisted and folded into complex and intricate three-dimensional structures that may contain more than one kind of protein, or incorporate other types of molecule, e.g. haemoglobin (Fig. 4.6). Such complex structures are stabilised by internal bonds between constituent amino acids, and the function of the protein will depend upon the three-dimensional shape it has been twisted into. One reason why changes in pH are so damaging to living tissues is that hydrogen ions disrupt these internal stabilising forces and change the shape of the protein (denaturing it), leaving it unable to function. Many important groups of biologically active substances are proteins, e.g.:

- carrier molecules, e.g. haemoglobin (p. 65)
- enzymes (p. 28)
- many hormones, e.g. insulin (p. 227)
- antibodies (pp. 381–2).

Proteins can also be used as an alternative energy source, usually in starvation. The main source of body protein is muscle tissue, so muscle wasting is a feature of starvation.

Lipids

The lipids are a diverse group of substances whose common property is an inability to mix with water (i.e. they are *hydrophobic*). They are made up mainly of carbon, hydrogen and oxygen atoms, and some contain additional elements, like nitrogen or phosphorus. The most important groups of lipids include:

- *phospholipids*, integral to cell membrane structure. They form a double layer, providing a water-repellant barrier separating the cell contents from its environment (p. 32)
- certain vitamins (p. 278). The fat-soluble vitamins are A, D, E and K
- *fats (triglycerides)*, stored in adipose tissue (p. 41) as an energy source. Fat also insulates the body and protects internal organs. A molecule of fat contains three fatty acids attached to a molecule of glycerol (Fig. 2.9). When fat is broken down under optimal conditions, more energy is released than when glucose is fully broken down.

Fats are classified as *saturated* or *unsaturated*, depending on the chemical nature of the fatty acids present. Saturated fat tends to be solid, whereas unsaturated fats are fluid.

- *prostaglandins* are important chemicals derived from fatty acids and are involved in inflammation (p. 377) and other processes.
- *steroids*, including important hormones produced by the gonads (the ovaries and testes, p. 455 and p. 459) and adrenal glands (p. 244). *Cholesterol* is a steroid that stabilises cell membranes and is the precursor of the hormones mentioned above, as well as being used to make bile salts for digestion.

Nucleotides

Nucleic acids

These are the largest molecules in the body and are built from nucleotides. They include deoxyribonucleic acid (DNA, p. 438) and ribonucleic acid (RNA, p. 441).

Adenosine triphosphate (ATP)

ATP is a nucleotide built from ribose (the sugar unit), adenine (the base) and three phosphate groups attached to the ribose (Fig. 2.10A). It is sometimes called the energy

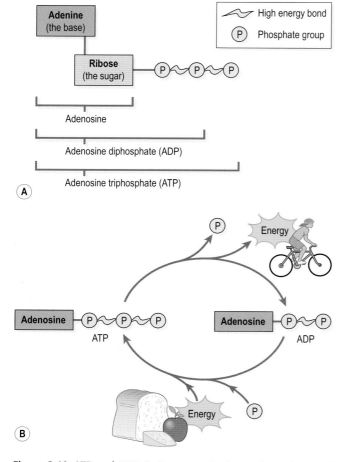

Figure 2.10 ATP and ADP. A. Structures. **B.** Conversion cycle.

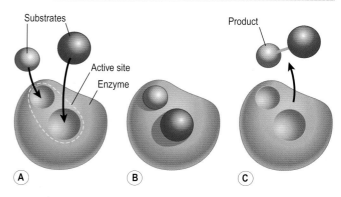

Figure 2.11 Action of an enzyme. A. Enzyme and substrates. **B.** Enzyme–substrate complex. **C.** Enzyme and product.

currency of the body, which implies that the body has to 'earn' (synthesise) it before it can 'spend' it. Many of the body's huge number of reactions release energy, e.g. the breakdown of sugars in the presence of O_2. The body captures the energy released by these reactions, using it to make ATP from adenosine diphosphate (ADP). When the cells need chemical energy to fuel metabolic activities, ATP is broken down again into ADP, releasing water, a phosphate group, and energy from the splitting of the high-energy phosphate bond (Fig. 2.10B). Energy generated from ATP breakdown fuels muscle contraction, motility of spermatozoa, anabolic reactions and the transport of materials across membranes.

Enzymes

Many of the body's chemical reactions can be reproduced in a test-tube. Surprisingly, the rate at which the reactions then occur usually plummets to the extent that, for all practical purposes, chemical activity ceases. The cells of the body have developed a solution to this apparent problem – they are equipped with a huge array of enzymes. Enzymes are proteins that act as *catalysts* for

biochemical reactions – that is, they speed the reaction up but are not themselves changed by it, and therefore can be used over and over again. Enzymes are very selective and will usually catalyse only one specific reaction. The molecule(s) entering the reaction is called the *substrate* and it binds to a very specific site on the enzyme, called the *active site*. Whilst the substrate(s) is bound to the active site the reaction proceeds, and once it is complete the product(s) of the reaction breaks away from the enzyme and the active site is ready for use again (Fig. 2.11).

Enzyme action is reduced or stopped altogether if conditions are unsuitable. Increased or decreased temperature is likely to reduce activity, as is any change in pH. Some enzymes require the presence of a *cofactor*, an ion or small molecule that allows the enzyme to bind its substrate(s). Some vitamins act as cofactors.

Enzymes can catalyse both synthetic and breakdown reactions, and their names (almost always!) end in ~ase. When an enzyme catalyses the combination of two or more substrates into a larger product, this is called an *anabolic reaction*. *Catabolic reactions* involve the breakdown of the substrate into smaller products, as occurs during the digestion of foods.

Movement of substances within body fluids

Learning outcomes

After studying this section, you should be able to:

- compare and contrast the processes of osmosis and diffusion

- using these concepts, describe how molecules move within and between body compartments.

Movement of substances within and between body fluids, sometimes across a barrier such as the cell membrane, is essential in normal physiology.

In liquids or gases, molecules distribute from an area of high concentration to one of low concentration, assuming that there is no barrier in the way. Between two such areas, there exists a *concentration gradient* and movement of substances occurs *down* the concentration gradient, or downhill, until the molecules are evenly spread throughout, i.e. equilibrium is reached. No energy is required for such movement, so this process is described as *passive*.

There are many examples in the body of substances moving *uphill*, i.e. against the concentration gradient; in this case, energy is required, usually from the breakdown of ATP. These processes are described as *active*. Movement of substances across cell membranes by active transport is described on page 37.

Passive movement of substances in the body proceeds usually in one of two main ways – *diffusion* or *osmosis*. ▓ **2.3**

Diffusion

Diffusion refers to the movement of molecules from an area of high concentration to an area of low concentration, and occurs mainly in gases, liquids and solutions. Sugar molecules heaped at the bottom of a cup of coffee that has not been stirred will, in time, become evenly distributed throughout the liquid by diffusion (Fig. 2.12). The process of diffusion is speeded up if the temperature rises and/or the concentration of the diffusing substance is increased.

Diffusion can also occur across a semipermeable membrane, such as the plasma membrane or the capillary wall. Only molecules small or soluble enough to cross the membrane can diffuse through. For example, oxygen diffuses freely through the walls of the alveoli (airsacs in the lungs), where oxygen concentrations are high, into the bloodstream, where oxygen concentrations are low. However, blood cells and large protein molecules in the plasma are too large to cross and so remain in the blood.

Osmosis

While diffusion of molecules across a semipermeable membrane results in equal concentrations on both sides of the membrane, *osmosis* refers specifically to diffusion of water down its concentration gradient. This is usually because any other molecules present are too large to pass through the pores in the membrane. The force with which this occurs is called the *osmotic pressure*. Imagine two solutions of sugar separated by a semipermeable membrane whose pores are too small to let the sugar molecules through. On one side, the sugar solution is twice as concentrated as on the other. After a period of time, the concentration of sugar molecules will have equalised on both sides of the membrane, not because sugar molecules have diffused across the membrane, but because osmotic pressure across the membrane 'pulls' water from the dilute solution into the concentrated solution, i.e. water has moved down its concentration gradient. Osmosis proceeds until equilibrium is reached, at which point the solutions on each side of the membrane are of the same concentration and are said to be *isotonic*. The importance of careful control of solute concentrations in the body fluids can be illustrated by looking at what happens to a cell (e.g. a red blood cell) when it is exposed to solutions that differ from normal physiological conditions.

Plasma osmolarity is maintained within a very narrow range because if the plasma water concentration rises, i.e. the plasma becomes more dilute than the intracellular fluid within the red blood cells, then water will move down its concentration gradient across their membranes and into the red blood cells. This may cause the red blood cells to swell and burst. In this situation, the plasma is said to be *hypotonic*. Conversely, if the plasma water concentration falls so that the plasma becomes more concentrated than the intracellular fluid within the red blood cells (the plasma becomes *hypertonic*), water passively moves by osmosis from the blood cells into the plasma and the blood cells shrink (Fig. 2.13).

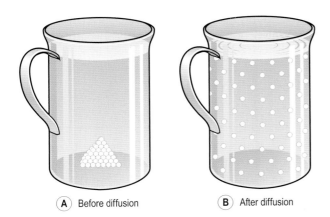

(A) Before diffusion   (B) After diffusion

Figure 2.12 The process of diffusion: a spoonful of sugar in a cup of coffee.

⚬ = solute molecule

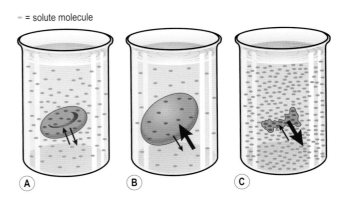

(A)   (B)   (C)

Figure 2.13 The process of osmosis. Net water movement when a red blood cell is suspended in solutions of varying concentrations (tonicity): **A.** Isotonic solution. **B.** Hypotonic solution. **C.** Hypertonic solution.

Body fluids

Learning outcomes

After studying this section, you should be able to:

■ define the terms intra- and extracellular fluid

■ using examples, explain why homeostatic control of the composition of these fluids is vital to body function.

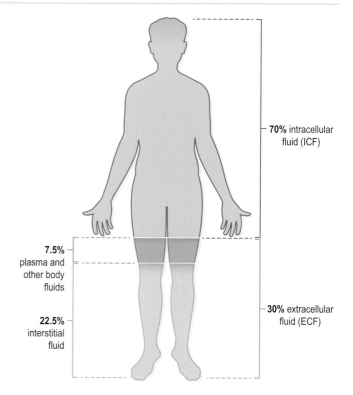

Figure 2.14 Distribution of body water in a 70 kg person.

70% intracellular fluid (ICF)

30% extracellular fluid (ECF)

7.5% plasma and other body fluids

22.5% interstitial fluid

The total body water in adults of average build is about 40L, around 60% of body weight. This proportion is higher in babies and young people and in adults below average weight. It is lower in the elderly and in obesity in all age groups. About 22% of body weight is extracellular water and about 38% is intracellular water. It is also lower in females than males, because females have proportionately more adipose than muscle tissue than males, and adipose tissue is only 10% water compared to 75% of muscle tissue.

Most of our total body water is found inside cells (about 70%, or 28L of the average 40L). The remaining 30% (12L) is extracellular, mostly in the interstitial fluid bathing the tissues, with nearly all the remainder found in plasma (Fig. 2.14).

Extracellular fluid

The extracellular fluid (ECF) consists mainly of blood, plasma, lymph, cerebrospinal fluid and fluid in the interstitial spaces of the body. Other extracellular fluids are present in very small amounts; their role is mainly in lubrication, and they include joint (synovial) fluid, pericardial fluid (around the heart) and pleural fluid (around the lungs).

Interstitial or intercellular fluid (tissue fluid) bathes all the cells of the body except the outer layers of skin. It is the medium through which substances diffuse from blood to body cells, and from cells to blood. Every body cell in contact with ECF is directly dependent upon the composition of that fluid for its well-being. Even slight changes can cause permanent damage, therefore, ECF composition is closely regulated. For example, a fall in plasma potassium levels may cause muscle weakness and cardiac arrhythmia, because of increased excitability of muscle and nervous tissue. Rising blood potassium also interferes with cardiac function, and can even cause the heart to stop beating. Potassium levels in the blood are only one of the many parameters under constant, careful adjustment by the homeostatic mechanisms of the body.

Intracellular fluid

The composition of intracellular fluid (ICF) is largely controlled by the cell itself, because there are selective uptake and discharge mechanisms present in the cell membrane. In some respects, the composition of ICF is very different from ECF. For example, sodium levels are nearly 10 times higher in the ECF than in the ICF. This concentration difference occurs because, although sodium diffuses into the cell down its concentration gradient, there is a pump in the membrane that selectively pumps it back out again. This concentration gradient is essential for the function of excitable cells (mainly nerve and muscle). Conversely, many substances are found inside the cell in significantly higher amounts than outside, e.g. ATP, protein and potassium. Water, however, passes freely in both directions across the cell membrane, and changes in water concentration of the ECF therefore have immediate consequences for intracellular water levels (Fig. 2.13).

 For a range of self-assessment exercises on the topics in this chapter, visit Evolve online resources: https://evolve.elsevier.com/Waugh/anatomy/

The cells, tissues and organisation of the body

ANIMATIONS

Cells are the body's smallest functional units. They are grouped together to form *tissues*, each of which has a specialised function, e.g. blood, muscle, bone. Different tissues are grouped together to form *organs*, e.g. the heart, stomach and brain. Organs are grouped together to form *systems*, each of which performs a particular function that maintains homeostasis and contributes to the health of the individual (see Fig. 1.2, p. 5). For example, the digestive system is responsible for taking in, digesting and absorbing food, which involves a number of organs, including the stomach and intestines. The structure and functions of cells and types of tissue are explored in this chapter.

The terminology used to describe the anatomical relationships between body parts, the skeleton and the cavities within the body are then considered.

The final section considers features of benign and malignant tumours, their causes and how they grow and may spread.

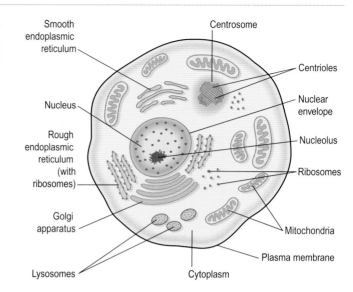

Figure 3.1 The simple cell.

The cell: structure and functions

Learning outcomes

After studying this section, you should be able to:

- describe the structure of the plasma membrane

- explain the functions of the principal organelles

- outline the process of mitosis

- compare and contrast active, passive and bulk transport of substances across cell membranes.

The human body develops from a single cell called the *zygote*, which results from the fusion of the ovum (female egg cell) and the spermatozoon (male sex cell). Cell division follows and, as the fetus grows, cells with different structural and functional specialisations develop, all with the same genetic make-up as the zygote. Individual cells are too small to be seen with the naked eye. However, they can be seen when thin slices of tissue are stained in the laboratory and magnified using a microscope.

A cell consists of a *plasma membrane* enclosing a number of *organelles* suspended in a watery fluid called *cytosol* (Fig. 3.1). Organelles, literally 'small organs', have individual and highly specialised functions, and are often enclosed in their own membrane within the cytosol. They include: the nucleus, mitochondria, ribosomes, endoplasmic reticulum, Golgi apparatus, lysosomes and the cytoskeleton. The cell contents, excluding the nucleus, is the *cytoplasm*, i.e. the cytosol and other organelles.

Plasma membrane

The plasma membrane (Fig. 3.2) consists of two layers of *phospholipids* (see p. 27) with proteins and sugars embedded in them. In addition to phospholipids, the lipid *cholesterol* is also present. The phospholipid molecules have a head, which is electrically charged and *hydrophilic* (meaning 'water loving'), and a tail which has no charge and is *hydrophobic* (meaning 'water hating', Fig. 3.2A). The phospholipid bilayer is arranged like a sandwich with the hydrophilic heads aligned on the outer surfaces of the membrane and the hydrophobic tails forming a central water-repelling layer. These differences influence the transfer of substances across the membrane.

Membrane proteins

Those proteins that extend all the way through the membrane provide channels that allow the passage of, for example, electrolytes and non-lipid soluble substances. Protein molecules on the surface of the plasma membrane are shown in Figure 3.2B. The membrane proteins perform several functions:

- branched carbohydrate molecules attached to the outside of some membrane protein molecules give the cell its immunological identity
- they can act as receptors (specific recognition sites) for hormones and other chemical messengers
- some are enzymes (p. 28)
- transmembrane proteins form channels that are filled with water and allow very small, water-soluble ions to cross the membrane
- some are involved in pumps that transport substances across the membrane.

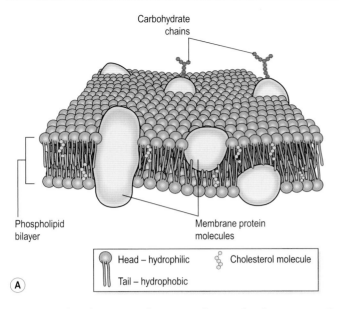

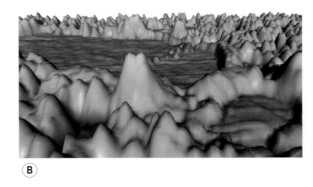

Figure 3.2 The plasma membrane. A. Diagram showing structure. **B.** Coloured atomic force micrograph of the surface showing plasma proteins.

Organelles ▓3.1

Nucleus

All body cells have a nucleus, with the exception of mature erythrocytes (red blood cells). Skeletal muscle fibres and some other cells contain several nuclei. The nucleus is the largest organelle and is contained within the nuclear envelope, a membrane similar to the plasma membrane but with tiny pores through which some substances can pass between it and the cytoplasm.

The nucleus contains the body's genetic material, in the form of deoxyribonucleic acid (DNA, p. 438); this directs all its metabolic activities. In a non-dividing cell DNA is present as a fine network of threads called *chromatin*, but when the cell prepares to divide the chromatin forms distinct structures called *chromosomes* (Fig. 17.1, p. 439). A related substance, ribonucleic acid (RNA) is also found in the nucleus. There are different types of RNA, not all found in the nucleus, but which are in general involved in protein synthesis.

Within the nucleus is a roughly spherical structure called the *nucleolus*, which is involved in synthesis (manufacture) and assembly of the components of ribosomes.

Mitochondria

Mitochondria are membranous, sausage-shaped structures in the cytoplasm, sometimes described as the 'power house' of the cell (Fig. 3.3). They are central to aerobic respiration, the processes by which chemical energy is made available in the cell. This is in the form of ATP, which releases energy when the cell breaks it down (see Fig. 2.10, p. 28). Synthesis of ATP is most efficient in the final stages of aerobic respiration, a process which requires oxygen (p. 315). The most active cell types have

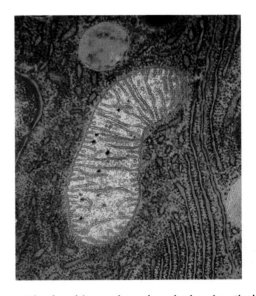

Figure 3.3 Mitochondrion and rough endoplasmic reticulum. False colour transmission electron micrograph showing mitochondrion (orange) and rough endoplasmic reticulum (turquoise) studded with ribosomes (dots).

the greatest number of mitochondria, e.g. liver, muscle and spermatozoa.

Ribosomes

These are tiny granules composed of RNA and protein. They synthesise proteins from amino acids, using RNA as the template (see Fig. 17.5, p. 441). When present in free units or in small clusters in the cytoplasm, the ribosomes make proteins for use within the cell. These include the enzymes required for metabolism. Metabolic pathways

33

consist of a series of steps, each driven by a specific enzyme. Ribosomes are also found on the outer surface of the nuclear envelope and rough endoplasmic reticulum (see Fig. 3.3 and below) where they manufacture proteins for export from the cell.

Endoplasmic reticulum (ER)

Endoplasmic reticulum is an extensive series of interconnecting membranous canals in the cytoplasm (Fig. 3.3). There are two types: smooth and rough. Smooth ER synthesises lipids and steroid hormones, and is also associated with the detoxification of some drugs. Some of the lipids are used to replace and repair the plasma membrane and membranes of organelles. Rough ER is studded with ribosomes. These are the site of synthesis of proteins, some of which are 'exported' from cells, i.e. enzymes and hormones that leave the parent cell by exocytosis (p. 37) to be used by cells elsewhere.

Golgi apparatus

The Golgi apparatus consists of stacks of closely folded flattened membranous sacs (Fig. 3.4). It is present in all cells but is larger in those that synthesise and export proteins. The proteins move from the endoplasmic reticulum to the Golgi apparatus where they are 'packaged' into membrane-bound *vesicles*. The vesicles are stored and, when needed, they move to the plasma membrane and fuse with it. The contents are expelled (secreted) from the cell. This process is called *exocytosis* (p. 37).

Lysosomes

Lysosomes are small membranous vesicles pinched off from the Golgi apparatus. They contain a variety of enzymes involved in breaking down fragments of organelles and large molecules (e.g. RNA, DNA, carbohydrates, proteins) inside the cell into smaller particles that are either recycled, or extruded from the cell as waste material.

Lysosomes in white blood cells contain enzymes that digest foreign material such as microbes.

Cytoskeleton

This consists of an extensive network of tiny protein fibres (Fig. 3.5).

Microfilaments. These are the smallest fibres. They provide structural support, maintain the characteristic shape of the cell and permit contraction, e.g. actin in muscle cells (p. 421).

Microtubules. These are larger contractile protein fibres that are involved in movement of:

- organelles within the cell
- chromosomes during cell division
- cell extensions (see below).

Centrosome. This directs organisation of microtubules within the cell. It consists of a pair of *centrioles* (small clusters of microtubules) and plays an important role in cell division.

Cell extensions. These project from the plasma membrane in some types of cell and their main components are microtubules, which allow movement. They include:

- microvilli – tiny projections that contain microfilaments. They cover the exposed surface of certain types of cell, e.g. absorptive cells that line the small intestine (see Fig. 3.6). By greatly increasing the surface area, microvilli make the structure of these cells ideal for their function – maximising absorption of nutrients from the small intestine.
- cilia – microscopic hair-like projections containing microtubules that lie along the free borders of some cells (see Fig. 10.12, p. 249). They beat in unison,

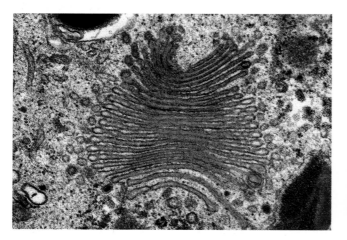

Figure 3.4 Coloured transmission electron micrograph showing the Golgi apparatus (green).

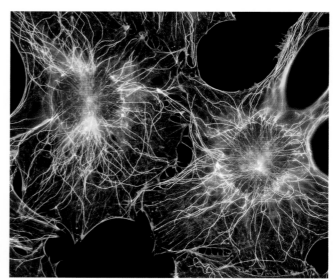

Figure 3.5 Fibroblasts. Fluorescent light micrograph showing their nuclei (purple) and cytoskeletons (yellow and blue).

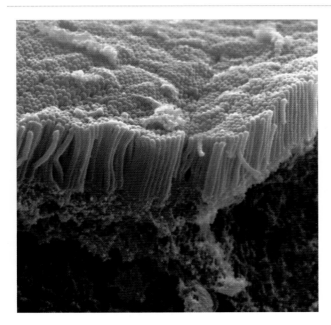

Figure 3.6 Coloured scanning electron micrograph of microvilli in small intestine.

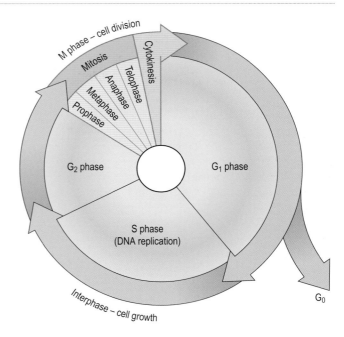

Figure 3.7 The cell cycle.

moving substances along the surface, e.g. mucus upwards in the respiratory tract.

- flagella – single, long whip-like projections, containing microtubules, which form the 'tails' of spermatozoa (see Fig. 1.19, p. 15) that propel them through the female reproductive tract.

The cell cycle

Many damaged, dead, and worn out cells can be replaced by growth and division of other similar cells. The frequency with which cell division occurs varies with different types of tissue (p. 44). This is normally carefully regulated to allow effective maintenance and repair of body tissues. At the end of their natural lifespan, ageing cells are programmed to 'self destruct' and their components are removed by phagocytosis; a process known as *apoptosis* (p. 54).

Cells with nuclei have 46 chromosomes and divide by *mitosis,* a process that results in two new genetically identical daughter cells. The only exception to this is the formation of *gametes* (sex cells), i.e. ova and spermatozoa, which takes place by *meiosis* (p. 442).

The period between two cell divisions is known as the *cell cycle,* which has two phases that can be seen on light microscopy: mitosis (M phase) and *interphase* (Fig. 3.7).

Interphase

This is the longer phase and three separate stages are recognised:

- first gap phase (G_1) – the cell grows in size and volume. This is usually the longest phase and most variable in length. Sometimes cells do not continue

round the cell cycle but enter a resting phase (G_0); during this time cells carry out their specific functions, e.g. secretion, absorption.
- synthesis of DNA (S phase) – the chromosomes replicate forming two identical copies of DNA (see p. 442). Therefore, following the S phase, the cell now has 92 chromosomes, i.e. enough DNA for two cells and is nearly ready to divide by mitosis.
- second gap phase – (G_2) there is further growth and preparation for cell division.

Mitosis (Figs 3.8 and 3.9) ▓ 3.2

This is a continuous process involving four distinct stages visible by light microscopy.

Prophase. During this stage the replicated chromatin becomes tightly coiled and easier to see under the microscope. Each of the original 46 chromosomes (called a *chromatid* at this stage) is paired with its copy in a double chromosome unit. The two chromatids are joined to each other at the *centromere* (Fig. 3.8). The *mitotic apparatus* appears; this consists of two *centrioles* separated by the *mitotic spindle,* which is formed from microtubules. The centrioles migrate, one to each end of the cell, and the nuclear envelope disappears.

Metaphase. The chromatids align on the centre of the spindle, attached by their centromeres.

Anaphase. The centromeres separate, and one of each pair of sister chromatids (now called chromosomes again) migrates to each end of the spindle as the microtubules that form the mitotic spindle contract.

35

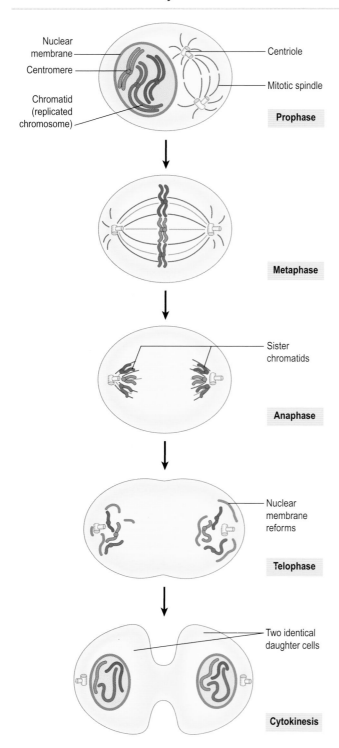

Figure 3.8 The stages of mitosis.

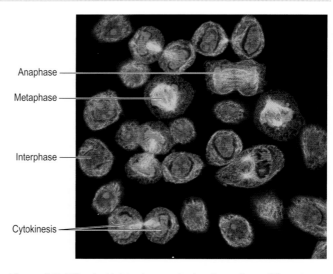

Figure 3.9 Mitosis. Light micrograph showing cells at different stages of reproduction with chromatin/chromatids shown in pink.

Transport of substances across cell membranes

The structure of the plasma membrane provides it with the property of *selective permeability,* meaning that not all substances can cross it. Those that can, do so in different ways depending on their size and characteristics (see Fig. 1.3, p. 6). ▓ **3.3**

Passive transport

This occurs when substances can cross the semipermeable plasma and organelle membranes and move down the concentration gradient (downhill) without using energy. ▓ **3.4**

Diffusion

This was described on page 29. Small molecules diffuse down their concentration gradient:

- lipid-soluble materials, e.g. oxygen, carbon dioxide, fatty acids and steroids, cross the membrane by dissolving in the lipid part of the membrane
- water-soluble materials, e.g. sodium, potassium and calcium, cross the membrane by passing through water-filled channels.

Facilitated diffusion

This passive process is used by some substances that are unable to diffuse through the semipermeable membrane unaided, e.g. glucose, amino acids. Specialised protein carrier molecules in the membrane have specific sites that attract and bind substances to be transferred, like a lock and key mechanism. The carrier then changes its shape and deposits the substance on the other side of the

Telophase. The mitotic spindle disappears, the chromosomes uncoil and the nuclear envelope reforms.

Following telophase, *cytokinesis* occurs: the cytosol, intracellular organelles and plasma membrane split forming two identical daughter cells.

membrane (Fig. 3.10). The carrier sites are specific and can be used by only one substance. As there are a finite number of carriers, there is a limit to the amount of a substance which can be transported at any time. This is known as the *transport maximum*.

Osmosis

Osmosis is passive movement of water down its concentration gradient towards equilibrium across a semipermeable membrane and is explained on page 29.

Active transport ▮ 3.5

This is the transport of substances up their concentration gradient (uphill), i.e. from a lower to a higher concentration. Chemical energy in the form of ATP (p. 27) drives

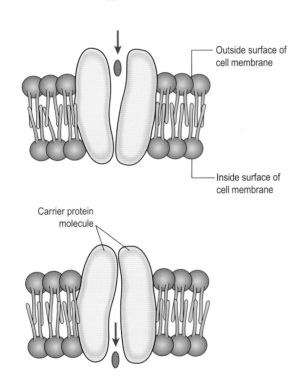

Figure 3.10 Specialised protein carrier molecules involved in facilitated diffusion and active transport.

Outside surface of cell membrane

Inside surface of cell membrane

Carrier protein molecule

specialised protein carrier molecules that transport substances across the membrane in either direction (see Fig. 3.10). The carrier sites are specific and can be used by only one substance; therefore the rate at which a substance is transferred depends on the number of sites available.

The sodium–potassium pump

All cells possess this pump, which indirectly supports other transport mechanisms such as glucose uptake, and is essential in maintaining the electrical gradient needed to generate action potentials in nerve and muscle cells.

This active transport mechanism maintains the unequal concentrations of sodium (Na^+) and potassium (K^+) ions on either side of the plasma membrane. It may use up to 30% of cellular ATP (energy) requirements.

Potassium levels are much higher inside the cell than outside – it is the principal intracellular cation. Sodium levels are much higher outside the cell than inside – it is the principal extracellular cation. These ions tend to diffuse down their concentration gradients, K^+ outwards and Na^+ into the cell. In order to maintain their concentration gradients, excess Na^+ is constantly pumped out across the cell membrane in exchange for K^+.

Bulk transport (Fig. 3.11)

Transfer of particles too large to cross cell membranes occurs by *pinocytosis* ('cell-drinking') or *phagocytosis* ('cell-eating'). These particles are engulfed by extensions of the cytoplasm (see Fig. 15.1, p. 376) which enclose them, forming a membrane-bound vacuole. Pinocytosis allows the cell to bring in fluid. In phagocytosis larger particles (e.g. cell fragments, foreign materials, microbes) are taken into the cell. Lysosomes then adhere to the vacuole membrane, releasing enzymes which digest the contents.

Extrusion of waste material by the reverse process through the plasma membrane is called *exocytosis*. Vesicles formed by the Golgi apparatus usually leave the cell in this way, as do any indigestible residues of phagocytosis.

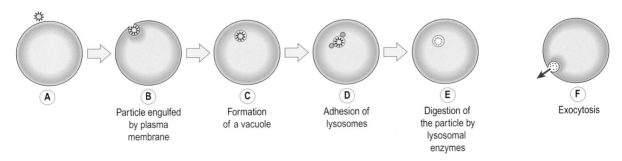

A

B
Particle engulfed by plasma membrane

C
Formation of a vacuole

D
Adhesion of lysosomes

E
Digestion of the particle by lysosomal enzymes

F
Exocytosis

Figure 3.11 Bulk transport across plasma membranes. A–E. Phagocytosis. **F.** Exocytosis.

Tissues

Learning outcomes

After studying this section, you should be able to:

■ describe the structure and functions of epithelial, connective and muscle tissue

■ outline the structure and functions of epithelial and synovial membranes

■ compare and contrast the structure and functions of exocrine and endocrine glands.

Tissues consist of large numbers of the same type of cells and are classified according to the size, shape and functions of their constituent cells. There are four main types of tissue each with subtypes. They are:

- epithelial tissue or epithelium
- connective tissue
- muscle tissue
- nervous tissue.

Epithelial tissue (Fig. 3.12)

This tissue type covers the body and lines cavities, hollow organs and tubes. It is also found in glands. The structure of epithelium is closely related to its functions, which include:

- protection of underlying structures from, for example, dehydration, chemical and mechanical damage
- secretion
- absorption.

The cells are very closely packed and the intercellular substance, the *matrix*, is minimal. The cells usually lie on a *basement membrane*, which is an inert connective tissue made by the epithelial cells themselves. Epithelial tissue may be:

- *simple*: a single layer of cells
- *stratified*: several layers of cells.

Simple epithelium

Simple epithelium consists of a single layer of identical cells and is divided into three main types. It is usually found on absorptive or secretory surfaces, where the single layer enhances these processes, and seldom on surfaces subject to stress. The types are named according to the shape of the cells, which differs according to their functions. The more active the tissue, the taller the cells.

Squamous (pavement) epithelium

This is composed of a single layer of flattened cells (Fig. 3.12A). The cells fit closely together like flat stones, forming a thin and very smooth membrane across which diffusion occurs easily. It forms the lining of the following structures:

- heart – where it is known as endocardium
- blood vessels ⎫ where it is also known
- lymph vessels ⎭ as endothelium
- alveoli of the lungs
- lining the collecting ducts of nephrons in the kidneys (see Fig. 13.8, p. 341).

Cuboidal epithelium

This consists of cube-shaped cells fitting closely together lying on a basement membrane (Fig. 3.12B). It forms the kidney tubules and is found in some glands such as the thyroid (see Fig. 9.9, p. 223). Cuboidal epithelium is actively involved in secretion, absorption and/or excretion.

Columnar epithelium

This is formed by a single layer of cells, rectangular in shape, on a basement membrane (Fig. 3.12C). It lines many organs and often has adaptations that make it well suited to a specific function. The lining of the stomach is formed from simple columnar epithelium without surface structures. The free surface of the columnar epithelium lining the small intestine is covered with microvilli (Fig. 3.6). Microvilli provide a very large surface area for absorption of nutrients from the small intestine. In the trachea, columnar epithelium is ciliated (see Fig. 10.12, p. 249) and also contains goblet cells that secrete mucus

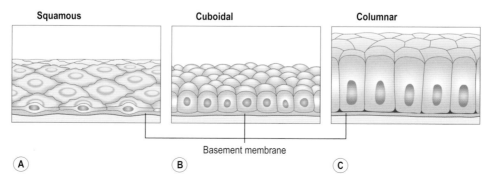

| Squamous | Cuboidal | Columnar |

Basement membrane

Ⓐ   Ⓑ   Ⓒ

Figure 3.12 Simple epithelium. A. Squamous. **B.** Cuboidal. **C.** Columnar.

(see Fig. 12.5, p. 290). This means that inhaled particles that stick to the mucus layer are moved towards the throat by cilia in the respiratory tract. In the uterine tubes, ova are propelled along by ciliary action towards the uterus.

Stratified epithelia

Stratified epithelia consist of several layers of cells of various shapes. Continual cell division in the lower (basal) layers pushes cells above nearer and nearer to the surface, where they are shed. Basement membranes are usually absent. The main function of stratified epithelium is to protect underlying structures from mechanical wear and tear. There are two main types: stratified squamous and transitional.

Stratified squamous epithelium (Fig. 3.13)

This is composed of several layers of cells. In the deepest layers the cells are mainly columnar and, as they grow towards the surface, they become flattened and are then shed.

Keratinised stratified epithelium. This is found on dry surfaces subjected to wear and tear, i.e. skin, hair and nails. The surface layer consists of dead epithelial cells that have lost their nuclei and contain the protein *keratin*. This forms a tough, relatively waterproof protective layer that prevents drying of the live cells underneath. The surface layer of skin is rubbed off and is replaced from below (see Figs 1.16 and 14.4).

Non-keratinised stratified epithelium. This protects moist surfaces subjected to wear and tear, and prevents them from drying out, e.g. the conjunctiva of the eyes, the lining of the mouth, the pharynx, the oesophagus and the vagina (Fig. 3.14).

Transitional epithelium (Fig. 3.15)

This is composed of several layers of pear-shaped cells. It lines several parts of the urinary tract including the bladder and allows for stretching as the bladder fills.

Connective tissue

Connective tissue is the most abundant tissue in the body. The connective tissue cells are more widely separated from each other than in epithelial tissues, and intercellular substance (matrix) is present in considerably larger amounts. There are usually fibres present in the matrix, which may be of a semisolid jelly-like consistency or

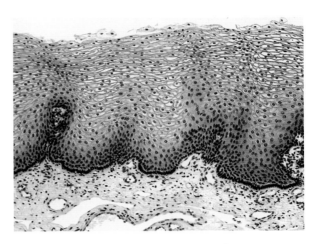

Figure 3.14 Section of non-keratinised stratified squamous epithelial lining of the vagina (magnified × 100).

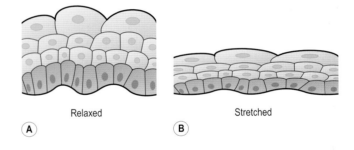

Relaxed   Stretched

(A)   (B)

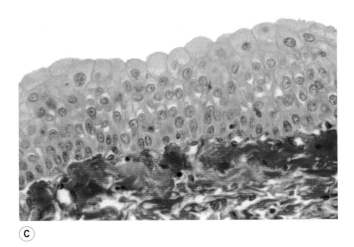

(C)

Figure 3.15 Transitional epithelium. A. Relaxed. **B.** Stretched. **C.** Light micrograph of bladder wall showing transitional epithelium (pink) above smooth muscle and connective tissue layer (red).

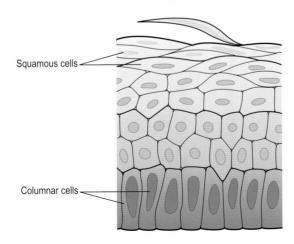

Squamous cells

Columnar cells

Figure 3.13 Stratified epithelium.

dense and rigid, depending upon the position and function of the tissue. The fibres form a supporting network for the cells to attach to. Most types of connective tissue have a good blood supply. Major functions of connective tissue are:

- binding and structural support
- protection
- transport
- insulation.

Cells in connective tissue

Connective tissue, excluding blood (see Ch. 4), is found in all organs supporting the specialised tissue. The different types of cell involved include: fibroblasts, fat cells, macrophages, leukocytes and mast cells.

Fibroblasts. Fibroblasts are large cells with irregular processes (Fig. 3.5). They manufacture *collagen* and *elastic fibres* and a matrix of extracellular material. Collagen fibres are shown in Figure 3.16. Very fine collagen fibres, sometimes called *reticulin fibres*, are found in highly active tissue, such as the liver and reticular tissue. Fibroblasts are particularly active in tissue repair (wound healing) where they may bind together the cut surfaces of wounds or form *granulation tissue* following tissue destruction (see p. 368). The collagen fibres formed during wound healing shrink as they age, sometimes interfering with the functions of the organ involved and with adjacent structures.

Fat cells. Also known as *adipocytes*, these cells occur singly or in groups in many types of connective tissue and are especially abundant in adipose tissue (see Fig. 3.19B). They vary in size and shape according to the amount of fat they contain.

Macrophages. These are large irregular-shaped cells with granules in the cytoplasm. Some are fixed, i.e. attached to connective tissue fibres, and others are motile. They are an important part of the body's defence mechanisms because they are actively phagocytic, engulfing and digesting cell debris, bacteria and other foreign bodies. Their activities are typical of those of the monocyte–macrophage defence system, e.g. monocytes in blood, Kupffer cells in liver sinusoids, sinus-lining cells in lymph nodes and spleen, and microglial cells in the brain (see Fig. 4.13, p. 70).

Leukocytes. White blood cells (p. 67) are normally found in small numbers in healthy connective tissue but *neutrophils* migrate in significant numbers during infection when they play an important part in tissue defence. *Plasma cells* develop from B-lymphocytes, a type of white blood cell (see p. 70). They synthesise and secrete specific defensive *antibodies* into the blood and tissues (see Ch. 15).

Mast cells. These are similar to basophil leukocytes (see p. 69). They are found in loose connective tissue, under the fibrous capsule of some organs, e.g. liver and spleen, and in considerable numbers round blood vessels. Their cytoplasm is packed with granules containing *heparin*, *histamine* and other substances, which are released when the cells are damaged by disease or injury (Fig. 3.17). Release of the granular contents is called *degranulation*. Histamine is involved in local and general inflammatory reactions, it stimulates secretion of gastric juice and is associated with development of allergies and hypersensitivity states (see p. 385). Heparin prevents coagulation of blood, which helps to maintain blood flow through inflamed tissues, supplying cells with oxygen and glucose and bringing additional protective leukocytes to the area.

Loose (areolar) connective tissue (Fig. 3.18)

This is the most generalised type of connective tissue. The matrix is semisolid with many fibroblasts and some fat

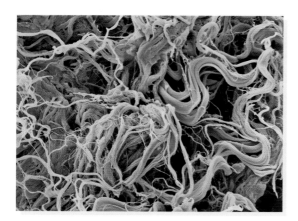

Figure 3.16 Coloured scanning electron micrograph of collagen fibres.

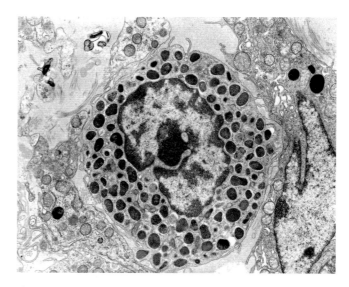

Figure 3.17 Mast cell. Coloured transmission electron micrograph showing nucleus (pink and brown) and cytoplasm (green) packed with granules (brown).

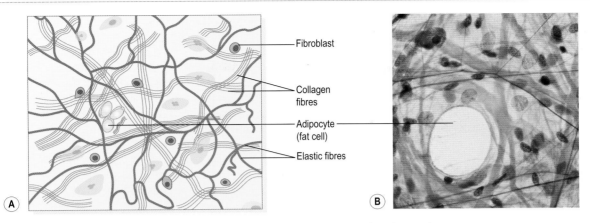

Figure 3.18 Loose (areolar) connective tissue. A. Diagram of basic structure. **B.** Light micrograph.

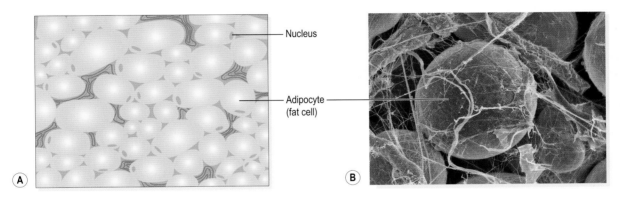

Figure 3.19 Adipose tissue. A. Diagram of basic structure. **B.** Coloured scanning electron micrograph of fat cells surrounded by strands of connective tissue.

cells (adipocytes), mast cells and macrophages widely separated by elastic and collagen fibres. It is found in almost every part of the body, providing elasticity and tensile strength. It connects and supports other tissues, for example:

- under the skin
- between muscles
- supporting blood vessels and nerves
- in the alimentary canal
- in glands supporting secretory cells.

Adipose tissue (Fig. 3.19)

Adipose tissue consists of fat cells (adipocytes), containing large fat globules, in a matrix of areolar tissue (Fig. 3.19). There are two types: white and brown.

White adipose tissue. This makes up 20–25% of body weight in adults with a normal body mass index (BMI, Ch. 11); more is present in obesity and less in those who are underweight. Adipose tissue secretes the hormone *leptin* (p. 284). The kidneys and eyeballs are supported by adipose tissue, which is also found between muscle fibres and under the skin, where it acts as a thermal insulator and energy store.

Brown adipose tissue. This is present in the newborn. It has a more extensive capillary network than white adipose tissue. When brown tissue is metabolised, it produces less energy and considerably more heat than other fat, contributing to the maintenance of body temperature. Sometimes small amounts are present in adults.

Reticular tissue (Fig. 3.20)

Reticular tissue has a semisolid matrix with fine branching reticulin fibres. It contains reticular cells and white

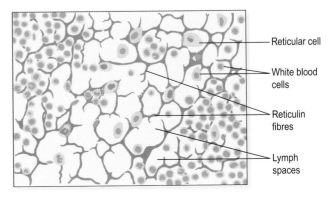

Figure 3.20 Reticular tissue.

blood cells (*monocytes* and *lymphocytes*). Reticular tissue is found in lymph nodes and all organs of the lymphatic system (see Fig. 6.1, p. 134).

Dense connective tissue

This contains more fibres and fewer cells than loose connective tissue.

Fibrous tissue (Fig. 3.21A)
This tissue is made up mainly of closely packed bundles of collagen fibres (Fig. 3.16) with very little matrix. Fibrocytes (old and inactive fibroblasts) are few in number and lie in rows between the bundles of fibres. Fibrous tissue is found:

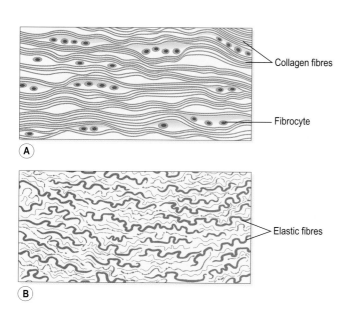

(A)

(B)

Figure 3.21 Dense connective tissue. A. Fibrous tissue. **B.** Elastic tissue.

- forming *ligaments*, which bind bones together
- as an outer protective covering for bone, called *periosteum*
- as an outer protective covering of some organs, e.g. the kidneys, lymph nodes and the brain
- forming muscle sheaths, called *muscle fascia* (see Fig. 16.61, p. 426), which extend beyond the muscle to become the *tendon* that attaches the muscle to bone.

Elastic tissue (Fig. 3.21B)
Elastic tissue is capable of considerable extension and recoil. There are few cells and the matrix consists mainly of masses of elastic fibres secreted by fibroblasts. It is found in organs where stretching or alteration of shape is required, e.g. in large blood vessel walls, the trachea and bronchi, and the lungs.

Blood

This is a fluid connective tissue that is described in detail in Chapter 4.

Cartilage

Cartilage is firmer than other connective tissues. The cells (*chondrocytes*) are sparse and lie embedded in matrix reinforced by collagen and elastic fibres. There are three types: hyaline cartilage, fibrocartilage and elastic fibrocartilage.

Hyaline cartilage (Fig. 3.22A)
Hyaline cartilage is a smooth bluish-white tissue. The chondrocytes are arranged in small groups within cell nests and the matrix is solid and smooth. Hyaline cartilage provides flexibility, support and smooth surfaces for movement at joints. It is found:

- on the ends of long bones that form joints
- forming the costal cartilages, which attach the ribs to the sternum
- forming part of the larynx, trachea and bronchi.

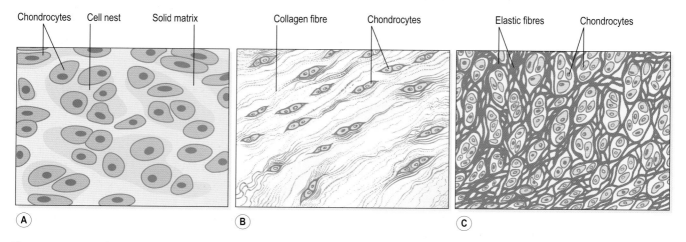

(A)   (B)   (C)

Figure 3.22 Cartilage. A. Hyaline cartilage. **B.** Fibrocartilage. **C.** Elastic fibrocartilage.

Fibrocartilage (Fig. 3.22B)

This consists of dense masses of white collagen fibres in a matrix similar to that of hyaline cartilage with the cells widely dispersed. It is a tough, slightly flexible, supporting tissue found:

- as pads between the bodies of the vertebrae, the *intervertebral discs*
- between the articulating surfaces of the bones of the knee joint, called *semilunar cartilages*
- on the rim of the bony sockets of the hip and shoulder joints, deepening the cavities without restricting movement.

Elastic fibrocartilage (Fig. 3.22C)

This flexible tissue consists of yellow elastic fibres lying in a solid matrix with chondrocytes lying between the fibres. It provides support and maintains shape of, e.g. the pinna or lobe of the ear, the epiglottis and part of the tunica media of blood vessel walls.

Bone

Bone cells (*osteocytes*) are surrounded by a matrix of collagen fibres strengthened by inorganic salts, especially calcium and phosphate. This provides bones with their characteristic strength and rigidity. Bone also has considerable capacity for growth in the first two decades of life, and for regeneration throughout life. Two types of bone can be identified by the naked eye:

- *compact bone* – solid or dense appearance
- *spongy* or *cancellous bone* –'spongy' or fine honeycomb appearance.

These are described in detail in Chapter 16.

Muscle tissue

This tissue is able to contract and relax, providing movement within the body and of the body itself. Muscle contraction requires a blood supply that will provide sufficient oxygen, calcium and nutrients and remove waste products. There are three types of specialised contractile cells, also known as *fibres*: skeletal muscle, smooth muscle and cardiac muscle.

Skeletal muscle (Fig. 3.23)

This type is described as skeletal because it forms those muscles that move the bones (of the skeleton), *striated* because striations (stripes) can be seen on microscopic examination and *voluntary* as it is under conscious control. Although most skeletal muscle moves bones, the diaphragm is made from this type of muscle to accommodate a degree of voluntary control in breathing. In reality, many movements can be finely coordinated, e.g. writing, but may also be controlled subconsciously. For example, maintaining an upright posture does not normally require

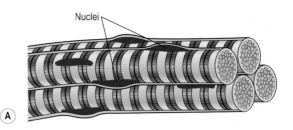

Nuclei

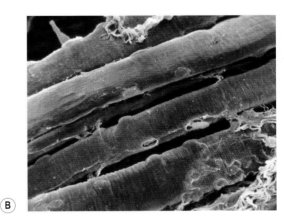

Figure 3.23 Skeletal muscle fibres. A. Diagram. **B.** Coloured scanning electron micrograph of skeletal muscle fibres and connective tissue fibres (bottom right).

thought unless a new locomotor skill is being learned, e.g. skating or cycling, and the diaphragm maintains breathing while asleep.

These fibres (cells) are cylindrical, contain several nuclei and can be up to 35 cm long. Skeletal muscle contraction is stimulated by motor nerve impulses originating in the brain or spinal cord and ending at the neuromuscular junction (see p. 422). The properties and functions of skeletal muscle are explained in detail in Chapter 16.

Smooth muscle (Fig. 3.24)

Smooth muscle is also described as *non-striated, visceral* or *involuntary*. It does not have striations and is not under conscious control. Some smooth muscle has the intrinsic ability to initiate its own contractions (*automaticity*), e.g. peristalsis (p. 289). It is innervated by the autonomic nervous system (p. 173). Additionally, autonomic nerve impulses, some hormones and local metabolites stimulate its contraction. A degree of muscle tone is always present, meaning that smooth muscle is only completely relaxed for short periods. Contraction of smooth muscle is slower and more sustained than skeletal muscle. It is found in the walls of hollow organs:

- regulating the diameter of blood vessels and parts of the respiratory tract
- propelling contents along, e.g. the ureters, ducts of glands and the alimentary tract
- expelling contents of the urinary bladder and uterus.

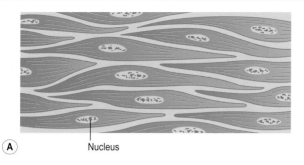

(A) Nucleus

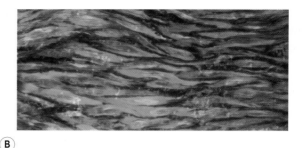

(B)

Figure 3.24 Smooth muscle. A. Diagram. **B.** Fluorescent light micrograph showing actin, a contractile muscle protein (green), nuclei (blue) and capillaries (red).

When examined under a microscope, the cells are seen to be spindle shaped with only one central nucleus. Bundles of fibres form sheets of muscle, such as those found in the walls of the above structures.

Cardiac muscle (Fig. 3.25)

This is only found only in the heart wall. It is not under conscious control but, when viewed under a microscope, cross-stripes (striations) characteristic of skeletal muscle can be seen. Each fibre (cell) has a nucleus and one or more branches. The ends of the cells and their branches are in very close contact with the ends and branches of adjacent cells. Microscopically these 'joints', or *intercalated discs*, appear as lines that are thicker and darker than the ordinary cross-stripes. This arrangement gives cardiac muscle the appearance of a sheet of muscle rather than a very large number of individual fibres. This is significant when the heart contracts as a wave of contraction spreads from cell to cell across the intercalated discs, which means that the cardiac muscle fibres do not need to be stimulated individually.

The heart has an intrinsic pacemaker system, which means that it beats in a coordinated manner without external nerve stimulation, although the rate at which it beats is influenced by autonomic nerve impulses, some hormones, local metabolites and other substances (see Ch. 5).

Nervous tissue

Two types of tissue are found in the nervous system:

- excitable cells – these are called *neurones* and they initiate, receive, conduct and transmit information
- non-excitable cells – also known as *glial cells*, these support the neurones.

These are described in detail in Chapter 7.

Tissue regeneration

The extent to which regeneration is possible depends on the normal rate of turnover of particular types of cell. Those with a rapid turnover regenerate most effectively. There are three general categories:

- tissues in which cell replication is a continuous process regenerate quickly – these include epithelial cells of, for example, the skin, mucous membrane, secretory glands, uterine lining and reticular tissue
- other tissues retain the ability to replicate, but do so infrequently; these include the liver, kidney, fibroblasts and smooth muscle cells. These tissues take longer to regenerate
- some cells are normally unable to replicate including nerve cells (neurones) and skeletal and cardiac muscle cells meaning that damaged tissue cannot be replaced.

Extensively damaged tissue is usually replaced by fibrous tissue, meaning that the functions of the original tissue are lost.

Membranes

Epithelial membranes

These membranes are sheets of epithelial tissue and supporting connective tissue that cover or line many internal

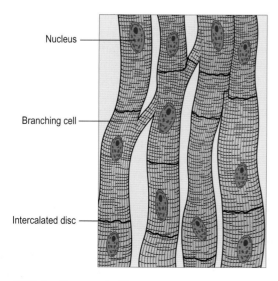

Nucleus

Branching cell

Intercalated disc

Figure 3.25 Cardiac muscle fibres.

structures or cavities. The main ones are mucous membrane, serous membrane and the skin (cutaneous membrane, see Ch. 14).

Mucous membrane ▦ 3.6

This is the moist lining of the alimentary, respiratory and genitourinary tracts and is sometimes referred to as the *mucosa*. The membrane surface consists of epithelial cells, some of which produce a secretion called *mucus*, a slimy tenacious fluid. As it accumulates the cells become distended and finally burst, discharging the mucus onto the free surface. As the cells fill up with mucus they have the appearance of a goblet or flask and are known as *goblet cells* (see Fig. 12.5, p. 290). Organs lined by mucous membrane have a moist slippery surface. Mucus protects the lining membrane from drying, and mechanical and chemical injury. In the respiratory tract it traps inhaled particles, preventing them from entering the alveoli of the lungs.

Serous membrane ▦ 3.7

Serous membranes, or *serosa*, secrete serous watery fluid. They consist of a double layer of loose areolar connective tissue lined by simple squamous epithelium. The *parietal* layer lines a cavity and the *visceral* layer surrounds organs (the viscera) within the cavity. The two layers are separated by *serous fluid* secreted by the epithelium. There are three sites where serous membranes are found:

- the *pleura* lining the thoracic cavity and surrounding the lungs (p. 252)
- the *pericardium* lining the pericardial cavity and surrounding the heart (p. 89)
- the *peritoneum* lining the abdominal cavity and surrounding abdominal organs (p. 288).

The serous fluid between the visceral and parietal layers enables an organ to glide freely within the cavity without being damaged by friction between it and adjacent organs. For example, the heart changes its shape and size during each beat and friction damage is prevented by the arrangement of pericardium and its serous fluid.

Synovial membrane ▦ 3.8

This membrane lines the cavities of moveable joints and surrounds tendons that could be injured by rubbing against bones, e.g. over the wrist joint. It is not an epithelial membrane, but instead consists of areolar connective tissue and elastic fibres.

Synovial membrane secretes clear, sticky, oily *synovial fluid*, which lubricates and nourishes the joints (see Ch. 16).

Glands

Glands are groups of epithelial cells that produce specialised secretions. Those that discharge their secretion onto

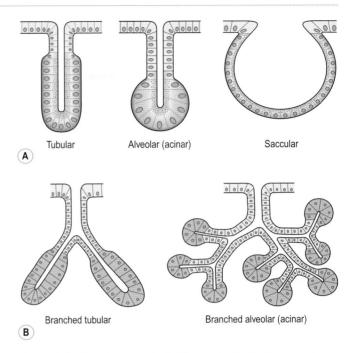

Tubular   Alveolar (acinar)   Saccular

(A)

Branched tubular   Branched alveolar (acinar)

(B)

Figure 3.26 Exocrine glands. A. Simple glands. **B.** Compound (branching) glands.

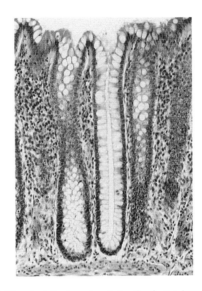

Figure 3.27 Simple tubular glands in the large intestine. A stained photograph (magnified × 50).

the epithelial surface of hollow organs, either directly or through a *duct*, are called *exocrine glands* and vary considerably in size, shape and complexity, as shown in Figure 3.26. Their secretions include mucus, saliva, digestive juices and earwax; Figure 3.27 shows simple tubular glands of the large intestine.

Other glands discharge their secretions into blood and lymph. These are called *endocrine glands* (ductless glands) and they secrete *hormones* (see Ch. 9).

Organisation of the body

Learning outcomes

After studying this section, you should be able to:

- define common anatomical terms
- identify the principal bones of the axial skeleton and the appendicular skeleton
- state the boundaries of the four body cavities
- list the contents of the body cavities.

This part of the chapter explains the anatomical terminology used to ensure that relationships between body structures are described consistently. An overview of the bones forming the skeleton is provided and the contents of the body cavities are explored.

Anatomical terms

The anatomical position. The position is used in all anatomical descriptions to ensure accuracy and consistency. The body is in the upright position with the head facing forward, the arms at the sides with the palms of the hands facing forward and the feet together.

Directional terms. These paired terms are used to describe the location of body parts in relation to others, and are explained in Table 3.1.

Regional terms. These are used to describe parts of the body (Fig. 3.28).

Body planes (Fig. 3.29)

There are three body planes, which lie at right angles to each other. These divide the body into sections and are used to visualise or describe its internal arrangement from different perspectives. The anatomical position (see above) is used as the reference position in descriptions using body planes.

Median plane. When the body is divided longitudinally through the midline into right and left halves it has been divided in the median plane, e.g. Figure 3.40. A *sagittal section* is any section made parallel to the median plane.

Coronal plane. A coronal or frontal section divides the body longitudinally into its anterior (front) and posterior (back) sections, e.g. Figure 7.19.

Transverse plane. A transverse or horizontal section provides a cross section dividing the body or body part into upper and lower parts. This may be at any level e.g. through the cranial cavity, thorax, abdomen, a limb or an organ, e.g. Figure 7.28.

Anatomical reference icons used in this book

These icons have been used to clarify relationships between body parts; many figures have a compass-like icon labelled with anatomical directions corresponding to the paired directional terms shown in Table 3.1 (see

Table 3.1 Paired directional terms used in anatomy

Directional term	Meaning
Medial	Structure is nearer to the midline. *The heart is medial to the humerus*
Lateral	Structure is further from the midline or at the side of the body. *The humerus is lateral to the heart*
Proximal	Nearer to a point of attachment of a limb, or origin of a body part. *The femur is proximal to the fibula*
Distal	Further from a point of attachment of a limb, or origin of a body part. *The fibula is distal to the femur*
Anterior or ventral	Part of the body being described is nearer the front of the body. *The sternum is anterior to the vertebrae*
Posterior or dorsal	Part of the body being described is nearer the back of the body. *The vertebrae are posterior to the sternum*
Superior	Structure nearer the head. *The skull is superior to the scapulae*
Inferior	Structure further from the head. *The scapulae are inferior to the skull*

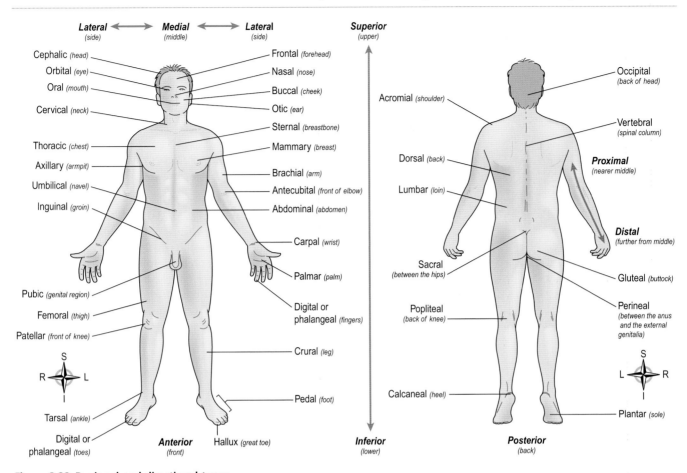

Figure 3.28 Regional and directional terms.

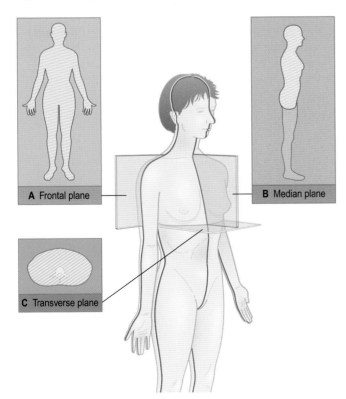

Figure 3.29 Body planes.

e.g. Fig. 3.28). A full description of all the icons used in the book is shown on page vi.

The skeleton

The skeleton (Fig. 3.30) is the bony framework of the body. It forms the cavities and fossae (depressions or hollows) that protect some structures, forms the joints and gives attachment to muscles. A detailed description of the bones is given in Chapter 16. Table 16.1, page 395 lists the terminology related to the skeleton.

The skeleton is described in two parts: *axial* and *appendicular* (the appendages attached to the axial skeleton).

Axial skeleton

The axial skeleton (axis of the body) consists of the skull, vertebral column, sternum (breast bone) and the ribs.

Skull

The skull is described in two parts, the *cranium*, which contains the brain, and the *face*. It consists of several bones, which develop separately but fuse together as they mature. The only movable bone is the mandible or lower

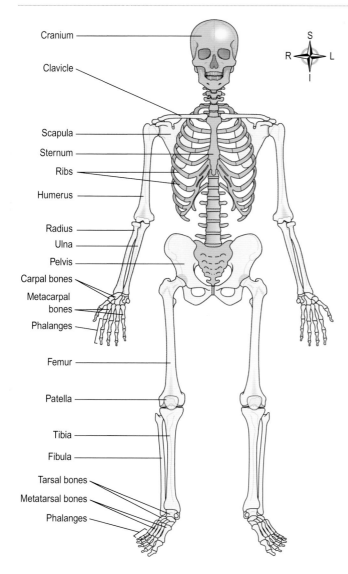

Cranium

Clavicle

Scapula

Sternum

Ribs

Humerus

Radius

Ulna

Pelvis

Carpal bones

Metacarpal bones

Phalanges

Femur

Patella

Tibia

Fibula

Tarsal bones

Metatarsal bones

Phalanges

Figure 3.30 Anterior view of the skeleton. Axial skeleton – gold, appendicular skeleton – light brown.

jaw. The names and positions of the individual bones of the skull can be seen in Figure 3.31.

Functions

The various parts of the skull have specific and different functions (see p. 401) and are, in summary:

- protection of delicate structures including the brain, eyes and inner ears
- maintaining patency of the nasal passages enabling breathing
- eating – the teeth are embedded in the mandible and maxilla; and movement of the mandible allows chewing.

Vertebral column 3.9

This consists of 24 movable bones (vertebrae) plus the sacrum and coccyx. The bodies of the bones are separated from each other by *intervertebral discs*, consisting of fibrocartilage. The vertebral column is described in five parts and the bones of each part are numbered from above downwards (Fig. 3.32):

- 7 cervical
- 12 thoracic
- 5 lumbar
- 1 sacrum (5 fused bones)
- 1 coccyx (4 fused bones).

The first cervical vertebra, called the *atlas*, forms a joint (*articulates*) with the skull. Thereafter each vertebra forms a joint with the vertebrae immediately above and below. More movement is possible in the cervical and lumbar regions than in the thoracic region.

The *sacrum* consists of five vertebrae fused into one bone that articulates with the fifth lumbar vertebra above, the coccyx below and an innominate (pelvic or hip) bone at each side.

The *coccyx* consists of the four terminal vertebrae fused into a small triangular bone that articulates with the sacrum above.

Functions

The vertebral column has several important functions:

- it protects the spinal cord. In each vertebra is a hole, the *vertebral foramen*, and collectively the foramina form a canal in which the spinal cord lies
- adjacent vertebrae form openings (intervertebral foramina), which protect the spinal nerves as they pass from the spinal cord (see Fig. 16.26, p. 404)
- in the thoracic region the ribs articulate with the vertebrae forming joints that allow movement of the ribcage during respiration.

Thoracic cage

The thoracic cage (Fig. 3.33) is formed by:

- 12 thoracic vertebrae
- 12 pairs of ribs
- 1 sternum or breast bone.

Functions

The thoracic cage:

- protects the contents of the thorax including the heart, lungs and large blood vessels
- forms joints between the upper limbs and the axial skeleton. The upper part of the sternum, the *manubrium*, articulates with the clavicles forming the only joints between the upper limbs and the axial skeleton
- gives attachment to the muscles of respiration:
  - *intercostal muscles* occupy the spaces between the ribs and when they contract the ribs move

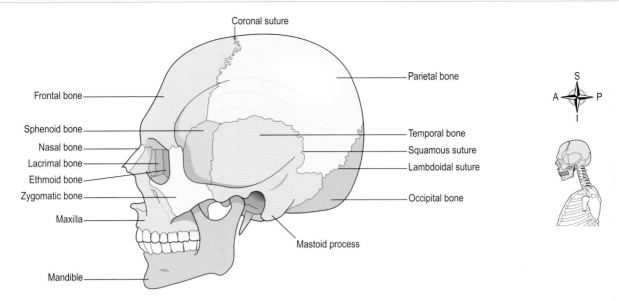

Figure 3.31 The skull: bones of the cranium and face.

upwards and outwards, increasing the capacity of the thoracic cage, and inspiration occurs
- the *diaphragm* is a dome-shaped muscle which separates the thoracic and abdominal cavities; when it contracts it assists with inspiration
• enables breathing to take place.

Appendicular skeleton

The appendicular skeleton consists of the shoulder girdles and upper limbs, and the pelvic girdle and lower limbs (Fig. 3.30).

The shoulder girdles and upper limbs. Each shoulder girdle consists of a clavicle and a scapula. Each upper limb comprises:

• 1 humerus
• 1 radius
• 1 ulna
• 8 carpal bones
• 5 metacarpal bones
• 14 phalanges.

The pelvic girdle and lower limbs. The bones of the pelvic girdle are the two innominate bones and the sacrum. Each lower limb consists of:

• 1 femur
• 1 tibia
• 1 fibula
• 1 patella
• 7 tarsal bones
• 5 metatarsal bones
• 14 phalanges.

Functions
The appendicular skeleton has two main functions.

• *Voluntary movement.* The bones, muscles and joints of the limbs are involved in movement of the skeleton. This ranges from very fine finger movements needed for writing to the coordinated movement of all the limbs associated with running and jumping.

• *Protection of blood vessels and nerves.* These delicate structures along the length of bones of the limbs and are protected from injury by the associated muscles and skin. They are most vulnerable where they cross joints and where bones can be felt immediately below the skin.

Cavities of the body

The body organs are contained and protected within four cavities: cranial, thoracic, abdominal and pelvic.

Cranial cavity

The cranial cavity contains the brain, and its boundaries are formed by the bones of the skull (Fig. 3.34):

Anteriorly – 1 frontal bone
Laterally – 2 temporal bones
Posteriorly – 1 occipital bone
Superiorly – 2 parietal bones
Inferiorly – 1 sphenoid and 1 ethmoid bone and parts of the frontal, temporal and occipital bones.

Thoracic cavity

This cavity is situated in the upper part of the trunk. Its boundaries are formed by the thoracic cage (Fig. 3.33) and supporting muscles (Fig. 3.35):

Anteriorly – the sternum and costal cartilages of the ribs
Laterally – 12 pairs of ribs and the intercostal muscles
Posteriorly – the thoracic vertebrae
Superiorly – the structures forming the root of the neck
Inferiorly – the diaphragm, a dome-shaped muscle.

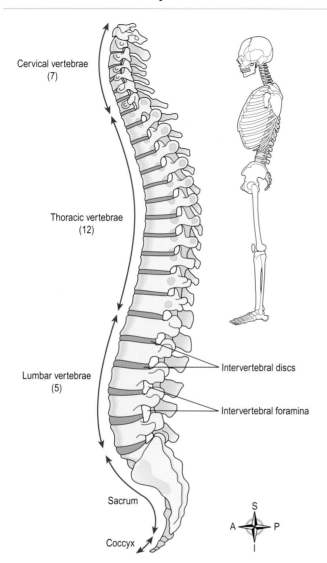

Figure 3.32 **The vertebral column.** Lateral view.

Contents of the thoracic cavity

The main organs and structures contained in the thoracic cavity are shown in Figure 5.10, page 88. These include:

- the trachea, 2 bronchi, 2 lungs
- the heart, aorta, superior and inferior vena cavae, numerous other blood vessels
- the oesophagus

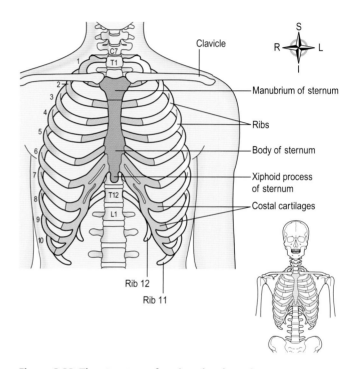

Figure 3.33 **The structures forming the thoracic cage.**

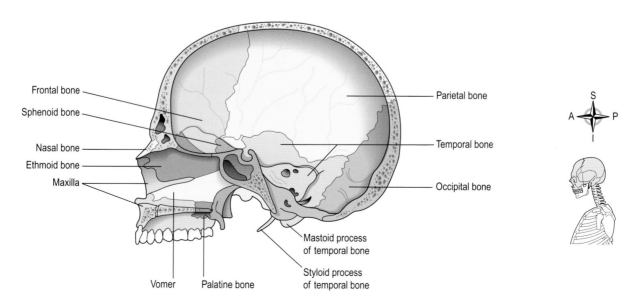

Figure 3.34 **Bones forming the right half of the cranium and the face.** Viewed from the left.

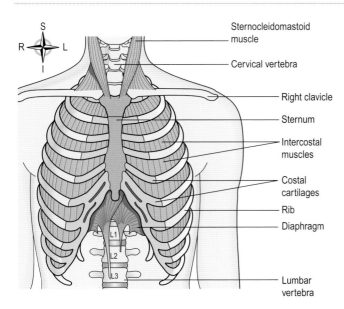

Figure 3.35 Structures forming the walls of the thoracic cavity and associated structures.

- lymph vessels and lymph nodes
- some important nerves.

The *mediastinum* is the space between the lungs including the structures found there, such as the heart, oesophagus and blood vessels.

Abdominal cavity 3.10

This is the largest body cavity and is oval in shape (Figs 3.36 and 3.37). It occupies most of the trunk and its boundaries are:

Superiorly – the diaphragm, which separates it from the thoracic cavity

Anteriorly – the muscles forming the anterior abdominal wall

Posteriorly – the lumbar vertebrae and muscles forming the posterior abdominal wall

Laterally – the lower ribs and parts of the muscles of the abdominal wall

Inferiorly – it is continuous with the pelvic cavity.

By convention, the abdominal cavity is divided into the nine regions shown in Figure 3.38. This facilitates the description of the positions of the organs and structures it contains.

Contents

Most of the abdominal cavity is occupied by the organs and glands of the digestive system (Figs 3.36 and 3.37). These are:

- the stomach, small intestine and most of the large intestine
- the liver, gall bladder, bile ducts and pancreas.

Other structures include:

- the spleen
- 2 kidneys and the upper part of the ureters
- 2 adrenal (suprarenal) glands
- numerous blood vessels, lymph vessels, nerves
- lymph nodes.

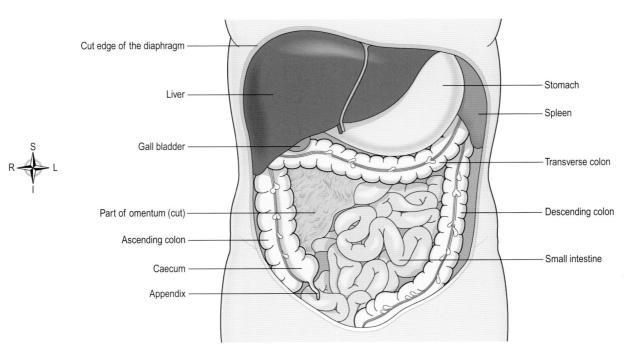

Figure 3.36 Organs occupying the anterior part of the abdominal cavity and the diaphragm (cut).

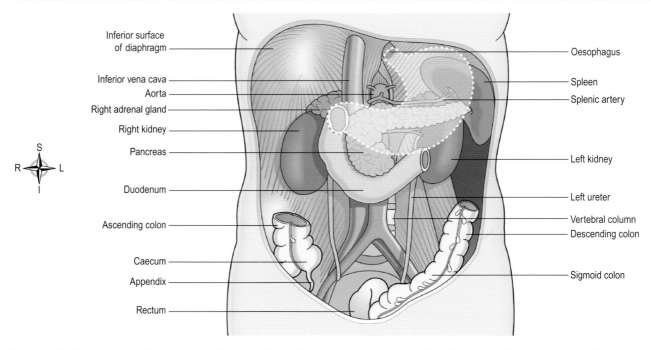

Figure 3.37 Organs occupying the posterior part of the abdominal and pelvic cavities. The broken line shows the position of the stomach.

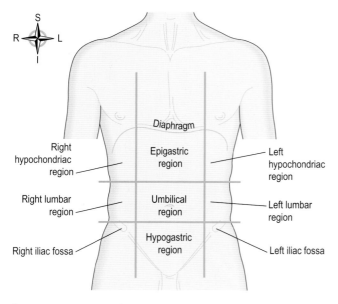

Figure 3.38 Regions of the abdominal cavity.

Pelvic cavity

The pelvic cavity is roughly funnel shaped and extends from the lower end of the abdominal cavity (Figs 3.39 and 3.40). The boundaries are:

Superiorly – it is continuous with the abdominal cavity
Anteriorly – the pubic bones

Posteriorly – the sacrum and coccyx
Laterally – the innominate bones
Inferiorly – the muscles of the pelvic floor.

Contents

The pelvic cavity contains the following structures:

- sigmoid colon, rectum and anus
- some loops of the small intestine
- urinary bladder, lower parts of the ureters and the urethra
- in the female, the organs of the reproductive system: the uterus, uterine tubes, ovaries and vagina (Fig. 3.39)
- in the male, some of the organs of the reproductive system: the prostate gland, seminal vesicles, spermatic cords, deferent ducts (vas deferens), ejaculatory ducts and the urethra (common to the reproductive and urinary systems) (Fig. 3.40).

Changes in cell size and number

The earlier part of this chapter explored characteristics typical of normal cells and tissues, but these may be affected by physiological and/or pathological changes.

Cells may enlarge, known as *hypertrophy* (Fig. 3.41) in response to additional demands, e.g skeletal muscle cells hypertrophy in response to fitness training, increasing the

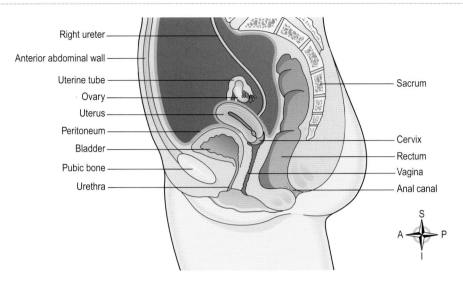

Figure 3.39 Female reproductive organs and other structures in the pelvic cavity.

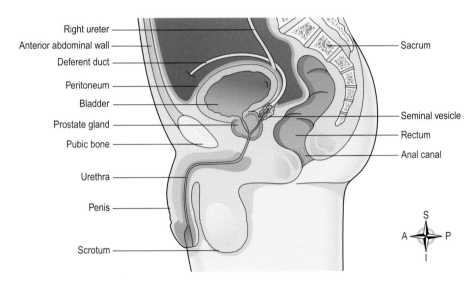

Figure 3.40 The pelvic cavity and reproductive structures in the male.

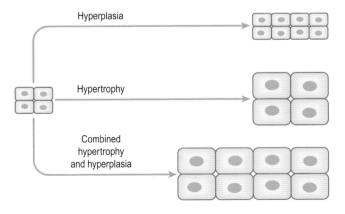

Figure 3.41 Hyperplasia and hypertrophy.

bulk and tone of the exercised muscle. A decrease in cell size or the number of cells is referred to as *atrophy*. Without use, muscle fibres atrophy (and muscle mass also decreases), e.g. those of a limb in a plaster cast applied to immobilise a fracture. Impaired nutrient or oxygen supply can also lead to atrophy.

Hyperplasia (Fig. 3.41) occurs when cells divide more quickly than previously, increasing cell numbers (and size of the tissue/organ), e.g. the glandular milk-producing tissue of the breasts during pregnancy and breast feeding. Abnormal hyperplasia can lead to development of tumours when mitosis is no longer controlled and the daughter cells may show abnormal internal characteristics (see cell differentiation, p. 56).

Cell death

Two different mechanisms are recognised.

Apoptosis

This is normal genetically programmed cell death where an ageing cell at the end of its life cycle shrinks and its remaining fragments are phagocytosed without any inflammatory reaction. In later life, fewer cells lost by apoptosis are replaced, contributing to the general reduction in tissue mass and organ sizes in older adults.

Necrosis

This is cell death resulting from lack of oxygen (*ischaemia*), injury or a pathological process. The plasma membrane ruptures releasing the intracellular contents, triggering the inflammatory response. Inflammation is the first stage of tissue repair and is needed to clear the area of cell debris before healing and tissue repair can progress (Ch. 14).

Neoplasms or tumours

Learning outcomes

After studying this section, you should be able to:

- outline the common causes of tumours

- explain the terms 'well differentiated' and 'poorly differentiated'

- outline causes of death in malignant disease

- compare and contrast the effects of benign and malignant tumours.

A tumour or *neoplasm* (literally meaning 'new growth') is a mass of tissue that grows faster than normal in an uncoordinated manner, and continues to grow after the initial stimulus has ceased.

Tumours are classified as benign or malignant although a clear distinction is not always possible (see Table 3.2). Benign tumours only rarely change their character and become malignant. Tumours, whether malignant or benign, may be classified according to their tissue of origin, e.g. *adeno-* (glandular) or, *sarco-* (connective tissue); the latter may be further distinguished e.g. *myo-* (muscle), *osteo-* (bone). Malignant tumours are further classified according to their origins; for example, a *carcinoma*, the commonest form of malignancy, originates from epithelial tissue and a *sarcoma* arises from connective tissue. Hence, an *adenoma* is a benign tumour of glandular tissue but an *adenocarcinoma* is a malignant tumour of the epithelial component of glands; a benign bone tumour is an *osteoma*, a malignant bone tumour an *osteosarcoma*.

Table 3.2 Typical differences between benign and malignant tumours

Benign	Malignant
Slow growth	Rapid growth
Cells well differentiated (resemble tissue of origin)	Cells poorly differentiated (may not resemble tissue of origin)
Usually encapsulated	Not encapsulated
No distant spread (metastases)	Spreads (metastasises): – by local infiltration – via lymph – via blood – via body cavities
Recurrence is rare	Recurrence is common

Causes of neoplasms

There are more than 200 different types of cancer, but all are caused by mutations within the cell's genetic material. Some mutations are spontaneous, i.e. happen by chance during cell division, others are related to exposure to a mutagenic agent (a *carcinogen*) and a small proportion are inherited. Advancing knowledge in the area has led to identification of many specific genes/chromosome mutations associated directly with particular cancers. Cell growth is regulated by genes that inhibit cell growth (*tumour suppressor genes*) and genes that stimulate cell growth (*proto-oncogenes*). One important tumour suppressor gene, *p53*, is thought to be defective in 50–60% of cancers. A proto-oncogene that becomes abnormally activated and allows uncontrolled cell growth can also cause cancers and is then referred to as an *oncogene*.

Carcinogens

These cause malignant changes in cells by irreversibly damaging a cell's DNA. It is impossible to specify a maximum 'safe dose' of a carcinogen. A small dose may initiate change but this may not be enough to cause malignancy unless there are repeated doses over time that have a cumulative effect. In addition, there are widely varying latent periods between exposure and signs of malignancy.

Chemical carcinogens
Examples include:

- cigarette smoke, which is the main risk factor for lung (bronchial) cancer (p. 269)
- aniline dyes, which predispose to bladder cancer (p. 356)
- asbestos, which is associated with pleural mesothelioma (p. 270).

Ionising radiation
Exposure to ionising radiation including X-rays, radioactive isotopes, environmental radiation and ultraviolet rays in sunlight may cause malignant changes in some cells and kill others. Cells are affected during mitosis so those normally undergoing frequent division are most susceptible. These labile tissues include skin, mucous membrane, bone marrow, reticular tissue and gametes in the ovaries and testes. For example, repeated episodes of sunburn (caused by exposure to ultraviolet rays in sunlight) predispose to development of skin cancer (see malignant melanoma, p. 373).

Oncogenic viruses
Some viruses cause malignant changes. Such viruses enter cells and incorporate their DNA or RNA into the host cell's genetic material, which causes mutation. The mutant cells may be malignant. Examples include

hepatitis B virus, which can cause liver cancer (p. 334) and human papilloma virus (HPV), which is associated with cervical cancer (p. 467).

Host factors

Individual characteristics can influence susceptibility to tumours. Some are outwith individual control e.g. race, increasing age and inherited (genetic) factors. Others can be modified and are referred to as *lifestyle factors*; these include eating a healthy balanced diet, cigarette smoking, taking sufficient exercise and avoiding obesity. Making healthy lifestyle choices where possible is important as these factors are thought to be involved in the development of nearly half of all malignant tumours. Tumours of specific tissues and organs are described in later chapters.

Growth of tumours

Normally cells divide in an orderly manner. Neoplastic cells have escaped from the normal controls and multiply in a disorderly and uncontrolled manner forming a tumour. Blood vessels grow with the proliferating cells, providing them with a good supply of oxygen and nutrients that promotes their growth. In some malignant tumours the blood supply does not keep pace with growth and *ischaemia* (lack of blood supply) leads to tumour cell death. If the tumour is near the body surface, this may result in skin ulceration and infection. In deeper tissues there is fibrosis; e.g. retraction of the nipple in breast cancer is due to the shrinkage of fibrous tissue in a necrotic tumour.

Cell differentiation

Differentiation into specialised cell types with particular structural and functional characteristics occurs at an early stage in fetal development, e.g. epithelial cells develop different characteristics from lymphocytes. Later, when cell replacement occurs, daughter cells have the same appearance, functions and genetic make-up as the parent cell. In benign tumours the cells from which they originate are easily recognised, i.e. tumour cells are *well differentiated*. Tumours with well-differentiated cells are usually benign but some may be malignant. Malignant tumours grow beyond their normal boundaries and show varying levels of differentiation:

- *mild dysplasia* – the tumour cells retain most of their normal features and their parent cells can usually be identified
- *anaplasia* – the tumour cells have lost most of their normal features and their parent cells cannot be identified.

Encapsulation and spread of tumours

Most benign tumours are contained within a fibrous capsule derived partly from the surrounding tissues and partly from the tumour. They neither invade local tissues nor spread to other parts of the body, even when they are not encapsulated.

Malignant tumours are not encapsulated. They spread locally by growing into and infiltrating nearby tissue (known as *invasion*). Tumour fragments may spread to other parts of the body in blood or lymph. Some of the spreading tumour cells may be recognised as 'non-self' and phagocytosed by macrophages or destroyed by defence cells of the immune system, e.g. cytotoxic T-cells and natural killer cells (see Ch. 15). Others may escape detection and lodge in tissues away from the primary site and grow into *secondary tumours* (metastases). Metastases are often multiple and Table 3.3 shows common sites of primary tumours and their metastases.

The likely prognosis may by assessed using *staging,* a process that assesses the size and spread of the tumour. A commonly used example is the *TMN system* where T is tumour size, N indicates affected regional lymph nodes and M identifies metastatic sites. For most tumours, large size and extensive spread suggest a poorer prognosis.

Local spread

Benign tumours enlarge and may cause pressure damage to local structures but they do not spread to other parts of the body.

Benign or malignant tumours may:

- damage nerves, causing pain and loss of nerve control of other tissues and organs supplied by the damaged nerves
- compress adjacent structures causing e.g. ischaemia (lack of blood), necrosis (death of tissue), blockage of ducts, organ dysfunction or displacement, or pain due to pressure on nerves.

Additionally, *malignant tumours* invade surrounding tissues and may also erode blood and lymph vessel walls, causing spread of tumour cells to distant parts of the body.

Table 3.3 Common sites of primary tumours and their metastases

Primary tumour	Metastatic tumours
Bronchi	Adrenal glands, brain
Alimentary tract	Abdominal and pelvic structures, especially liver
Prostate gland	Pelvic bones, vertebrae
Thyroid gland	Pelvic bones, vertebrae
Breast	Vertebrae, brain, bone
Many organs	Lungs

Body cavities spread

This occurs when a tumour penetrates the wall of a cavity. The peritoneal cavity is most frequently involved. If, for example, a malignant tumour in an abdominal organ invades the visceral peritoneum, tumour cells may metastasise to folds of peritoneum or any abdominal or pelvic organ. Where there is less scope for the movement of fragments within a cavity, the tumour tends to bind layers of tissue together, e.g. a pleural tumour binds the visceral and parietal layers together, limiting expansion of the lung.

Lymphatic spread

This occurs when malignant tumours invade nearby lymph vessels. Groups of tumour cells break off and are carried to lymph nodes where they lodge and may grow into secondary tumours. There may be further spread through the lymphatic system and to blood because lymph drains into the subclavian veins.

Blood spread

This occurs when a malignant tumour erodes the walls of a blood vessel. A *thrombus* (blood clot) may form at the site and *emboli* consisting of fragments of tumour and blood clot enter the bloodstream. These emboli block small blood vessels, causing *infarcts* (areas of dead tissue) and development of metastatic tumours. Phagocytosis of tumour cells in the emboli is unlikely to occur because these are protected by the blood clot. Single tumour cells can also lodge in the capillaries of other body organs. Division and subsequent growth of secondary tumours, or *metastases*, may then occur. The sites of blood-spread metastases depend on the location of the original tumour and the anatomy of the circulatory system in the area. The most common sites of these metastases are bone, the lungs, the brain and the liver.

Effects of tumours

Pressure effects

Both benign and malignant tumours may compress and damage adjacent structures, especially if in a confined space. The effects depend on the site of the tumour but are most marked in areas where there is little space for expansion, e.g. inside the skull, under the periosteum of bones, in bony sinuses and respiratory passages. Compression of adjacent structures may cause ischaemia, necrosis, blockage of ducts, organ dysfunction or displacement, pain due to invasion of nerves or pressure on nerves.

Hormonal effects

Tumours of endocrine glands may secrete hormones, producing the effects of hypersecretion. The extent of cell dysplasia is an important factor. Well-differentiated benign tumours are more likely to secrete hormones than markedly dysplastic malignant tumours. High levels of hormones are found in the bloodstream as secretion occurs in the absence of the normal stimulus and homeostatic control mechanism. Some malignant tumours produce uncharacteristic hormones, e.g. some lung tumours produce insulin. Endocrine glands may be destroyed by invading tumours, causing hormone deficiency.

Cachexia

This is the severe weight loss accompanied by progressive weakness, loss of appetite, wasting and anaemia that is usually associated with advanced metastatic cancer. The severity is usually indicative of the stage of the disease. The causes are not clear.

Causes of death in malignant disease

Infection

Acute infection is a common cause of death when superimposed on advanced malignancy. Predisposition to infection is increased by prolonged immobility or bedrest, and by depression of the immune system by cytotoxic drugs and radiotherapy or radioactive isotopes used in treatment. The most common infections are pneumonia, septicaemia, peritonitis and pyelonephritis.

Organ failure

A tumour may destroy so much healthy tissue that an organ cannot function. Severe damage to vital organs, such as lungs, brain, liver and kidneys, are common causes of death.

Carcinomatosis

This is the presence of widespread metastatic disease and is usually associated with cachexia. Increasingly severe physiological and biochemical disruption follows causing death.

Haemorrhage

This occurs when a tumour grows into and ruptures the wall of a vein or artery. The most common sites are the gastrointestinal tract, brain, lungs and the peritoneal cavity.

 For a range of self-assessment exercises on the topics in this chapter, visit Evolve online resources: https://evolve.elsevier.com/Waugh/anatomy/

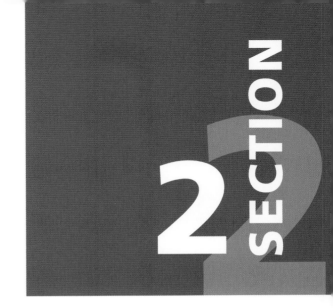

SECTION 2

Communication

The blood

ANIMATIONS

Blood is a fluid connective tissue. It circulates constantly around the body, allowing constant communication between tissues distant from each other. It transports:

- oxygen
- nutrients
- hormones
- heat
- protective substances
- clotting factors.

Blood is composed of a clear, straw-coloured, watery fluid called *plasma* in which several different types of blood cell are suspended. Plasma normally constitutes 55% of the volume of blood and the cell fraction 45%. Blood cells and plasma can be separated by centrifugation (spinning) or by gravity when blood is allowed to stand (Fig. 4.1A). The cells are heavier than plasma and sink to the bottom of any sample.

Blood makes up about 7% of body weight (about 5.6 litres in a 70 kg man). This proportion is less in women and considerably greater in children, gradually decreasing until the adult level is reached.

Blood in the blood vessels is always in motion because of the pumping action of the heart. The continual flow maintains a fairly constant environment for body cells. Blood volume and the concentration of its many constituents are kept within narrow limits by homeostatic mechanisms. Heat produced from metabolically active organs, such as working skeletal muscles and the liver, is distributed around the body by the bloodstream, contributing to maintenance of core body temperature.

The first part of the chapter describes normal blood physiology, and the later sections are concerned with some disorders of the blood. Effects of ageing on white blood cell function are described in Chapter 15.

Plasma

Learning outcomes

After studying this section, you should be able to:

- list the constituents of plasma
- describe their functions

The constituents of plasma are water (90–92%) and dissolved and suspended substances, including:

- plasma proteins
- inorganic salts
- nutrients, principally from digested foods
- waste materials
- hormones
- gases.

Plasma proteins

Plasma proteins, which make up about 7% of plasma, are normally retained within the blood, because they are too big to escape through the capillary pores into the tissues. They are largely responsible for creating the osmotic pressure of blood (p. 86), which keeps plasma fluid within the circulation. If plasma protein levels fall, because of either reduced production or loss from the blood vessels, osmotic pressure is also reduced, and fluid moves into the tissues (oedema) and body cavities.

Plasma viscosity (thickness) is due to plasma proteins, mainly albumin and fibrinogen. Plasma proteins, with the exception of immunoglobulins, are formed in the liver.

Albumins. These are the most abundant plasma proteins (about 60% of total) and their main function is to maintain normal plasma osmotic pressure. Albumins also act as carrier molecules for free fatty acids, some drugs and steroid hormones.

Globulins. Their main functions are:

- as *antibodies* (immunoglobulins), which are complex proteins produced by lymphocytes that play an important part in immunity. They bind to, and neutralise, foreign materials (antigens) such as microorganisms (see also p. 381).
- transportation of some hormones and mineral salts, e.g. thyroglobulin, carries the hormone thyroxine and transferrin carries the mineral iron
- inhibition of some proteolytic enzymes, e.g. α_2 macroglobulin inhibits trypsin activity.

Clotting factors. These are responsible for coagulation of blood (p. 71). *Serum* is plasma from which clotting factors have been removed (Fig. 4.1B). The most abundant clotting factor is *fibrinogen*.

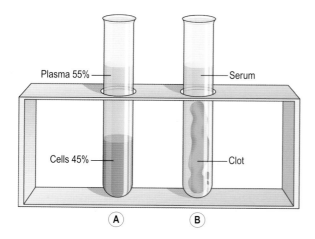

Plasma 55%

Serum

Cells 45%

Clot

(A) (B)

Figure 4.1 A. The proportions of blood cells and plasma in whole blood separated by gravity. **B.** A blood clot in serum.

Electrolytes

These have a range of functions, including muscle contraction (e.g. Ca^{2+}), transmission of nerve impulses (e.g. Ca^{2+} and Na^+), and maintenance of acid–base balance (e.g. phosphate, PO_4^{3-}). The pH of blood is maintained between 7.35 and 7.45 (slightly alkaline) by an ongoing buffering system (p. 25).

Nutrients

The products of digestion, e.g. glucose, amino acids, fatty acids and glycerol, are absorbed from the alimentary tract. Together with mineral salts and vitamins they are used by body cells for energy, heat, repair and replacement, and for the synthesis of other blood components and body secretions.

Waste products

Urea, creatinine and uric acid are the waste products of protein metabolism. They are formed in the liver and carried in blood to the kidneys for excretion. Carbon dioxide from tissue metabolism is transported to the lungs for excretion.

Hormones (see Ch. 9)

These are chemical messengers synthesised by endocrine glands. Hormones pass directly from the endocrine cells into the blood, which transports them to their target tissues and organs elsewhere in the body, where they influence cellular activity.

Gases

Oxygen, carbon dioxide and nitrogen are transported round the body dissolved in plasma. Oxygen and carbon dioxide are also transported in combination with haemoglobin in red blood cells (p. 65). Most oxygen is carried in combination with haemoglobin and most carbon dioxide as bicarbonate ions dissolved in plasma (p. 260). Atmospheric nitrogen enters the body in the same way as other gases and is present in plasma but it has no physiological function.

Cellular content of blood 4.1

Learning outcomes

After studying this section, you should be able to:

- discuss the structure, function and formation of red blood cells, including the systems used in medicine to classify the different types

- discuss the functions and formation of the different types of white blood cell

- outline the role of platelets in blood clotting.

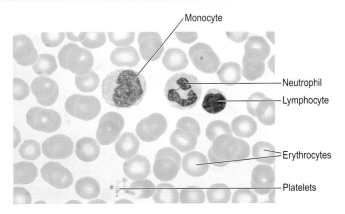

Figure 4.2 A blood smear, showing erythrocytes, a monocyte, a neutrophil, a lymphocyte and a platelet.

There are three types of blood cell (Fig. 4.2).

- erythrocytes (red cells)
- platelets (thrombocytes)
- leukocytes (white cells).

Blood cells are synthesised mainly in red bone marrow. Some lymphocytes, additionally, are produced in lymphoid tissue. In the bone marrow, all blood cells originate from *pluripotent* (i.e. capable of developing into one of a number of cell types) *stem cells* and go through several developmental stages before entering the blood. Different types of blood cell follow separate lines of development. The process of blood cell formation is called *haemopoiesis* (Fig. 4.3).

For the first few years of life, red marrow occupies the entire bone capacity and, over the next 20 years, is gradually replaced by fatty yellow marrow that has no haemopoietic function. In adults, haemopoiesis in the skeleton is confined to flat bones, irregular bones and the ends (*epiphyses*) of long bones, the main sites being the sternum, ribs, pelvis and skull.

Erythrocytes (red blood cells) 4.2

Red blood cells are by far the most abundant type of blood cell; 99% of all blood cells are erythrocytes (Fig. 4.2). They are biconcave discs with no nucleus, and their diameter is about 7 μm (Fig. 4.4). Their main function is in gas transport, mainly of oxygen, but they also carry some carbon dioxide. Their characteristic shape is suited to their purpose; the biconcavity increases their surface area for gas exchange, and the thinness of the central portion allows fast entry and exit of gases. The cells are flexible so they can squeeze through narrow capillaries, and contain no intracellular organelles, leaving more room for haemoglobin, the large pigmented protein responsible for gas transport.

Measurements of red cell numbers, volume and haemoglobin content are routine and useful assessments

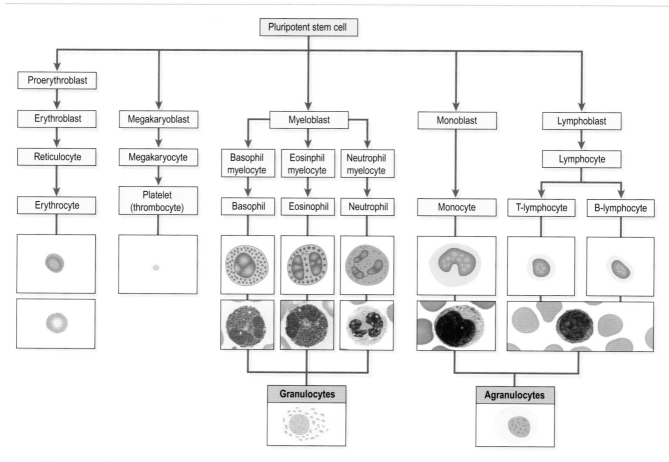

Figure 4.3 Haemopoiesis: stages in the development of blood cells.

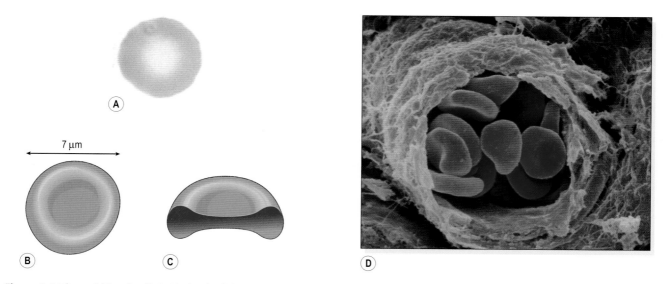

Figure 4.4 The red blood cell. A. Under the light microscope. **B.** Drawn from the front. **C.** Drawn in section. **D.** Coloured scanning electron micrograph of a group of red blood cells travelling along an arteriole.

Table 4.1 Erythrocytes – normal values

Measure	Normal values
Erythrocyte count – number of erythrocytes per litre, or cubic millilitre, (mm³) of blood	Male: 4.5×10^{12}/L to 6.5×10^{12}/L (4.5–6.5 million/mm³) Female: 3.8×10^{12}/L to 5.8×10^{12}/L (3.8–5.8 million/mm³)
Packed cell volume (PCV, haematocrit) – the volume of red cells in 1 L or mm³ of blood	0.40–0.55 L/L
Mean cell volume (MCV) – the volume of an average cell, measured in femtolitres (1 fL = 10^{-15} litre)	80–96 fL
Haemoglobin – the weight of haemoglobin in whole blood, measured in grams/100 mL blood	Male: 13–18 g/100 mL Female: 11.5–16.5 g/100 mL
Mean cell haemoglobin (MCH) – the average amount of haemoglobin per cell, measured in picograms (1 pg = 10^{-12} gram)	27–32 pg/cell
Mean cell haemoglobin concentration (MCHC) – the weight of haemoglobin in 100 mL of red cells	30–35 g/100 mL of red cells

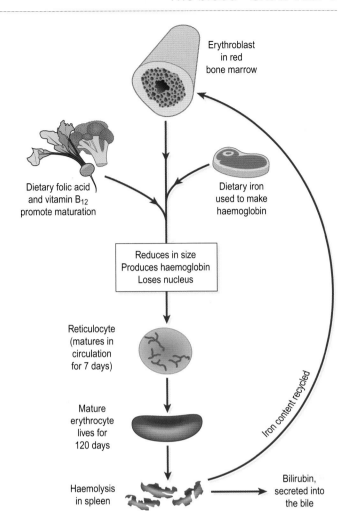

Figure 4.5 Life cycle of the erythrocyte.

made in clinical practice (Table 4.1). The symbols in brackets are the abbreviations commonly used in laboratory reports.

Life span and function of erythrocytes

Because they have no nucleus, erythrocytes cannot divide and so need to be continually replaced by new cells from the red bone marrow, which is present in the ends of long bones and in flat and irregular bones. They pass through several stages of development before entering the blood. Their life span in the circulation is about 120 days. There are approximately 30 trillion (10^{14}) red blood cells in the average human body, about 25% of the body's total cell count, and around 1%, mainly older cells, are cleared and destroyed daily.

The process of development of red blood cells from stem cells takes about 7 days and is called *erythropoiesis* (Fig. 4.3). The immature cells are released into the bloodstream as reticulocytes, and mature into erythrocytes over a day or two within the circulation. During this time, they lose their nucleus and therefore become incapable of division (Fig. 4.5).

Both vitamin B_{12} and folic acid are required for red blood cell synthesis. They are absorbed in the intestines, although vitamin B_{12} must be bound to intrinsic factor (p. 300) to allow absorption to take place. Both vitamins are present in dairy products, meat and green vegetables. The liver usually contains substantial stores of vitamin B_{12}, several years' worth, but signs of folic acid deficiency appear within a few months. The life cycle of the erythrocyte is shown in Figure 4.5.

Haemoglobin

Haemoglobin is a large, complex molecule containing a globular protein (globin) and a pigmented iron-containing complex called haem. Each haemoglobin molecule contains four globin chains and four haem units, each with one atom of iron (Fig. 4.6). As each atom of iron can combine with an oxygen molecule, this means that a single haemoglobin molecule can carry up to four molecules of oxygen. An average red blood cell carries about 280 million haemoglobin molecules, giving each cell a

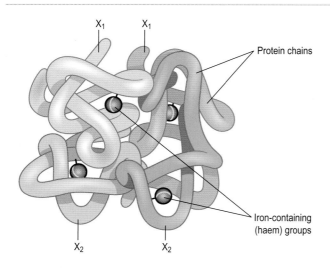

Figure 4.6 The haemoglobin molecule.

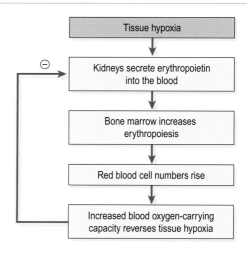

Figure 4.7 Control of erythropoiesis: the role of erythropoietin.

theoretical oxygen-carrying capacity of over a billion oxygen molecules!

Iron is carried in the bloodstream bound to its transport protein, *transferrin*, and stored in the liver. Normal red cell production requires a steady supply of iron. Absorption of iron from the alimentary canal is very slow, even if the diet is rich in iron, meaning that iron deficiency can readily occur if losses exceed intake.

Oxygen transport

When all four oxygen-binding sites on a haemoglobin molecule are full, it is described as *saturated*. Haemoglobin binds reversibly to oxygen to form oxyhaemoglobin, according to the equation:

$$\text{Haemoglobin} + \text{oxygen} \leftrightarrow \text{oxyhaemoglobin}$$
$$(\text{Hb}) \qquad\qquad (\text{O}_2) \qquad\quad (\text{HbO})$$

As the oxygen content of blood increases, its colour changes too. Blood rich in oxygen (usually arterial blood) is bright red because of the high levels of oxyhaemoglobin it contains, compared with blood with lower oxygen levels (usually venous blood), which is dark bluish in colour because it is not saturated.

The association of oxygen with haemoglobin is a loose one, so that oxyhaemoglobin releases its oxygen readily, especially under certain conditions.

Low pH Metabolically active tissues, e.g. exercising muscle, release acid waste products, and so the local pH falls. Under these conditions, oxyhaemoglobin readily breaks down, giving up additional oxygen for tissue use.

Low oxygen levels (hypoxia) Where oxygen levels are low, oxyhaemoglobin breaks down, releasing oxygen. In the tissues, which constantly consume oxygen, oxygen levels are always low. This encourages oxyhaemoglobin to release its oxygen to the cells. In addition, the lower

the tissue oxygen level, the more oxygen is released, meaning that as tissue oxygen demand rises, so does the supply to match it. On the other hand, when oxygen levels are high, as they are in the lungs, oxyhaemoglobin formation is favoured.

Temperature Actively metabolising tissues, which have higher than normal oxygen needs, are warmer than less active ones, which drive the equation above to the left, increasing oxygen release. This ensures that very active tissues receive a higher oxygen supply than less active ones. In the lungs, where the alveoli are exposed to inspired air, the temperature is lower, favouring oxyhaemoglobin formation.

Control of erythropoiesis

Red cell numbers remain fairly constant, because the bone marrow produces erythrocytes at the rate at which they are destroyed. This is due to a homeostatic negative feedback mechanism. The hormone that regulates red blood cell production is *erythropoietin*, produced mainly by the kidney.

The primary stimulus to increased erythropoiesis is *hypoxia*, i.e. deficient oxygen supply to body cells.

Hypoxia can result from anaemia, low blood volume, poor blood flow, reduced oxygen content of inspired air (as at altitude) or lung disease. Each of these leads to erythropoietin production in an attempt to restore oxygen supplies to the tissues.

Erythropoietin stimulates an increase in the production of proerythroblasts and the release of more reticulocytes into the blood. It also speeds up reticulocyte maturation. These changes increase the oxygen-carrying capacity of the blood and reverse tissue hypoxia, the original stimulus. When the tissue hypoxia is overcome, erythropoietin production declines (Fig. 4.7). When erythropoietin levels are low, red cell formation does not take place even in the presence of hypoxia, and anaemia (the inability of the blood to carry adequate oxygen for body needs) develops.

Destruction of erythrocytes

The life span of erythrocytes (Fig. 4.5) is about 120 days and their breakdown, or *haemolysis*, is carried out by *phagocytic reticuloendothelial cells*. These cells are found in many tissues but the main sites of haemolysis are the spleen, bone marrow and liver. As erythrocytes age, their cell membranes become more fragile and so more susceptible to haemolysis. Iron released by haemolysis is retained in the body and reused in the bone marrow to form new haemoglobin molecules. *Biliverdin* is formed from the haem part of the haemoglobin. It is almost completely reduced to the yellow pigment *bilirubin*, before being bound to plasma globulin and transported to the liver (Fig. 4.5, see also Fig. 12.37, p. 311). In the liver it is changed from a fat-soluble to a water-soluble form to be excreted as a constituent of bile.

Blood groups 4.3

Early attempts to transfuse blood from one person to another or from animals to humans were only rarely successful, the recipient of the blood usually becoming very ill or dying. It is now known that the surface of red blood cells carries a range of different proteins (called antigens) that can stimulate an immune response if transferred from one individual (the donor) into the bloodstream of an incompatible individual. These antigens, which are inherited, determine the individual's *blood group*. In addition, individuals can make antibodies to these antigens, but not to their own type of antigen, since if they did the antigens and antibodies would react, causing a potentially fatal *transfusion reaction*.

If individuals are transfused with blood of the same group, i.e. possessing the same antigens on the surface of the cells, their immune system will not recognise them as foreign and will not reject them. However, if they are given blood from an individual of a different blood type, i.e. with a different type of antigen on the red cells, their immune system will generate antibodies to the foreign antigens and destroy the transfused cells. This is the basis of the transfusion reaction; the two blood types, the donor and the recipient, are *incompatible*.

There are many different collections of red cell surface antigens, but the most important are the ABO and the Rhesus systems.

The ABO system

About 55% of the population has either A-type antigens (blood group A), B-type antigens (blood group B) or both (blood group AB) on their red cell surface. The remaining 45% have neither A nor B type antigens (blood group O). The corresponding antibodies are called anti-A and anti-B. Blood group A individuals cannot make anti-A (and therefore do not have these antibodies in their plasma), since otherwise a reaction to their own cells would occur; they can, however, make anti-B. Blood group B individuals, for the same reasons, can make only anti-A. Blood group AB make neither, and blood group O make both anti-A and anti-B (Fig. 4.8).

Because blood group AB people make neither anti-A nor anti-B antibodies, they are sometimes known as *universal recipients*: transfusion of either type A or type B blood into these individuals is likely to be safe, since there are no antibodies to react with them. Conversely, group O people have neither A nor B antigens on their red cell membranes, and their blood may be safely transfused into A, B, AB or O types; group O is sometimes known as the *universal donor*. The terms *universal donor* and *universal recipient* are misleading, however, since they imply that the ABO system is the only one that needs to be considered. In practice, although the ABO systems may be compatible, other antigen systems on donor/recipient cells may be incompatible, and cause a transfusion reaction (p. 76). For this reason, prior to transfusion, cross-matching is still required to ensure that there is no reaction between donor and recipient bloods. Inheritance of ABO blood groups is described in Chapter 17 (p. 444).

The Rhesus system 4.4

The red blood cell membrane antigen important here is the Rhesus (Rh) antigen, or Rhesus factor. About 85% of people have this antigen; they are Rhesus positive (Rh$^+$) and do not therefore make anti-Rhesus antibodies. The remaining 15% have no Rhesus antigen (they are Rhesus negative, or Rh$^-$). Rh$^-$ individuals are capable of making anti-Rhesus antibodies, but are stimulated to do so only in certain circumstances, e.g. in pregnancy (p. 75), or as the result of an incompatible blood transfusion.

Leukocytes (white blood cells) 4.5

These cells have an important function in defence and immunity. They detect foreign or abnormal (antigenic) material and destroy it, through a range of defence mechanisms described below and in Chapter 15. Leukocytes are the largest blood cells but they account for only about 1% of the blood volume. They contain nuclei and some have granules in their cytoplasm (Table 4.2 and Fig. 4.2). There are two main types:

- *granulocytes* (polymorphonuclear leukocytes) – neutrophils, eosinophils and basophils
- *agranulocytes* – monocytes and lymphocytes.

Rising white cell numbers in the bloodstream usually indicate a physiological problem, e.g. infection, trauma or malignancy.

Blood group	Antigen + antibody(ies) present		As donor, is	As recipient, is
A	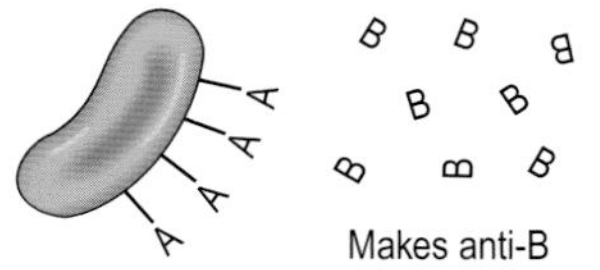 Antigen A	Makes anti-B	Compatible with: A and AB Incompatible with: B and O, because both make anti-A antibodies that will react with A antigens	Compatible with: A and O Incompatible with: B and AB, because type A makes anti-B antibodies that will react with B antigens
B	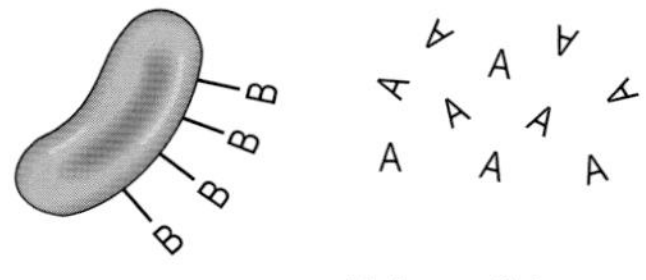 Antigen B	Makes anti-A	Compatible with: B and AB Incompatible with: A and O, because both make anti-B antibodies that will react with B antigens	Compatible with: B and O Incompatible with: A and AB, because type B makes anti-A antibodies that will react with A antigens
AB	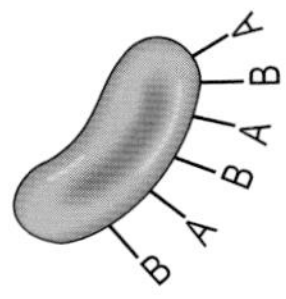 Antigens A and B	Makes neither anti-A nor anti-B	Compatible with: AB only Incompatible with: A, B and O, because all three make antibodies that will react with AB antigens	Compatible with all groups **UNIVERSAL RECIPIENT** AB makes no antibodies and therefore will not react with any type of donated blood
O	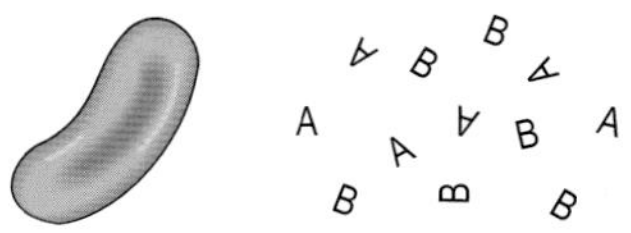 Neither A nor B antigen	Makes both anti-A and anti-B	Compatible with all groups **UNIVERSAL DONOR** O red cells have no antigens, and will therefore not stimulate anti-A or anti-B antibodies	Compatible with: O only Incompatible with: A, AB and B, because type O makes anti-A and anti-B antibodies

Figure 4.8 The ABO system of blood grouping: antigens, antibodies and compatibility.

Table 4.2 Normal leukocyte counts in adult blood		
	Number $\times 10^9$/L	Percentage of total
Granulocytes		
Neutrophils	2.5 to 7.5	40 to 75
Eosinophils	0.04 to 0.44	1 to 6
Basophils	0.015 to 0.1	< 1
Agranulocytes		
Monocytes	0.2 to 0.8	2 to 10
Lymphocytes	1.5 to 3.5	20 to 50
Total	5 to 9	100

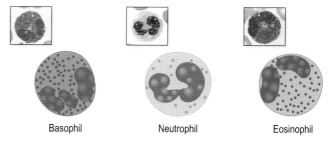

Basophil   Neutrophil   Eosinophil

Figure 4.9 The granulocytes (granular leukocytes).

when stained in the laboratory. Eosinophils take up the red acid dye, eosin; basophils take up alkaline methylene blue; and neutrophils are purple because they take up both dyes.

Neutrophils

These small, fast and active scavengers protect the body against bacterial invasion, and remove dead cells and debris from damaged tissues. They are attracted in large numbers to any area of infection by chemicals called *chemotaxins*, released by damaged cells. Neutrophils are highly mobile, and squeeze through the capillary walls in the affected area by *diapedesis* (Fig. 4.10). Their numbers rise very quickly in an area of damaged or infected tissue. Once there, they engulf and kill bacteria by *phagocytosis*

Granulocytes (polymorphonuclear leukocytes)

During their formation, *granulopoiesis*, they follow a common line of development through *myeloblast* to *myelocyte* before differentiating into the three types (Figs 4.3 and 4.9). All granulocytes have multilobed nuclei in their cytoplasm. Their names represent the dyes they take up

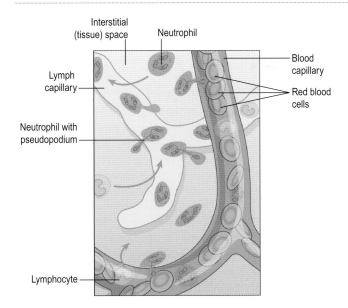

Figure 4.10 Diapedesis of leukocytes.

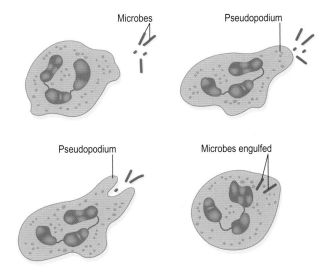

Figure 4.11 Phagocytic action of neutrophils.

(Fig. 4.11 and Fig. 15.1). Their nuclei are characteristically complex, with up to six lobes (Fig. 4.2), and their granules are *lysosomes* containing enzymes to digest engulfed material. Neutrophils live on average 6–9 hours in the bloodstream. Pus that may form in an infected area consists of dead tissue cells, dead and live microbes, and phagocytes killed by microbes.

Eosinophils

Eosinophils, although capable of phagocytosis, are less active in this than neutrophils; their specialised role appears to be in the elimination of parasites, such as worms, which are too big to be phagocytosed. They are equipped with certain toxic chemicals, stored in their

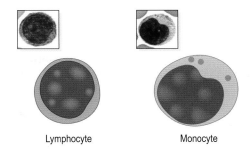

Figure 4.12 The agranulocytes.

granules, which they release when the eosinophil binds to an infecting organism.

Local accumulation of eosinophils may occur in allergic inflammation, such as the asthmatic airway and skin allergies. There, they promote tissue inflammation by releasing their array of toxic chemicals, but they may also dampen down the inflammatory process through the release of other chemicals, such as *histaminase*, an enzyme that breaks down histamine (p. 378).

Basophils

Basophils, which are closely associated with allergic reactions, contain cytoplasmic granules packed with heparin (an anticoagulant), histamine (an inflammatory agent) and other substances that promote inflammation. Usually the stimulus that causes basophils to release the contents of their granules is an *allergen* (an antigen that causes allergy) of some type. This binds to antibody-type receptors on the basophil membrane. A cell type very similar to basophils, except that it is found in the tissues, not in the circulation, is the *mast cell*. Mast cells release their granule contents within seconds of binding an allergen, which accounts for the rapid onset of allergic symptoms following exposure to, for example, pollen in hay fever (p. 385).

Agranulocytes

The *monocytes* and *lymphocytes* make up 25 to 50% of the total leukocyte count (Figs 4.3 and 4.12). They have a large nucleus and no cytoplasmic granules.

Monocytes

These are the largest of the white blood cells (Fig. 4.2). Some circulate in the blood and are actively motile and phagocytic while others migrate into the tissues where they develop into *macrophages*. Both types of cell produce *interleukin* 1, which:

- acts on the hypothalamus, causing the rise in body temperature associated with microbial infections
- stimulates the production of some globulins by the liver
- enhances the production of activated T-lymphocytes.

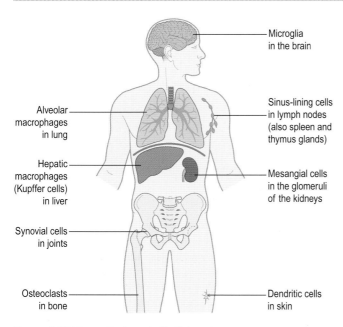

Microglia
in the brain

Alveolar
macrophages
in lung

Sinus-lining cells
in lymph nodes
(also spleen and
thymus glands)

Hepatic
macrophages
(Kupffer cells)
in liver

Mesangial cells
in the glomeruli
of the kidneys

Synovial cells
in joints

Osteoclasts
in bone

Dendritic cells
in skin

Figure 4.13 The reticuloendothelial system.

Macrophages have important functions in inflammation (p. 376) and immunity (Ch. 15).

The monocyte–macrophage system. This is sometimes called the *reticuloendothelial system*, and consists of the body's complement of monocytes and macrophages. Some macrophages are mobile, whereas others are fixed, providing effective defence at key body locations.

The main collections of fixed macrophages are shown in Figure 4.13.

Macrophages have a diverse range of protective functions. They are actively phagocytic (their name means 'big eaters') and are much more powerful and longer-lived than the smaller neutophils. They synthesise and release an array of biologically active chemicals, called *cytokines*, including interleukin 1 mentioned earlier. They also have a central role linking the non-specific and specific (immune) systems of body defence (Ch. 15), and produce factors important in inflammation and repair. They can 'wall off' indigestible pockets of material, isolating them from surrounding normal tissue. In the lungs, for example, resistant bacteria such as tuberculosis bacilli and inhaled inorganic dusts can be sealed off in such capsules.

Lymphocytes

Lymphocytes are smaller than monocytes and have large nuclei. Some circulate in the blood but most are found in tissues, including lymphatic tissue such as lymph nodes and the spleen. Lymphocytes develop from pluripotent stem cells in red bone marrow and from precursors in lymphoid tissue.

Although all lymphocytes originate from only one type of stem cell, the final steps in their development lead to the production of two distinct types of lymphocyte – *T-lymphocytes* and *B-lymphocytes*. The specific functions of these two cell types are discussed in Chapter 15.

Platelets (thrombocytes) ▉ 4.6

These are very small discs, 2–4 μm in diameter, derived from the cytoplasm of megakaryocytes in red bone marrow (Figs 4.2 and 4.3). Although they have no nucleus, their cytoplasm is packed with granules containing a variety of substances that promote blood clotting, which causes *haemostasis* (cessation of bleeding).

The normal blood platelet count is between $200 \times 10^9/\text{L}$ and $350 \times 10^9/\text{L}$ ($200\,000$–$350\,000/\text{mm}^3$). The mechanisms that regulate platelet numbers are not fully understood, but the hormone *thrombopoeitin* from the liver stimulates platelet production.

The life span of platelets is between 8 and 11 days and those not used in haemostasis are destroyed by macrophages, mainly in the spleen. About a third of platelets are stored within the spleen rather than in the circulation; this is an emergency store that can be released as required to control excessive bleeding.

Haemostasis

When a blood vessel is damaged, loss of blood is stopped and healing occurs in a series of overlapping processes, in which platelets play a vital part. The more badly damaged the vessel wall is, the faster coagulation begins, sometimes as quickly as 15 seconds after injury.

1. Vasoconstriction. When platelets come into contact with a damaged blood vessel, their surface becomes sticky and they adhere to the damaged wall. They then release *serotonin* (5-hydroxytryptamine), which constricts (narrows) the vessel, reducing or stopping blood flow through it. Other chemicals that cause vasoconstriction, e.g. thromboxanes, are released by the damaged vessel itself.

2. Platelet plug formation. The adherent platelets clump to each other and release other substances, including *adenosine diphosphate* (ADP), which attract more platelets to the site. Passing platelets stick to those already at the damaged vessel and they too release their chemicals. This is a positive feedback system by which many platelets rapidly arrive at the site of vascular damage and quickly form a temporary seal – the platelet plug. Platelet plug formation is usually complete within 6 minutes of injury.

3. Coagulation (blood clotting). This is a complex process that also involves a positive feedback system and only a few stages are included here. The factors involved are listed in Table 4.3. Their numbers represent the order in which they were discovered and not the order of participation in the clotting process. These clotting factors

Table 4.3 Blood clotting factors

I	Fibrinogen
II	Prothrombin
III	Tissue factor (thromboplastin)
IV	Calcium (Ca^{2+})
V	Labile factor, proaccelerin, Ac-globulin
VII	Stable factor, proconvertin
VIII	Antihaemophilic globulin (AHG), antihaemophilic factor A
IX	Christmas factor, plasma thromboplastin component (PTA), antihaemophilic factor B
X	Stuart Prower factor
XI	Plasma thromboplastin antecedent (PTA), antihaemophilic factor C
XII	Hageman factor
XIII	Fibrin stabilising factor

(There is no factor VI)
Vitamin K is essential for synthesis of factors II, VII, IX and X.

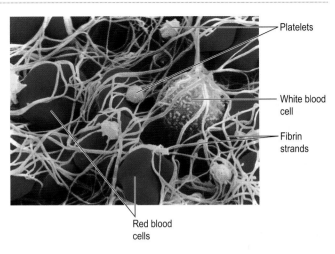

Figure 4.15 Scanning electron micrograph of a blood clot, showing the fibrin meshwork (pink strands), red blood cells, platelets and a white blood cell.

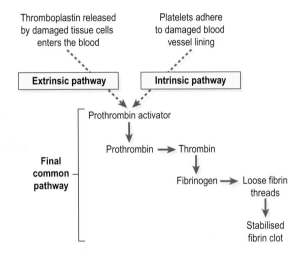

Figure 4.14 Stages of blood clotting (coagulation).

activate each other in a specific order, eventually resulting in the formation of *prothrombin activator*, which is the first step in the *final common pathway*. Prothrombin activates the enzyme *thrombin*, which converts inactive *fibrinogen* to insoluble threads of *fibrin* (Fig. 4.14). As clotting proceeds, the platelet plug is progressively stabilised by increasing amounts of fibrin laid down in a three-dimensional meshwork within it. The maturing blood clot traps blood cells and other plasma proteins including *plasminogen* (which will eventually destroy the clot), and is much stronger than the rapidly formed platelet plug.

The final common pathway can be initiated by two processes which often occur together: the extrinsic and intrinsic pathways (Fig. 4.14). The *extrinsic pathway* is activated rapidly (within seconds) following tissue damage. Damaged tissue releases a complex of chemicals called *thromboplastin* or tissue factor, which initiates coagulation. The *intrinsic pathway* is slower (3–6 minutes) and is

triggered when blood comes into contact with damaged blood vessel lining (endothelium).

After a time the clot shrinks (*retracts*) because the platelets contract, squeezing out serum, a clear sticky fluid that consists of plasma from which clotting factors have been removed. Clot shrinkage pulls the edges of the damaged vessel together, reducing blood loss and closing off the hole in the vessel wall.

Figure 4.15 shows a scanning electron micrograph of a blood clot. The fibrin strands (pink) have trapped red blood cells, platelets and a white blood cell.

4. Fibrinolysis. After the clot has formed, the process of removing it and healing the damaged blood vessel begins. The breakdown of the clot, or *fibrinolysis*, is the first stage. Plasminogen, trapped within the clot as it forms, is converted to the enzyme *plasmin* by activators released from the damaged endothelial cells. Plasmin breaks down fibrin to soluble products that are treated as waste material and removed by phagocytosis. As the clot is removed, the healing process restores the integrity of the blood vessel wall.

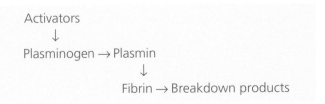

Control of coagulation
The process of blood clotting relies heavily on several self-perpetuating processes – that is, once started, a positive feedback mechanism promotes their continuation. For example, thrombin is a powerful stimulator of its own production. The body therefore possesses several mechanisms to control and limit the coagulation cascade;

otherwise once started the clotting process would spread throughout the circulatory system, instead of being limited to the local area where it is needed. The main controls are:

- the perfect smoothness of normal blood vessel lining prevents platelet adhesion in healthy, undamaged blood vessels

- activated clotting factors remain active for only a short time because they are inhibited by natural anticoagulants such as heparin and antithrombin III, which interrupt the clotting cascade.

Erythrocyte disorders

Learning outcomes

After studying this section, you should be able to:

■ define the term anaemia

■ compare and contrast the causes and effects of iron deficiency, megaloblastic, aplastic, hypoplastic and haemolytic anaemias

■ explain why polycythaemia occurs.

Anaemias

Anaemia is the inability of the blood to carry enough oxygen to meet body needs. Usually this is because there are low levels of haemoglobin in the blood, but sometimes it is due to production of faulty haemoglobin.

Anaemia is classified depending on the cause:

• production of insufficient or defective erythrocytes.

If the number of red blood cells being released is too low or the red blood cells are defective in some way, anaemia may result. Important causes include iron deficiency, vitamin B_{12}/folic acid deficiency and bone marrow failure.

• blood loss or excessive erythrocyte breakdown (haemolysis).

If erythrocytes are lost from the circulation, either through loss of blood in haemorrhage or by accelerated haemolysis, anaemia can result.

Anaemia can cause abnormal changes in red cell size or colour, detectable microscopically. Characteristic changes are listed in Table 4.4. Anaemia may be associated with a normal red cell count and no abnormalities of erythrocyte structure (normochromic normocytic anaemia). For example, following sudden haemorrhage, the red cells in the bloodstream are normal in shape and colour, but their numbers are fewer.

Signs and symptoms of anaemia relate to the inability of the blood to supply body cells with enough oxygen, and may represent adaptive measures. Examples include:

• tachycardia; the heart rate increases to improve blood supply and speed up circulation

• palpitations (an awareness of the heartbeat), or angina pectoris (p. 127); these are caused by the increased effort of the overworked heart muscle

• breathlessness on exertion; when oxygen requirements increase, respiratory rate and effort rise in an effort to meet the greater demand.

Iron deficiency anaemia

This is the most common form of anaemia in many parts of the world. Dietary iron comes mainly from red meat and highly coloured vegetables. Daily iron requirement in men is about 1–2 mg. Women need 3 mg daily because of blood loss during menstruation and to meet the needs of the growing fetus during pregnancy. Children require more than adults to meet their growth requirements.

In iron deficiency anaemia, the red blood cell count is often normal, but the cells are small, pale, of variable size and contain less haemoglobin than normal.

The amount of haemoglobin in each cell is regarded as below normal when the mean cell haemoglobin (MCH) is less than 27 pg/cell (Table 4.1). The anaemia is regarded as severe when the haemoglobin level is below 9 g/dL blood.

Iron deficiency anaemia can result from deficient intake, unusually high iron requirements, or poor absorption from the alimentary tract.

Deficient intake

Because of the relative inefficiency of iron absorption, deficiency occurs frequently, even in individuals whose requirements are normal. It generally develops slowly over a prolonged period of time, and symptoms only appear once the anaemia is well established. The risk of deficiency increases if the daily diet is restricted in some way, as in poorly planned vegetarian diets, or in weight-reducing diets where the range of foods eaten is small. Babies dependent on milk may also suffer mild iron deficiency anaemia if weaning on to a mixed diet is delayed much past the first year, since the liver carries only a few months' store and milk is a poor source of iron. Other at-risk groups include older adults and the alcohol-dependent, whose diet can be poor.

Table 4.4 Terms used to describe red blood cell characteristics

Term	Definition
Normochromic	Cell colour normal
Normocytic	Cells normal sized
Microcytic	Cells smaller than normal
Macrocytic	Cells bigger than normal
Hypochromic	Cells paler than normal
Haemolytic	Rate of cell destruction raised
Megaloblastic	Cells large and immature

High requirements

In pregnancy iron requirements are increased both for fetal growth and to support the additional load on the mother's cardiovascular system. Iron requirements also rise when there is chronic blood loss, the causes of which include peptic ulcers (p. 323), heavy menstrual bleeding (menorrhagia), haemorrhoids, regular aspirin ingestion or carcinoma of the GI tract (pp. 324, 329).

Malabsorption

Iron absorption is usually increased following haemorrhage, but may be reduced in abnormalities of the stomach, duodenum or jejunum. Because iron absorption is dependent on an acid environment in the stomach, an increase in gastric pH may reduce it; this may follow excessive use of antacids, removal of part of the stomach, or in pernicious anaemia (see below), where the acid-releasing (parietal) cells of the stomach are destroyed. Loss of surface area for absorption in the intestine, e.g. after surgical removal, can also cause deficiency.

Vitamin B$_{12}$/folic acid deficiency anaemias

Deficiency of vitamin B$_{12}$ and/or folic acid impairs erythrocyte maturation (Fig. 4.5) and abnormally large erythrocytes (*megaloblasts*) are found in the blood. During normal erythropoiesis (Fig. 4.3) several cell divisions occur and the daughter cells at each stage are smaller than the parent cell because there is not much time for cell enlargement between divisions. When deficiency of vitamin B$_{12}$ and/or folic acid occurs, the rate of DNA and RNA synthesis is reduced, delaying cell division. The cells therefore grow larger than normal between divisions. Circulating cells are immature, larger than normal and some are nucleated (mean cell volume (MCV) > 94 fL). The haemoglobin content of each cell is normal or raised. The cells are fragile and their life span is reduced to between 40 and 50 days. Depressed production and early lysis cause anaemia.

Vitamin B$_{12}$ deficiency anaemia

Pernicious anaemia

This is the most common form of vitamin B$_{12}$ deficiency anaemia. It is commonest in females over 50. It is an autoimmune disease in which autoantibodies destroy intrinsic factor (IF) and parietal cells in the stomach (p. 299).

Dietary deficiency of vitamin B$_{12}$

Vitamin B$_{12}$ is widely available in animal-derived foodstuffs, including dairy products, meat and eggs, so deficiency is rare except in strict vegans, who eat no animal products at all. The liver has extensive stores of the vitamin, so deficiency can take several years to appear.

Other causes of vitamin B$_{12}$ deficiency

These include the following.

- *Gastrectomy* (removal of all or part or the stomach) – this leaves fewer cells available to produce IF.
- *Chronic gastritis, malignant disease and ionising radiation* – these damage the gastric mucosa including the parietal cells that produce IF.
- *Malabsorption* – if the terminal ileum is removed or inflamed, e.g. in Crohn's disease, the vitamin cannot be absorbed.

Complications of vitamin B$_{12}$ deficiency anaemia

These may appear before the signs of anaemia. Because vitamin B$_{12}$ is used in myelin production, deficiency leads to irreversible neurological damage, commonly in the spinal cord (p. 187). Mucosal abnormalities, such as glossitis (inflammation of the tongue) are also common, although they are reversible.

Folic acid deficiency anaemia

Deficiency of folic acid causes a form of megaloblastic anaemia identical to that seen in vitamin B$_{12}$ deficiency, but not associated with neurological damage. It may be due to:

- dietary deficiency, e.g. in infants if there is delay in establishing a mixed diet, in alcoholism, in anorexia and in pregnancy
- malabsorption from the jejunum caused by, e.g., coeliac disease, tropical sprue or anticonvulsant drugs
- interference with folate metabolism by, e.g., cytotoxic and anticonvulsant drugs.

Aplastic anaemia

Aplastic (hypoplastic) anaemia results from bone marrow failure. Erythrocyte numbers are reduced. Since the bone marrow also produces leukocytes and platelets, *leukopenia* (low white cell count) and *thrombocytopenia* (low platelet count) are also likely. When all three cell types are low, the condition is called *pancytopenia*, and is accompanied by anaemia, diminished immunity and a tendency to bleed. The condition is occasionally (15% of cases) inherited. Usually no cause is identified, but the known causes include:

- drugs, e.g. cytotoxic therapy and, rarely, as an adverse reaction to anti-inflammatory and anticonvulsant drugs and some antibiotics
- ionising radiation
- some chemicals, e.g. benzene and its derivatives
- viral disease, including hepatitis.

The presenting symptoms are usually bleeding and bruising.

Haemolytic anaemias

These occur when circulating red cells are destroyed or are removed prematurely from the blood because the cells are abnormal or the spleen is overactive. Most haemolysis takes place in the liver or spleen and the normal erythrocyte life span of about 120 days can be considerably shortened. If the condition is relatively mild, red cell numbers may remain stable because the red bone marrow production of erythrocytes increases to compensate, so there may be ongoing haemolysis without anaemia. However, if the bone marrow cannot compensate, red blood cell numbers will fall and anaemia results.

Even in the absence of symptoms of anaemia (pallor, tiredness, dyspnoea, etc.), haemolytic anaemias can cause additional symptoms such as jaundice or splenomegaly.

Congenital haemolytic anaemias

In these diseases, genetic abnormality leads to the synthesis of abnormal haemoglobin and increased red cell membrane fragility, reducing their oxygen-carrying capacity and life span. The most common forms are sickle cell anaemia and thalassaemia.

Sickle cell anaemia

The abnormal haemoglobin molecules become misshapen when deoxygenated, making the erythrocytes sickle shaped (Fig. 4.16). If the cells contain a high proportion of abnormal Hb, sickling is permanent. The life span of cells is reduced by early haemolysis, which causes anaemia. Sickle cells do not move smoothly through the circulation. They obstruct blood flow, leading to intravascular clotting, tissue ischaemia and infarction. Acute episodes (sickle crises), caused by blockage of small vessels, cause acute pain in the affected area, often the hands and feet. Longer term problems arising from poor perfusion and anaemia include cardiac disease, kidney

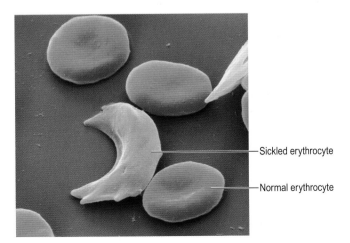

Figure 4.16 Scanning electron micrograph showing three normal and one sickled erythrocyte.

— Sickled erythrocyte

— Normal erythrocyte

failure, retinopathy, poor tissue healing and slow growth in children. Obstruction of blood flow to the brain greatly increases the risk of stroke and seizures, and both mother and child are at significant risk of complications in pregnancy.

Black people are more affected than others. Some affected individuals have a degree of immunity to malaria because the life span of the sickled cells is less than the time needed for the malaria parasite to mature inside the cells.

Complications. Pregnancy, infection and dehydration predispose to the development of 'sickle crises' due to intravascular clotting and ischaemia, causing severe pain in long bones, chest or the abdomen. Excessive haemolysis results in high levels of circulating bilirubin. This in turn frequently leads to gallstones (*cholelithiasis*) and inflammation of the gall bladder (*cholecystitis*) (p. 335).

Thalassaemia

This inherited condition, commonest in Mediterranean countries, causes abnormal haemoglobin production, which in turn reduces erythropoiesis and stimulates haemolysis. The resultant anaemia may present in a range of forms, from mild and asymptomatic to profound and life-threatening. Symptoms in moderate to severe thalassaemia include bone marrow expansion and splenomegaly, as production of red blood cells increases to correct the anaemia. In the most severe form of the disease, regular blood transfusions are required, which can lead to iron overload.

Haemolytic disease of the newborn

In this disorder, the mother's immune system makes antibodies to the baby's red blood cells, causing destruction of fetal erythrocytes. The antigen system involved is usually (but not always) the Rhesus (Rh) antigen.

A Rh⁻ mother carries no Rh antigen on her red blood cells, but she has the capacity to produce anti-Rh antibodies. If she conceives a child fathered by a Rh⁺ man, and the baby inherits the Rh antigen from him, the baby may also be Rh⁺, i.e. different from the mother. During pregnancy, the placenta protects the baby from the mother's immune system, but at delivery a few fetal red blood cells may enter the maternal circulation. Because they carry an antigen (the Rh antigen) foreign to the mother, her immune system will be stimulated to produce neutralising antibodies to it. The red cells of second and subsequent Rh⁺ babies are attacked by these maternal antibodies, which can cross the placenta and enter the fetal circulation (Fig. 4.17). In the most severe cases, the baby dies in the womb from profound anaemia. In less serious circumstances, the baby is born with some degree of anaemia, which is corrected with blood transfusions.

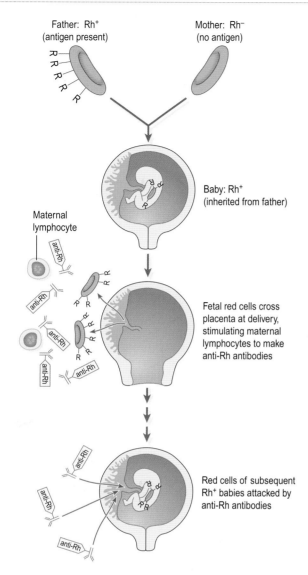

Figure 4.17 The immunity of haemolytic disease of the newborn.

The disease is much less common than it used to be, because it was discovered that if a Rh⁻ mother is given an injection of anti-Rh antibodies within 72 hours of the delivery of a Rh⁺ baby, her immune system does not make its own anti-Rh antibodies to the fetal red cells. Subsequent pregnancies are therefore not affected. The anti-Rh antibodies given to the mother bind to, and neutralise, any fetal red cells present in her circulation before her immune system becomes sensitised to them.

Acquired haemolytic anaemias

In this context, 'acquired' means haemolytic anaemia in which no familial or racial factors have been identified. There are several causes.

Chemical agents

These substances cause early or excessive haemolysis, for example:

- some drugs, especially when taken long term in large doses, e.g. sulphonamides
- chemicals encountered in the general or work environment, e.g. lead, arsenic compounds
- toxins produced by microbes, e.g. *Streptococcus pyogenes, Clostridium perfringens.*

Autoimmunity

In autoimmunity, individuals make antibodies to their own red cell antigens, causing haemolysis. It may be acute or chronic and primary or secondary to other diseases, e.g. carcinoma, viral infection or other autoimmune diseases.

Blood transfusion reactions

Individuals do not normally produce antibodies to their own red blood cell antigens; if they did, the antigens and antibodies would react, causing clumping and lysis of the erythrocytes (see Fig. 4.8). However, if individuals receive a transfusion of blood carrying antigens different from their own, their immune system will recognise them as foreign, make antibodies to them and destroy them (transfusion reaction). This adverse reaction between the blood of incompatible recipients and donors leads to haemolysis within the cardiovascular system. The breakdown products of haemolysis lodge in and block the filtering mechanism of the nephron, impairing kidney function. Other principal signs of a transfusion reaction include fever, chills, lumbar pain and shock.

Polycythaemia

This means an abnormally large number of erythrocytes in the blood. This increases blood viscosity, slows blood flow and increases the risk of intravascular clotting, ischaemia and infarction.

Relative increase in erythrocyte count

This occurs when the erythrocyte count is normal but the blood volume is reduced by fluid loss, e.g. excessive serum exudate from extensive burns.

True increase in erythrocyte count

Physiological. Prolonged hypoxia stimulates erythropoiesis and the number of reticulocytes released into the normal volume of blood is increased. This occurs naturally in people living at high altitudes where the oxygen tension in the air is low and the partial pressure of oxygen in the alveoli of the lungs is correspondingly low. Each cell carries less oxygen so more cells are needed to meet the body's oxygen needs. Other causes of hypoxia, such as heart or lung disease or heavy smoking can also cause polycythaemia.

Pathological. Some cancers increase red blood cell production, although the reason is not always known.

Leukocyte disorders

Learning outcomes

After studying this section, you should be able to:

- define the terms leukopenia and leukocytosis
- review the physiological importance of abnormally increased and decreased leukocyte numbers in the blood
- discuss the main forms of leukaemia, including the causes, signs and symptoms of the disease.

Leukopenia

In this condition, the total blood leukocyte count is less than $4 \times 10^9/L$ ($4000/mm^3$).

Granulocytopenia (neutropenia)

This is a general term used to indicate an abnormal reduction in the numbers of circulating granulocytes (polymorphonuclear leukocytes), commonly called neutropenia because 40–75% of granulocytes are neutrophils. A reduction in the number of circulating granulocytes occurs when production does not keep pace with the normal removal of cells or when the life span of the cells is reduced. Extreme shortage or the absence of granulocytes is called *agranulocytosis*. A temporary reduction occurs in response to inflammation but the numbers are usually quickly restored. Inadequate granulopoiesis may be caused by:

- drugs, e.g. cytotoxic drugs, phenothiazines, some sulphonamides and antibiotics
- irradiation damage to granulocyte precursors in the bone marrow, e.g. radiotherapy
- diseases of red bone marrow, e.g. leukaemias, some anaemias
- severe microbial infections.

In conditions where the spleen is enlarged, excessive numbers of granulocytes are trapped, reducing the number in circulation. Neutropenia predisposes to severe infections that can lead to septicaemia and death. Septicaemia is the presence of significant numbers of active pathogens in the blood.

Leukocytosis

An increase in the number of circulating leukocytes occurs as a normal protective reaction in a variety of pathological conditions, especially infections. When the infection subsides the leukocyte count returns to normal.

Pathological leukocytosis exists when a blood leukocyte count of more than $11 \times 10^9/L$ ($11\,000/mm^3$) is sustained and is not consistent with the normal protective function. One or more of the different types of cell is involved.

Leukaemia

Leukaemia is a malignant proliferation of white blood cell precursors by the bone marrow. It results in the uncontrolled increase in the production of leukocytes and/or their precursors. As the tumour cells enter the blood the total leukocyte count is usually raised but in some cases it may be normal or even low. The proliferation of immature leukaemic blast cells crowds out other blood cells formed in bone marrow, causing anaemia, thrombocytopenia and leukopenia (pancytopenia). Because the leukocytes are immature when released, immunity is reduced and the risk of infection high.

Causes of leukaemia

Some causes of leukaemia are known but many cases cannot be accounted for. Some people may have a genetic predisposition that is triggered by environmental factors, including viral infection. Other known causes include:

Ionising radiation. Radiation such as that produced by X-rays and radioactive isotopes causes malignant changes in the precursors of white blood cells. The DNA of the cells may be damaged and some cells die while others reproduce at an abnormally rapid rate. Leukaemia may develop at any time after irradiation, even 20 or more years later.

Chemicals. Some chemicals encountered in the general or work environment alter the DNA of the white blood cell precursors in the bone marrow. These include benzene and its derivatives, asbestos, cytotoxic drugs, chloramphenicol.

Genetic factors. Identical twins of leukaemia sufferers have a much higher risk than normal of developing the disease, suggesting involvement of genetic factors.

Types of leukaemia

Leukaemias are usually classified according to the type of cell involved, the maturity of the cells and the rate at which the disease develops (see Fig. 4.3).

Acute leukaemias

These types usually have a sudden onset and affect the poorly differentiated and immature 'blast' cells (Fig. 4.3). They are aggressive tumours that reach a climax within a few weeks or months. The rapid progress of bone marrow invasion causes rapid bone marrow failure and culminates in anaemia, haemorrhage and susceptibility to infection. The mucous membranes of the mouth and upper gastrointestinal tract are most commonly affected.

Leukocytosis is usually present in acute leukaemia. The bone marrow is packed with large numbers of immature and abnormal cells.

Acute myeloblastic leukaemia (AML). Involves proliferation of myeloblasts (Fig. 4.3), and is most common in adults between the ages of 25 and 60, the risk gradually increasing with age. The disease can often be cured, or long-term remission achieved.

Acute lymphoblastic leukaemia (ALL). Seen mainly in children, who have a better prognosis than adults, with up to 70% achieving cure. The cell responsible here is a primitive B-lymphocyte.

Chronic leukaemias

These conditions are less aggressive than the acute forms and the leukocytes are more differentiated, i.e. at the 'cyte' stage (Fig. 4.3).

Leukocytosis is a feature of chronic leukaemia, with crowding of the bone marrow with immature and abnormal leukocytes, although this varies depending upon the form of the disease.

Chronic myeloid leukaemia (CML). Occurs at all ages and, although its onset is gradual, in most patients it eventually transforms into a rapidly progressive stage similar to AML and proves fatal although it sometimes progresses to ALL and its better prognosis. Death usually occurs within 5 years.

Chronic lymphocytic leukaemia (CLL). Involves proliferation of B-lymphocytes, and is usually less aggressive than CML. It is most often seen in the elderly; disease progression is usually slow, and survival times can be as long as 25 years.

Haemorrhagic diseases

Learning outcomes

After studying this section, you should be able to:

- indicate the main causes and effects of thrombocytopenia

- outline how vitamin K deficiency relates to clotting disorders

- explain the term disseminated intravascular coagulation, including its principal causes

- describe the physiological deficiencies present in the haemophilias.

Thrombocytopenia

This is defined as a blood platelet count below $150 \times 10^9/L$ ($150\,000/mm^3$) but spontaneous capillary bleeding does not usually occur unless the count falls below $30 \times 10^9/L$ ($30\,000/mm^3$). It may be due to a reduced rate of platelet production or increased rate of destruction.

Reduced platelet production

This is usually due to bone marrow deficiencies, and therefore production of erythrocytes and leukocytes is also reduced, giving rise to pancytopenia. It is often due to:

- platelets being crowded out of the bone marrow in bone marrow diseases, e.g. leukaemias, pernicious anaemia, malignant tumours
- ionising radiation, e.g. X-rays or radioactive isotopes, which damage the rapidly dividing precursor cells in the bone marrow
- drugs that can damage bone marrow, e.g. cytotoxic drugs, chloramphenicol, chlorpromazine, sulphonamides.

Increased platelet destruction

A reduced platelet count occurs when production of new platelets does not keep pace with destruction of damaged and worn out ones. This occurs in disseminated intravascular coagulation (see below) and autoimmune thrombocytopenic purpura.

Autoimmune thrombocytopenic purpura. This condition, which usually affects children and young adults, may be triggered by a viral infection such as measles. Antiplatelet antibodies are formed that coat platelets, leading to platelet destruction and their removal from the circulation. A significant feature of this disease is the presence of purpura, which are haemorrhages into the skin ranging in size from pinpoints to large blotches. The severity of the disease varies from mild bleeding into the skin to severe haemorrhage. When the platelet count is very low there may be severe bruising, haematuria, gastrointestinal or intracranial haemorrhages.

Vitamin K deficiency

Vitamin K is required by the liver for the synthesis of many clotting factors and therefore deficiency predisposes to abnormal clotting.

Haemorrhagic disease of the newborn

Spontaneous haemorrhage from the umbilical cord and intestinal mucosa occurs in babies when the stored vitamin K obtained from the mother before birth has been used up and the intestinal bacteria needed for its synthesis in the infant's bowel are not yet established. This is most likely to occur when the baby is premature.

Deficiency in adults

Vitamin K is fat soluble and bile salts are required in the colon for its absorption. Deficiency may occur when there is liver disease, prolonged obstruction to the biliary tract or in any other disease where fat absorption is impaired, e.g. coeliac disease (p. 331). Dietary deficiency is rare because a sufficient supply of vitamin K is usually synthesised in the intestine by bacterial action. However, it may occur during treatment with drugs that sterilise the bowel.

Disseminated intravascular coagulation (DIC)

In DIC, the coagulation system is activated within blood vessels, leading to formation of intravascular clots and deposition of fibrin in the tissues. Because of this consumption of clotting factors and platelets, there is a consequent tendency to haemorrhage. DIC is a common complication of a number of other disorders, including:

- infection, such as septicaemia, when endotoxins are released by Gram-negative bacteria
- severe trauma
- premature separation of placenta when amniotic fluid enters maternal blood
- acute pancreatitis when digestive enzymes are released into the blood
- advanced cancer
- transfusion of very large volumes of blood.

Congenital disorders

The haemophilias

The haemophilias are a group of inherited clotting disorders, carried by genes present on the X-chromosome (i.e. inheritance is sex linked, p. 444). The faulty genes code for abnormal clotting factors (factor VIII and Christmas factor), and if inherited by a male child always leads to expression of the disease. Women inheriting one copy are carriers, but, provided their second X chromosome bears a copy of the normal gene, their blood clotting is normal. It is possible, but unusual, for a woman to inherit two copies of the abnormal gene and have haemophilia.

Those who have haemophilia experience repeated episodes of severe and prolonged bleeding at any site, even in the absence of trauma. Recurrent bleeding into joints is common, causing severe pain and, in the long term, cartilage is damaged. The disease ranges in severity from mild forms, where the defective factor has partial activity, to extreme forms where bleeding can take days or weeks to control.

The two main forms of haemophilia differ only in the clotting factor involved; the clinical picture in both is identical:

- haemophilia A. In this disease, factor VIII is abnormal and is less biologically active than normal
- haemophilia B (Christmas disease). This is less common and factor IX is deficient, resulting in deficiency of thromboplastin (clotting factor III).

von Willebrand disease

In this disease, a deficiency in von Willebrand factor causes low levels of factor VIII. As its inheritance is not sex linked, haemorrhages due to impaired clotting occur equally in males and females.

For a range of self-assessment exercises on the topics in this chapter, visit Evolve online resources: https://evolve.elsevier.com/Waugh/anatomy/

The cardiovascular system

The cardiovascular (cardio – heart, vascular – blood vessels) system is divided for descriptive purposes into two main parts:

- the *heart*, whose pumping action ensures constant circulation of the blood
- the *blood vessels*, which form a lengthy network through which the blood flows.

The *lymphatic system* is closely connected, both structurally and functionally, with the cardiovascular system and is discussed in Chapter 6.

The heart pumps blood into two anatomically separate systems of blood vessels (Fig. 5.1):

- the pulmonary circulation
- the systemic circulation.

The right side of the heart pumps blood to the lungs (the pulmonary circulation) where gas exchange occurs, i.e. the blood collects oxygen from the airsacs and excess carbon dioxide diffuses into the airsacs for exhalation. The left side of the heart pumps blood into the systemic circulation, which supplies the rest of the body. Here, tissue wastes are passed into the blood for excretion, and body cells extract nutrients and oxygen.

The cardiovascular system ensures a continuous flow of blood to all body cells, and its function is subject to continual physiological adjustments to maintain an adequate blood supply. Should the supply of oxygen and nutrients to body cells become inadequate, tissue damage occurs and cell death may follow.

Cardiovascular function normally declines with age, which is discussed on p. 117. Disease of the cardiovascular system is likely to have significant consequences, not only for the heart and blood vessels, but also for other body systems, which is discussed from page 118.

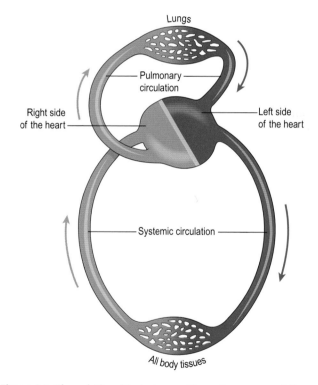

Figure 5.1 The relationship between the pulmonary and the systemic circulations.

Blood vessels

Blood vessels vary in structure, size and function, and there are several types: arteries, arterioles, capillaries, venules and veins (Fig. 5.2). **5.1**

Arteries and arterioles

These blood vessels transport blood away from the heart. They vary considerably in size and their walls consist of three layers of tissue (Fig. 5.3):

- *tunica adventitia* or outer layer of fibrous tissue
- *tunica media* or middle layer of smooth muscle and elastic tissue
- *tunica intima* or inner lining of squamous epithelium called *endothelium*.

The amount of muscular and elastic tissue varies in the arteries depending upon their size and function. In the large arteries, including the aorta, sometimes called elastic arteries, the tunica media contains more elastic tissue and less smooth muscle. This allows the vessel wall to stretch, absorbing the pressure wave generated by the heart as it beats. These proportions gradually change as the arteries branch many times and become smaller until in the *arterioles* (the smallest arteries) the tunica media consists almost entirely of smooth muscle. This enables their diameter to be precisely controlled, which regulates the pressure within them. Systemic blood pressure is mainly determined by the resistance these tiny arteries offer to blood flow, and for this reason they are called *resistance vessels*.

Arteries have thicker walls than veins to withstand the high pressure of arterial blood.

Anastomoses and end-arteries

Anastomoses are arteries that form a link between main arteries supplying an area, e.g. the arterial supply to the palms of the hand (p. 107) and soles of the feet, the brain, the joints and, to a limited extent, the heart muscle. If one artery supplying the area is occluded, anastomotic arteries provide a *collateral circulation*. This is most likely to provide an adequate blood supply when the occlusion occurs gradually, giving the anastomotic arteries time to dilate.

An *end-artery* is an artery that is the sole source of blood to a tissue, e.g. the branches from the circulus arteriosus (circle of Willis) in the brain or the central artery to the retina of the eye. When an end-artery is occluded the tissues it supplies die because there is no alternative blood supply.

Capillaries and sinusoids

The smallest arterioles break up into a number of minute vessels called *capillaries*. Capillary walls consist of a single layer of endothelial cells sitting on a very thin basement membrane, through which water and other small molecules can pass. Blood cells and large molecules such as plasma proteins do not normally pass through capillary walls. The capillaries form a vast network of tiny vessels that link the smallest arterioles to the smallest venules. Their diameter is approximately that of an erythrocyte (7 μm). The capillary bed is the site of exchange of substances between the blood and the tissue fluid, which

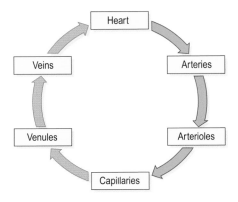

Figure 5.2 The relationship between the heart and the different types of blood vessel.

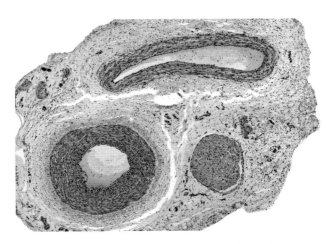

Figure 5.3 Light micrograph of an artery, a vein and an associated nerve.

bathes the body cells and, with the exception of those on the skin surface and in the cornea of the eye, every body cell lies close to a capillary.

Entry to capillary beds is guarded by rings of smooth muscle (*precapillary sphincters*) that direct blood flow. Hypoxia (low levels of oxygen in the tissues), or high levels of tissue wastes, indicating high levels of activity, dilate the sphincters and increase blood flow through the affected beds.

In certain places, including the liver (p. 309) and bone marrow, the capillaries are significantly wider and leakier than normal. These capillaries are called *sinusoids* and because their walls are incomplete and their lumen is much larger than usual, blood flows through them more slowly under less pressure and can come directly into contact with the cells outside the sinusoid wall. This allows much faster exchange of substances between the blood and the tissues, useful, for example, in the liver, which regulates the composition of blood arriving from the gastrointestinal tract.

Capillary refill time

When an area of skin is pressed firmly with a finger, it turns white (blanches) because the blood in the capillaries under the finger has been squeezed out. Normally it should take less than two seconds for the capillaries to refill once the finger is removed, and for the skin to turn pink again. Although the test may produce unreliable results, particularly in adults, its use in children can be useful and a prolonged capillary refill time suggests poor perfusion or dehydration.

Veins and venules

Veins return blood at low pressure to the heart. The walls of the veins are thinner than arteries but have the same three layers of tissue (Fig. 5.3). They are thinner because there is less muscle and elastic tissue in the tunica media, as veins carry blood at a lower pressure than arteries. When cut, the veins collapse while the thicker-walled arteries remain open. When an artery is cut blood spurts at high pressure while a slower, steady flow of blood escapes from a vein.

Some veins possess *valves*, which prevent backflow of blood, ensuring that it flows towards the heart (Fig. 5.4). They are formed by a fold of tunica intima and strengthened by connective tissue. The cusps are *semilunar* in shape with the concavity towards the heart. Valves are abundant in the veins of the limbs, especially the lower limbs where blood must travel a considerable distance against gravity when the individual is standing. They are absent in very small and very large veins in the thorax and abdomen. Valves are assisted in maintaining one-way flow by skeletal muscles surrounding the veins (p. 95).

The smallest veins are called *venules*.

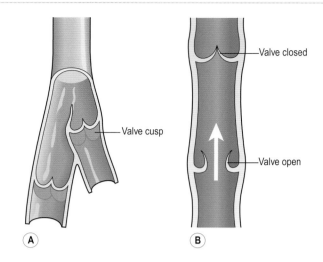

Figure 5.4 Interior of a vein. A. The valves and cusps. **B.** The direction of blood flow through a valve.

Veins are called *capacitance vessels* because they are distensible, and therefore have the capacity to hold a large proportion of the body's blood. At any one time, about two-thirds of the body's blood is in the venous system. This allows the vascular system to absorb (to an extent) sudden changes in blood volume, such as in haemorrhage; the veins can constrict, helping to prevent a sudden fall in blood pressure.

Blood supply

The outer layers of tissue of thick-walled blood vessels receive their blood supply via a network of blood vessels called the *vasa vasorum*. Thin-walled vessels and the endothelium of the others receive oxygen and nutrients by diffusion from the blood passing through them.

Control of blood vessel diameter

The smooth muscle in the tunica media of veins and arteries is supplied by nerves of the *autonomic nervous system*. These nerves arise from the *vasomotor centre* in the *medulla oblongata* and they change the diameter of blood vessels, controlling the volume of blood they contain.

The blood vessels most closely regulated by this nervous mechanism are the arterioles, since they contain proportionally more smooth muscle in their walls than any other blood vessel. The walls of large arteries such as the aorta contain mainly elastic tissue and so they tend to passively expand and recoil, depending on how much blood is passing through them. Veins also respond to nerve stimulation, although they have only a little smooth muscle in their tunica media.

Blood vessel diameter and blood flow

Resistance to flow of fluids along a tube is determined by three factors: the diameter of the tube; the length of the tube; and the viscosity of the fluid. The most important factor determining how easily the blood flows through blood vessels is the first of these variables, that is, the diameter of the resistance vessels (the *peripheral resistance*). The length of the vessels and viscosity of blood also contribute to peripheral resistance, but in health these are constant and are therefore not significant determinants of changes in blood flow. Peripheral resistance is a major factor in blood pressure regulation, which is further discussed on page 96.

Blood vessel diameter is regulated by the smooth muscle of the tunica media, which is supplied by sympathetic nerves of the autonomic nervous system (p. 173). There is no parasympathetic nerve supply to most blood vessels and therefore the diameter of the vessel lumen and the tone of the smooth muscle are determined by the degree of sympathetic activity. Sympathetic activity generally constricts blood vessel smooth muscle and therefore narrows the vessel (*vasoconstriction*), increasing the pressure inside. A degree of resting sympathetic activity maintains a constant baseline tone in the vessel wall and prevents pressure falling too low (Fig. 5.5). Decreased nerve stimulation relaxes the smooth muscle, thinning the vessel wall and enlarging the lumen (*vasodilation*). This results in increased blood flow under less pressure.

Constant adjustment of blood vessel diameter helps to regulate peripheral resistance and systemic blood pressure.

Although most arterioles respond to sympathetic stimulation with vasoconstriction, the response is much less marked in some arteriolar beds, e.g. in skeletal muscle and the brain. This is important so that in a stress response, such as the flight or fight response (p. 176), when sympathetic activity is very high, these essential tissues receive the extra oxygen and nutrients they need.

Local regulation of blood flow

Tissues' oxygen and nutrient requirements vary depending on their activities, so it is important that blood flow is regulated locally to ensure that blood flow matches tissue needs. The ability of an organ to control its own blood flow according to need is called *autoregulation*. Some organs, including the central nervous system, liver and kidneys receive proportionately higher blood flow as a matter of course. Other tissues, such as resting skeletal muscle, receive much less, but their blood supply can increase by as much as 20-fold during heavy exercise. Other examples include blood flow through the gastrointestinal tract increasing after a meal to allow for increased activity in the tract, and adjustments to blood flow through the skin in the control of body temperature (p. 367). Blood flow through individual organs is increased by vasodilation of the vessels supplying it, and decreased through vasoconstriction. The main mechanisms associated with this local control of blood flow include:

- release of metabolic waste products, e.g. CO_2 and lactic acid. Active tissues release more wastes than resting tissues, and increased levels of waste increase blood flow into the area
- tissue temperature: a rise in metabolic activity increases tissue temperature, which in turn causes vasodilation
- hypoxia, or lack of oxygen, stimulates vasodilation and a rise in blood flow through the affected tissue
- release of vasodilator chemicals. Inflamed and metabolically active tissues produce a number of vasodilators, which increase blood supply to the area. One important vasodilator is *nitric oxide*, which is very short lived, but which is important in opening up the larger arteries supplying an organ. Other agents include substances released in the inflammatory response, such as histamine and bradykinin (p. 378)
- action of vasoconstrictors. The sympathetic hormone adrenaline (epinephrine), released from the adrenal medulla, is a powerful vasoconstrictor. Others include angiotensin 2 (p. 343).

Capillary exchange

Exchange of gases

Internal respiration (Fig. 5.6) is the process by which gases are exchanged between capillary blood and local body cells.

Oxygen is carried from the lungs to the tissues in combination with haemoglobin (p. 66) as *oxyhaemoglobin*.

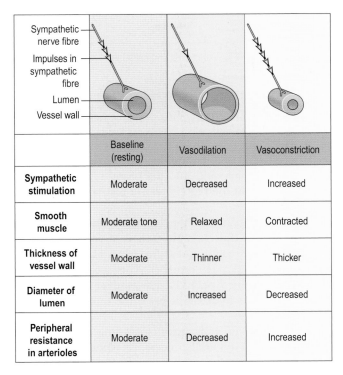

	Baseline (resting)	Vasodilation	Vasoconstriction
Sympathetic stimulation	Moderate	Decreased	Increased
Smooth muscle	Moderate tone	Relaxed	Contracted
Thickness of vessel wall	Moderate	Thinner	Thicker
Diameter of lumen	Moderate	Increased	Decreased
Peripheral resistance in arterioles	Moderate	Decreased	Increased

Figure 5.5 The relationship between sympathetic stimulation and blood vessel diameter.

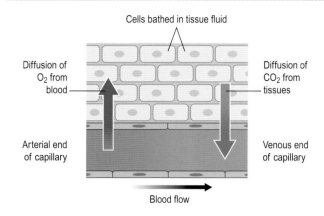

Figure 5.6 The exchange of gases in internal respiration.

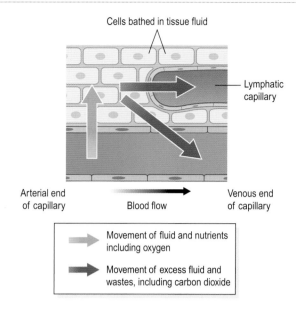

Figure 5.7 Diffusion of fluid, nutrients and waste products between capillaries and cells.

Exchange in the tissues takes place between blood at the arterial end of the capillaries and the tissue fluid and then between the tissue fluid and the cells. Oxygen diffuses down its concentration gradient, from the oxygen-rich arterial blood, into the tissues, where oxygen levels are lower because of constant tissue consumption.

Oxyhaemoglobin is an unstable compound and breaks up (dissociates) easily to liberate oxygen. Factors that increase dissociation are discussed on page 66.

Carbon dioxide is one of the waste products of cell metabolism and, towards the venous end of the capillary, it diffuses into the blood down the concentration gradient. Blood transports carbon dioxide to the lungs for excretion by three different mechanisms:

- dissolved in the water of the blood plasma – 7%
- in chemical combination with sodium in the form of sodium bicarbonate – 70%
- remainder in combination with haemoglobin – 23%.

Exchange of other substances

The nutrients, including glucose, amino acids, fatty acids, vitamins and mineral salts required by all body cells are transported round the body in the blood plasma. They diffuse through the semipermeable capillary walls into the tissues (Fig. 5.7). Water exchanges freely between the plasma and tissue fluid by osmosis. Diffusion and osmosis are described on p. 29.

Capillary fluid dynamics

The two main forces determining overall fluid movement across the capillary wall are the *hydrostatic pressure* (blood pressure), which tends to push fluid out of the bloodstream, and the *osmotic pressure* of the blood, which tends to pull it back in, and is due mainly to the presence of plasma proteins, especially albumin (Fig. 5.8).

At *the arterial end*, the hydrostatic pressure is about 5 kPa (35 mmHg), and the opposing osmotic pressure of the blood is only 3 kPa (25 mmHg). The overall force at

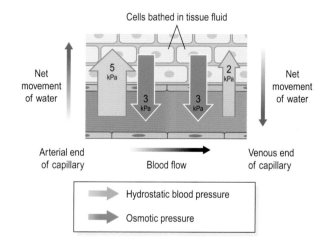

Figure 5.8 Effect of capillary pressures on water movement between capillaries and cells.

the arterial end of the capillary therefore drives fluid out of the capillary and into the tissue spaces. This net loss of fluid from the bloodstream must be reclaimed in some way.

At *the venous end* of the capillary, the situation is reversed. Blood flow is slower than at the arterial end because the hydrostatic pressure drops along the capillary to only 2 kPa (15 mmHg). The osmotic pressure remains unchanged at 3 kPa (25 mmHg) and, because this now exceeds hydrostatic pressure, fluid moves back into the capillary.

This transfer of substances, including water, to the tissue spaces is a dynamic process. As blood flows slowly through the large network of capillaries from the arterial to the venous end, there is constant change. Not all the water and cell waste products return to the blood capillaries. Of the 24 litres or so of fluid that moves out of the blood across capillary walls every day, only about 21 litres returns to the bloodstream at the venous end of the capillary bed. The excess is drained away from the tissue spaces in the minute lymph capillaries which originate as blind-end tubes with walls similar to, but more permeable than, those of the blood capillaries (Fig. 5.7). Extra tissue fluid and some cell waste materials enter the lymph capillaries and are eventually returned to the bloodstream (Ch. 6).

Heart

Learning outcomes

After studying this section, you should be able to:

- describe the structure of the heart and its position within the thorax
- trace the circulation of the blood through the heart and the blood vessels of the body
- outline the conducting system of the heart
- relate the electrical activity of the cardiac conduction system to the cardiac cycle
- describe the main factors determining heart rate and cardiac output.

The heart is a roughly cone-shaped hollow muscular organ. It is about 10 cm long and is about the size of the owner's fist. It weighs about 225 g in women and is heavier in men (about 310 g).

Position 5.2

The heart lies in the thoracic cavity (Fig. 5.9) in the mediastinum (the space between the lungs). It lies obliquely, a little more to the left than the right, and presents a base above, and an *apex* below. The apex is about 9 cm to the left of the midline at the level of the 5th intercostal space, i.e. a little below the nipple and slightly nearer the midline. The base extends to the level of the 2nd rib.

Organs associated with the heart (Fig. 5.10)

Inferiorly – the apex rests on the central tendon of the diaphragm

Superiorly – the great blood vessels, i.e. the aorta, superior vena cava, pulmonary artery and pulmonary veins

Posteriorly – the oesophagus, trachea, left and right bronchus, descending aorta, inferior vena cava and thoracic vertebrae

Laterally – the lungs – the left lung overlaps the left side of the heart

Anteriorly – the sternum, ribs and intercostal muscles.

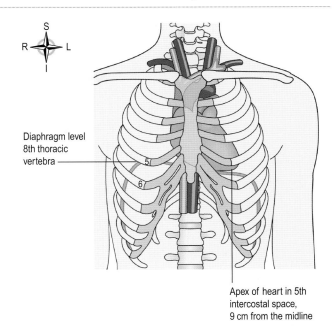

Diaphragm level 8th thoracic vertebra

Apex of heart in 5th intercostal space, 9 cm from the midline

Figure 5.9 Position of the heart in the thorax.

Structure

The heart wall

The heart wall is composed of three layers of tissue (Fig. 5.11A): pericardium, myocardium and endocardium.

Pericardium

The pericardium is the outermost layer and is made up of two sacs. The outer sac (the fibrous pericardium) consists of fibrous tissue and the inner (the serous pericardium) of a continuous double layer of serous membrane.

The fibrous pericardium is continuous with the tunica adventitia of the great blood vessels above and is adherent to the diaphragm below. Its inelastic, fibrous nature prevents overdistension of the heart.

The outer layer of the serous pericardium, the *parietal pericardium*, lines the fibrous pericardium. The inner layer, the *visceral pericardium*, which is continuous with the parietal pericardium, is adherent to the heart muscle. A similar arrangement of a double membrane forming a closed space is seen also with the pleura, the membrane enclosing the lungs (see Fig. 10.15, p. 250).

The serous membrane consists of flattened epithelial cells. It secretes serous fluid, called *pericardial fluid*, into the space between the visceral and parietal layers, which allows smooth movement between them when the heart beats. The space between the parietal and visceral pericardium is only a *potential space*. In health the two layers lie closely together, with only the thin film of pericardial fluid between them.

87

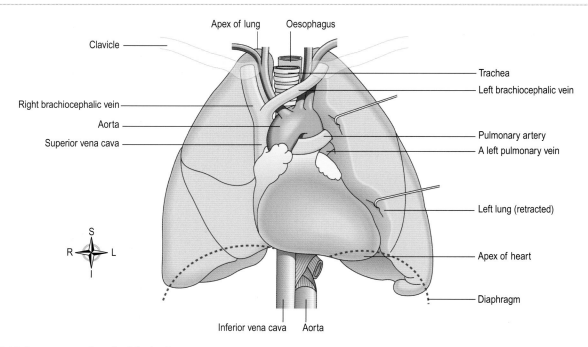

Figure 5.10 Organs associated with the heart.

Myocardium

The myocardium is composed of specialised cardiac muscle found only in the heart (Fig. 5.11B and C). It is striated, like skeletal muscle, but is not under voluntary control. Each fibre (cell) has a nucleus and one or more branches. The ends of the cells and their branches are in very close contact with the ends and branches of adjacent cells. Microscopically these 'joints', or *intercalated discs*, are thicker, darker lines than the striations. This arrangement gives cardiac muscle the appearance of being a sheet of muscle rather than a very large number of individual cells. Because of the end-to-end continuity of the fibres, each one does not need to have a separate nerve supply. When an impulse is initiated it spreads from cell to cell via the branches and intercalated discs over the whole 'sheet' of muscle, causing contraction. The 'sheet' arrangement of the myocardium enables the atria and ventricles to contract in a coordinated and efficient manner.

Running through the myocardium is also the network of specialised conducting fibres responsible for transmitting the heart's electrical signals. The myocardium is thickest at the apex and thins out towards the base (Fig. 5.12). This reflects the amount of work each chamber contributes to the pumping of blood. It is thickest in the left ventricle, which has the greatest workload.

Specialised muscle cells in the walls of the atria secrete atrial natriuretic peptide (ANP, p. 228).

Fibrous tissue in the heart. The myocardium is supported by a network of fine fibres that run through all the heart muscle. This is called the *fibrous skeleton* of the heart. In addition, the atria and the ventricles are separated by a ring of fibrous tissue, which does not conduct electrical impulses. Consequently, when a wave of electrical activity passes over the atrial muscle, it can only spread to the ventricles through the conducting system that bridges the fibrous ring from atria to ventricles (p. 90).

Endocardium

This lines the chambers and valves of the heart. It is a thin, smooth membrane to ensure smooth flow of blood through the heart. It consists of flattened epithelial cells, and it is continuous with the endothelium lining the blood vessels.

Interior of the heart 5.3, 5.4

The heart is divided into a right and left side by the *septum* (Fig. 5.12), a partition consisting of myocardium covered by endocardium. After birth, blood cannot cross the septum from one side to the other. Each side is divided by an *atrioventricular valve* into the upper atrium and the ventricle below. The atrioventricular valves are formed by double folds of endocardium strengthened by a little fibrous tissue. The right atrioventricular valve (tricuspid valve) has three flaps or cusps and the left atrioventricular valve (mitral valve, Fig. 5.13) has two cusps. Flow of blood in the heart is one way; blood enters the heart via the atria and passes into the ventricles below.

The valves between the atria and ventricles open and close passively according to changes in pressure in the chambers (Fig. 5.13A and B). They open when the pressure in the atria is greater than that in the ventricles. During *ventricular systole* (contraction) the pressure in the ventricles rises above that in the atria and the valves snap shut, preventing backward flow of blood. The valves are

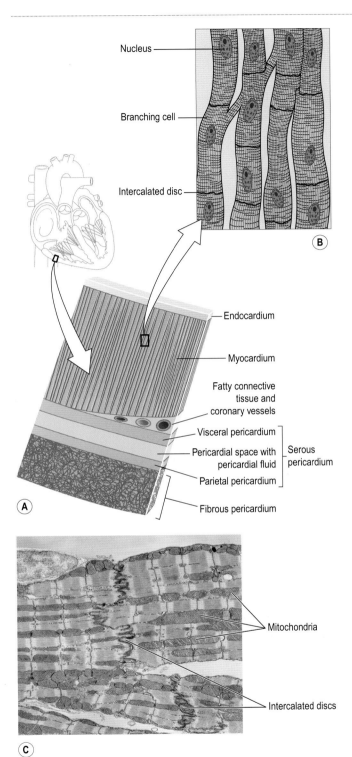

prevented from opening upwards into the atria by tendinous cords, called *chordae tendineae* (Fig. 5.13C), which extend from the inferior surface of the cusps to little projections of myocardium into the ventricles, covered with endothelium, called *papillary muscles* (Fig. 5.13).

Flow of blood through the heart

(Fig. 5.14) ▓ **5.5**

The two largest veins of the body, the *superior* and *inferior venae cavae*, empty their contents into the right atrium. This blood passes via the right atrioventricular valve into the right ventricle, and from there is pumped into the *pulmonary artery* or *trunk* (the only artery in the body which carries deoxygenated blood). The opening of the pulmonary artery is guarded by the *pulmonary valve*, formed by three *semilunar cusps*. This valve prevents the backflow of blood into the right ventricle when the ventricular muscle relaxes. After leaving the heart the pulmonary artery divides into *left* and *right pulmonary arteries*, which carry the venous blood to the lungs where exchange of gases takes place: carbon dioxide is excreted and oxygen is absorbed.

Two *pulmonary veins* from each lung carry *oxygenated blood* back to the *left atrium*. Blood then passes through the left atrioventricular valve into the left ventricle, and from there it is pumped into the aorta, the first artery of the general circulation. The opening of the aorta is guarded by the *aortic valve*, formed by three *semilunar cusps* (Fig. 5.15).

From this sequence of events it can be seen that the blood passes from the right to the left side of the heart via the lungs, or pulmonary circulation (Fig. 5.16). However, it should be noted that both atria contract at the same time and this is followed by the simultaneous contraction of both ventricles.

The muscle layer of the walls of the atria is thinner than that of the ventricles (Fig. 5.12). This is consistent with the amount of work they do. The atria, usually assisted by gravity, pump the blood only through the atrioventricular valves into the ventricles, whereas the more powerful ventricles pump the blood to the lungs and round the whole body.

The pulmonary trunk leaves the heart from the upper part of the right ventricle, and the aorta leaves from the upper part of the left ventricle.

Blood supply to the heart (the coronary circulation) ▓ **5.6**

Arterial supply (Fig. 5.17)**.** The heart is supplied with arterial blood by the *right* and *left coronary arteries*, which branch from the aorta immediately distal to the aortic valve (Figs 5.15 and 5.17). The coronary arteries receive about 5% of the blood pumped from the heart, although the heart comprises a small proportion of body weight.

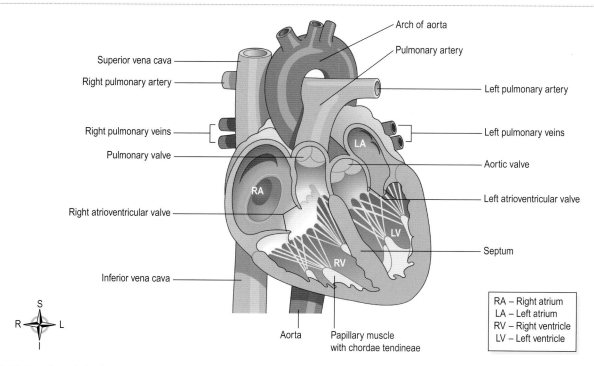

Figure 5.12 Interior of the heart.

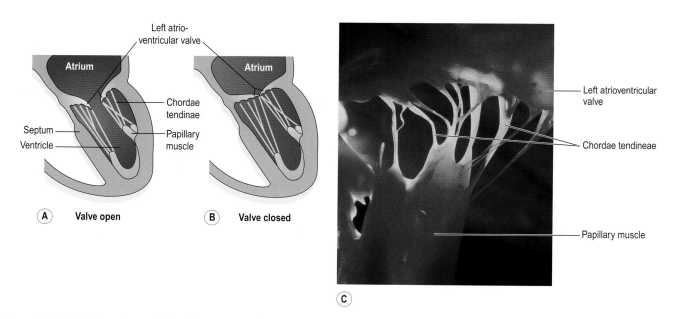

Figure 5.13 The left atrioventricular (mitral) valve. A. Valve open. **B.** Valve closed. **C.** Photograph of the chordae tendinae.

This large blood supply, of which a large proportion goes to the left ventricle, highlights the importance of the heart to body function. The coronary arteries traverse the heart, eventually forming a vast network of capillaries.

Venous drainage. Most of the venous blood is collected into a number of *cardiac veins* that join to form the *coronary sinus*, which opens into the right atrium. The remainder passes directly into the heart chambers through little venous channels.

Conducting system of the heart
(Fig. 5.18) █ 5.7

The heart possesses the property of *autorhythmicity*, which means it generates its own electrical impulses and beats independently of nervous or hormonal control, i.e. it is not reliant on external mechanisms to initiate each heartbeat. However, it is supplied with both sympathetic and parasympathetic nerve fibres, which increase and

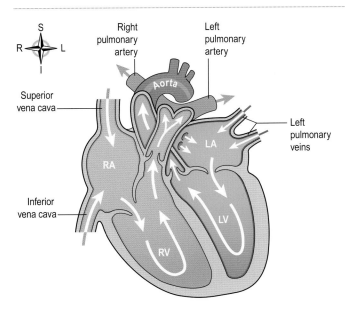

Figure 5.14 Direction of blood flow through the heart.

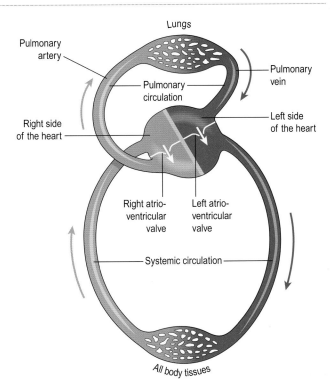

Figure 5.16 Circulation of blood through the heart and the pulmonary and systemic circulations.

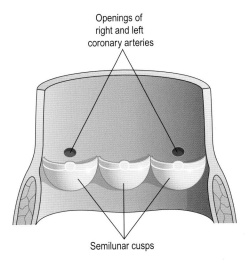

Figure 5.15 The aorta cut open to show the semilunar cusps of the aortic valve.

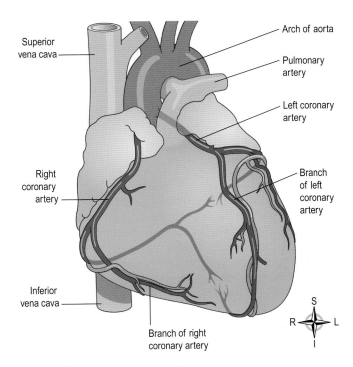

Figure 5.17 The coronary arteries.

decrease respectively the intrinsic heart rate. In addition, the heart responds to a number of circulating hormones, including adrenaline (epinephrine) and thyroxine.

Small groups of specialised neuromuscular cells in the myocardium initiate and conduct impulses, causing coordinated and synchronised contraction of the heart muscle.

Sinoatrial node (SA node)

This small mass of specialised cells lies in the wall of the right atrium near the opening of the superior vena cava.

The sinoatrial cells generate these regular impulses because they are electrically unstable. This instability leads them to discharge (*depolarise*) regularly, usually between 60 and 80 times a minute. This depolarisation is

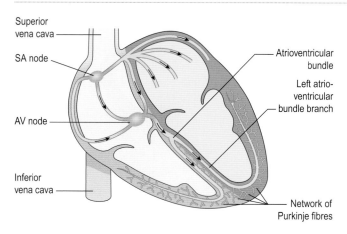

Figure 5.18 The conducting system of the heart.

followed by recovery (*repolarisation*), but almost immediately their instability leads them to discharge again, setting the heart rate. Because the SA node discharges faster than any other part of the heart, it normally sets the heart rate and is called the *pacemaker* of the heart. Firing of the SA node triggers atrial contraction.

Atrioventricular node (AV node)

This small mass of neuromuscular tissue is situated in the wall of the atrial septum near the atrioventricular valves. Normally, the AV node merely transmits the electrical signals from the atria into the ventricles. There is a delay here; the electrical signal takes 0.1 of a second to pass through into the ventricles. This allows the atria to finish contracting before the ventricles start.

The AV node also has a secondary pacemaker function and takes over this role if there is a problem with the SA node itself, or with the transmission of impulses from the atria. Its intrinsic firing rate, however, is slower than that set by the SA node (40–60 beats per minute).

Atrioventricular bundle (AV bundle or bundle of His)

This mass of specialised fibres originates from the AV node. The AV bundle crosses the fibrous ring that separates atria and ventricles then, at the upper end of the ventricular septum, it divides into *right* and *left bundle branches*. Within the ventricular myocardium the branches break up into fine fibres, called the *Purkinje fibres*. The AV bundle, bundle branches and Purkinje fibres transmit electrical impulses from the AV node to the apex of the myocardium where the wave of ventricular contraction begins, then sweeps upwards and outwards, pumping blood into the pulmonary artery and the aorta.

Nerve supply to the heart

As mentioned earlier, the heart is influenced by autonomic (sympathetic and parasympathetic) nerves

originating in the *cardiovascular centre* in the *medulla oblongata*.

The *vagus nerve* (parasympathetic) supplies mainly the SA and AV nodes and atrial muscle. Vagal stimulation reduces the rate at which impulses are produced, decreasing the rate and force of the heartbeat.

Sympathetic nerves supply the SA and AV nodes and the myocardium of atria and ventricles, and stimulation increases the rate and force of the heartbeat.

Factors affecting heart rate

The most important ones are listed in Box 5.1, and explained in more detail on page 95.

The cardiac cycle

At rest, the healthy adult heart is likely to beat at a rate of 60–80 beats per minute (b.p.m.). During each heartbeat, or *cardiac cycle* (Fig. 5.19), the heart contracts (systole) and then relaxes (diastole).

Stages of the cardiac cycle

Taking 74 b.p.m. as an example, each cycle lasts about 0.8 of a second and consists of:

- *atrial systole* – contraction of the atria
- *ventricular systole* – contraction of the ventricles
- *complete cardiac diastole* – relaxation of the atria and ventricles.

It does not matter at which stage of the cardiac cycle a description starts. For convenience the period when the atria are filling has been chosen.

The superior vena cava and the inferior vena cava transport deoxygenated blood into the right atrium *at the same time* as the four pulmonary veins bring oxygenated blood into the left atrium. The atrioventricular valves are open and blood flows passively through to the ventricles. The SA node triggers a wave of contraction that spreads over the myocardium of both atria, emptying the atria and completing ventricular filling (atrial systole 0.1 s; Fig. 5.19A). When the electrical impulse reaches the AV node it is slowed down, delaying atrioventricular transmission. This delay means that the mechanical result of atrial stimulation, atrial contraction, lags behind the electrical activity by a fraction of a second. This allows the atria to finish emptying into the ventricles before the

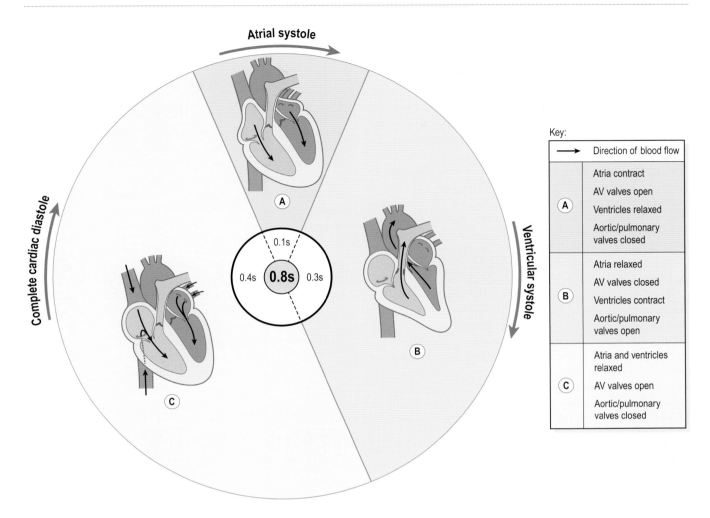

Figure 5.19 The cardiac cycle.

ventricles begin to contract. After this brief delay, the AV node triggers its own electrical impulse, which quickly spreads to the ventricular muscle via the AV bundle, the bundle branches and Purkinje fibres. This results in a wave of contraction which sweeps upwards from the apex of the heart and across the walls of both ventricles pumping the blood into the pulmonary artery and the aorta (ventricular systole 0.3 s; Fig. 5.19B). The high pressure generated during ventricular contraction forces the atrioventricular valves to close, preventing backflow of blood into the atria.

After contraction of the ventricles there is *complete cardiac diastole*, a period of *0.4 seconds*, when atria and ventricles are relaxed. During this time the myocardium recovers ready for the next heartbeat, and the atria refill ready for the next cycle (Fig. 5.19C).

The valves of the heart and of the great vessels open and close according to the pressure within the chambers of the heart. The AV valves are open while the ventricular muscle is relaxed during atrial filling and systole. When the ventricles contract there is a rapid increase in the pressure in these chambers, and when it rises above atrial pressure the atrioventricular valves close. When the ventricular pressure rises above that in the pulmonary artery and in the aorta, the pulmonary and aortic valves open and blood flows into these vessels. When the ventricles relax and the pressure within them falls, the reverse process occurs. First the pulmonary and aortic valves close, then the atrioventricular valves open and the cycle begins again. This sequence of opening and closing valves ensures that the blood flows in only one direction.

Heart sounds

The individual is not usually conscious of their heartbeat, but if the ear, or the diaphragm of a stethoscope, is placed on the chest wall a little below the left nipple and slightly nearer the midline the heartbeat can be heard (Fig. 5.9).

There are four heart sounds, each corresponding to a particular event in the cardiac cycle. The first two are most easily distinguished, and sound through the stethoscope like 'lub dup'. The first sound, *'lub'*, is fairly loud and is due to the closure of the atrioventricular valves.

This corresponds with the start of ventricular systole. The second sound, '*dup*', is softer and is due to the closure of the aortic and pulmonary valves. This corresponds with ventricular diastole.

Electrical changes in the heart ▮5.8

The body tissues and fluids conduct electricity well, so the electrical activity in the heart can be recorded on the skin surface using electrodes positioned on the limbs and/or the chest. This recording, called an electrocardiogram (ECG) shows the spread of the electrical signal generated by the SA node as it travels through the atria, the AV node and the ventricles. The normal ECG tracing shows five waves which, by convention, have been named P, Q, R, S and T (Fig. 5.20).

The P wave arises when the impulse from the SA node sweeps over the atria (atrial depolarisation).

The QRS complex represents the very rapid spread of the impulse from the AV node through the AV bundle and the Purkinje fibres and the electrical activity of the ventricular muscle (ventricular depolarisation). Note the delay between the completion of the P wave and the onset of the QRS complex. This represents the conduction of the impulse through the AV node (p. 92), which is much slower than conduction elsewhere in the heart, and allows atrial contraction to finish completely before ventricular contraction starts.

The T wave represents the relaxation of the ventricular muscle (ventricular repolarisation). Atrial repolarisation occurs during ventricular contraction, and so is not seen because of the larger QRS complex.

The ECG described above originates from the SA node and is called *sinus rhythm*. The rate of sinus rhythm is 60–100 b.p.m. A faster heart rate is called *tachycardia* and a slower heart rate, *bradycardia*.

By examining the pattern of waves and the time interval between cycles and parts of cycles, information about the state of the myocardium and the cardiac conduction system is obtained.

Cardiac output

The cardiac output is the amount of blood ejected from each ventricle every minute. The amount expelled by each contraction of each ventricle is the *stroke volume*. Cardiac output is expressed in litres per minute (L/min) and is calculated by multiplying the stroke volume by the heart rate (measured in beats per minute):

Cardiac output = Stroke volume × Heart rate.

In a healthy adult at rest, the stroke volume is approximately 70 mL and if the heart rate is 72 per minute, the cardiac output is 5 L/minute. This can be greatly increased to meet the demands of exercise to around 25 L/minute, and in athletes up to 35 L/minute. This increase during exercise is called the *cardiac reserve*.

When increased blood supply is needed to meet increased tissue requirements of oxygen and nutrients, heart rate and/or stroke volume can be increased (see Box 5.2).

Stroke volume

The stroke volume is determined by the volume of blood in the ventricles immediately before they contract, i.e. the *ventricular end-diastolic volume* (VEDV), sometimes called *preload*. In turn, preload depends on the amount of blood returning to the heart through the superior and inferior venae cavae (the *venous return*). Increased preload leads to stronger myocardial contraction, and more blood is expelled. In turn the stroke volume and cardiac output rise. In this way, the heart, within physiological limits, always pumps out all the blood that it receives, allowing it to adjust cardiac output to match body needs. This capacity to increase the stroke volume with increasing preload is finite, and when the limit is reached, i.e. venous return to the heart exceeds cardiac

---

Box 5.2 Summary of factors affecting cardiac output

Cardiac output = Stroke volume × Heart rate

Factors affecting stroke volume:
- VEDV (ventricular end-diastolic volume – preload)
- Venous return
  - position of the body
  - skeletal muscle pump
  - respiratory pump
- Strength of myocardial contraction
- Blood volume

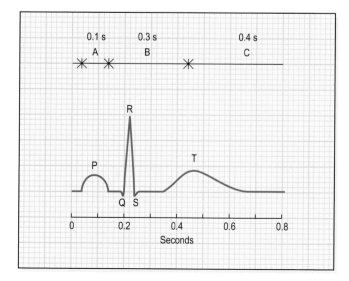

Figure 5.20 Electrocardiogram of one cardiac cycle. A, B and **C** correspond to the phases of the cardiac cycle shown in Figure 5.19.

output (i.e. more blood is arriving in the atria than the ventricles can pump out), cardiac output decreases and the heart begins to fail (p. 126). Other factors that increase the force and rate of myocardial contraction include increased sympathetic nerve activity and circulating hormones, e.g. adrenaline (epinephrine), noradrenaline (norepinephrine) and thyroxine.

Arterial blood pressure. This affects the stroke volume as it creates resistance to blood being pumped from the ventricles into the great arteries. This resistance (sometimes called *afterload*) is determined by the distensibility, or *elasticity*, of the large arteries and the peripheral resistance of arterioles (p. 85). Increasing afterload increases the workload of the ventricles, because it increases the pressure against which they have to pump. This may actually reduce stroke volume if systemic blood pressure becomes significantly higher than normal.

Blood volume. This is normally kept constant by the kidneys. Should blood volume fall, e.g. through sudden haemorrhage, this can cause stroke volume, cardiac output and venous return to fall. However, the body's compensatory mechanisms (p. 96) will tend to return these values towards normal, unless the blood loss is too sudden or severe for compensation (see Shock, p. 118).

Venous return

Venous return is the major determinant of cardiac output and, normally, the heart pumps out all blood returned to it. The force of contraction of the left ventricle ejecting blood into the aorta is not sufficient to push the blood through the arterial and venous circulation and back to the heart. Other factors are involved.

The position of the body. Gravity assists venous return from the head and neck when standing or sitting and offers less resistance to venous return from the lower parts of the body when lying flat.

Muscular contraction. Backflow of blood in veins of the limbs, especially when standing, is prevented by valves (Fig. 5.4). The contraction of skeletal muscles surrounding the deep veins compresses them, pushing blood towards the heart (Fig. 5.21). In the lower limbs, this is called the *skeletal muscle pump*.

The respiratory pump. During inspiration, the expansion of the chest creates a negative pressure within the thorax, assisting flow of blood towards the heart. In addition, when the diaphragm descends during inspiration, the increased intra-abdominal pressure pushes blood towards the heart.

Heart rate

The heart rate is a major determinant of cardiac output. If heart rate rises, cardiac output increases, and if it falls,

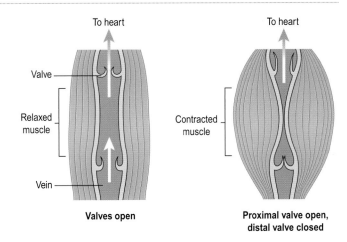

Figure 5.21 The skeletal muscle pump.

cardiac output falls too. The main factors determining heart rate are outlined below.

Autonomic nervous system. The intrinsic rate at which the heart beats is a balance between sympathetic and parasympathetic activity and this is the most important factor in determining heart rate.

Circulating chemicals. The hormones adrenaline (epinephrine) and noradrenaline (norepinephrine), secreted by the adrenal medulla, have the same effect as sympathetic stimulation, i.e. they increase the heart rate. Other hormones, including thyroxine, increase heart rate. Hypoxia and elevated carbon dioxide levels stimulate heart rate. Electrolyte imbalances may affect it, e.g. hyperkalaemia depresses cardiac function and leads to bradycardia (slow heart rate). Some drugs, such as β-receptor antagonists (e.g. atenolol) used in hypertension, can also cause bradycardia.

Position. When upright, the heart rate is usually faster than when lying down.

Exercise. Active muscles need more blood than resting muscles and this is achieved by an increased heart rate and local vasodilation.

Emotional states. During excitement, fear or anxiety the heart rate is increased. Other effects mediated by the sympathetic nervous system may be present (see Fig. 7.43, p. 174).

Gender. The heart rate is faster in women than men.

Age. In babies and small children the heart rate is more rapid than in older children and adults.

Temperature. The heart rate rises and falls with body temperature.

Baroreceptor reflex. See page 97.

A summary of the factors that alter CO is shown in Box 5.2.

Blood pressure

Learning outcomes

After studying this section, you should be able to:

- define the term blood pressure
- describe the factors that influence blood pressure
- explain the two main mechanisms that control blood pressure.

Blood pressure is the force or pressure that the blood exerts on the walls of blood vessels. Systemic arterial blood pressure maintains the essential flow of blood into and out of the organs of the body. Keeping blood pressure within normal limits is very important. If it becomes too high, blood vessels can be damaged, causing clots or bleeding from sites of blood vessel rupture. If it falls too low, then blood flow through tissue beds may be inadequate. This is particularly dangerous for essential organs such as the heart, brain or kidneys.

The systemic arterial blood pressure, usually called simply arterial blood pressure, is the result of the discharge of blood from the left ventricle into the already full aorta.

Blood pressure varies according to the time of day, the posture, gender and age of the individual. Blood pressure falls at rest and during sleep. It increases with age and is usually higher in women than in men.

Systolic and diastolic pressures. When the left ventricle contracts and pushes blood into the aorta, the pressure produced within the arterial system is called the *systolic blood pressure*. In adults it is about 120 mmHg or 16 kPa.

In complete cardiac diastole when the heart is resting following the ejection of blood, the pressure within the arteries is much lower and is called *diastolic blood pressure*. In an adult this is about 80 mmHg or 11 kPa. The difference between systolic and diastolic blood pressures is the *pulse pressure*.

Arterial blood pressure (BP) is measured with a *sphygmomanometer* and is usually expressed with the systolic pressure written above the diastolic pressure:

$$BP = \frac{120}{80} \text{ mmHg} \quad \text{or} \quad BP = \frac{16}{11} \text{ kPa}$$

Elasticity of arterial walls. There is a considerable amount of elastic tissue in the arterial walls, especially in large arteries. Therefore, when the left ventricle ejects blood into the already full aorta, the aorta expands to accommodate it, and then recoils because of the elastic tissue in the wall. This pushes the blood forwards, into the systemic circulation. This distension and recoil occurs throughout the arterial system. During cardiac diastole the elastic recoil of the arteries maintains the diastolic pressure.

Factors determining blood pressure

Blood pressure is determined by *cardiac output* and *peripheral resistance*. Change in either of these parameters tends to alter systemic blood pressure, although the body's compensatory mechanisms usually adjust for any significant change.

$$\text{Blood pressure} = \frac{\text{Cardiac}}{\text{output}} \times \frac{\text{Peripheral}}{\text{resistance}}$$

Cardiac output

Cardiac output is determined by the stroke volume and the heart rate (p. 94). Factors that affect the heart rate and stroke volume are described above, and they may increase or decrease cardiac output and, in turn, blood pressure. An increase in cardiac output raises both systolic and diastolic pressures. An increase in stroke volume increases systolic pressure more than diastolic pressure.

Peripheral or arteriolar resistance

Arterioles, the smallest arteries, have a tunica media composed almost entirely of smooth muscle, which responds to nerve and chemical stimulation. Constriction and dilation of the arterioles are the main determinants of peripheral resistance (p. 85). Vasoconstriction causes blood pressure to rise and vasodilation causes it to fall.

When elastic tissue in the tunica media is replaced by inelastic fibrous tissue as part of the ageing process, blood pressure rises.

Autoregulation

Systemic blood pressure continually rises and falls, according to levels of activity, body position, etc. However, the body organs are capable of adjusting blood flow and blood pressure in their own local vessels independently of systemic blood pressure. This property is called *autoregulation*, and protects the tissues against swings in systemic pressures. It is especially important in the kidneys, which can be damaged by increased pressure in their delicate glomerular capillary beds (p. 339), and in the brain, which is very sensitive to even slight increases in levels of cellular waste.

Control of blood pressure (BP)

Blood pressure is controlled in two ways:

- short-term control, on a moment-to-moment basis, which mainly involves the baroreceptor reflex, discussed below, and also chemoreceptors and circulating hormones
- long-term control, which involves regulation of blood volume by the kidneys and the renin–angiotensin–aldosterone system (p. 343).

Table 5.1 The effects of the autonomic nervous system on the heart and blood vessels

	Sympathetic stimulation	Parasympathetic stimulation
Heart	↑rate ↑strength of contraction	↓rate ↓strength of contraction
Blood vessels	Most constrict, but arteries supplying skeletal muscle and brain dilate	Most blood vessels do not have a parasympathetic blood supply

Short-term blood pressure regulation

The cardiovascular centre (CVC) is a collection of interconnected neurones in the medulla and pons of the brain stem. The CVC receives, integrates and coordinates inputs from:

- baroreceptors (pressure receptors)
- chemoreceptors
- higher centres in the brain.

The CVC sends autonomic nerves (both sympathetic and parasympathetic [see Ch. 7]) to the heart and blood vessels (Table 5.1). It controls BP by slowing down or speeding up the heart rate and by dilating or constricting blood vessels. Activity in these fibres is essential for control of blood pressure (Fig. 5.22).

Baroreceptors

Within the wall of the aortic and carotid sinuses are *baroreceptors*, nerve endings sensitive to stretch (pressure) (Fig. 5.23), which are the body's principal moment-to-moment regulatory mechanism for controlling blood pressure. A rise in blood pressure in these arteries stimulates the baroreceptors, increasing their input to the CVC. The CVC responds by increasing parasympathetic nerve activity to the heart; this slows the heart down. At the same time, sympathetic stimulation to the blood vessels is inhibited, causing vasodilation. The net result is a fall in systemic blood pressure.

Conversely, if pressure within the aortic arch and carotid sinuses falls, the rate of baroreceptor discharge also falls. The CVC responds by increasing sympathetic drive to the heart to speed it up. Sympathetic activity in blood vessels is also increased, leading to vasoconstriction. Both these measures counteract the falling blood pressure. Baroreceptor control of blood pressure is also called the *baroreceptor reflex* (Fig. 5.23).

Chemoreceptors

These are nerve endings situated in the carotid and aortic bodies, and are primarily involved in control of respiration (p. 260). They are sensitive to changes in the levels of

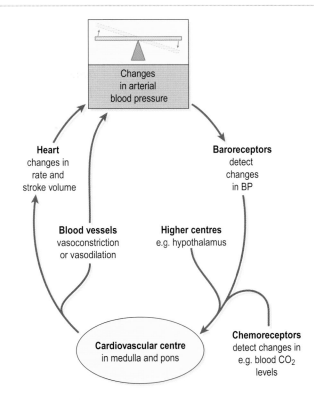

Figure 5.22 Summary of the main mechanisms in blood pressure control.

carbon dioxide, oxygen and the acidity of the blood (pH) (Fig. 5.24). Rising blood CO_2, falling blood O_2 levels and/or falling arterial blood pH all indicate failing tissue perfusion. When these changes are detected by the chemoreceptors, they send signals to the CVC, which then increases sympathetic drive to the heart and blood vessels, pushing blood pressure up to improve tissue blood supply. Because respiratory effort is also stimulated, blood oxygen levels rise as well.

Chemoreceptor input to the CVC influences its output only when severe disruption of respiratory function occurs or when arterial BP falls to less than 80 mmHg. Similar chemoreceptors are found on the brain surface in the medulla oblongata, and they measure carbon dioxide/oxygen levels and pH of the surrounding cerebrospinal fluid. Changes from normal activate responses similar to those described above for the aortic/carotid receptors.

Higher centres in the brain

Input to the CVC from the higher centres is influenced by emotional states such as fear, anxiety, pain and anger that may stimulate changes in blood pressure.

The hypothalamus in the brain controls body temperature and influences the CVC, which responds by adjusting the diameter of blood vessels in the skin. This important mechanism regulates conservation and loss of heat so that core body temperature remains in the normal range (p. 366).

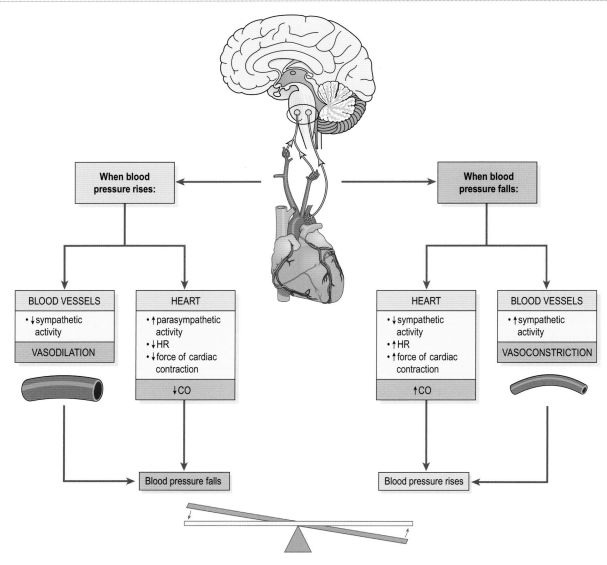

Figure 5.23 The baroreceptor reflex.

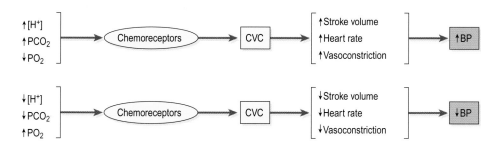

Figure 5.24 The relationship between stimulation of chemoreceptors and arterial blood pressure.

Long-term blood pressure regulation

Slower, longer lasting changes in blood pressure are effected by the *renin–angiotensin–aldosterone* system (RAAS, see p. 343) and the action of *antidiuretic hormone* (ADH, see p. 221). Both of these systems regulate blood volume, thus influencing blood pressure. In addition, *atrial natriuretic peptide* (ANP, p. 228), a hormone released by the heart itself, causes sodium and water loss from the kidney and reduces blood pressure, opposing the activities of both ADH and the RAAS.

Pressure in the pulmonary circulation

Pulmonary blood pressure is much lower than in the systemic circulation. This is because although the lungs receive the same amount of blood from the right ventricle as the rest of the body receives from the left ventricle, there are so many capillaries in the lungs that pressure is kept low. If pulmonary capillary pressure exceeds 25 mmHg, fluid is forced out of the bloodstream and into the airsacs (*pulmonary oedema*, p. 125), with very serious consequences. Autoregulation in the pulmonary circulation makes sure that blood flow through the vast network of capillaries is directed through well-oxygenated airsacs (p. 260).

Pulse

Learning outcomes

After studying this section, you should be able to:

■ define the term pulse

■ list the main sites on the body surface where the pulse is detected

■ describe the main factors affecting the pulse.

The pulse can be felt with gentle finger pressure in a superficial artery when its wall is distended by blood pumped from the left ventricle during contraction (systole). The wave passes quickly as the arterial wall recoils. Each contraction of the left ventricle forces about 60–80 millilitres of blood through the already full aorta and into the arterial system. The aortic pressure wave is transmitted through the arterial system and can be felt at any point where a superficial artery can be pressed firmly but gently against a bone (Fig. 5.25). The number of pulse b.p.m. normally represents the heart rate and varies considerably in different people and in the same person at different times. An average of 60–80 is common at rest. Information that may be obtained from the pulse includes:

- the rate at which the heart is beating
- the regularity of the heartbeat – the intervals between beats should be equal

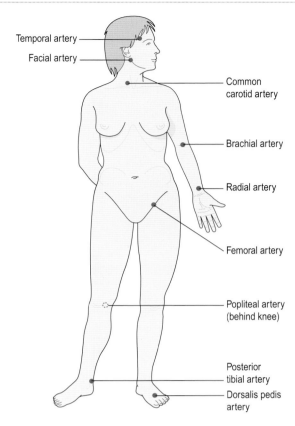

Figure 5.25 The main pulse points.

- the volume or strength of the beat – it should be possible to compress the artery with moderate pressure, stopping the flow of blood; the compressibility of the blood vessel gives some indication of the blood pressure and the state of the blood vessel wall
- the tension – the artery wall should feel soft and pliant under the fingers.

Factors affecting the pulse ▓ 5.9

In health, the pulse rate and the heart rate are identical. Factors influencing heart rate are summarised on page 95. In certain circumstances, the pulse may be less than the heart rate. This may occur, for example, if:

- the arteries supplying the peripheral tissues are narrowed or blocked and the blood therefore is not pumped through them with each heartbeat. Provided enough blood is reaching an extremity to nourish it, it will remain pink in colour and warm to touch, even if the pulse cannot be felt
- there is some disorder of cardiac contraction, e.g. atrial fibrillation (p. 129) and the heart is unable to generate enough force, with each contraction, to circulate blood to the peripheral arteries.

Circulation of the blood

Learning outcomes

After studying this section, you should be able to:

■ describe the circulation of the blood through the lungs, naming the main vessels involved

■ list the arteries supplying blood to all major body structures

■ describe the venous drainage involved in returning blood to the heart from the body

■ describe the arrangement of blood vessels relating to the portal circulation.

Although circulation of blood round the body is continuous (Fig. 5.16) it is convenient to describe it in two parts:

• pulmonary circulation
• systemic or general circulation (Figs 5.26 and 5.27).

Pulmonary circulation ▓ 5.10

This is the circulation of blood from the right ventricle of the heart to the lungs and back to the left atrium. In the lungs, carbon dioxide is excreted and oxygen is absorbed.

The pulmonary artery or trunk, carrying *deoxygenated blood*, leaves the upper part of the right ventricle of the heart. It passes upwards and divides into left and right pulmonary arteries at the level of the 5th thoracic vertebra.

The left pulmonary artery runs to the root of the left lung (p. 251) where it divides into two branches, one passing into each lobe.

The right pulmonary artery passes to the root of the right lung (p. 251) and divides into two branches. The larger branch carries blood to the middle and lower lobes, and the smaller branch to the upper lobe.

Within the lung these arteries divide and subdivide into smaller arteries, arterioles and capillaries. The exchange of gases takes place between capillary blood and air in the alveoli of the lungs (p. 259). In each lung the capillaries containing oxygenated blood merge into progressively larger venules, and eventually form two pulmonary veins.

Two pulmonary veins leave each lung, returning oxygenated blood to the left atrium of the heart. During atrial systole this blood is pumped into the left ventricle, and during ventricular systole it is forced into the aorta, the first artery of the general circulation.

Systemic or general circulation

The blood pumped out from the left ventricle is carried by the branches of the *aorta* around the body and returns to the right atrium of the heart by the *superior* and *inferior venae cavae*. Figure 5.26 shows the general positions of the aorta and the main arteries of the limbs. Figure 5.27 provides an overview of the venae cavae and the veins of the limbs.

The circulation of blood to the different parts of the body will be described in the order in which their arteries branch off the aorta.

Major blood vessels

The aorta is the largest artery of the body. The two largest veins, the superior and inferior venae cavae, return blood from all body parts to the heart.

Aorta (Fig. 5.28)

The aorta begins at the upper part of the left ventricle and, after passing upwards for a short way, it arches backwards and to the left. It then descends behind the heart through the thoracic cavity a little to the left of the thoracic vertebrae. At the level of the 12th thoracic vertebra it passes behind the diaphragm then downwards in the abdominal cavity to the level of the 4th lumbar vertebra, where it divides into the *right* and *left common iliac arteries*.

Throughout its length the aorta gives off numerous branches. Some of the branches are *paired*, i.e. there is a right and left branch of the same name, for instance, the right and left renal arteries supplying the kidneys, and some are single or *unpaired*, e.g. the coeliac artery.

The aorta will be described here according to its location:

• thoracic aorta (see below)
• abdominal aorta (p. 103).

Thoracic aorta (Fig. 5.28)

This part of the aorta lies above the diaphragm and is described in three parts:

• ascending aorta
• arch of the aorta
• descending aorta in the thorax (p. 103).

Ascending aorta. This is the short section of the aorta that rises from the heart. It is about 5 cm long and lies well protected behind the sternum.

The right and left coronary arteries are its only branches. They arise from the aorta just above the level of the aortic valve (Fig. 5.15) and supply the myocardium.

Arch of the aorta. This is a continuation of the ascending aorta. It begins behind the manubrium of the sternum

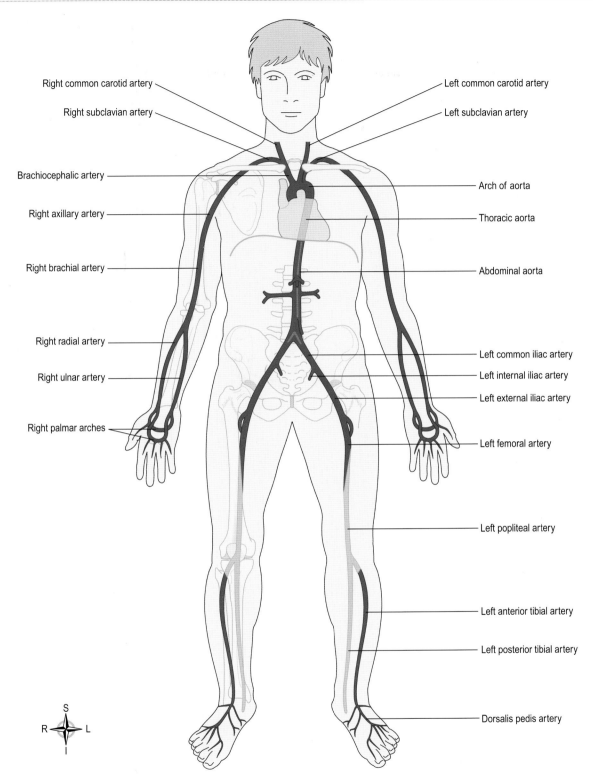

Right common carotid artery

Right subclavian artery

Brachiocephalic artery

Right axillary artery

Right brachial artery

Right radial artery

Right ulnar artery

Right palmar arches

Left common carotid artery

Left subclavian artery

Arch of aorta

Thoracic aorta

Abdominal aorta

Left common iliac artery

Left internal iliac artery

Left external iliac artery

Left femoral artery

Left popliteal artery

Left anterior tibial artery

Left posterior tibial artery

Dorsalis pedis artery

Figure 5.26 The aorta and the main arteries of the limbs.

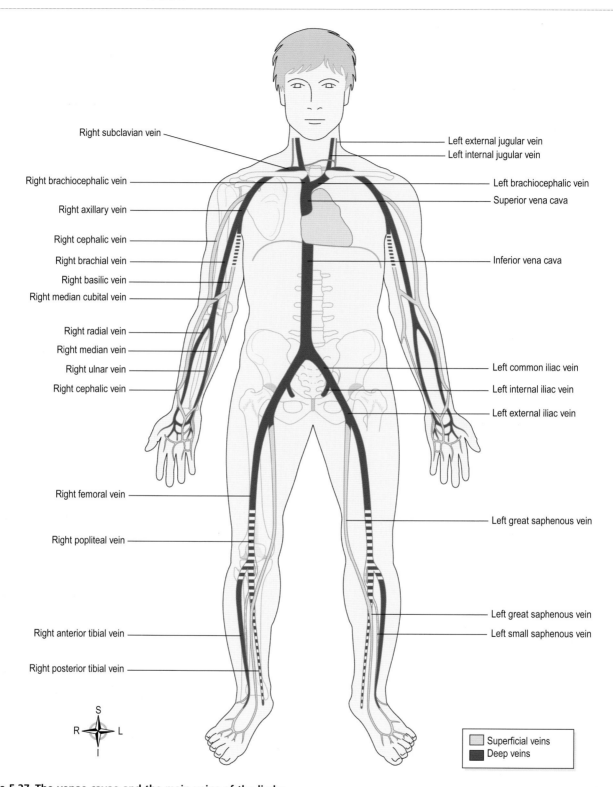

Right subclavian vein

Right brachiocephalic vein

Right axillary vein

Right cephalic vein

Right brachial vein

Right basilic vein

Right median cubital vein

Right radial vein

Right median vein

Right ulnar vein

Right cephalic vein

Right femoral vein

Right popliteal vein

Right anterior tibial vein

Right posterior tibial vein

Left external jugular vein

Left internal jugular vein

Left brachiocephalic vein

Superior vena cava

Inferior vena cava

Left common iliac vein

Left internal iliac vein

Left external iliac vein

Left great saphenous vein

Left great saphenous vein

Left small saphenous vein

S
R — L
I

Superficial veins
Deep veins

Figure 5.27 The venae cavae and the main veins of the limbs.

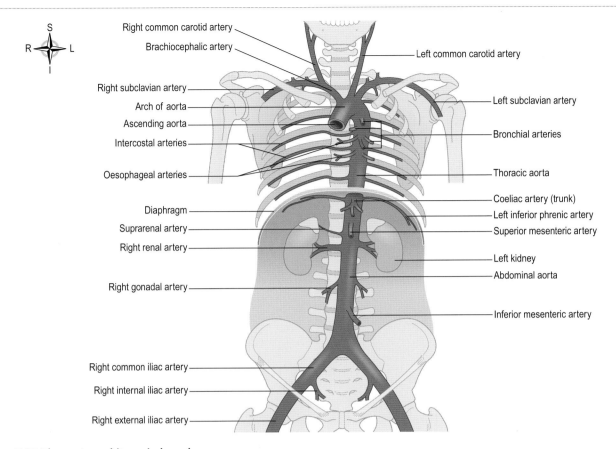

Figure 5.28 The aorta and its main branches.

and runs upwards, backwards and to the left in front of the trachea. It then passes downwards to the left of the trachea and is continuous with the descending aorta.

Three branches arise from its upper aspect:

- brachiocephalic artery or trunk
- left common carotid artery
- left subclavian artery.

The *brachiocephalic artery* is about 4 to 5 cm long and passes obliquely upwards, backwards and to the right. At the level of the sternoclavicular joint it divides into the *right common carotid artery* and the *right subclavian artery*.

Descending aorta in the thorax. This part is continuous with the arch of the aorta and begins at the level of the 4th thoracic vertebra. It extends downwards on the anterior surface of the bodies of the thoracic vertebrae to the level of the 12th thoracic vertebra, where it passes behind the diaphragm to become the abdominal aorta.

The descending aorta in the thorax gives off many paired branches which supply the walls and organs of the thoracic cavity (p. 108).

Abdominal aorta (Fig. 5.28)
The abdominal aorta is a continuation of the thoracic aorta. The name changes when the aorta enters the

abdominal cavity by passing behind the diaphragm at the level of the 12th thoracic vertebra. It descends in front of the vertebral column to the level of the 4th lumbar vertebra, where it divides into the *right* and *left common iliac arteries*.

Many branches arise from the abdominal aorta, some paired and some unpaired, supplying the abdominal structures and organs (p. 108).

Venae cavae (Fig. 5.29)

The superior and inferior venae cavae are the largest veins in the body and empty blood directly into the right atrium of the heart (Fig. 5.14). The superior vena cava drains all body structures lying above the diaphragm and the inferior vena cava drains blood from all structures below the diaphragm.

Superior vena cava
This is about 7 cm long and is formed by the union of the left and right brachiocephalic veins.

Inferior vena cava
This is formed at the level of the 5th lumbar vertebra by the union of the right and left common iliac veins, and

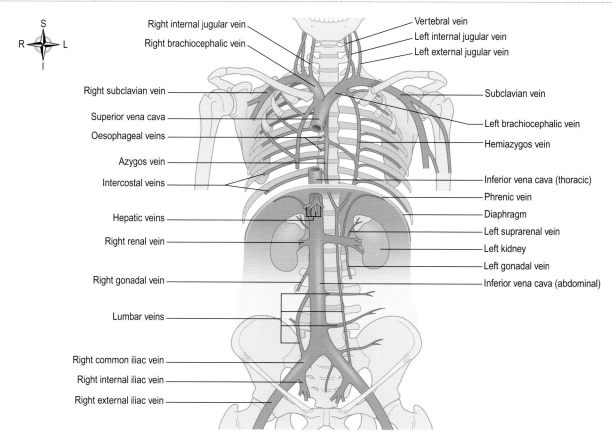

Figure 5.29 The venae cava and the main veins that form them.

ascends through the abdomen, lying close against the vertebral column and parallel to and just to the right of the descending abdominal aorta. It passes through the tendinous portion of the diaphragm into the thorax at the level of the 8th thoracic vertebra. As the inferior vena cava ascends through the abdomen, veins draining pelvic and abdominal organs empty into it (p. 110).

Circulation in the head and neck

Arterial supply

The paired arteries supplying the head and neck are the common carotid arteries and the vertebral arteries (Figs 5.30 and 5.32).

Carotid arteries. The *right common carotid artery* is a branch of the brachiocephalic artery. The *left common carotid artery* arises directly from the arch of the aorta. They pass upwards on either side of the neck and have the same distribution on each side. The common carotid arteries are embedded in fascia, called the *carotid sheath*. At the level of the upper border of the thyroid cartilage each divides into an *internal carotid artery* and an *external carotid artery*.

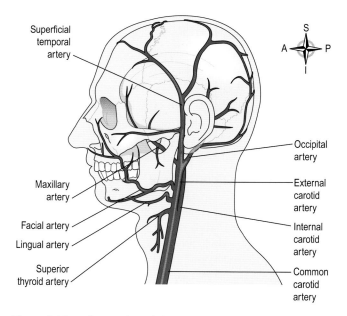

Figure 5.30 Main arteries of the left side of the head and neck.

The *carotid sinuses* are slight dilations at the point of division (bifurcation) of the common carotid arteries into their internal and external branches. The walls of the sinuses are thin and contain numerous nerve endings of the glossopharyngeal nerves. These nerve endings, or *baroreceptors*, are stimulated by changes in blood pressure in the carotid sinuses. The resultant nerve impulses initiate reflex adjustments of blood pressure through the vasomotor centre in the medulla oblongata (p. 159).

The carotid bodies are two small groups of *chemoreceptors*, one lying in close association with each common carotid artery at its bifurcation. They are supplied by the glossopharyngeal nerves and are stimulated by changes in the carbon dioxide and oxygen content of blood. The resultant nerve impulses initiate reflex adjustments of respiration through the respiratory centre in the medulla oblongata (p. 159).

External carotid artery (Fig. 5.30). This artery supplies the superficial tissues of the head and neck, via a number of branches:

- The *superior thyroid artery* supplies the thyroid gland and adjacent muscles.
- The *lingual artery* supplies the tongue, the membrane that lines the mouth, the structures in the floor of the mouth, the tonsil and the epiglottis.
- The *facial artery* passes outwards over the mandible just in front of the angle of the jaw and supplies the muscles of facial expression (p. 423) and structures in the mouth. A pulse can be felt where the artery crosses the jaw bone.
- The *occipital artery* supplies the posterior part of the scalp.
- The *temporal artery* passes upwards over the zygomatic process in front of the ear and supplies the frontal, temporal and parietal parts of the scalp. The temporal pulse can be felt in front of the upper part of the ear.
- The *maxillary artery* supplies the muscles of mastication and a branch of this artery, the *middle meningeal artery*, runs deeply to supply structures in the interior of the skull.

Internal carotid artery. This is a major contributor to the circulus arteriosus (circle of Willis) (Fig. 5.31), which supplies the greater part of the brain. It also has branches that supply the eyes, forehead and nose. It ascends to the base of the skull and passes through the carotid foramen in the temporal bone.

Circulus arteriosus (circle of Willis [Fig. 5.31]**).** The greater part of the brain is supplied with arterial blood by an arrangement of arteries called the *circulus arteriosus* or the *circle of Willis*. Four large arteries contribute to its formation: the two *internal carotid arteries* and the two *vertebral arteries* (Fig. 5.32). The vertebral arteries arise from the subclavian arteries, pass upwards through the

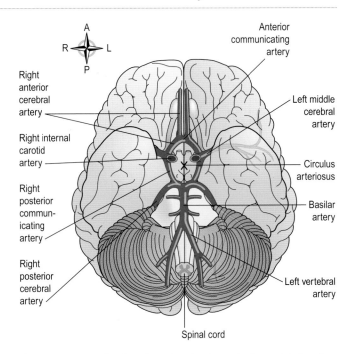

Figure 5.31 Arteries forming the circulus arteriosus (circle of Willis) and its main branches to the brain. Viewed from below.

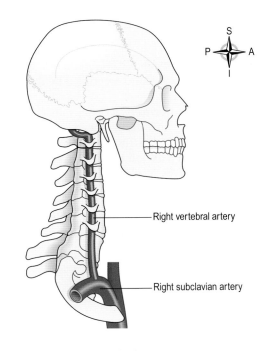

Figure 5.32 The right vertebral artery.

foramina in the transverse processes of the cervical vertebrae, enter the skull through the foramen magnum, then join to form the *basilar artery*. The arrangement in the circulus arteriosus is such that the brain as a whole receives an adequate blood supply even when a contributing artery is damaged and during extreme movements of the head and neck.

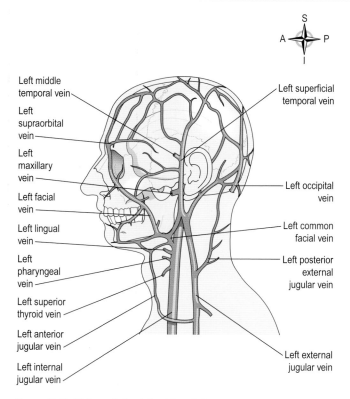

Figure 5.33 Veins of the left side of the head and neck.

Anteriorly, the two *anterior cerebral arteries* arise from the internal carotid arteries and are joined by the anterior *communicating artery.*

Posteriorly, the two *vertebral arteries* join to form the basilar artery. After travelling for a short distance the *basilar artery* divides to form two *posterior cerebral arteries*, each of which is joined to the corresponding internal carotid artery by a *posterior communicating artery,*

completing the circle. The circulus arteriosus is therefore formed by:

- 2 anterior cerebral arteries
- 2 internal carotid arteries
- 1 anterior communicating artery
- 2 posterior communicating arteries
- 2 posterior cerebral arteries
- 1 basilar artery.

From this circle, the *anterior cerebral arteries* pass forward to supply the anterior part of the brain, the *middle cerebral arteries* pass laterally to supply the sides of the brain, and the *posterior cerebral arteries* supply the posterior part of the brain.

Branches of the basilar artery supply parts of the brain stem.

Venous return

Venous blood from the head and neck is returned by deep and superficial veins.

Superficial veins with the same names as the branches of the external carotid artery return venous blood from the superficial structures of the face and scalp and unite to form the external jugular vein (Fig. 5.33).

The external jugular vein begins in the neck at the level of the angle of the jaw. It passes downwards in front of the sternocleidomastoid muscle, then behind the clavicle before entering the subclavian vein.

Venous blood from the deep areas of the brain is collected into channels called the *dural venous sinuses* (Figs 5.34 and 5.35), which are formed by layers of dura mater lined with endothelium. The dura mater is the outer protective covering of the brain (p. 152). The main venous sinuses are listed below:

- The *superior sagittal sinus* carries the venous blood from the superior part of the brain. It begins in the

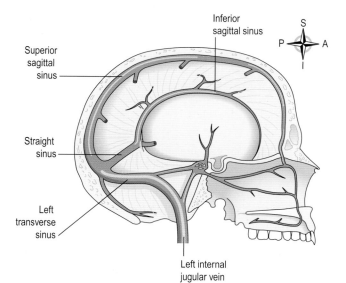

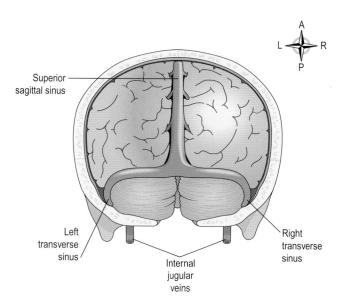

Figure 5.34 Venous sinuses of the brain viewed from the right.

Figure 5.35 Venous sinuses of the brain viewed from above.

frontal region and passes directly backwards in the midline of the skull to the occipital region where it turns to the right side and continues as the *right transverse sinus*.

- The *inferior sagittal sinus* lies deep within the brain and passes backwards to form the *straight sinus*.
- The *straight sinus* runs backwards and downwards to become the *left transverse sinus*.
- The *transverse sinuses* begin in the occipital region. They run forward and medially in a curved groove of the skull, to become continuous with the *sigmoid sinuses*.
- The *sigmoid sinuses* are a continuation of the transverse sinuses. Each curves downwards and medially and lies in a groove in the mastoid process of the temporal bone. Anteriorly only a thin plate of bone separates the sinus from the air cells in the mastoid process of the temporal bone. Inferiorly it continues as the internal jugular vein.

The *internal jugular veins* begin at the jugular foramina in the middle cranial fossa and each is the continuation of a sigmoid sinus. They run downwards in the neck behind the sternocleidomastoid muscles. Behind the clavicle they unite with the *subclavian veins*, carrying blood from the upper limbs, to form the *brachiocephalic veins*.

The brachiocephalic veins are situated one on each side in the root of the neck. Each is formed by the union of the internal jugular and the subclavian veins. The left brachiocephalic vein is longer than the right and passes obliquely behind the manubrium of the sternum, where it joins the right brachiocephalic vein to form the superior vena cava (Fig. 5.29).

The *superior vena cava*, which drains all the venous blood from the head, neck and upper limbs, is about 7 cm long. It passes downwards along the right border of the sternum and ends in the right atrium of the heart.

Circulation in the upper limb

Arterial supply

The subclavian arteries. The right subclavian artery arises from the brachiocephalic artery; the left branches from the arch of the aorta. They are slightly arched and pass behind the clavicles and over the first ribs before entering the axillae, where they continue as the *axillary arteries* (Fig. 5.36).

Before entering the axilla, each subclavian artery gives off two branches: the *vertebral artery*, which passes upwards to supply the brain (Fig. 5.32), and the *internal thoracic artery*, which supplies the breast and a number of structures in the thoracic cavity.

The *axillary artery* is a continuation of the subclavian artery and lies in the axilla. The first part lies deeply; then it runs more superficially to become the *brachial artery*.

The *brachial artery* is a continuation of the axillary artery. It runs down the medial aspect of the upper arm,

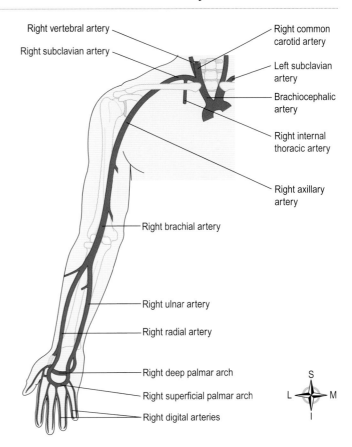

Figure 5.36 The main arteries of the right arm.

passes to the front of the elbow and extends to about 1 cm below the joint, where it divides into the *radial* and *ulnar arteries*.

The *radial artery* passes down the radial or lateral side of the forearm to the wrist. Just above the wrist it lies superficially and can be felt in front of the radius, as the radial pulse. The artery then passes between the first and second metacarpal bones and enters the palm of the hand.

The *ulnar artery* runs downwards on the ulnar or medial aspect of the forearm to cross the wrist and pass into the hand.

There are anastomoses between the radial and ulnar arteries, called the *deep* and *superficial palmar arches*, from which *palmar metacarpal* and *palmar digital arteries* arise to supply the structures in the hand and fingers.

Venous return

The upper limb is drained by both deep and superficial veins (Fig. 5.37). The deep veins follow the course of the arteries and have the same names:

- palmar metacarpal veins
- deep palmar venous arch
- ulnar and radial veins
- brachial vein
- axillary vein
- subclavian vein.

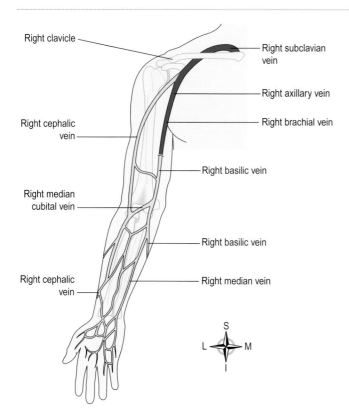

Right clavicle

Right subclavian vein

Right axillary vein

Right brachial vein

Right cephalic vein

Right basilic vein

Right median cubital vein

Right basilic vein

Right median vein

Right cephalic vein

S
L — M
I

Figure 5.37 The main veins of the right arm. Dark blue indicates deep veins.

The superficial veins begin in the hand and consist of the following:

- cephalic vein
- basilic vein
- median vein
- median cubital vein.

The *cephalic vein* begins at the back of the hand where it collects blood from a complex of superficial veins, many of which can be easily seen. It then winds round the radial side to the anterior aspect of the forearm. In front of the elbow it gives off a large branch, the *median cubital vein*, which slants upwards and medially to join the *basilic vein*. After crossing the elbow joint the cephalic vein passes up the lateral aspect of the arm and in front of the shoulder joint to end in the axillary vein. Throughout its length it receives blood from the superficial tissues on the lateral aspects of the hand, forearm and arm.

The *basilic vein* begins at the back of the hand on the ulnar aspect. It ascends on the medial side of the forearm and upper arm then joins the axillary vein. It receives blood from the medial aspect of the hand, forearm and arm. There are many small veins which link the cephalic and basilic veins.

The *median vein* is a small vein that is not always present. It begins at the palmar surface of the hand, ascends on the front of the forearm and ends in the basilic vein or the median cubital vein.

The brachiocephalic vein is formed when the subclavian and internal jugular veins unite. There is one on each side.

The *superior vena cava* is formed when the two brachiocephalic veins unite. It drains all the venous blood from the head, neck and upper limbs and terminates in the right atrium. It is about 7 cm long and passes downwards along the right border of the sternum.

Circulation in the thorax

Arterial supply
Branches of the thoracic aorta (Fig. 5.28) supply structures in the chest, including:

- *bronchial arteries*, which supply lung tissues not directly involved in gas exchange
- *oesophageal arteries*, which supply the oesophagus
- *intercostal arteries*, which run along the inferior border of each rib and supply the intercostal muscles, some muscles of the thorax, the ribs, skin and its underlying connective tissues.

Venous return
Most of the venous blood from the organs in the thoracic cavity is drained into the *azygos vein* and the *hemiazygos* vein (Fig. 5.29). Some of the main veins that join them are the *bronchial, oesophageal* and *intercostal veins*. The azygos vein joins the superior vena cava and the hemiazygos vein joins the left brachiocephalic vein. At the distal end of the oesophagus, some oesophageal veins join the azygos vein, and others the left gastric vein. A venous plexus is formed by anastomoses between the veins joining the azygos vein and those joining the left gastric veins, linking the general and portal circulations (see Fig. 12.46, p. 322).

Circulation in the abdomen

Arterial supply
Branches of the abdominal aorta (Fig. 5.28) supply structures in the abdomen.

Paired branches. These include:

- *phrenic arteries*, supplying the diaphragm
- *renal arteries*, which supply the kidneys
- *suprarenal arteries*, supplying the adrenal glands
- *gonadal arteries*, supplying the ovaries (female) and testes (male). These arteries are much longer than the other paired branches, because the gonads begin their development high in the abdominal cavity. As fetal development proceeds, they descend into the pelvis and their supplying arteries become correspondingly longer to maintain supply.

Unpaired branches. These include the:

- *coeliac artery* (sometimes called the *coeliac trunk*, Fig. 5.38), a short thick artery about 1.25 cm long.

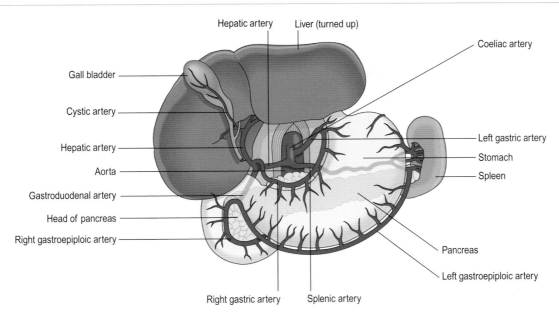

Hepatic artery

Liver (turned up)

Coeliac artery

Gall bladder

Cystic artery

Hepatic artery

Aorta

Gastroduodenal artery

Head of pancreas

Right gastroepiploic artery

Left gastric artery

Stomach

Spleen

Pancreas

Left gastroepiploic artery

Right gastric artery

Splenic artery

Figure 5.38 The coeliac artery and its branches, and the inferior phrenic arteries.

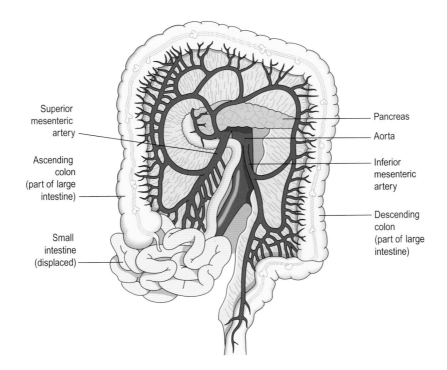

Superior
mesenteric
artery

Ascending
colon
(part of large
intestine)

Small
intestine
(displaced)

Pancreas

Aorta

Inferior
mesenteric
artery

Descending
colon
(part of large
intestine)

Figure 5.39 The superior and inferior mesenteric arteries and their branches.

It arises immediately below the diaphragm and divides into three branches:

- the *left gastric artery* supplying the stomach
- the *splenic artery* supplying the spleen and pancreas
- the *hepatic artery* supplying the liver, gall bladder and parts of the stomach, duodenum and pancreas

- *superior mesenteric artery* (Fig. 5.39), which branches from the aorta between the coeliac artery and the renal arteries. It supplies the entire small intestine and about half the proximal large intestine
- *inferior mesenteric artery* (Fig. 5.39), which arises from the aorta about 4 cm above its division into the common iliac arteries. It supplies the distal half of the large intestine and part of the rectum.

Venous return

Blood drains from some abdominal organs directly into the inferior vena cava via veins named as the corresponding arteries (Fig. 5.29). *Hepatic* veins drain the liver, *renal veins* drain the kidneys, *suprarenal veins* drain the adrenal glands, *lumbar veins* drain lower abdominal structures and *gonadal veins* drain the ovaries (female) and testes (male). However, most blood from the digestive organs in the abdomen is drained into the *hepatic portal vein* and passes through the liver before being emptied into the inferior vena cava (the *portal circulation*, see below).

Portal circulation ▓ 5.11

As a general rule, venous blood passes from the tissues to the heart by the most direct route through only one capillary bed. In the portal circulation, venous blood from the capillary beds of the abdominal part of the digestive system, the spleen and pancreas travels first to the liver. In the liver, it passes through a second capillary bed, the hepatic sinusoids, before entering the general circulation via the inferior vena cava. In this way, blood with a high concentration of nutrients, absorbed from the stomach and intestines, goes to the liver first. This supplies the liver with a rich source of nutrients for its extensive metabolic activities and ensures that the composition of blood leaving the alimentary tract can be appropriately regulated. It also ensures that unwanted and/or potentially toxic materials such as drugs are eliminated before the blood is returned into general circulation.

Portal vein. This is formed by the union of several veins (Figs 5.40 and 5.41), each of which drains blood from the area supplied by the corresponding artery:

- the *splenic vein* drains blood from the spleen, the pancreas and part of the stomach
- the *inferior mesenteric vein* returns the venous blood from the rectum, pelvic and descending colon of the large intestine. It joins the splenic vein
- the *superior mesenteric vein* returns venous blood from the small intestine and the proximal parts of the large intestine, i.e. the caecum, ascending and transverse colon. It unites with the splenic vein to form the portal vein
- the *gastric veins* drain blood from the stomach and the distal end of the oesophagus, then join the portal vein
- the *cystic vein,* which drains venous blood from the gall bladder, joins the portal vein.

After blood has passed through the hepatic portal circulation, it is then returned directly to the inferior vena cava through the hepatic veins.

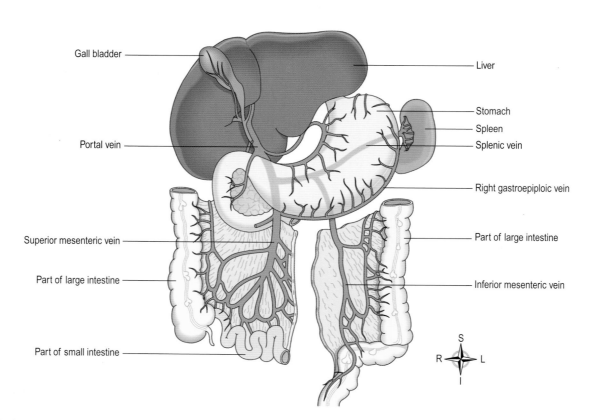

Gall bladder — Liver — Stomach — Spleen — Splenic vein — Right gastroepiploic vein — Portal vein — Superior mesenteric vein — Part of large intestine — Inferior mesenteric vein — Part of large intestine — Part of small intestine

Figure 5.40 Venous drainage from the abdominal organs, and the formation of the portal vein.

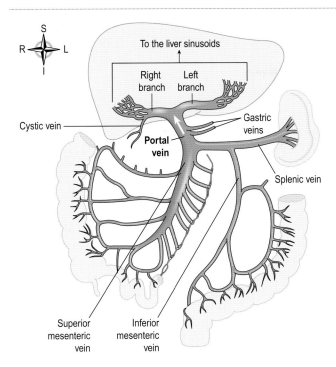

Figure 5.41 The portal vein: origin and termination.

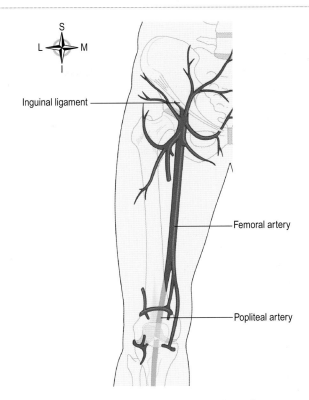

Figure 5.42 The femoral artery and its main branches.

Circulation in the pelvis and lower limb

Arterial supply

Common iliac arteries. The right and left common iliac arteries are formed when the abdominal aorta divides at the level of the 4th lumbar vertebra (Fig. 5.26). In front of the sacroiliac joint each divides into the internal and the external iliac arteries.

The *internal iliac artery* runs medially to supply the organs within the pelvic cavity. In the female, one of the largest branches is the uterine artery, which provides the main arterial blood supply to the reproductive organs.

The external iliac artery runs obliquely downwards and passes behind the inguinal ligament into the thigh where it becomes the femoral artery.

The *femoral artery* (Fig. 5.42) begins at the midpoint of the inguinal ligament and extends downwards in front of the thigh. The femoral pulse can be felt at the origin of the femoral artery. It then turns medially and eventually passes round the medial aspect of the femur to enter the popliteal space where it becomes the popliteal artery. It supplies blood to the structures of the thigh and some superficial pelvic and inguinal structures.

The *popliteal artery* (Fig. 5.43) passes through the popliteal fossa behind the knee, where the popliteal pulse can be felt. It supplies the structures in this area, including the knee joint. At the lower border of the popliteal fossa it divides into the anterior and posterior tibial arteries.

The *anterior tibial artery* (Fig. 5.43) passes forwards between the tibia and fibula and supplies the structures in the front of the leg. It lies on the tibia, runs in front of the ankle joint and continues over the dorsum (top) of the foot as the *dorsalis pedis artery.*

The *dorsalis pedis artery* is a continuation of the anterior tibial artery and passes over the dorsum of the foot, where the pulse can be felt, supplying arterial blood to the structures in this area. It ends by passing between the first and second metatarsal bones into the sole of the foot where it contributes to the formation of the plantar arch.

The *posterior tibial artery* (Fig. 5.43) runs downwards and medially on the back of the leg. Near its origin it gives off a large branch called the *peroneal artery*, which supplies the lateral aspect of the leg. In the lower part it becomes superficial and passes medial to the ankle joint to reach the sole of the foot, where it continues as the *plantar artery.*

The *plantar artery* supplies the structures in the sole of the foot. This artery, its branches and the dorsalis pedis artery form the *plantar arch* from which the digital branches arise to supply the toes.

Venous return

There are both deep and superficial veins in the lower limb (Fig. 5.27). Blood entering the superficial veins passes to the deep veins through *communicating veins.* Movement of blood towards the heart is partly dependent on contraction of skeletal muscles. Backward flow is prevented by a large number of valves. Superficial veins receive less support from surrounding tissues than deep veins.

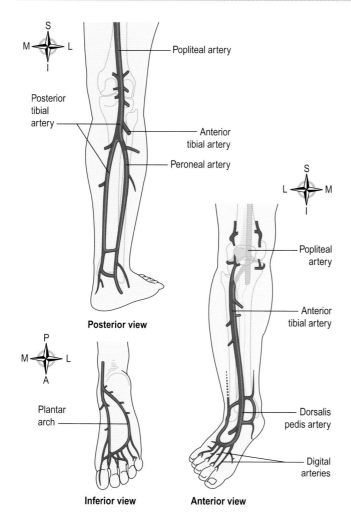

Figure 5.43 The right popliteal artery and its main branches.

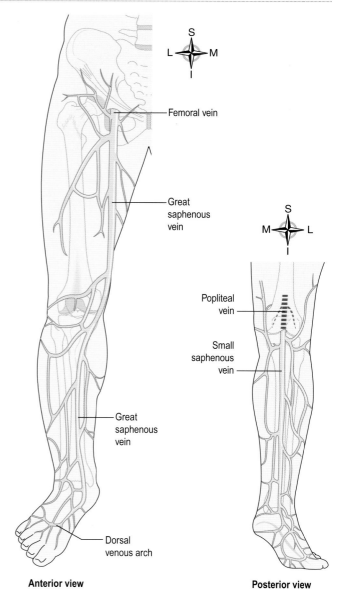

Figure 5.44 Superficial veins of the leg.

Deep veins. The deep veins accompany the arteries and their branches and have the same names. They are the:

- *femoral vein*, which ascends in the thigh to the level of the inguinal ligament, where it becomes the external iliac vein
- *external iliac vein*, the continuation of the femoral vein where it enters the pelvis lying close to the femoral artery. It passes along the brim of the pelvis, and at the level of the sacroiliac joint it is joined by the *internal iliac vein* to form the *common iliac vein*
- *internal iliac vein*, which receives tributaries from several veins draining the organs of the pelvic cavity
- *two common iliac veins*, which begin at the level of the sacroiliac joints. They ascend obliquely and end a little to the right of the body of the 5th lumbar vertebra by uniting to form the *inferior vena cava*.

Superficial veins (Fig. 5.44). The two main superficial veins draining blood from the lower limbs are the small and the great saphenous veins.

The *small saphenous vein* begins behind the ankle joint where many small veins which drain the dorsum of the foot join together. It ascends superficially along the back of the leg and in the popliteal space it joins the *popliteal vein* – a deep vein.

The *great saphenous vein* is the longest vein in the body. It begins at the medial half of the dorsum of the foot and runs upwards, crossing the medial aspect of the tibia and up the inner side of the thigh. Just below the inguinal ligament it joins the *femoral vein*.

Many communicating veins join the superficial veins, and the superficial and deep veins of the lower limb.

Summary of the main blood vessels (Fig. 5.45)

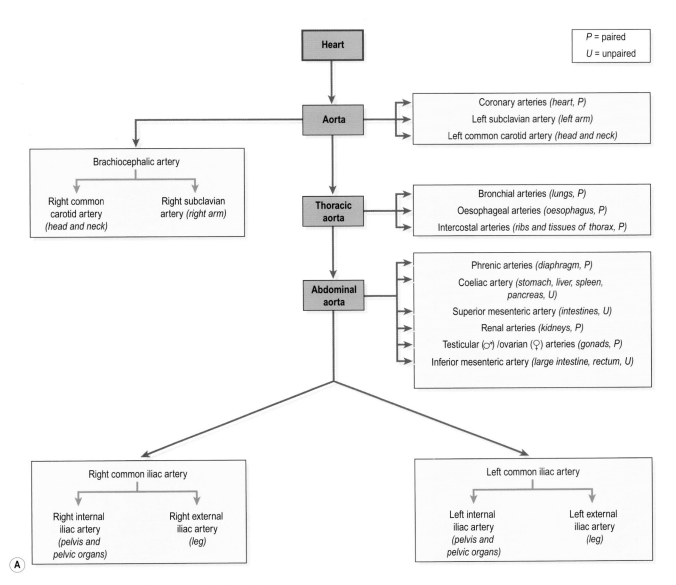

Figure 5.45 A. The aorta and main arteries of the body.

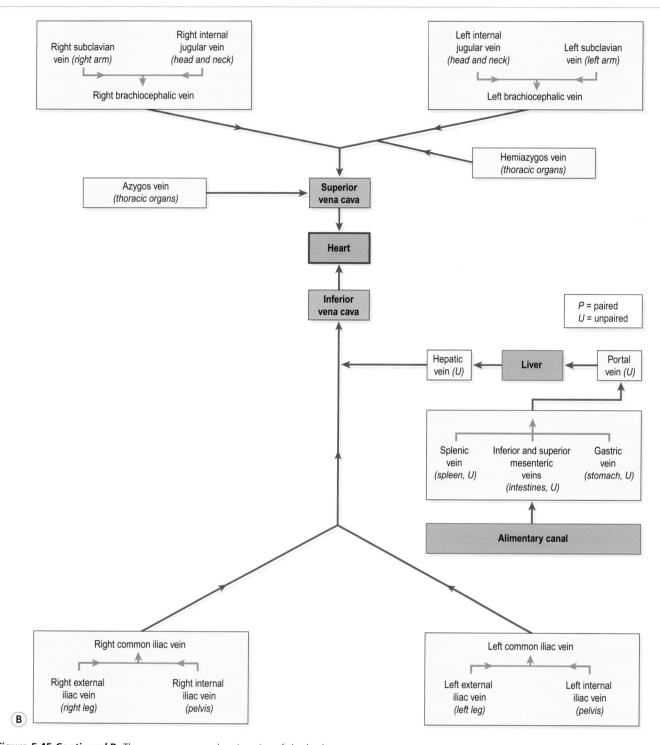

Figure 5.45 Continued B. The venae cavae and main veins of the body.

Fetal circulation

Features of the fetal circulation 5.12

The developing fetus obtains its oxygen and nutrients, and excretes its waste, via the mother's circulation. To this end, both maternal and fetal circulations develop specific adaptations unique to pregnancy. Because the lungs, gastrointestinal system and kidneys do not begin to function till after birth, certain modifications in the fetal circulation divert blood flow to meet pre-natal requirements.

Placenta

This is a temporary structure that provides an interface between the mother and fetus, and allows exchange of substances between their circulatory systems. It develops from the surface of the fertilized ovum embedded into the maternal uterine endometrium (Fig. 5.46). It is expelled from the uterus during the final stage of labour soon after birth, when it is no longer needed.

Structure

The mature placenta (Fig. 5.46A) is pancake-shaped, weighs around 500 g, has a diameter of 20 cm and is about 2.5 cm thick, although wide individual variations occur. The placenta is firmly attached to the uterine wall and consists of an extensive network of fetal capillaries bathed in maternal blood. Whilst the fetal capillaries are in very close proximity to the maternal blood supply, the two circulations are completely separate. The placenta is attached to the fetus by a cord (the *umbilical cord*), which is usually about 50 cm long and contains two *umbilical arteries* and one *umbilical vein* wrapped in a soft connective tissue coat (Fig. 5.46B). The cord enters the fetus at a spot on the abdomen called the *umbilicus*.

Functions

Placental functions include exchange of substances, protection of the fetus and maintenance of pregnancy.

Exchange of nutrients and wastes. Deoxygenated blood flows from the fetus into the placenta through the umbilical arteries, and travels through the network of fetal capillaries in the placenta. Because these capillaries are

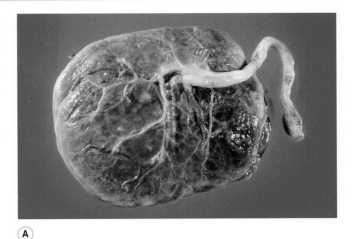

(A)

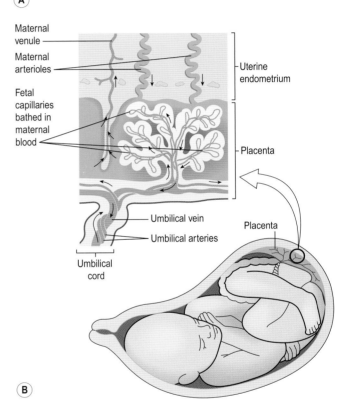

(B)

Figure 5.46 The placenta. A. The mature placenta. **B.** The relationship between the uterine wall and the placenta.

bathed in maternal blood, exchange of nutrients and gases takes place here and the blood that returns to the fetus in the umbilical vein has collected oxygen and nutrients and lost excess carbon dioxide and other wastes (Fig. 5.46).

Protection of the fetus. Temporary passive immunity (p. 383) lasting for a few months is provided by *maternal antibodies* that cross the placenta before birth.

Indirect exchange between the fetal and maternal circulations provides a 'barrier' to potentially harmful substances, including bacteria and drugs, although some may cross into the fetus, causing abnormal development.

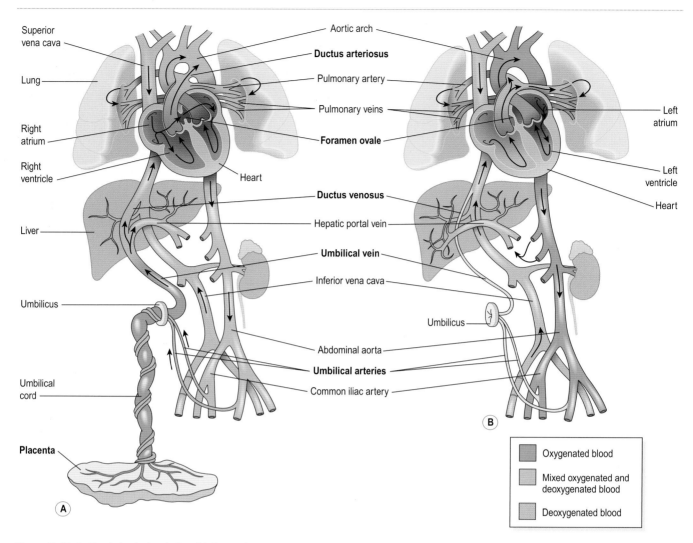

Figure 5.47 A. Fetal circulation before birth. **B.** Changes to the fetal circulation at birth.

Any substance causing abnormal fetal development is called a *teratogen*. Important teratogens include alcohol, certain drugs including some antibiotics and anticancer agents, ionising radiation and some infections, including the rubella (German measles) virus, cytomegalovirus and syphilis.

Maintenance of pregnancy. The placenta has an essential endocrine function and secretes the hormones that maintain pregnancy.

Human chorionic gonadotrophin (hCG). This hormone is secreted in early pregnancy, peaking at around 8 or 9 weeks and thereafter in smaller amounts. hCG stimulates the *corpus luteum* (Ch. 18) to continue secreting progesterone and oestrogen which prevent menstruation and maintain the uterine endometrium, sustaining pregnancy in the early weeks (see Fig. 18.10, p. 457).

Progesterone and oestrogen. As pregnancy progresses, the placenta takes over secretion of these

hormones from the corpus luteum, which degenerates after about 12 weeks. From 12 weeks until delivery, the placenta secretes increasing levels of oestrogen and progesterone. These hormones are essential for maintenance of pregnancy.

Fetal adaptations (Fig. 5.47A)

Ductus venosus. This is a continuation of the umbilical vein that returns blood directly into the fetal inferior vena cava, and most blood, therefore, bypasses the non-functional fetal liver.

Ductus arteriosus. This small vessel connects the pulmonary artery to the descending thoracic aorta and diverts more blood into the systemic circulation, meaning that very little blood passes through the fetal lungs (see Fig. 5.59).

Foramen ovale. This forms a valve-like opening (see Fig. 5.60) allowing blood to flow between the right and left atria, so that most blood bypasses the non-functional fetal lungs.

Changes at birth (Fig. 5.47B)

When the baby takes its first breath the lungs inflate for the first time, increasing pulmonary blood flow. Blood returning from the lungs increases the pressure in the left atrium, closing the flap over the foramen ovale and preventing blood flow between the atria. Blood entering the right atrium is therefore diverted into the right ventricle and into the pulmonary circulation through the pulmonary veins. As the pulmonary circulation is established (see Fig. 5.1) blood oxygen levels increase, causing constriction and closure of the ductus arteriosus. If these adaptations do not take place after birth, they become evident as congenital abnormalities (see Figs 5.59 and 5.60). When the placental circulation ceases, soon after birth, the umbilical vein, ductus venosus and umbilical arteries collapse, as they are no longer required.

Ageing and the cardiovascular system

Learning outcome

After studying this section, you should be able to:

■ Describe the effects of ageing on the cardiovascular system.

Ageing and the heart

As the heart gets older, its function generally declines; cardiac output falls and the conduction pathways become less efficient. Cardiac muscle cell numbers steadily reduce with age, but hypertrophy (cell enlargement) generally balances this and the ventricles of the heart in older adults are actually slightly larger than in younger people. The compliance (stretchability) of the heart falls with age, mainly because the fibrous skeleton (p. 88) of the heart stiffens, increasing the heart's workload. The ability of the heart muscle to respond to adrenaline and noradrenaline lessens, and the contractile strength of the heart and cardiac reserve are reduced. The older heart is therefore more prone to heart failure (p. 126).

These changes occur in the healthy ageing heart, and are not consequences of disease. It is notable that age-related decline in cardiovascular function is greatly slowed in individuals who take regular exercise, even in old age.

Ageing and blood vessels

Vasoconstriction and vasodilation responses are less efficient in ageing blood vessels, so regulation of blood flow to the tissues is less well controlled. Arterial and arteriolar walls become stiffer and less compliant, which raises blood pressure and increases the work of the left ventricle. Blood pressure tends to rise with age, even in the absence of any overt cardiovascular disease. The amount of smooth muscle in the walls of most arteries, including those of the heart, kidneys and brain, rises with age, which contributes to their stiffening. This means that the blood supply to most body organs tends to fall, but in healthy old age it does not cause problems because it is matched by a general reduction in metabolic rate.

The baroreceptor reflex (p. 97) becomes less brisk with age, not only because the heart and blood vessels are slower to respond, but also because of neuronal ageing. This may lead to postural hypotension (p. 132).

Shock

After studying this section, you should be able to:

- define the term shock
- describe the main physiological changes that occur during shock
- explain the underlying pathophysiology of the main causes of shock.

Shock (circulatory failure) occurs when the metabolic needs of cells are not being met because of inadequate blood flow. In effect, there is a reduction in circulating blood volume, in blood pressure and in cardiac output. This causes tissue hypoxia, an inadequate supply of nutrients and the accumulation of waste products. A number of different types of shock are described.

Hypovolaemic shock

This occurs when the blood volume is reduced by 15–25%. Cardiac output may fall because of low blood volume and hence low venous return, as a result of different situations:

- severe haemorrhage – whole blood is lost
- extensive burns – serum is lost
- severe vomiting and diarrhoea – water and electrolytes are lost.

Cardiogenic shock

This occurs in acute heart disease when damaged heart muscle cannot maintain an adequate cardiac output, e.g. in myocardial infarction.

Septic shock (bacteraemic, endotoxic)

This is caused by severe infections in which bacterial toxins are released into the circulation. These toxins trigger a massive inflammatory and immune response, and many powerful mediators are released. Because the response is not controlled, it can cause multiple organ damage, depression of myocardial contractility, poor tissue perfusion and tissue death (necrosis). Profound hypotension occurs because the inflammatory mediators cause profound vasodilation.

Neurogenic shock

The causes include sudden acute pain, severe emotional experience, spinal anaesthesia and spinal cord damage. These interfere with normal nervous control of blood vessel diameter, leading to hypotension.

Anaphylactic shock

Anaphylaxis (p. 385) is a severe allergic response that may be triggered in sensitive individuals by substances

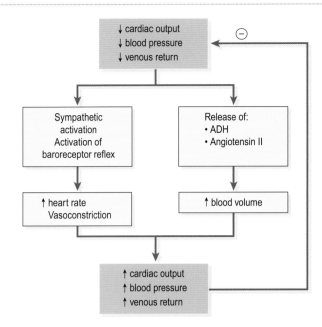

Figure 5.48 Compensatory mechanisms in shock.

like penicillin, peanuts or latex rubber. Vasodilation, provoked by systemic release of inflammatory mediators, e.g. histamine and bradykinin, causes venous pooling and hypotension. Severe bronchoconstriction leads to respiratory difficulty and hypoxia. Onset is usually sudden, and in severe cases can cause death in a matter of minutes if untreated.

Physiological changes during shock

In the short term, changes are associated with physiological attempts to restore an adequate blood circulation – *compensated shock* (Fig. 5.48). If the state of shock persists, the longer-term changes may be irreversible.

Compensated shock

As the blood pressure falls, a number of reflexes are stimulated and hormone secretions increased in an attempt to restore it. These raise blood pressure by increasing peripheral resistance, blood volume and cardiac output (Fig. 5.48).

Increased sympathetic stimulation increases heart rate and cardiac output, and also causes vasoconstriction, all of which increase blood pressure. Low blood volume and increased osmolarity of the blood cause secretion of ADH (p. 221) and activation of the renin–angiotensin–aldosterone system (p. 225). Consequent release of aldosterone reduces water and sodium excretion and promotes vasoconstriction. The veins also constrict, helping to reduce venous pooling and support venous return.

If these compensatory mechanisms, plus any medical interventions available, are sufficient then perfusion of the heart and brain can be maintained and the patient's condition may be stabilised.

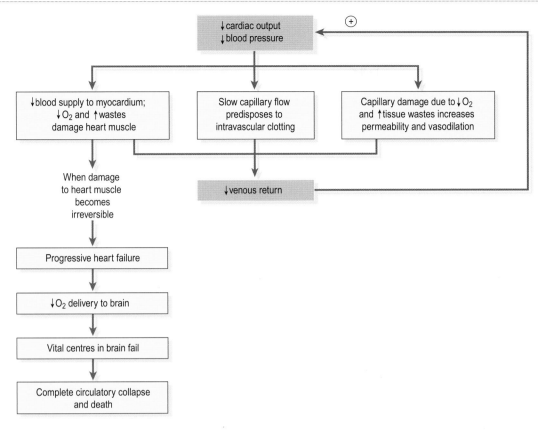

Figure 5.49 Uncompensated shock.

Uncompensated shock

If the insult is more severe, shock becomes a self-perpetuating sequence of deteriorating cardiovascular function – *uncompensated shock* (Fig. 5.49). Hypoxia causes cellular metabolism to switch to anaerobic pathways (p. 316), resulting in accumulation of lactic acid and progressive acidosis, which damages capillaries. The capillaries then become more permeable, leaking fluid from the vascular system into the tissues, further lowering blood pressure and tissue perfusion. Also, the accumulation of waste products causes vasodilation, making it harder for control mechanisms to support blood pressure. Organs, including the heart, are deprived of oxygen and may start to fail.

Eventually, the cardiovascular system reaches the stage when, although its compensatory mechanisms are running at maximum, it is unable to supply the brain's requirements. As the brain, including the cardiovascular and respiratory centres in the brain stem, becomes starved of oxygen and nutrients, it begins to fail and there is loss of central control of the body's compensatory mechanisms. Circulatory collapse follows. Finally, degenerating cardiovascular function leads to irreversible and progressive brain-stem damage, and death follows.

Thrombosis and embolism

Learning outcomes

After studying this section, you should be able to:

■ define the terms thrombosis, embolism and infarction

■ explain, in general terms, the effects of the above on the body

■ describe three risk factors for thrombosis formation.

Thrombosis

Thrombosis is the formation of a blood clot (thrombus) inside a blood vessel, interrupting blood supply to the tissues. The risk of a thrombus developing within a blood vessel is increased by:

Slow blood flow. This may happen in immobility, e.g. prolonged sitting or in bedrest, or if a blood vessel is compressed by an adjacent structure such as a tumour or tight clothing, or if there is a sustained fall in blood pressure, as in shock.

Box 5.3 Possible embolic materials

- Fragments of atheromatous plaques (p. 121)
- Fragments of vegetations from heart valves, e.g. in infective endocarditis (p. 128)
- Tumour fragments, which may cause metastases
- Amniotic fluid, during childbirth
- Fat, from bone fractures
- Air, from a punctured blood vessel, e.g. by a broken rib or during a clinical procedure
- Nitrogen bubbles in decompression sickness (the 'bends')
- Pus from an abscess

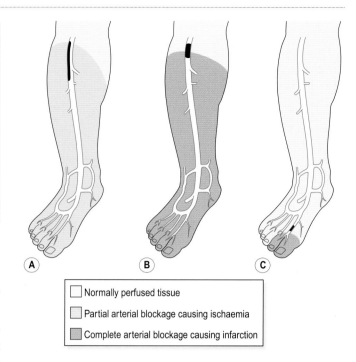

☐ Normally perfused tissue

☐ Partial arterial blockage causing ischaemia

☐ Complete arterial blockage causing infarction

Figure 5.50 Ischaemia and infarction. A. Partial blockage but normal perfusion. **B, C.** Complete blockage causes distal tissue ischaemia and infarction, dependent on the location of the blockage.

Damage to the blood vessel intima. This is usually associated with atherosclerosis (p. 121).

Increased blood coagulability. Dehydration, pregnancy and childbirth, blood clotting disorders, some malignant disease, the presence of an intravenous cannula and oestrogen (including when used as a contraceptive) all increase the risk of blood clots forming.

Embolism

Embolism is the blocking of a blood vessel by any mass of material (an *embolus*) travelling in the blood. This is usually a thrombus or a fragment of a thrombus, but other embolic materials are shown in Box 5.3.

Emboli originating in an artery travel away from the heart until they reach an artery too narrow to let them pass, and lodge there, partly or completely blocking blood supply to distal tissues. This is a common cause of stroke (p. 181), myocardial infarction (p. 127) and gangrenous limbs (Fig. 5.50). Emboli originating in veins (DVT, p. 123) travel towards the heart, and from there to the lungs in the pulmonary artery. They then lodge in the first branch narrower than they are (pulmonary embolism).

Pulmonary embolism. Where a pulmonary artery or one of its branches is blocked causing an immediate reduction in blood flow through the lung, is one of the most serious consequences of venous embolism. Massive pulmonary embolism blocks a main pulmonary artery and usually causes sudden collapse and death.

Infarction and ischaemia

Infarction is the term given to tissue death because of interrupted blood supply. The consequences of interrupting tissue blood supply depend of the size of the artery blocked and the functions of the tissue affected. *Ischaemia* means tissue damage because of reduced blood supply (Fig. 5.50).

Blood vessel pathology

Learning outcomes

After studying this section, you should be able to:

- discuss the main causes, effects and complications of arterial disease, including atheroma, arteriosclerosis and aneurysm

- discuss the underlying abnormality in varicose veins

- list the predisposing factors and the common sites of occurrence of varicose veins

- describe the main tumours that affect blood vessels.

Atheroma

Pathological changes

Atheromatous plaques are patchy changes that develop in the tunica intima of large and medium-sized arteries. Initial changes show a fatty streak in the artery wall. Mature plaques consist of accumulations of cholesterol and other lipids, excess smooth muscle and fat-filled monocytes (foam cells). The plaque is covered with a rough fibrous cap. As plaques grow and thicken they spread along the artery wall and protrude into the lumen. Eventually the whole thickness of the wall and long

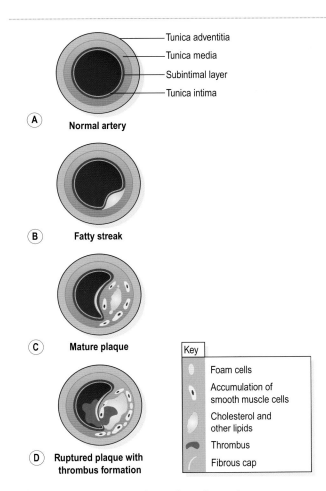

Figure 5.51 Stages in the formation of an atheromatous plaque.

(Labels in figure: Tunica adventitia, Tunica media, Subintimal layer, Tunica intima; A Normal artery; B Fatty streak; C Mature plaque; D Ruptured plaque with thrombus formation)

Box 5.4 Predisposing factors in atherosclerosis

(Modifiable factors are shown in green.)

- Heredity – family history
- Obesity
- Gender – males are more susceptible than females, until after the female menopause
- Diet – high in refined carbohydrates and/or saturated fats and cholesterol
- Increasing age
- Smoking cigarettes
- Diabetes mellitus
- Excessive emotional stress
- Hypertension
- Sedentary lifestyle
- Hyperlipidaemia, especially high levels of LDL (p. 227)
- Excessive alcohol consumption

Effects of atheroma 5.13

Atheromatous plaques may cause partial or complete obstruction of an artery (Fig. 5.50). The blockage may be complicated by clot formation. The consequences of this depend on the site and size of the artery involved and the extent of collateral circulation.

Narrowing of an artery

The tissues distal to the narrow point become ischaemic. The cells may receive enough blood to meet their minimum needs, but not enough to cope with an increase in metabolic rate, e.g. when muscle activity is increased. This causes acute cramp-like ischaemic pain, which disappears when exertion stops. Cardiac muscle and skeletal muscles of the lower limb are most commonly affected. Ischaemic pain in the heart is called *angina pectoris* (p. 127), and in the lower limbs, *intermittent claudication*.

Occlusion of an artery

When an artery is completely blocked, the tissues it supplies rapidly degenerate (ischaemia), which leads to infarction (p. 120). If a major artery supplying a large amount of tissue is affected, the consequences are likely to be more severe than if the obstruction occurs in a minor vessel. If the tissue is well provided with a collateral circulation (such as the circulus arteriosus provides in the brain), tissue damage is less than if there are few collateral vessels (which may be the case in the heart).

When a coronary artery is occluded *myocardial infarction* (p. 127) occurs. Occlusion of arteries in the brain causes cerebral ischaemia and this leads to *cerebral infarction* (stroke, p. 181).

Complications of atheroma

Thrombosis and infarction (p. 120)

If the fibrous cap overlying a plaque breaks down, platelets are activated by the damaged cells and an

sections of the vessel may be affected (Fig. 5.51). Plaques may rupture, exposing subintimal materials to the blood. This may cause thrombosis and vasospasm and will compromise blood flow.

Arteries most commonly involved are those in the heart, brain, kidneys, small intestine and lower limbs.

Causes of atheroma

The origin of atheromatous plaques is uncertain. *Fatty streaks* present in artery walls of infants are usually absorbed but their incomplete absorption may be the origin of atheromatous plaques in later life.

Atherosclerosis (the presence of plaques) is considered to be a disease of older people because it is usually in these age groups that clinical signs appear. Plaques, however, start to form in childhood in developed countries.

The incidence of atheroma is widespread in developed countries. Why atheromatous plaques develop is not clearly understood, but the predisposing factors appear to exert their effects over a long period. This may mean that the development of atheroma can be delayed or even arrested by a change in lifestyle (Box 5.4).

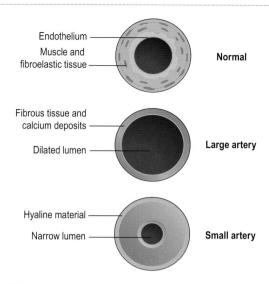

Figure 5.52 Arteriosclerotic arteries.

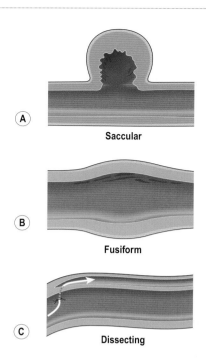

Figure 5.53 Types of aneurysm. A. Saccular. **B.** Fusiform. **C.** Dissecting.

intravascular blood clot forms (thrombosis), blocking the artery and causing ischaemia and infarction. Emboli may break off, travel in the bloodstream and lodge in small arteries distal to the clot, causing small infarcts.

Haemorrhage

Plaques may become calcified, making the artery brittle, rigid and more prone to aneurysm formation, increasing the risk of rupture and haemorrhage.

Aneurysm

When the arterial wall is weakened by spread of the plaque between the layers of tissue, a local dilation (aneurysm) may develop (see below). This may lead to thrombosis and embolism, or the aneurysm may rupture causing severe haemorrhage. The most common sites affected by atheroma are the aorta and the abdominal and pelvic arteries.

Arteriosclerosis

This is a progressive degeneration of arterial walls, associated with ageing and accompanied by hypertension.

In large and medium-sized arteries, the tunica media is infiltrated with fibrous tissue and calcium. This causes the vessels to become dilated, inelastic and tortuous (Fig. 5.52). Loss of elasticity increases systolic blood pressure, and the *pulse pressure* (the difference between systolic and diastolic pressure).

When small arteries (arterioles) are involved, their lumen is narrowed because of a deposition of a substance called *hyaline material*, which reduces the elasticity of the vessel wall. Because arterioles control peripheral resistance (p. 84), this narrowing increases peripheral resistance and blood pressure. Damage to small vessels has a disproportionate effect on blood flow, leading to

ischaemia of tissues supplied by affected arteries. In the limbs, the resultant ischaemia predisposes to gangrene, which is particularly serious in people with diabetes mellitus. If arteries supplying the brain are affected, cerebral ischaemia can result in progressive deterioration of higher order functions (p. 181).

Aneurysms

Aneurysms are abnormal local dilations of arteries, which vary considerably in size (Fig. 5.53). Predisposing factors include atheroma, hypertension and defective formation of collagen in the arterial wall.

If an aneurysm ruptures, haemorrhage follows, the consequences of which depend on the site and extent of the bleed. Rupture of the aorta is likely to be fatal, while bleeding into the subarachnoid space can also cause death, or permanent disability. Bleeding in the brain can cause symptoms of stroke. An aneurysm damages the blood vessel endothelium, making it rougher than usual, which increases the risk of clot formation. Clots may block circulation locally, or elsewhere if they travel in the bloodstream as emboli. In addition, the swelling associated with the distended artery can cause pressure on local structures such as other blood vessels, nerves or organs.

Types of aneurysm

Saccular aneurysms (Fig. 5.53A) bulge out on one side of the artery. When they occur in the relatively thin-walled arteries of the circulus arteriosus (circle of Willis, p. 105)

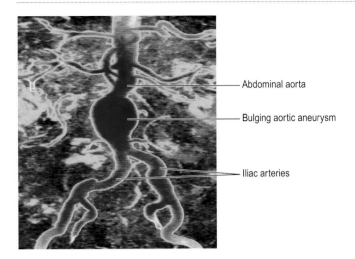

Figure 5.54 Abdominal aortic aneurysm.

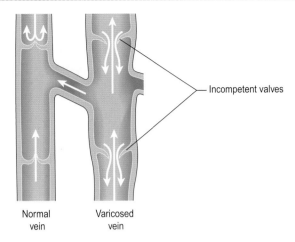

Figure 5.55 Anastomatic connection between superficial and varicosed vein (right) and deeper unaffected vein (left).

in the brain they are sometimes called 'berry' aneurysms. They may be congenital, or be associated with defective collagen production or with atheroma.

Fusiform or spindle-shaped distensions (Fig. 5.53B) occur mainly in the abdominal aorta. They are usually associated with atheroma.

Dissecting aneurysms (Fig. 5.53C) occur mainly in the arch of the aorta. They are caused by infiltration of blood between the endothelium and tunica media, beginning at a site of endothelial damage.

Figure 5.54 shows the bulging abdominal aortic wall caused by an aneurysm.

Venous thrombosis

The risk factors predisposing to a clot developing within a vein are discussed on page 119.

Venous thrombosis may be *superficial thrombophlebitis*, which usually resolves spontaneously, or *deep vein thrombosis*.

Superficial thrombophlebitis

If a thrombus forms in a superficial vein, the tissue around the affected vein becomes inflamed, red and painful. The most common causes are intravenous infusion and varicosities in the saphenous vein.

Deep vein thrombosis (DVT)

DVT usually affects the lower limb, pelvic or iliac veins, but occasionally the upper limb veins. It may be accompanied by local pain and swelling, but is often asymptomatic. Risk factors for DVT include varicose veins, surgery, pregnancy and prolonged immobility, e.g. long journeys with restricted leg room ('economy class syndrome'). It carries a significant risk of death (often from pulmonary embolism (p. 120) if a clot fragment travels to the lungs).

Varicosed veins

Blood pooling in a vein stretches and damages its soft walls and the vein becomes inelastic, dilated and coiled. Generally, superficial veins with little support are involved. The valves then cannot close properly because the vein is distended, and pooling and engorgement get worse. Venous return is maintained because superficial veins are usually connected into the network of deeper veins, which are better supported by surrounding tissues and less likely to become varicosed (Fig. 5.55).

Sites and effects of varicose veins

Varicose veins of the legs

Blood in the veins of the leg is constantly subject to gravity, which can lead to sluggish venous return and accumulation of blood in these veins. If the valves become incompetent, pooling gets worse, and the leg veins become chronically dilated, twisted and lengthened. The superficial veins are more prone to this than deeper ones, because there is less support from surrounding tissues such as muscle, and the varicose veins become clearly visible (Fig. 5.56A). The great and small saphenous veins and the anterior tibial veins are most commonly affected, causing aching and fatigue of the legs, especially during long periods of standing. These dilated, inelastic veins rupture easily if injured, and haemorrhage occurs.

The skin over a varicose vein may become poorly nourished due to stasis of blood, leading to *varicose ulcer*, usually on the medial aspects of the leg just above the ankle.

Risk factors include increasing age, obesity, pregnancy, standing for long periods, wearing constricting clothing, family history and female gender.

Haemorrhoids

Sustained pressure on distended veins at the junction of the rectum and anus leads to increased venous pressure,

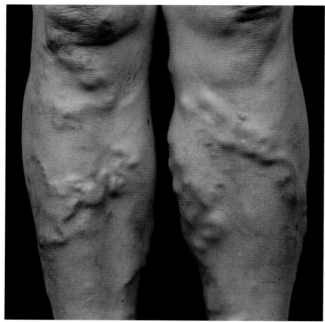

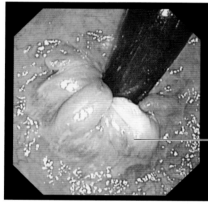

Varicosed rectal veins
(haemorrhoids)

Figure 5.56 Varicosed veins. A. Of the leg. **B.** In the rectum (haemorrhoids).

valvular incompetence and the development of haemorrhoids (piles; Fig. 5.56B). The most common causes are chronic constipation, and the increased pressure in the pelvis towards the end of pregnancy. Slight bleeding may occur each time stools are passed and, in time, may cause anaemia. Severe haemorrhage is rare.

Scrotal varicocele

Each spermatic cord is surrounded by a plexus of veins that may become varicosed, especially in men whose work involves standing for long periods. If the varicocele is bilateral, the increased temperature due to venous congestion may depress spermatogenesis and cause infertility.

Oesophageal varices

Raised pressure in the lower oesophageal veins can rupture them, leading to a potentially fatal haemorrhage (p. 321).

Tumours of blood and lymph vessels

Angiomas

Angiomas are benign tumours of either blood vessels (haemangiomas) or lymph vessels (lymphangiomas). The latter rarely occur, so angioma is usually taken to mean haemangioma.

Haemangiomas. These are not true tumours, but are sufficiently similar to be classified as such. They consist of an excessive growth of blood vessels arranged in an uncharacteristic manner and interspersed with collagen fibres.

Capillary haemangiomas. Excess capillary growth interspersed with collagen in a localised area makes a dense, plexus-like network of tissue. Each haemangioma is supplied by only one blood vessel and if it thromboses, the haemangioma atrophies and disappears.

They are usually present at birth and are seen as a purple or red mole or birthmark. They may be quite small at birth but grow at an alarming rate in the first few months, keeping pace with the growth of the child. After 1–3 years, atrophy may begin, and after 5 years about 80% have disappeared.

Oedema

Learning outcomes

After studying this section, you should be able to:

■ define the term oedema

■ describe the main causes of oedema

■ relate the causes of oedema to relevant clinical problems

■ explain the causes and consequences of excess fluid collecting in body cavities.

In oedema, excess tissue fluid accumulates, causing swelling. It may occur either in superficial tissues or deeper organs.

Sites of oedema

Oedema of the superficial tissues causes *pitting*, i.e. an indentation remains after firm finger pressure has been applied. Oedema develops at different sites depending on body position and gravity. When standing or sitting, the oedema develops in the lower limbs, beginning in the feet and ankles. Patients on bedrest tend to develop oedema in the sacral area. This is called *dependent oedema*.

In *pulmonary oedema*, venous congestion in the lungs or increased pulmonary vessel permeability results in accumulation of fluid in the tissue spaces and in the alveoli. This reduces the area available for gaseous exchange and results in *dyspnoea* (breathlessness), cyanosis and coughing up (expectoration) of frothy sputum. The most common causes of pulmonary oedema are cardiac failure, inflammation or irritation of the lungs and excessive infusion of intravenous fluids.

Causes of oedema

Fluid accumulates in the tissues when some aspect of normal capillary fluid dynamics (Fig. 5.57A and see also p. 85) is deranged.

Increased venous hydrostatic (blood) pressure

Congestion of the venous circulation increases venous hydrostatic pressure, reducing the net effect of osmotic pressure that draws fluid back into the capillary at the venous end. Excess fluid then remains in the tissues. This may be caused by heart failure, kidney disease or compression of a limb due to prolonged sitting or tight clothes.

Decreased plasma osmotic pressure

When plasma protein levels fall, less fluid returns to the circulation at the venous end of the capillary (Fig. 5.57B). Causes include excessive protein loss in kidney disease (p. 351), and reduced plasma protein levels caused by, for example, liver failure or a protein-deficient diet.

Impaired lymphatic drainage

Some fluid returns to the circulation via the lymphatic system and when flow is impaired, oedema develops (Fig. 5.57C). Causes include malignancy that blocks lymph drainage, surgical removal of lymph nodes or lymph node destruction by chronic inflammation.

Increased small-vessel permeability

In inflammation (p. 377), chemical mediators increase small vessel permeability in the affected area. Plasma proteins then leave the circulation (Fig. 5.57D) and the resultant increased tissue osmotic pressure draws fluid into the area causing swelling of the affected tissue. This type of oedema also occurs in allergic reactions (p. 385), e.g. anaphylaxis, asthma or hay fever.

Effusions and ascites

Abnormal accumulation of excess fluid in body spaces, e.g. the pericardial sac or a joint space, is often associated with inflammatory, infective or obstructive conditions and is generally referred to as an *effusion*.

Pleural effusion. This is excess serous fluid in the pleural cavity. This is usually due to infection or inflammation of

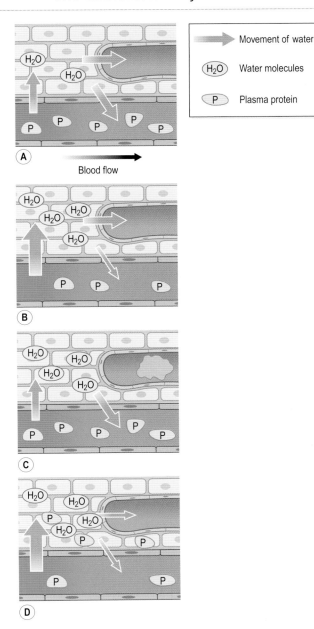

Figure 5.57 Capillary fluid dynamics. A. Normal. **B.** Effect of reduced plasma proteins. **C.** Effect of impaired lymphatic drainage. **D.** Effect of increased capillary permeability. Arrows indicate direction of movement of water.

the pleura (p. 250), or to left ventricular failure, which increases pressure in the pulmonary circulation because the left ventricle is not able to pump out all the blood returning to it from the lungs.

Ascites. This is accumulation of excess fluid in the peritoneal cavity. The most common causes include liver failure (when plasma protein synthesis is reduced), obstruction of abdominal lymph nodes draining the peritoneal cavity, or inflammatory conditions. This includes malignant disease, because many tumours release pro-inflammatory mediators.

Diseases of the heart

Learning outcomes

After studying this section, you should be able to:

■ describe the consequences of failure of either or both sides of the heart

■ the compensatory mechanisms that occur in heart failure

■ explain the causes and consequences of faulty heart valve function

■ define the term ischaemic heart disease

■ discuss the main conditions associated with ischaemic heart disease

■ describe rheumatic heart disease and its effects on cardiac function

■ explain the underlying pathophysiology of pericarditis

■ describe, with reference to standard ECG trace, the main cardiac arrhythmias

■ describe the principal congenital cardiac abnormalities.

Heart (cardiac) failure

The heart is described as *failing* when the cardiac output is unable to circulate sufficient blood to meet the needs of the body. In mild cases, cardiac output is adequate at rest and becomes inadequate only when tissue needs are increased, e.g. in exercise. Heart failure may affect either side of the heart, but since both sides of the heart are part of one circuit, when one half of the pump begins to fail it frequently leads to increased strain on, and eventual failure of, the other side. The main clinical manifestations depend on which side of the heart is most affected. Left ventricular failure is more common than right, because of the greater workload of the left ventricle.

Compensatory mechanisms in heart failure

In acute heart failure, the body has little time to make compensatory changes, but if the heart fails over a period of time the following changes are likely to occur in an attempt to maintain cardiac output and tissue perfusion, especially of vital organs:

● the cardiac muscle mass increases (hypertrophy), which makes the walls of the chambers thicker
● the heart chambers enlarge
● decreased renal blood flow activates the renin–angiotensin–aldosterone system (p. 225), which leads to salt and water retention. This increases

blood volume and cardiac workload. The direct vasoconstrictor action of angiotensin 2 increases peripheral resistance and puts further strain on the failing heart.

Acute heart failure

If heart failure occurs abruptly, the supply of oxygenated blood to body tissues is suddenly and catastrophically reduced and there is no time for significant compensation to take place. Death may follow if the brain's vital centres are starved of oxygen. Even if the acute phase is survived, myocardial damage may lead to chronic heart failure. Common causes include:

● myocardial infarction (p. 127)
● pulmonary embolism, blocking blood flow through the pulmonary circulation – the heart fails if it cannot pump hard enough to overcome the obstruction
● life-threatening cardiac arrhythmia, when the pumping action of the heart is badly impaired or stopped
● rupture of a heart chamber or valve cusp; both greatly increase the cardiac effort required to maintain adequate output
● severe malignant hypertension, which greatly increases resistance to blood flow.

Chronic heart failure

This develops gradually and in the early stages there may be no symptoms because compensatory changes occur as described above. When further compensation is not possible, myocardial function gradually declines. Underlying causes include degenerative heart changes with advancing age, and many chronic conditions, e.g. anaemia, lung disease, hypertension or cardiac disease.

Right-sided (congestive cardiac) failure

The right ventricle fails when the pressure developed within it by the contracting myocardium is insufficient to push blood through the lungs.

When compensation has reached its limit, and the ventricle can no longer empty completely, the right atrium and venae cavae become congested with blood and this is followed by congestion throughout the venous system. The organs affected first are the liver, spleen and kidneys. *Oedema* (p. 124) of the limbs and *ascites* (excess fluid in the peritoneal cavity) usually follow.

This problem may be caused by increased vascular resistance in the lungs or weakness of the myocardium.

Resistance to blood flow through the lungs. When this is increased the right ventricle has more work to do. The two commonest causes are pulmonary embolism and left ventricular failure, when the pulmonary circulation is congested because the left ventricle is not clearing all the blood flowing into it.

Weakness of the myocardium. This is caused by myocardial damage following ischaemia or infarction.

Left-sided (left ventricular) failure

This occurs when the pressure developed in the left ventricle by the contracting myocardium is not enough to force blood into the aorta and the ventricle cannot then pump out all the blood it receives. Causes include ischaemic heart disease, which reduces the efficiency of the myocardium, and hypertension, when the heart's workload is increased because of raised systemic resistance. Disease of the mitral (left atrioventricular) and/or aortic valves may prevent efficient emptying of the heart chambers, so that myocardial workload is increased.

Failure of the left ventricle leads to dilation of the atrium and an increase in pulmonary blood pressure. This is followed by a rise in the blood pressure in the right side of the heart and eventually systemic venous congestion.

Exercise tolerance becomes progressively reduced as the condition worsens and is accompanied by cough caused by pulmonary oedema. The sufferer is easily tired and is likely to have poorly perfused peripheral tissues and low blood pressure.

Congestion in the lungs leads to pulmonary oedema and dyspnoea, often most severe at night. This paroxysmal *nocturnal dyspnoea* may be due to raised blood volume as fluid from peripheral oedema is reabsorbed when the patient slips down in bed during sleep.

Disorders of heart valves ▨ 5.14

The heart valves prevent backflow of blood in the heart during the cardiac cycle. The mitral and aortic valves are subject to greater pressures than those on the right side and are therefore more susceptible to damage.

Distinctive heart sounds arise when the valves close during the cardiac cycle (p. 93). Damaged valves generate abnormal heart sounds called *murmurs*. A severe valve disorder causes heart failure. The most common causes of valve defects are rheumatic fever, fibrosis following inflammation and congenital abnormalities.

Stenosis

This is the narrowing of a valve opening, impeding blood flow through the valve. It occurs when inflammation and encrustations roughen the edges of the cusps so that they stick together, narrowing the valve opening. When healing occurs, fibrous tissue is formed which shrinks as it ages, increasing the stenosis and leading to incompetence.

Incompetence

Sometimes called *regurgitation*, this is a functional defect caused by failure of a valve to close completely, allowing blood to flow backwards.

Ischaemic heart disease

This is due to ischaemia, usually caused by atheromatous plaques narrowing or occluding of one or more branches of the coronary arteries. Occlusion may be by plaques alone, or plaques complicated by thrombosis. The overall effect depends on the size of the coronary artery involved and whether it is only narrowed or completely blocked. Narrowing of an artery leads to angina pectoris, and occlusion to myocardial infarction.

When atheroma develops slowly, a *collateral arterial blood supply* may have time to develop and effectively supplement or replace the original. This consists of the dilation of normally occurring anastomotic arteries joining adjacent arteries. When sudden severe narrowing or occlusion of an artery occurs, the anastomotic arteries dilate but may not be able to supply enough blood to meet myocardial needs.

Angina pectoris

This is sometimes called *angina of effort* because the increased cardiac output required during extra physical effort causes severe chest pain, which may also radiate to the arms, neck and jaw. Other precipitating factors for angina include cold weather and emotional states.

A narrowed coronary artery may supply sufficient blood to the myocardium to meet its needs during rest or moderate exercise but not when greatly increased cardiac output is needed, e.g. walking may be tolerated but not running. The thick, inflexible atheromatous artery wall is unable to dilate to allow for the increased blood flow needed by the more active myocardium, which then becomes ischaemic. In the early stages of angina, the chest pain stops when the cardiac output returns to its resting level soon after the extra effort stops.

Myocardial infarction

The myocardium may infarct (p. 120) when a branch of a coronary artery is blocked. The commonest cause is an atheromatous plaque complicated by thrombosis. The damage is permanent because cardiac muscle cannot regenerate, and the dead muscle is replaced with non-functional fibrous tissue. Speedy restoration of blood flow through the blocked artery using clot-dissolving (thrombolytic) drugs can greatly reduce the extent of the permanent damage and improve prognosis, but treatment must be started within a few hours of the infarction occurring. The effects and complications are greatest when the left ventricle is involved.

Myocardial infarction is usually accompanied by very severe crushing chest pain behind the sternum which, unlike angina pectoris, continues even when the individual is at rest. It is a significant cause of death in the developed world.

Complications

These may be fatal and include:

- severe and sometimes life-threatening arrhythmias, especially *ventricular fibrillation* (p. 129), due to disruption of the cardiac conducting system
- acute heart failure (p. 126), caused by impaired contraction of the damaged myocardium and, in severe cases, cardiogenic shock
- rupture of a ventricle wall, usually within 2 weeks of the original episode
- pulmonary or cerebral embolism originating from a mural clot within a ventricle, i.e. a clot that forms inside the heart over the infarct
- pericarditis
- angina pectoris (p. 127)
- recurrence.

Rheumatic heart disease

Rheumatic fever is an inflammatory illness that sometimes follows streptococcal throat infections, most commonly in children and young adults. It is an autoimmune disorder; the antibodies produced to combat the original infection damage connective tissues, including the heart, joints (p. 432) and skin.

Death rarely occurs in the acute phase, but after recovery there may be permanent damage to the heart valves, eventually leading to disability and possibly cardiac failure.

Acute rheumatic heart disease. In the acute stages, all layers of the heart wall are inflamed (*pancarditis*, 'pan-' meaning 'all of'). The heart valves, especially the mitral valve, are frequently affected. Fibrotic nodules develop on their cusps, which shrink as they age, distorting the cusp and causing stenosis and incompetence of the valve. The inflamed myocardium can fail, leading to signs of heart failure, including tachycardia, breathlessness and cardiac enlargement. Inflammation of the pericardium can lead to friction within the pericardial cavity as the heart beats, pain behind the sternum and interference with the pumping action of the heart. Permanent fibrotic damage may fuse the visceral and parietal layers of the serous pericardium together, restricting the heart's action.

Chronic rheumatic heart disease. Inflamed tissue becomes fibrous as it heals, and this fibrous tissue interferes with the action of the myocardium and the heart valves. At least half of acute cases develop chronic valvular incompetence following recovery. The great majority of these patients have mitral valve damage, but the aortic valve is frequently affected too. Chronic fibrotic changes in the pericardium and myocardium cause heart failure.

Sometimes rheumatic valvular disease presents with no history of acute rheumatic fever or streptococcal infection.

Infective endocarditis

Pathogenic organisms (usually bacteria or fungi) in the blood may colonise any part of the endocardium, but the most common sites are on or near the heart valves and round the margins of congenital heart defects. These areas are susceptible to infection because they are exposed to fast-flowing blood that may cause mild trauma. This illness, which may be acute or subacute, is serious and sometimes fatal without treatment.

The main predisposing factors are bacteraemia, depressed immune response and heart abnormalities.

Bacteraemia

Microbes in the bloodstream, if not destroyed by phagocytes or antibodies, tend to adhere to platelets and form tiny infected emboli. Inside the heart, the emboli are most likely to settle on already damaged endocardium. Vegetations consisting of platelets and fibrin surround the microbes and seem to protect them from normal body defences and antibiotics. Because of this, infection may be caused by a wide range of bacteria, including some that do not normally cause clinical infection. They normally originate from the skin or the mouth.

Depressed immune response

This enables low-virulence bacteria, viruses, yeasts and fungi to become established and cause infection. These are organisms always present in the body and the environment. Depression of the immune systems may be caused by HIV infection, malignant disease, cytotoxic drugs, radiotherapy or steroid therapy.

Heart abnormalities

The sites most commonly infected are already abnormal in some way. Pathogenic organisms present in the bloodstream cannot adhere to healthy endothelium, but if the endothelial lining of the cardiovascular system is damaged, infection is more likely. Often, the cardiac valves are involved, especially if damaged by rheumatic disease or congenital malformation. Other likely sites of infection include regions of cardiac abnormality, such as ventricular septal defect (p. 130) and patent ductus arteriosus (p. 130). Prosthetic (artificial) valves can also be a focus for infective growths.

Cardiac arrhythmias

The heart rate is normally determined by intrinsic impulses generated in the SA node. The rhythm is determined by the route of impulse transmission through the conducting system. The heart rate is usually measured as the pulse, but to determine the rhythm, an electrocardiogram (ECG) is required (Fig. 5.58A). A *cardiac arrhythmia* is any disorder of heart rate or rhythm, and is the result of abnormal generation or conduction of impulses. The

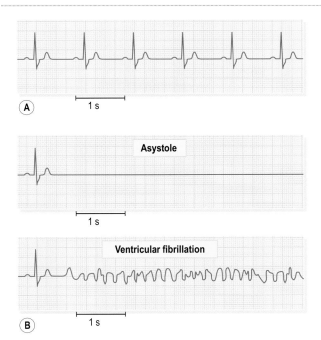

Figure 5.58 ECG traces. A. Normal sinus rhythm.
B. Life-threatening arrhythmias.

normal cardiac cycle (p. 92) gives rise to *normal sinus rhythm*, which has a rate of between 60 and 100 b.p.m.

Sinus bradycardia. This is normal sinus rhythm below 60 b.p.m. This may occur during sleep and is common in athletes. It is an abnormality when it follows myocardial infarction or accompanies raised intracranial pressure (p. 179).

Sinus tachycardia. This is normal sinus rhythm above 100 b.p.m. when the individual is at rest. This accompanies exercise and anxiety, but is an indicator of some disorders, e.g. fever, hyperthyroidism, some cardiac conditions.

Asystole

This occurs when there is no electrical activity in the ventricles and therefore no cardiac output. The ECG shows a flat line (Fig. 5.58B). Ventricular fibrillation and asystole cause sudden and complete loss of cardiac output, i.e. *cardiac arrest* and death.

Fibrillation

This is the contraction of the cardiac muscle fibres in a disorderly sequence. The chambers do not contract as a coordinated unit and the pumping action is disrupted.

In *atrial fibrillation* (AF), contraction of the atria is uncoordinated and rapid, pumping is ineffective and stimulation of the AV node is disorderly. AF is very common, especially in older adults. It may be asymptomatic, because although atrial function is disordered, most ventricular filling happens passively and atrial contraction only tops it up, so cardiac output is maintained. However, common symptoms include unpleasant palpitations, breathlessness and fatigue. The pulse is irregular and there are no discernible P waves on the ECG. Often the cause is unknown but AF can develop as a result of many forms of heart disease, thyrotoxicosis (p. 231), alcoholism and lung disease.

Ventricular fibrillation is a medical emergency that will swiftly lead to death if untreated, because the chaotic electrical activity within the ventricular walls cannot coordinate effective pumping action (cardiac arrest).

Blood is not pumped from the heart into either the pulmonary or the systemic circulation. No pulses can be felt; consciousness is lost and breathing stops. The ECG shows an irregular chaotic trace with no recognisable wave pattern (Fig. 5.58B).

Heart block

Heart block occurs when normal impulse transmission is blocked or impaired. A common form involves obstruction of impulse transmission through the AV node, but (less commonly) conducting tissue in the atria or ventricles can also be affected. When the AV node is involved, the delay between atrial and ventricular contraction is increased. The severity depends on the extent of loss of stimulation of the AV node.

In *complete heart block*, ventricular contraction is entirely independent of impulses initiated by the SA node. Freed from the normal pacing action of the SA node, the ventricles are driven by impulses generated by the pacemaker activity of the AV node, resulting in slow, regular ventricular contractions and a heart rate of about 30 to 40 b.p.m. In this state the heart is unable to respond quickly to a sudden increase in demand by, for example, muscular exercise. The most common causes are:

- acute ischaemic heart disease
- myocardial fibrosis following repeated infarctions or myocarditis
- drugs used to treat heart disease, e.g. digitalis, propranolol.

When heart block develops gradually there is some degree of adjustment in the body to reduced cardiac output but, if progressive, it eventually leads to death from cardiac failure and cerebral anoxia.

Congenital abnormalities

Abnormalities in the heart and great vessels at birth may be due to intrauterine developmental errors or to the failure of the heart and blood vessels to adapt to extrauterine life. Sometimes, there are no symptoms in early life

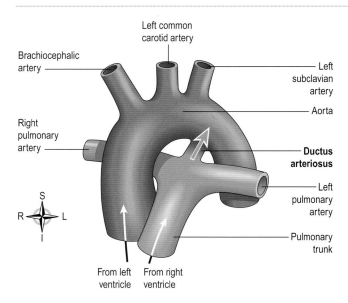

Figure 5.59 **The ductus arteriosus in the fetus.** The arrow indicates the direction of flow of blood from the pulmonary circulation into the aorta.

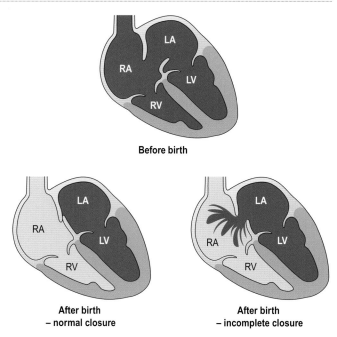

Figure 5.60 **Atrioseptal valve:** normal and incomplete closure after birth.

and the abnormality is recognised only when complications appear.

Patent ductus arteriosus

In the fetus, the ductus arteriosis (p. 116) bypasses the non-functional lungs (Fig. 5.59). At birth, when the pulmonary circulation is established, the ductus arteriosus should close completely. If it remains patent, blood regurgitates from the aorta to the pulmonary artery where the pressure is lower, reducing the volume entering the systemic circulation and increasing the volume of blood in the pulmonary circulation. This leads to pulmonary congestion and eventually cardiac failure.

Atrial septal defect

This is commonly known as 'hole in the heart'. After birth, when the pulmonary circulation is established and the pressure in the left atrium exceeds that in the right atrium, the atrioseptal valve closes. Later the closure becomes permanent due to fibrosis (Fig. 5.60).

When the membranes do not overlap, an opening between the atria remains patent after birth. In many cases it is too small to cause symptoms in early life but they may appear later. In severe cases blood flows back to the right atrium from the left. This increases the right ventricular and pulmonary pressure, causing hypertrophy of the myocardium and eventually cardiac failure. As pressure in the right atrium rises, blood flow through the defect may be reversed, but this is not an improvement because deoxygenated blood gains access to the general circulation.

Coarctation of the aorta

The most common site of coarctation (narrowing) of the aorta is between the left subclavian artery and ductus arteriosus. This leads to hypertension in the upper body (which is supplied by arteries arising from the aorta proximal to the narrowing) because increased force of contraction of the heart is needed to push the blood through the coarctation. There may be systemic hypotension.

Fallot's tetralogy

This is a characteristic combination of four congenital cardiac abnormalities, which causes cyanosis, growth retardation and exercise intolerance in babies and young children. The four abnormalities are:

- stenosis of the pulmonary artery at its point of origin, which increases right ventricular workload
- ventricular septal defect, i.e. an abnormal communicating hole between the two ventricles, just below the atrioventricular valves
- aortic misplacement, i.e. the origin of the aorta is displaced to the right so that it is immediately above the septal defect
- right ventricular hypertrophy to counteract the pulmonary stenosis.

Cardiac function is inadequate to meet the needs of the growing child; surgical correction carries a good prognosis.

Disorders of blood pressure

Learning outcomes

After studying this section, you should be able to:

■ explain the term hypertension

■ define essential and secondary hypertension and list the main causes of the latter

■ discuss the effects of prolonged hypertension on the body, including elevated blood pressure in the lungs

■ describe the term hypotension.

Hypertension

The term hypertension is used to describe a level of blood pressure that, taking all other cardiovascular risk factors into account, would benefit the patient if reduced. Blood pressure readings where systolic and diastolic values fall below 130/85 respectively are considered normal. Readings that indicate hypertension are listed in Table 5.2. Blood pressure tends to rise naturally with age. Arteriosclerosis (p. 122) may contribute to this, but is not the only factor.

Hypertension is classified as *essential* (primary, idiopathic) or *secondary* to other diseases. Irrespective of the cause, hypertension commonly affects the kidneys (p. 352).

Essential hypertension

Essential hypertension (hypertension of unknown cause) is very common in the Western world and accounts for 95% of all cases of hypertension. Treatment aims to prevent complications, which can be serious, primarily cardiovascular and renal disease. Sometimes complications, such as heart failure, cerebrovascular accident or myocardial infarction are the first indication of hypertension, but often the condition is symptomless and is only discovered during a routine examination.

Risk factors. Risk factors for hypertension include obesity, diabetes mellitus, family history, cigarette smoking, a sedentary lifestyle and high intakes of salt or alcohol. Stress may increase blood pressure, and there is a well-documented link between low birth weight and incidence of hypertension in later life.

Malignant (accelerated) hypertension

This is a rapid and aggressive acceleration of hypertensive disease. Diastolic pressure in excess of 120 mmHg is common. The effects are serious and quickly become apparent, e.g. haemorrhages into the retina, papilloedema (oedema around the optic disc), encephalopathy (cerebral oedema) and progressive renal disease, leading to cardiac failure.

Secondary hypertension

Hypertension resulting from other diseases accounts for 5% of all cases.

Some causes of secondary hypertension are listed in Box 5.5.

Effects and complications of hypertension

The effects of long-standing and progressively rising blood pressure are serious. Hypertension predisposes to atherosclerosis and has specific effects on particular organs.

Heart. The rate and force of cardiac contraction are increased to maintain the cardiac output against a sustained rise in arterial pressure. The left ventricle hypertrophies and begins to fail when compensation has reached its limit. This is followed by back pressure and accumulation of blood in the lungs (pulmonary congestion), hypertrophy of the right ventricle and eventually

---

Table 5.2 Hypertension: indicative blood pressure readings. British Hypertension Society/NICE guidelines, 2011

Grade	Systolic reading (mmHg)	Diastolic reading (mmHg)
1, mild	140–59	90–99
2, moderate	160–179	100–109
3, severe	≥180	≥ 110

Box 5.5 Some causes of secondary hypertension

Causes of secondary hypertension

- Kidney disease (p. 352)
- Adrenal gland disorders
  - excessive steroid secretion (Conn's syndrome, Cushing's syndrome, p. 233)
  - excessive adrenaline secretion, e.g. phaeochromocytoma (p. 235)
- Thyrotoxicosis (p. 231)
- Stricture of the aorta
- Alcohol
- Obesity
- Pregnancy
- Drug treatment, e.g. oral contraceptives containing oestrogen, corticosteroids

to right ventricular failure. Hypertension also predisposes to ischaemic heart disease (p. 127) and aneurysm formation (p. 122).

Brain. Stroke, caused by cerebral haemorrhage, is common, the effects depending on the position and size of the ruptured vessel. When a series of small blood vessels rupture, e.g. microaneurysms, at different times, there is progressive disability. Rupture of a large vessel causes extensive loss of function or death.

Kidneys. Hypertension causes kidney damage. If sustained for only a short time recovery may be complete. Otherwise the kidney damage causes further hypertension owing to activation of the renin–angiotensin–aldosterone system (p. 343), progressive loss of kidney function and kidney failure.

Blood vessels. High blood pressure damages blood vessels. The walls of small arteries become hardened, and in larger arteries, atheroma is accelerated. If other risk factors for vascular disease are present, such as diabetes or smoking, damage is more extensive. The vessel wall may become so badly weakened by these changes that an aneurysm develops, and as the blood vessels become progressively damaged and less elastic, hypertension worsens.

The capillaries of the retina and the kidneys are particularly susceptible to the effects of chronic hypertension, leading to retinal bleeding and reduced renal function.

Pulmonary hypertension

Normally, the pulmonary circulation is a low-pressure system, to prevent fluid being forced out of the pulmonary capillaries into the alveoli. When blood pressure rises, alveoli begin to fill with fluid, which blocks gas exchange. Rising pulmonary blood pressure may result from left-sided heart failure (p. 127), or other problems with left ventricular function, when blood accumulates in the pulmonary circulation because the left ventricle is not pumping efficiently. Lung disease can also increase in pulmonary blood pressure because of destruction of lung capillaries, e.g. in emphysema. Primary pulmonary hypertension, where there is no identifiable cause, is rare.

Hypotension

This usually occurs as a complication of other conditions, such as shock (p. 118) or Addison's disease (p. 235). Low blood pressure leads to inadequate blood supply to the brain. Depending on the cause, unconsciousness may be brief (fainting) or more prolonged, possibly causing death.

Postural hypotension is an abrupt fall in blood pressure on standing up suddenly from a sitting or lying position. It causes dizziness and occasionally syncope (fainting).

For a range of self-assessment exercises on the topics in this chapter, visit Evolve online resources: https://evolve.elsevier.com/Waugh/anatomy/

The lymphatic system

ANIMATIONS

The body cells are bathed in *interstitial (tissue) fluid*, which leaks constantly out of the bloodstream through the permeable walls of blood capillaries. It is therefore very similar in composition to blood plasma. Some tissue fluid returns to the capillaries at their venous end and the remainder diffuses through the more permeable walls of the lymph capillaries, forming *lymph*.

Lymph passes through vessels of increasing size and a varying number of *lymph nodes* before returning to the blood. The lymphatic system (Fig. 6.1) consists of:

- lymph
- lymph vessels
- lymph nodes
- lymph organs, e.g. spleen and thymus
- diffuse lymphoid tissue, e.g. tonsils
- bone marrow.

The first sections of this chapter explore the structures and functions of the organs listed above. In the final section, the consequences of disorders of the immune system are considered. The main effects of ageing on the lymphatic system relate to declining immunity, described in Chapter 15 (p. 384).

Functions of the lymphatic system

Tissue drainage

Every day, around 21 litres of fluid from plasma, carrying dissolved substances and some plasma protein, escape from the arterial end of the capillaries and into the tissues. Most of this fluid is returned directly to the bloodstream via the capillary at its venous end, but the excess, about 3–4 litres of fluid, is drained away by the lymphatic

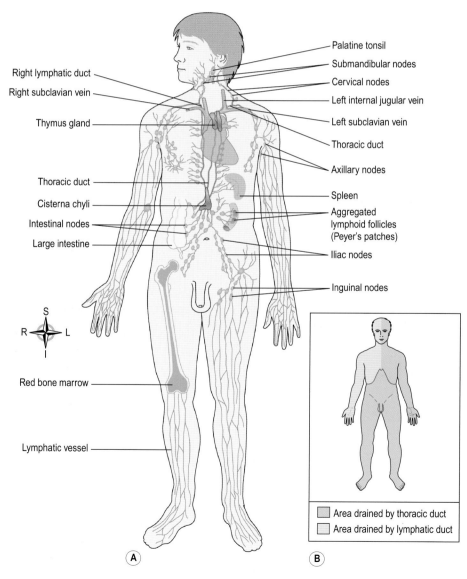

Figure 6.1 **The lymphatic system. A.** Major parts of the lymphatic system. **B.** Regional drainage of lymph.

vessels. Without this, the tissues would rapidly become waterlogged, and the cardiovascular system would begin to fail as the blood volume falls.

Absorption in the small intestine (Ch. 12)

Fat and fat-soluble materials, e.g. the fat-soluble vitamins, are absorbed into the central lacteals (lymphatic vessels) of the villi.

Immunity (Ch. 15)

The lymphatic organs are concerned with the production and maturation of lymphocytes, the white blood cells responsible for immunity. Bone marrow is therefore considered to be lymphatic tissue, since lymphocytes are produced there.

Lymph and lymph vessels

Learning outcomes

After studying this section, you should be able to:

■ describe the composition and the main functions of lymph ▮ 6.1

■ identify the locations and functions of the main lymphatic vessels of the body.

Lymph

Lymph is a clear watery fluid, similar in composition to plasma, with the important exception of plasma proteins, and identical in composition to interstitial fluid. Lymph transports the plasma proteins that seep out of the capillary beds back to the bloodstream. It also carries away larger particles, e.g. bacteria and cell debris from damaged tissues, which can then be filtered out and destroyed by the lymph nodes. Lymph contains lymphocytes (defence cells, p. 380), which circulate in the lymphatic system allowing them to patrol the different regions of the body. In the lacteals of the small intestine, fats absorbed into the lymphatics give the lymph (now called *chyle*), a milky appearance.

Lymph capillaries

These originate as blind-end tubes in the interstitial spaces (Fig. 6.2). They have the same structure as blood capillaries, i.e. a single layer of endothelial cells, but their walls are more permeable to all interstitial fluid constituents, including proteins and cell debris. The tiny capillaries join up to form larger lymph vessels.

Nearly all tissues have a network of lymphatic vessels, important exceptions being the central nervous system, the cornea of the eye, the bones and the most superficial layers of the skin.

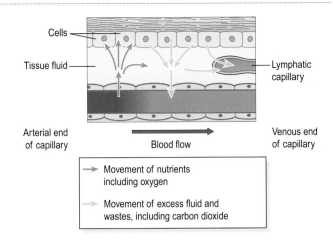

Figure 6.2 The origin of a lymph capillary.

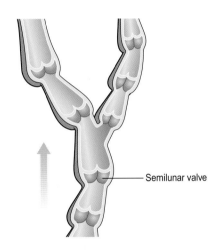

Figure 6.3 A lymph vessel cut open to show valves.

Larger lymph vessels

Lymph vessels are often found running alongside the arteries and veins serving the area. Their walls are about the same thickness as those of small veins and have the same layers of tissue, i.e. a fibrous covering, a middle layer of smooth muscle and elastic tissue and an inner lining of endothelium. Like veins, lymph vessels have numerous cup-shaped valves to ensure that lymph flows in a one-way system towards the thorax (Fig. 6.3). There is no 'pump', like the heart, involved in the onward movement of lymph, but the muscle layer in the walls of the large lymph vessels has an intrinsic ability to contract rhythmically (the lymphatic pump).

In addition, lymph vessels are compressed by activity in adjacent structures, such as contraction of muscles and the regular pulsation of large arteries. This 'milking' action on the lymph vessel wall helps to push lymph along.

Lymph vessels become larger as they join together, eventually forming two large ducts, the *thoracic duct* and *right lymphatic duct*, which empty lymph into the subclavian veins. █ **6.2**

Thoracic duct

This duct begins at the *cisterna chyli*, which is a dilated lymph channel situated in front of the bodies of the first two lumbar vertebrae. The duct is about 40 cm long and opens into the left subclavian vein in the root of the neck. It drains lymph from both legs, the pelvic and abdominal cavities, the left half of the thorax, head and neck and the left arm (Fig. 6.1A and B).

Right lymphatic duct

This is a dilated lymph vessel about 1 cm long. It lies in the root of the neck and opens into the right subclavian vein. It drains lymph from the right half of the thorax, head and neck and the right arm (Fig. 6.1A and B).

Lymphatic organs and tissues

Learning outcomes

After studying this section, you should be able to:

- compare and contrast the structure and functions of a typical lymph node with that of the spleen

- describe the location, structure and function of the thymus gland

- describe the location, structure and function of mucosa-associated lymphatic tissue (MALT).

Lymph nodes █ 6.3

Lymph nodes are oval or bean-shaped organs that lie, often in groups, along the length of lymph vessels. The lymph drains through a number of nodes, usually 8–10, before returning to the venous circulation. These nodes vary considerably in size: some are as small as a pin head and the largest are about the size of an almond.

Structure

Lymph nodes (Fig. 6.4) have an outer capsule of fibrous tissue that dips down into the node substance forming partitions, or *trabeculae*. The main substance of the node consists of reticular and lymphatic tissue containing many lymphocytes and macrophages. Reticular cells produce the network of fibres that provide internal structure within the lymph node. The lymphatic tissue contains immune and defence cells, including lymphocytes and macrophages.

As many as four or five afferent lymph vessels may enter a lymph node while only one efferent vessel carries

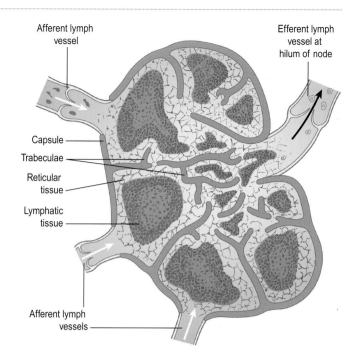

Figure 6.4 Section through a lymph node. Arrows indicate the direction of lymph flow.

lymph away from the node. Each node has a concave surface called the hilum where an artery enters and a vein and the efferent lymph vessel leave.

The large numbers of lymph nodes situated in strategic positions throughout the body are arranged in deep and superficial groups.

Lymph from the head and neck passes through deep and superficial *cervical nodes* (Fig. 6.5).

Lymph from the upper limbs passes through nodes situated in the elbow region, then through the deep and superficial *axillary nodes*.

Lymph from organs and tissues in the thoracic cavity drains through groups of nodes situated close to the mediastinum, large airways, oesophagus and chest wall. Most of the lymph from the breast passes through the axillary nodes.

Lymph from the pelvic and abdominal cavities passes through many lymph nodes before entering the cisterna chyli. The abdominal and pelvic nodes are situated mainly in association with the blood vessels supplying the organs and close to the main arteries, i.e. the aorta and the external and internal iliac arteries.

The lymph from the lower limbs drains through deep and superficial nodes including groups of nodes behind the knee and in the groin (inguinal nodes).

Functions

Filtering and phagocytosis

Lymph is filtered by the reticular and lymphatic tissue as it passes through lymph nodes. Particulate matter may

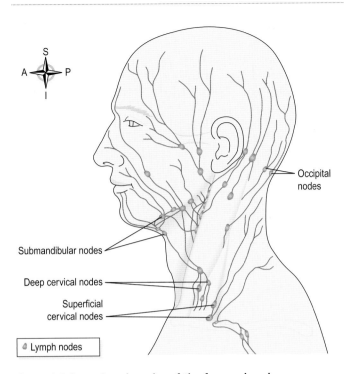

Figure 6.5 Some lymph nodes of the face and neck.

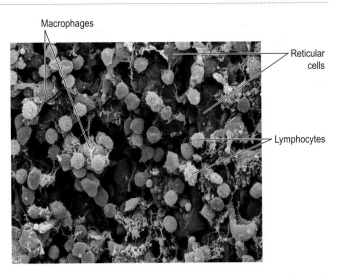

Figure 6.6 Colour scanning electron micrograph of lymph node tissue. Cell population includes reticular cells (brown), macrophages (pink) and lymphocytes (yellow).

include bacteria, dead and live phagocytes containing ingested microbes, cells from malignant tumours, worn-out and damaged tissue cells and inhaled particles. Organic material is destroyed in lymph nodes by macrophages and antibodies. Some inorganic inhaled particles cannot be destroyed by phagocytosis. These remain inside the macrophages, either causing no damage or killing the cell. Material not filtered out and dealt with in one lymph node passes on to successive nodes and by the time lymph enters the blood it has usually been cleared of foreign matter and cell debris. In some cases where phagocytosis of bacteria is incomplete they may stimulate inflammation and enlargement of the node (*lymphadenopathy*).

Proliferation of lymphocytes

Activated T- and B-lymphocytes multiply in lymph nodes. Antibodies produced by sensitised B-lymphocytes enter lymph and blood draining the node.

Figure 6.6 shows a scanning electron micrograph of lymph node tissue, with reticular cells, white blood cells and macrophages.

Spleen ▦ 6.4

The spleen (Figs 6.7 and 4.13) contains reticular and lymphatic tissue and is the largest lymph organ.

The spleen lies in the left hypochondriac region of the abdominal cavity between the fundus of the stomach and the diaphragm. It is purplish in colour and varies in size in different individuals, but is usually about 12 cm long, 7 cm wide and 2.5 cm thick. It weighs about 200 g.

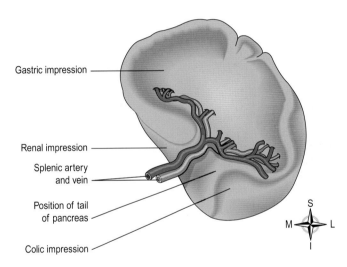

Figure 6.7 The spleen.

Organs associated with the spleen

Superiorly and posteriorly – diaphragm
Inferiorly – left colic flexure of the large intestine
Anteriorly – fundus of the stomach
Medially – pancreas and the left kidney
Laterally – separated from the 9th, 10th and 11th ribs and the intercostal muscles by the diaphragm

Structure (Fig. 6.8)

The spleen is slightly oval in shape with the hilum on the lower medial border. The anterior surface is covered with peritoneum. It is enclosed in a fibroelastic capsule that dips into the organ, forming trabeculae. The cellular material, consisting of lymphocytes and macrophages, is called *splenic pulp*, and lies between the trabeculae. *Red pulp* is the part suffused with blood and *white pulp* consists of areas of lymphatic tissue where there are sleeves of lymphocytes and macrophages around blood vessels.

The structures entering and leaving the spleen at the hilum are:

- splenic artery, a branch of the coeliac artery
- splenic vein, a branch of the portal vein
- lymph vessels (efferent only)
- nerves.

Blood passing through the spleen flows in sinusoids (p. 83), which have distinct pores between the endothelial cells, allowing it to come into close association with splenic pulp. This is essential for the spleen's function in removing ageing or damaged cells from the bloodstream.

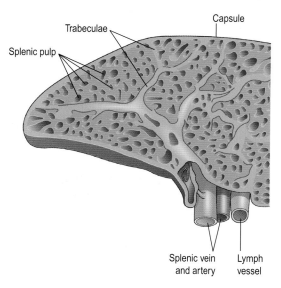

Figure 6.8 A section through the spleen.

Functions

Phagocytosis

As described previously (p. 68), old and abnormal erythrocytes are mainly destroyed in the spleen, and the breakdown products, bilirubin (Fig. 12.37) and iron, are transported to the liver via the splenic and portal veins. Other cellular material, e.g. leukocytes, platelets and bacteria, is phagocytosed in the spleen.

Unlike lymph nodes, the spleen has no afferent lymphatics entering it, so it is not exposed to diseases spread by lymph.

Storage of blood

The spleen contains up to 350 mL of blood, and in response to sympathetic stimulation can rapidly return most of this volume to the circulation, e.g. in haemorrhage.

Immune response

The spleen contains T- and B-lymphocytes, which are activated by the presence of antigens, e.g. in infection. Lymphocyte proliferation during serious infection can cause enlargement of the spleen (*splenomegaly*).

Erythropoiesis

The spleen and liver are important sites of fetal blood cell production, and the spleen can also fulfil this function in adults in times of great need.

Thymus gland 6.5

The thymus gland lies in the upper part of the mediastinum behind the sternum and extends upwards into the root of the neck (Fig. 6.9). It weighs about 10 to 15 g at birth and grows until puberty, when it begins to atrophy. Its maximum weight, at puberty, is between 30 and 40 g and by middle age it has returned to approximately its weight at birth.

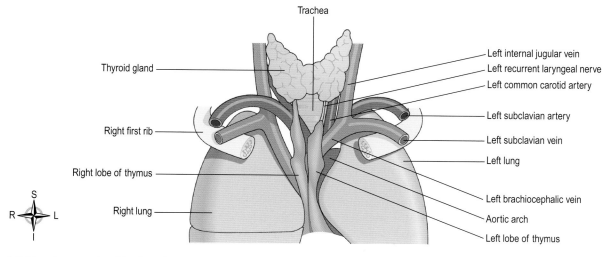

Figure 6.9 The thymus gland in the adult, and related structures.

Organs associated with the thymus

Anteriorly – sternum and upper four costal cartilages
Posteriorly – aortic arch and its branches, brachiocephalic veins, trachea
Laterally – lungs
Superiorly – structures in the root of the neck
Inferiorly – heart

Structure

The thymus consists of two lobes joined by areolar tissue. The lobes are enclosed by a fibrous capsule which dips into their substance, dividing them into lobules that consist of an irregular branching framework of epithelial cells and lymphocytes.

Function

Lymphocytes originate from stem cells in red bone marrow (p. 64). Those that enter the thymus develop into activated T-lymphocytes (p. 380).

Thymic processing produces mature T-lymphocytes that can distinguish 'self' tissue from foreign tissue, and also provides each T-lymphocyte with the ability to react to only one specific antigen from the millions it will encounter (p. 380). T-lymphocytes then leave the thymus and enter the blood. Some enter lymphoid tissues and others circulate in the bloodstream. T-lymphocyte production, although most prolific in youth, probably continues throughout life from a resident population of thymic stem cells.

The maturation of the thymus and other lymphoid tissue is stimulated by *thymosin*, a hormone secreted by the epithelial cells that form the framework of the thymus gland. Shrinking of the gland begins in adolescence and, with increasing age, the effectiveness of the T-lymphocyte response to antigens declines.

Mucosa-associated lymphoid tissue (MALT)

Throughout the body, at strategically placed locations, are collections of lymphoid tissue which, unlike the spleen and thymus, are not enclosed within a capsule. They contain B- and T-lymphocytes, which have migrated from bone marrow and the thymus, and are important in the early detection of invaders. However, as they have no afferent lymphatic vessels, they do not filter lymph, and are therefore not exposed to diseases spread by lymph. MALT is found throughout the gastrointestinal tract, in the respiratory tract and in the genitourinary tract, all systems of the body exposed to the external environment.

The main groups of MALT are the tonsils and aggregated lymphoid follicles (Peyer's patches).

Tonsils. These are located in the mouth and throat, and will therefore destroy swallowed and inhaled antigens (see also p. 245).

Aggregated lymphoid follicles (Peyer's patches). These large collections of lymphoid tissue are found in the small intestine, and intercept swallowed antigens (Fig. 12.25).

Lymph vessel pathology

Learning outcomes

After studying this section, you should be able to:

■ explain the role of lymphatic vessels in the spread of infectious and malignant disease

■ discuss the main causes and consequences of lymphatic obstruction.

The main involvements of lymph vessels are in relation to the spread of disease in the body, and the effects of lymphatic obstruction. Table 6.1 defines some common terms used when describing lymphatic system pathology.

Spread of disease

The materials most commonly spread via the lymph vessels from their original site to the circulating blood are fragments of tumours and infected material.

Malignant disease

Malignant tumours shed cells into the surrounding interstitial fluid, which drains into local lymphatic vessels and carries the tumour cells to the nearest set of lymph nodes. Here, if tumour cells arrive in sufficient numbers, they can establish secondary growths (metastases). From local lymph nodes, the tumour usually spreads to further lymph nodes and/or via the bloodstream to distant organs.

Infection

Infectious material may enter lymph vessels from infected tissues. If phagocytosis is not effective the infection may spread from node to node, and eventually reach the bloodstream.

Lymphangitis. This occurs in some acute bacterial infections in which the microbes in the lymph draining from the area infect and spread along the walls of lymph vessels, e.g. in acute *Streptococcus pyogenes* infection of the hand, a red line may be seen extending from the hand to the axilla. This is caused by an inflamed superficial lymph vessel and adjacent tissues. The infection may be stopped at the first lymph node or spread through the lymph drainage network to the blood.

Lymphatic obstruction

When a lymph vessel is obstructed, lymph accumulates distal to the obstruction (*lymphoedema*). The amount of resultant swelling and the size of the area affected depend on the size of the vessel involved. Lymphoedema usually leads to low-grade inflammation and fibrosis of the lymph vessel and further lymphoedema. The most common causes are tumours and following surgical removal of lymph nodes.

Tumours

A tumour may grow into, and block, a lymph vessel or node, obstructing the flow of lymph. A large tumour outside the lymphatic system may also cause sufficient pressure to stop the flow of lymph.

Surgery

In some surgical procedures lymph nodes are removed because cancer cells may have already spread to them. This aims to prevent growth of secondary tumours in local lymph nodes and further spread of the disease via the lymphatic system, e.g. axillary nodes may be removed during mastectomy (breast removal), but it can lead to obstruction of lymph drainage.

Table 6.1 Common terms used in lymphatic system pathology

Term	Definition
Lymphangitis	Inflammation of lymph vessels
Lymphadenitis	Infection of lymph nodes
Lymphadenopathy	Enlargement of lymph nodes
Splenomegaly	Enlargement of the spleen
Lymphoedema	Swelling in tissues whose lymphatic drainage has been obstructed in some way

Diseases of lymph nodes

Learning outcomes

After studying this section, you should be able to:

■ describe the term lymphadenitis, listing its primary causes

■ describe the effects of the two main forms of lymphoma

■ explain why secondary disease of the lymph nodes is commonly found in individuals with cancer.

Lymphadenitis

Acute lymphadenitis (acute infection of lymph nodes) is usually caused by microbes transported in lymph from other areas of infection. The nodes become inflamed, enlarged and congested with blood, and chemotaxis attracts large numbers of phagocytes. If lymph node defences (phagocytes and antibody production) are overwhelmed, the infection can cause abscess formation within the node. Adjacent tissues may become involved, and infected materials transported through other nodes and into the blood.

Acute lymphadenitis is secondary to a number of conditions.

Infectious mononucleosis (glandular fever)

This is a highly contagious viral infection, usually of young adults, spread by direct contact. During the incubation period of 7–10 days, viruses multiply in the epithelial cells of the pharynx. They subsequently spread to cervical lymph nodes, then to lymphoid tissue throughout the body.

Clinical features include tonsillitis, lymphadenopathy and splenomegaly. A common complication is myalgic encephalitis (chronic fatigue syndrome, p. 185). Clinical or subclinical infection confers lifelong immunity.

Other diseases

Minor lymphadenitis accompanies many infections and indicates the mobilisation of normal protective mechanisms, e.g. proliferation of defence cells. More serious infection occurs in, e.g. measles, typhoid and cat-scratch fever, and wound or skin infections. Chronic lymphadenitis occurs following unresolved acute infections, in tuberculosis, syphilis and some low-grade infections.

Lymphomas

These are malignant tumours of lymphoid tissue and are classified as either Hodgkin's or non-Hodgkin's lymphomas.

Hodgkin's disease

In this disease there is progressive, painless enlargement of lymph nodes throughout the body, as lymphoid tissue within them proliferates. The superficial lymph nodes in the neck are often the first to be noticed. The disease is malignant and the cause is unknown. The prognosis varies considerably but the pattern of spread is predictable because the disease spreads to adjacent nodes and to other tissues in a consistent way. The effectiveness of treatment depends largely on the stage of the disease at which it begins. The disease leads to reduced immunity, because lymphocyte function is depressed, and recurrent infection is therefore common. As lymph nodes enlarge, they may compress adjacent tissues and organs. Anaemia

and changes in leukocyte numbers occur if the bone marrow is involved.

Non-Hodgkin's lymphoma (NHL)

NHL is associated with immunodeficiency states and certain viral infections including HIV (p. 386). NHL includes *multiple myeloma* and *Burkitt's lymphoma* and may occur in any lymphoid tissue or in bone marrow. They are classified according to the type of cell involved and the degree of malignancy, i.e. low, intermediate or high grade. Low-grade tumours consist of well-differentiated cells and slow progress of the disease, death occurring after a period of years. High-grade lymphomas consist of poorly differentiated cells and rapid progress of the disease, death occurring in weeks or months. Some low- or intermediate-grade tumours change their status to high grade with increased rate of progress.

The expanding lymph nodes may compress adjacent tissues and organs. Immunological deficiency leads to increased incidence of infections, and if the bone marrow or spleen (or both) is involved there may be varying degrees of anaemia and leukopenia.

Disorders of the spleen

Learning outcome

After studying this section, you should be able to:

- identify the main causes of splenomegaly.

Splenomegaly

This is enlargement of the spleen, and is usually secondary to other conditions, e.g. infections, circulatory disorders, blood diseases, malignant neoplasms.

Infections

The spleen may be infected by blood-borne microbes or by local spread of infection. The red pulp becomes congested with blood and there is an accumulation of phagocytes and plasma cells. Acute infections are rare.

Chronic infections. Some chronic non-pyogenic infections cause splenomegaly, but this is usually less severe than in the case of acute infections. The most commonly occurring primary infections include:

- tuberculosis (p. 268)
- typhoid fever (p. 325)
- malaria
- infectious mononucleosis (see above).

Circulatory disorders

Splenomegaly due to congestion of blood occurs when the flow of blood through the liver is impeded by, e.g., fibrosis in liver cirrhosis, or portal venous congestion in right-sided heart failure.

Blood disease

Splenomegaly may be caused by blood disorders. The spleen enlarges to deal with the extra workload associated with removing damaged, worn out and abnormal blood cells in, e.g., haemolytic and macrocytic anaemia, polycythaemia and chronic myeloid leukaemia (Ch. 4).

Splenomegaly may itself cause blood disorders. When the spleen is enlarged for any reason, especially in portal hypertension, excessive and premature haemolysis of red cells or phagocytosis of normal white cells and platelets leads to marked anaemia, leukopenia and thrombocytopenia.

Tumours

Benign and primary malignant tumours of the spleen are rare but blood-spread tumour fragments from elsewhere in the body may cause metastases. Splenomegaly caused by infiltration of malignant cells is characteristic of some conditions, especially chronic leukaemia, Hodgkin's disease and non-Hodgkin's lymphoma.

Diseases of the thymus gland

Learning outcome

After studying this section, you should be able to:

■ describe the principal disorders of the thymus gland.

Enlargement of the gland is associated with some autoimmune diseases, such as thyrotoxicosis and Addison's disease.

Tumours are rare, although pressure caused by enlargement of the gland may damage or interfere with the functions of adjacent structures, e.g. the trachea, oesophagus or veins in the neck.

In myasthenia gravis (p. 435), most patients have either thymic hyperplasia (the majority) or thymoma (a minority), although the role of thymic function in this disorder is not understood.

 For a range of self-assessment exercises on the topics in this chapter, visit Evolve online resources: https://evolve.elsevier .com/Waugh/anatomy/

The nervous system

The nervous system detects and responds to changes inside and outside the body. Together with the endocrine system, it coordinates and controls vital aspects of body function and maintains homeostasis. To this end the nervous system provides an immediate response while endocrine activity (Ch. 9) is, usually, slower and more prolonged.

The nervous system consists of the brain, the spinal cord and peripheral nerves (see Fig. 1.10, p. 10). The structure and organisation of the tissues that form these components enables rapid communication between all parts of the body.

For descriptive purposes the parts of the nervous system are grouped as follows:

- the *central nervous system* (CNS), consisting of the brain and the spinal cord
- the *peripheral nervous system* (PNS), consisting of all the nerves outside the brain and spinal cord. **7.1**

The PNS comprises paired cranial and sacral nerves – some of these are sensory (afferent) transmitting impulses to the CNS, some are motor (efferent) transmitting impulses from the CNS and others are mixed. It is useful to consider two functional parts within the PNS:

- the sensory division
- the motor division (Fig. 7.1).

The motor division has two parts:

- the *somatic nervous system*, which controls voluntary movement of skeletal muscles
- the *autonomic nervous system*, controlling involuntary processes such as heartbeat, peristalsis (p. 289) and glandular activity. The autonomic nervous system has two divisions: *sympathetic* and *parasympathetic*.

In summary, the CNS receives sensory information about its internal and external environments from afferent nerves. The CNS integrates and processes this input and responds, when appropriate, by sending nerve impulses through motor nerves to the effector organs: muscles and glands. For example, responses to changes in the internal environment regulate essential involuntary body functions such as respiration and blood pressure; responses to changes in the external environment maintain posture and other voluntary activities.

The first sections of this chapter explore the structure and functions of the components of the nervous system including the impact of ageing, while the final one considers the effects on body function when its structures do not function normally.

Cells and tissues of the nervous system

Learning outcomes

After studying this section, you should be able to:

- compare and contrast the structure and functions of myelinated and unmyelinated neurones

- state the functions of sensory and motor nerves

- explain the events that occur following release of a neurotransmitter at a synapse

- briefly describe the functions of four types of neuroglial cells

- outline the response of nervous tissue to injury.

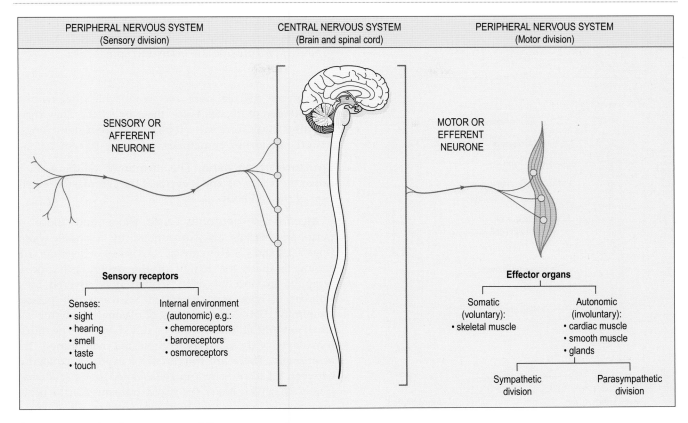

| PERIPHERAL NERVOUS SYSTEM (Sensory division) | CENTRAL NERVOUS SYSTEM (Brain and spinal cord) | PERIPHERAL NERVOUS SYSTEM (Motor division) |

SENSORY OR AFFERENT NEURONE

MOTOR OR EFFERENT NEURONE

Sensory receptors

Senses:
• sight
• hearing
• smell
• taste
• touch

Internal environment (autonomic) e.g.:
• chemoreceptors
• baroreceptors
• osmoreceptors

Effector organs

Somatic (voluntary):
• skeletal muscle

Autonomic (involuntary):
• cardiac muscle
• smooth muscle
• glands

Sympathetic division   Parasympathetic division

Figure 7.1 Functional components of the nervous system.

There are two types of nervous tissue, neurones and neuroglia. *Neurones* (nerve cells) are the working units of the nervous system that generate and transmit *nerve impulses*. Neurones are supported by connective tissue, collectively known as *neuroglia*, which is formed from different types of *glial cells*. There are vast numbers of both cell types, 1 trillion (10^{12}) glial cells and 10 times fewer (10^{11}) neurones.

Neurones (Fig. 7.2) ■ 7.2

Each neurone (Fig. 7.2) consists of a *cell body* and its processes, one *axon* and many *dendrites*. Neurones are commonly referred to as nerve cells. Bundles of axons bound together are called *nerves*. Neurones cannot divide, and for survival they need a continuous supply of oxygen and glucose. Unlike many other cells, neurones can synthesise chemical energy (ATP) only from glucose.

Neurones generate and transmit electrical impulses called *action potentials*. The initial strength of the impulse is maintained throughout the length of the neurone. Some neurones initiate nerve impulses while others act as 'relay stations' where impulses are passed on and sometimes redirected.

Nerve impulses can be initiated in response to stimuli from:

• outside the body, e.g. touch, light waves
• inside the body, e.g. a change in the concentration of carbon dioxide in the blood alters respiration; a thought may result in voluntary movement.

Transmission of nerve signals is both electrical and chemical. The action potential travelling down the nerve axon is an electrical signal, but because nerves do not come into direct contact with each other, the signal between a nerve cell and the next cell in the chain is nearly always chemical (p. 148).

Cell bodies

Nerve cells vary considerably in size and shape but they are all too small to be seen by the naked eye. Cell bodies form the *grey matter* of the nervous system and are found at the periphery of the brain and in the centre of the spinal cord. Groups of cell bodies are called *nuclei* in the central nervous system and *ganglia* in the peripheral nervous system. An important exception is the basal ganglia (nuclei) situated within the cerebrum (p. 156).

Axons and dendrites

Axons and dendrites are extensions of cell bodies and form the *white matter* of the nervous system. Axons are

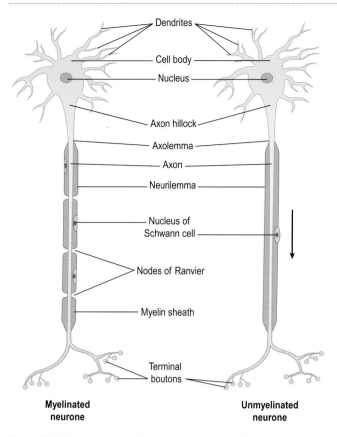

Figure 7.2 The structure of neurones. Arrow indicates direction of impulse conduction.

found deep in the brain and in groups, called *tracts*, at the periphery of the spinal cord. They are referred to as *nerves* or *nerve fibres* outside the brain and spinal cord.

Axons

Each nerve cell has only one axon, which begins at a tapered area of the cell body, the *axon hillock*. They carry impulses away from the cell body and are usually longer than the dendrites, sometimes as long as 100 cm.

Structure of an axon. The membrane of the axon is called the *axolemma* and it encloses the cytoplasmic extension of the cell body.

Myelinated neurones Large axons and those of peripheral nerves are surrounded by a *myelin sheath* (Figs 7.3A and C). This consists of a series of *Schwann cells* arranged along the length of the axon. Each one is wrapped around the axon so that it is covered by a number of concentric layers of Schwann cell plasma membrane. Between the layers of plasma membrane is a small amount of fatty substance called *myelin*. The outermost layer of the Schwann cell plasma membrane is the *neurilemma*. There are tiny areas of exposed axolemma between adjacent Schwann cells, called *nodes of Ranvier* (Fig. 7.2), which assist the rapid transmission of nerve impulses in myelinated neurones. Figure 7.4 shows a section through a nerve fibre at a node of Ranvier where the area without myelin can be clearly seen.

Unmyelinated neurones Postganglionic fibres and some small fibres in the central nervous system are *unmyelinated*. In this type a number of axons are embedded in one Schwann cell (Fig. 7.3B). The adjacent Schwann cells are in close association and there is no

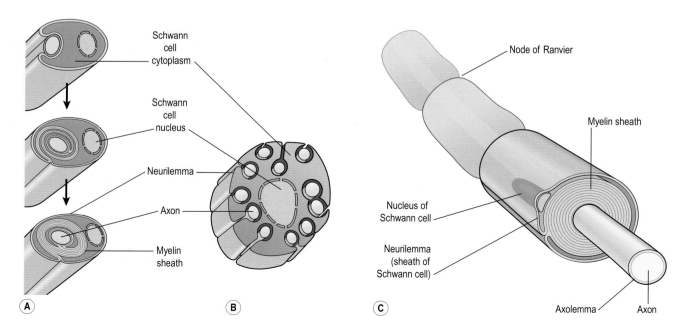

Figure 7.3 Arrangement of myelin. A. Myelinated neurone. **B.** Unmyelinated neurone. **C.** Length of myelinated axon.

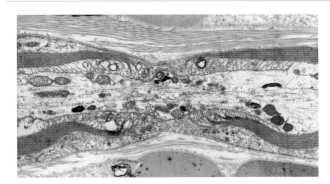

Figure 7.4 Node of Ranvier. A colour transmission electron micrograph of a longitudinal section of a myelinated nerve fibre. Nerve tissue is shown in blue and myelin in red.

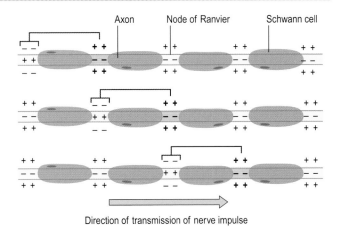

Direction of transmission of nerve impulse

Figure 7.5 Saltatory conduction of an impulse in a myelinated nerve fibre.

exposed axolemma. The speed of transmission of nerve impulses is significantly slower in unmyelinated fibres.

Dendrites

These are the many short processes that receive and carry incoming impulses towards cell bodies. They have the same structure as axons but are usually shorter and branching. In motor neurones dendrites form part of synapses (see Fig. 7.7) and in sensory neurones they form the sensory receptors that respond to specific stimuli.

The nerve impulse (action potential) ◼7.3

An impulse is initiated by stimulation of sensory nerve endings or by the passage of an impulse from another nerve. Transmission of the impulse, or action potential, is due to movement of ions across the nerve cell membrane. In the resting state the nerve cell membrane is *polarised* due to differences in the concentrations of ions across the plasma membrane. This means that there is a different electrical charge on each side of the membrane, which is called the *resting membrane potential*. At rest the charge on the outside is positive and inside it is negative. The principal ions involved are:

- sodium (Na^+), the main extracellular cation
- potassium (K^+), the main intracellular cation.

In the resting state there is a continual tendency for these ions to diffuse along their concentration gradients, i.e. K^+ outwards and Na^+ into cells. When stimulated, the permeability of the nerve cell membrane to these ions changes. Initially Na^+ floods into the neurone from the extracellular fluid causing *depolarisation*, creating a *nerve impulse* or *action potential*. Depolarisation is very rapid, enabling the conduction of a nerve impulse along the entire length of a neurone in a few milliseconds. It passes from the point of stimulation in one direction only, i.e. away from the point of stimulation towards the area of resting potential. The one-way direction of transmission is ensured because following depolarisation it takes time for *repolarisation* to occur.

Almost immediately following the entry of Na^+, K^+ floods out of the neurone and the movement of these ions returns the membrane potential to its resting state. This is called the *refractory period* during which restimulation is not possible. The action of the *sodium–potassium pump* expels Na^+ from the cell in exchange for K^+ (see p. 37) returning levels of Na^+ and K^+ to the original resting state, repolarizing the neurone.

In myelinated neurones, the insulating properties of the myelin sheath prevent the movement of ions. Therefore electrical changes across the membrane can only occur at the gaps in the myelin sheath, i.e. at the nodes of Ranvier (see Fig. 7.2). When an impulse occurs at one node, depolarisation passes along the myelin sheath to the next node so that the flow of current appears to 'leap' from one node to the next. This is called *saltatory conduction* (Fig. 7.5).

The speed of conduction depends on the diameter of the neurone: the larger the diameter, the faster the conduction. In addition, myelinated fibres conduct impulses faster than unmyelinated fibres because saltatory conduction is faster than continuous conduction, or *simple propagation* (Fig. 7.6). The fastest fibres can conduct impulses to, e.g., skeletal muscles at a rate of 130 metres per second while the slowest impulses travel at 0.5 metres per second.

The synapse and neurotransmitters ◼7.4

There is always more than one neurone involved in the transmission of a nerve impulse from its origin to its destination, whether it is sensory or motor. There is no physical contact between two neurones. The point at which the nerve impulse passes from the *presynaptic neurone* to the *postsynaptic neurone* is the *synapse* (Fig. 7.7). At its free end, the axon of the presynaptic neurone breaks up into minute branches that terminate in small swellings called *synaptic knobs*, or terminal boutons. These are in close proximity to the dendrites and the cell body of the

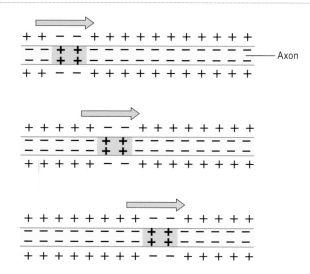

Figure 7.6 Simple propagation of an impulse in an unmyelinated nerve fibre. Arrows indicate the direction of impulse transmission.

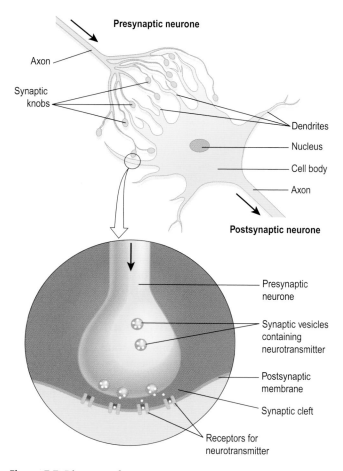

Figure 7.7 Diagram of a synapse. Arrows show direction of nerve impulse.

postsynaptic neurone. The space between them is the *synaptic cleft*. Synaptic knobs contain spherical membrane bound *synaptic vesicles*, which store a chemical, the *neurotransmitter* that is released into the synaptic cleft. Neurotransmitters are synthesised by nerve cell bodies, actively transported along the axons and stored in the synaptic vesicles. They are released by exocytosis in response to the action potential and diffuse across the synaptic cleft. They act on specific receptor sites on the postsynaptic membrane. Their action is short lived, because immediately they have acted on the postsynaptic cell such as a muscle fibre, they are either inactivated by enzymes or taken back into the synaptic knob. Some important drugs mimic, neutralise (antagonise) or prolong neurotransmitter activity. Neurotransmitters usually have an excitatory effect on postsynaptic receptors but they are sometimes inhibitory.

There are more than 50 neurotransmitters in the brain and spinal cord including noradrenaline (norepinephrine), adrenaline (epinephrine), dopamine, histamine, serotonin, gamma aminobutyric acid (GABA) and acetylcholine. Other substances, such as enkephalins, endorphins and substance P, have specialised roles in, for example, transmission of pain signals. Figure 7.8 summarises the main neurotransmitters of the peripheral nervous system.

Somatic nerves carry impulses directly to the synapses at skeletal muscles, the *neuromuscular junctions* (p. 422) stimulating contraction. In the autonomic nervous system (see p. 173), efferent impulses travel along two neurones (preganglionic and postganglionic) and across two synapses to the effector tissue, i.e. cardiac muscle, smooth muscle and glands, in both the sympathetic and the parasympathetic divisions.

Nerves

A nerve consists of numerous neurones collected into bundles (bundles of nerve fibres in the central nervous system are known as *tracts*). For example large nerves such as the sciatic nerves (p. 169) contain tens of thousands of axons. Each bundle has several coverings of protective connective tissue (Fig. 7.9):

- *endoneurium* is a delicate tissue, surrounding each individual fibre, which is continuous with the septa that pass inwards from the perineurium
- *perineurium* is a smooth connective tissue, surrounding each *bundle* of fibres
- *epineurium* is the fibrous tissue which surrounds and encloses a number of bundles of nerve fibres. Most large nerves are covered by epineurium.

Sensory or afferent nerves

Sensory nerves carry information from the body to the spinal cord (Fig. 7.1). The impulses may then pass to the

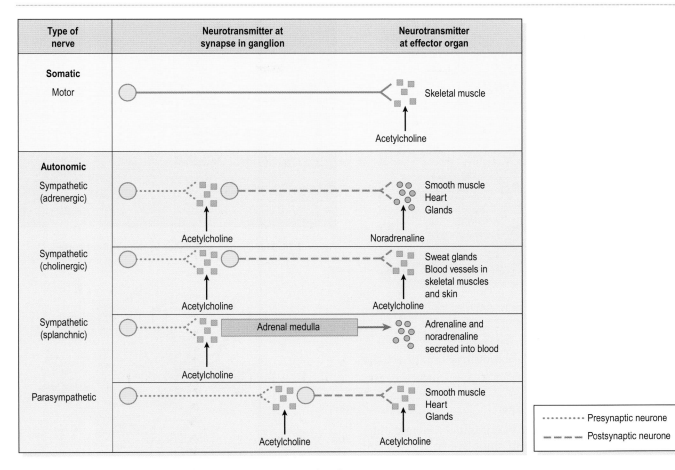

Type of nerve	Neurotransmitter at synapse in ganglion	Neurotransmitter at effector organ
Somatic Motor		Skeletal muscle Acetylcholine
Autonomic Sympathetic (adrenergic)	Acetylcholine	Smooth muscle Heart Glands Noradrenaline
Sympathetic (cholinergic)	Acetylcholine	Sweat glands Blood vessels in skeletal muscles and skin Acetylcholine
Sympathetic (splanchnic)	Acetylcholine — Adrenal medulla	Adrenaline and noradrenaline secreted into blood
Parasympathetic	Acetylcholine	Smooth muscle Heart Glands Acetylcholine

- - - - - - - Presynaptic neurone

— — — Postsynaptic neurone

Figure 7.8 Main neurotransmitters at synapses in the peripheral nervous system.

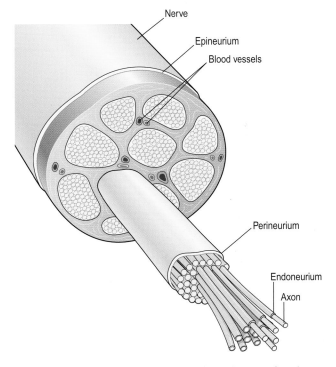

Figure 7.9 Transverse section of a peripheral nerve showing the protective connective tissue coverings.

Labels: Nerve, Epineurium, Blood vessels, Perineurium, Endoneurium, Axon

brain or to connector neurones of reflex arcs in the spinal cord (see p. 164).

Sensory receptors

Specialised endings of sensory neurones respond to different stimuli (changes) inside and outside the body.

Somatic, cutaneous or common senses. These originate from the skin. They are: pain, touch, heat and cold. Sensory nerve endings in the skin are fine branching filaments without myelin sheaths (see Fig. 14.4, p. 364). When stimulated, an impulse is generated and transmitted by the sensory nerves to the brain where the sensation is perceived.

Proprioceptor senses. These originate in muscles and joints. Impulses sent to the brain enable perception of the position of the body and its parts in space maintaining posture and balance (see Ch. 16).

Special senses. These are sight, hearing, balance, smell and taste (see Ch. 8).

Autonomic afferent nerves. These originate in internal organs, glands and tissues, e.g. baroreceptors involved in the control of blood pressure (Ch. 5), chemoreceptors involved in the control of respiration (Ch. 10), and are

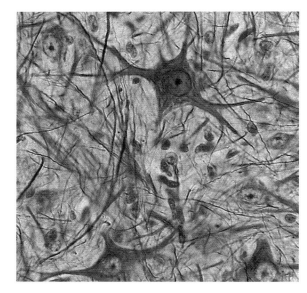

Figure 7.10 Neurones and glial cells. A stained light micrograph of neurones (gold) and nuclei of the more numerous glial cells (blue).

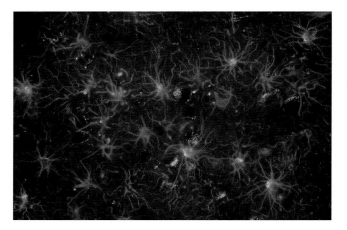

Figure 7.11 Star-shaped astrocytes in the cerebral cortex.

associated with reflex regulation of involuntary activity and visceral pain.

Motor or efferent nerves

Motor nerves originate in the brain, spinal cord and autonomic ganglia. They transmit impulses to the effector organs: muscles and glands (Fig. 7.1). There are two types:

- *somatic nerves* – involved in voluntary and reflex skeletal muscle contraction
- *autonomic nerves* (sympathetic and parasympathetic) – involved in cardiac and smooth muscle contraction and glandular secretion.

Mixed nerves

In the spinal cord, sensory and motor nerves are arranged in separate groups, or *tracts*. Outside the spinal cord, when sensory and motor nerves are enclosed within the same sheath of connective tissue they are called *mixed nerves*.

Neuroglia

The neurones of the central nervous system are supported by non-excitable *glial cells* that greatly outnumber the neurones (Fig. 7.10). Unlike nerve cells, which cannot divide, glial cells continue to replicate throughout life. There are four types: *astrocytes, oligodendrocytes, ependymal cells* and *microglia*.

Astrocytes

These cells form the main supporting tissue of the central nervous system (Fig. 7.11). They are star shaped with

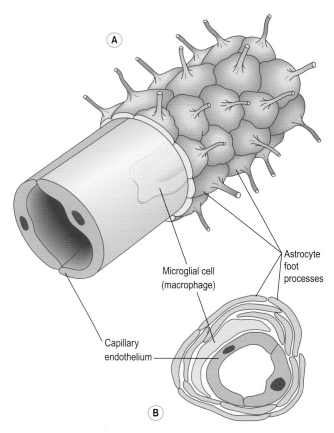

Figure 7.12 Blood–brain barrier. A. Longitudinal section. **B.** Transverse section.

fine branching processes and they lie in a mucopolysaccharide ground substance. At the free ends of some of the processes are small swellings called *foot processes*. Astrocytes are found in large numbers adjacent to blood vessels with their foot processes forming a sleeve round them. This means that the blood is separated from the neurones by the capillary wall and a layer of astrocyte foot processes which together constitute the *blood–brain barrier* (Fig. 7.12).

The blood–brain barrier is a selective barrier that protects the brain from potentially toxic substances and chemical variations in the blood, e.g. after a meal. Oxygen, carbon dioxide, glucose and other lipid-soluble substances, e.g. alcohol, quickly cross the barrier into the brain. Some large molecules, many drugs, inorganic ions and amino acids pass more slowly, if at all, from the blood to the brain.

Oligodendrocytes

These cells are smaller than astrocytes and are found in clusters round nerve cell bodies in grey matter, where they are thought to have a supportive function. They are found adjacent to, and along the length of, myelinated nerve fibres. Oligodendrocytes form and maintain myelin like Schwann cells in peripheral nerves.

Ependymal cells

These cells form the epithelial lining of the ventricles of the brain and the central canal of the spinal cord. Those cells that form the choroid plexuses of the ventricles secrete cerebrospinal fluid.

Microglia

The smallest and least numerous glial cells, these cells may be derived from monocytes that migrate from the blood into the nervous system before birth. They are found mainly in the area of blood vessels. They enlarge and become phagocytic, removing microbes and damaged tissue, in areas of inflammation and cell destruction.

Response of nervous tissue to injury

Neurones reach maturity a few weeks after birth and cannot be replaced.

Damage to neurones can either lead to rapid necrosis with sudden acute functional failure, or to slow atrophy with gradually increasing dysfunction. These changes are associated with:

- hypoxia and anoxia
- nutritional deficiencies
- poisons, e.g. organic lead
- trauma
- infections
- ageing
- hypoglycaemia.

Peripheral nerve regeneration (Fig. 7.13)

The axons of *peripheral nerves* can sometimes regenerate if the cell body remains intact. Distal to the damage, the axon and myelin sheath disintegrate and are removed by macrophages; the muscle supplied by the damaged fibre atrophies in the absence of nerve stimulation. The neurilemma then regenerates (about 1.5 mm per day) from the point of injury towards the effector along its original track provided the two parts of the neurilemma are in close apposition (Fig. 7.13A). New Schwann cells develop

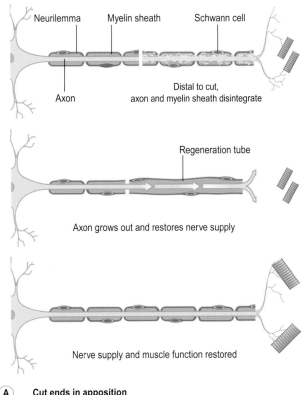

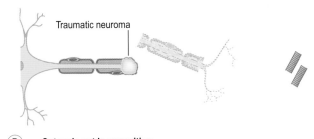

Figure 7.13 Regrowth of peripheral nerves following injury.

within the neurilemma providing a pathway within which the axon can regenerate.

Restoration of function depends on the re-establishment of satisfactory neural connections with the effector organ. When the neurilemma is out of position or destroyed, the sprouting axons and Schwann cells form a tumour-like cluster (*traumatic neuroma*) producing severe pain, e.g. following some fractures and amputation of limbs (Fig. 7.13B).

Neuroglial damage

Astrocytes. When these cells are damaged, their processes multiply forming a mesh or 'scar', which is thought to inhibit the regrowth of damaged CNS neurones.

Oligodendrocytes. These cells increase in number around degenerating neurones and are destroyed in demyelinating diseases such as *multiple sclerosis* (p. 185).

Microglia. Where there is inflammation and cell destruction the microglia increase in size and become phagocytic.

Central nervous system

The central nervous system consists of the brain and the spinal cord (see Fig. 7.1). These essential structures are both well protected from damage and injury; the brain is enclosed within the skull and the spinal cord by the vertebrae that form the spinal column. Membranous coverings known as the *meninges* provide further protection. The structure and functions of the meninges, brain and spinal cord are explored in this section.

The meninges and cerebrospinal fluid (CSF)

Learning outcomes

After studying this section, you should be able to:

■ describe the structure of the meninges

■ describe the flow of cerebrospinal fluid in the brain

■ list the functions of cerebrospinal fluid.

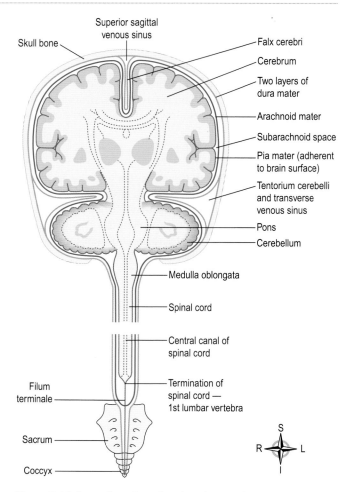

Figure 7.14 Frontal section showing the meninges covering the brain and spinal cord.

The meninges (Fig. 7.14)

The brain and spinal cord are completely surrounded by three layers of tissue, the *meninges*, lying between the skull and the brain, and between the vertebral foramina and the spinal cord. Named from outside inwards they are the:

- dura mater
- arachnoid mater
- pia mater.

The dura and arachnoid maters are separated by a potential space, the *subdural space*. The arachnoid and pia maters are separated by the *subarachnoid space*, containing *cerebrospinal fluid*.

Dura mater

The cerebral dura mater consists of two layers of dense fibrous tissue. The outer layer takes the place of the periosteum on the inner surface of the skull bones and the inner layer provides a protective covering for the brain. There is only a potential space between the two layers except where the inner layer sweeps inwards between the

cerebral hemispheres to form the *falx cerebri*; between the cerebellar hemispheres to form the *falx cerebelli*; and between the cerebrum and cerebellum to form the *tentorium cerebelli*.

Venous blood from the brain drains into venous sinuses between the two layers of dura mater. The *superior sagittal sinus* is formed by the falx cerebri, and the tentorium cerebelli forms the *straight* and *transverse sinuses* (see Figs 5.34 and 5.35, p. 106).

Spinal dura mater forms a loose sheath round the spinal cord, extending from the foramen magnum to the 2nd sacral vertebra. Thereafter it encloses the *filum terminale* and fuses with the periosteum of the coccyx. It is an extension of the inner layer of cerebral dura mater and is separated from the periosteum of the vertebrae and ligaments within the neural canal by the *epidural space* (see Fig. 7.26), containing blood vessels and areolar connective tissue. It is attached to the foramen magnum and by strands of fibrous tissue to the posterior longitudinal ligament at intervals along its length. Nerves entering and leaving the spinal cord pass through the epidural space. These attachments stabilise the spinal cord in the neural canal. Dyes, used for diagnostic purposes, and local anaesthetics or analgesics to relieve pain, may be injected into the epidural space.

Arachnoid mater

This is a layer of fibrous tissue that lies between the dura and pia maters. It is separated from the dura mater by the *subdural space* that contains a small amount of serous fluid, and from the pia mater by the *subarachnoid space*, which contains *cerebrospinal fluid*. The arachnoid mater passes over the convolutions of the brain and accompanies the inner layer of dura mater in the formation of the falx cerebri, tentorium cerebelli and falx cerebelli. It continues downwards to envelop the spinal cord and ends by merging with the dura mater at the level of the 2nd sacral vertebra.

Pia mater

This is a delicate layer of connective tissue containing many minute blood vessels. It adheres to the brain, completely covering the convolutions and dipping into each fissure. It continues downwards surrounding the spinal cord. Beyond the end of the cord it continues as the *filum terminale*, pierces the arachnoid tube and goes on, with the dura mater, to fuse with the periosteum of the coccyx.

Ventricles of the brain and the cerebrospinal fluid ▮7.5

The brain contains four irregular-shaped cavities, or *ventricles*, containing cerebrospinal fluid (CSF) (Fig. 7.15). They are:

- right and left lateral ventricles
- third ventricle
- fourth ventricle.

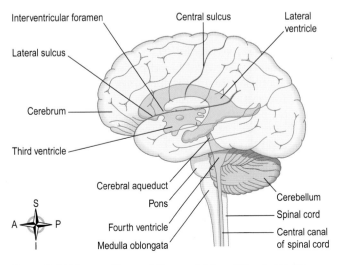

Interventricular foramen
Central sulcus
Lateral ventricle
Lateral sulcus
Cerebrum
Third ventricle
Cerebral aqueduct
Pons
Cerebellum
Spinal cord
Fourth ventricle
Central canal of spinal cord
Medulla oblongata

S
A — P
I

Figure 7.15 The positions of the ventricles of the brain (in blue) superimposed on its surface. Viewed from the left side.

The lateral ventricles

These cavities lie within the cerebral hemispheres, one on each side of the median plane just below the corpus callosum. They are separated from each other by a thin membrane, the septum lucidum, and are lined with ciliated epithelium. They communicate with the third ventricle by *interventricular foramina*.

The third ventricle

The third ventricle is a cavity situated below the lateral ventricles between the two parts of the thalamus. It communicates with the fourth ventricle by a canal, the *cerebral aqueduct*.

The fourth ventricle

The fourth ventricle is a diamond-shaped cavity situated below and behind the third ventricle, between the *cerebellum* and *pons*. It is continuous below with the *central canal* of the spinal cord and communicates with the subarachnoid space by foramina in its roof. Cerebrospinal fluid enters the subarachnoid space through these openings and through the open distal end of the central canal of the spinal cord.

Cerebrospinal fluid (CSF)

Cerebrospinal fluid is secreted into each ventricle of the brain by *choroid plexuses*. These are vascular areas where there is a proliferation of blood vessels surrounded by ependymal cells in the lining of ventricle walls. CSF passes back into the blood through tiny diverticula of arachnoid mater, called *arachnoid villi* (arachnoid granulations, Fig. 7.16), which project into the venous sinuses. The movement of CSF from the subarachnoid space to venous sinuses depends upon the difference in pressure on each side of the walls of the arachnoid villi, which act as one-way valves. When CSF pressure is higher than venous pressure, CSF is pushed into the blood and when the venous pressure is higher the arachnoid villi collapse, preventing the passage of blood constituents into the CSF. There may also be some reabsorption of CSF by cells in the walls of the ventricles.

From the roof of the fourth ventricle CSF flows through foramina into the subarachnoid space and completely surrounds the brain and spinal cord (Fig. 7.16). There is no intrinsic system of CSF circulation but its movement is aided by pulsating blood vessels, respiration and changes of posture.

CSF is secreted continuously at a rate of about 0.5 mL per minute, i.e. 720 mL per day. The volume remains fairly constant at about 150 mL, as absorption keeps pace with secretion. CSF pressure may be measured using a vertical tube attached to a *lumbar puncture* needle inserted into the subarachnoid space above or below the 4th lumbar vertebra (which is below the end of

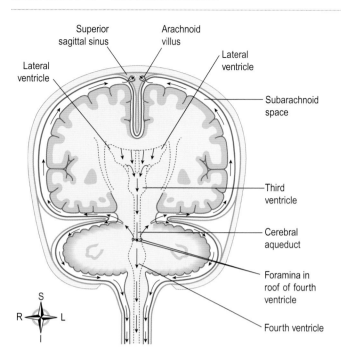

Figure 7.16 Frontal section of the skull with arrows showing the flow of cerebrospinal fluid.

the spinal cord). The pressure remains fairly constant at about 10 cm H_2O when lying on one side and about 30 cm H_2O when sitting up. If the brain is enlarged by, e.g., haemorrhage or tumour, some compensation is made by a reduction in the amount of CSF. When the volume of brain tissue is reduced, such as in degeneration or atrophy, the volume of CSF is increased. CSF is a clear, slightly alkaline fluid with a specific gravity of 1.005, consisting of:

- water
- mineral salts
- glucose
- plasma proteins: small amounts of albumin and globulin
- a few leukocytes
- creatinine ⎫
- urea   ⎬ small amounts

Functions of cerebrospinal fluid

CSF supports and protects the brain and spinal cord by maintaining a uniform pressure around these vital structures and acting as a cushion or shock absorber between the brain and the skull.

It keeps the brain and spinal cord moist and there may be exchange of nutrients and waste products between CSF and the interstitial fluid of the brain. CSF is thought to be involved in regulation of breathing as it bathes the surface of the medulla where the central respiratory chemoreceptors are located (Ch. 10).

Brain

> ### Learning outcomes
>
> After studying this section, you should be able to:
>
> - describe the blood supply to the brain
> - name the lobes and principal sulci of the brain
> - outline the functions of the cerebrum
> - identify the main sensory and motor areas of the cerebrum
> - outline the position and functions of the thalamus and hypothalamus
> - describe the position and functions of the midbrain, pons, medulla oblongata and reticular activating system
> - describe the structure and functions of the cerebellum.

The brain is a large organ weighing around 1.4 kg that lies within the cranial cavity. Its parts are (Fig. 7.17):

- cerebrum
- thalamus   ⎫
- hypothalamus   ⎬ the diencephalon
- midbrain
- pons   ⎫
- medulla oblongata ⎬ the brain stem
- cerebellum ▓ **7.6, 7.7**

Blood supply and venous drainage

The *circulus arteriosus* and its contributing arteries (see Fig. 5.31, p. 105) play a vital role in maintaining a constant supply of oxygen and glucose to the brain when the head is moved and also if a contributing artery is narrowed. The brain receives about 15% of the cardiac output, approximately 750 mL of blood per minute. Autoregulation keeps blood flow to the brain constant by adjusting the diameter of the arterioles across a wide range of arterial blood pressure (about 65–140 mmHg) with changes occurring only outside these limits.

Venous blood from the brain drains into the *dural venous sinuses* and then downwards into the *internal jugular veins* (see Figs 5.34 and 5.35, p. 106).

Cerebrum

This is the largest part of the brain and it occupies the anterior and middle cranial fossae (see Fig. 16.11, p. 398). It is divided by a deep cleft, the *longitudinal cerebral fissure*, into *right* and *left cerebral hemispheres*, each

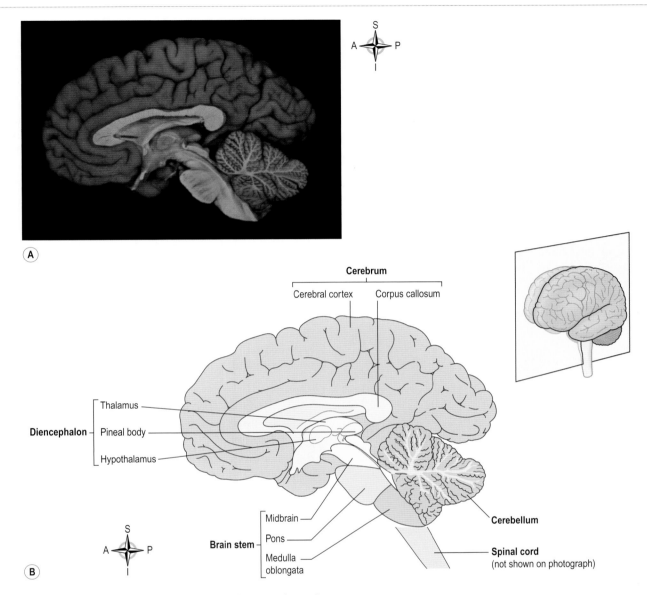

Figure 7.17 A midsaggital section of the brain showing the main parts.

containing one of the lateral ventricles. Deep within the brain, the hemispheres are connected by a mass of white matter (nerve fibres) called the *corpus callosum*. The falx cerebri is formed by the dura mater (see Fig. 7.14). It separates the two cerebral hemispheres and penetrates to the depth of the corpus callosum. The superficial part of the cerebrum is composed of nerve cell bodies (grey matter), forming the *cerebral cortex*, and the deeper layers consist of nerve fibres (axons, white matter).

The cerebral cortex shows many infoldings or furrows of varying depth. The exposed areas of the folds are the *gyri* (convolutions) and these are separated by *sulci* (fissures). These convolutions greatly increase the surface area of the cerebrum.

For descriptive purposes each hemisphere of the cerebrum is divided into *lobes* which take the names of the bones of the cranium under which they lie:

- frontal
- parietal
- temporal
- occipital.

The boundaries of the lobes are marked by deep sulci. These are the *central*, *lateral* and *parieto-occipital sulci* (Fig. 7.18).

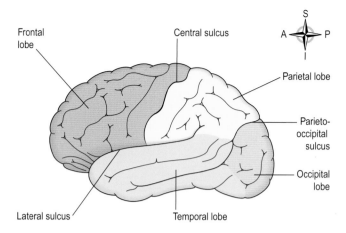

Figure 7.18 The lobes and principal sulci of the cerebrum. Viewed from the left side.

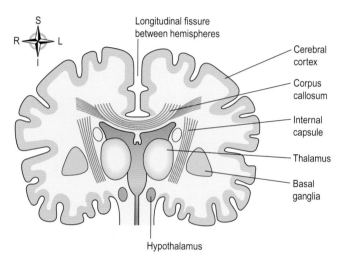

Figure 7.19 A frontal section of the cerebrum. Important tracts are shown in dark brown.

Cerebral tracts and basal ganglia (Fig. 7.19)

The surface of the cerebral cortex is composed of grey matter (nerve cell bodies). Within the cerebrum the lobes are connected by masses of nerve fibres, or *tracts*, which make up the white matter of the brain. The afferent and efferent fibres linking the different parts of the brain and spinal cord are as follows.

- *Association (arcuate) tracts* are most numerous and connect different parts of a cerebral hemisphere by extending from one gyrus to another, some of which are adjacent and some distant.
- *Commissural tracts* connect corresponding areas of the two cerebral hemispheres; the largest and most important commissure is the *corpus callosum*.
- *Projection tracts* connect the cerebral cortex with grey matter of lower parts of the brain and with the spinal cord, e.g. the internal capsule.

The *internal capsule* (Fig. 7.19) is an important projection tract that lies deep within the brain between the basal ganglia and the thalamus. Many nerve impulses passing to and from the cerebral cortex are carried by fibres that form the internal capsule. Motor fibres within the internal capsule form the *pyramidal tracts* (corticospinal tracts) that cross over (decussate) at the medulla oblongata and are the main pathway to skeletal muscles. Those motor fibres that do not pass through the internal capsule form the *extrapyramidal tracts* and have connections with many parts of the brain including the basal ganglia, thalamus and cerebellum.

Basal ganglia

The basal ganglia are groups of cell bodies that lie deep within the brain and form part of the extrapyramidal tracts. They act as relay stations with connections to many parts of the brain including motor areas of the cerebral cortex and thalamus. Their functions include initiation and fine control of complex movement and learned coordinated activities, such as posture and walking. If control is inadequate or absent, movements are jerky, clumsy and uncoordinated.

Functions of the cerebral cortex

There are three main types of activity associated with the cerebral cortex:

- higher order functions, i.e. the mental activities involved in memory, sense of responsibility, thinking, reasoning, moral decision making and learning
- sensory perception, including the perception of pain, temperature, touch, sight, hearing, taste and smell
- initiation and control of skeletal muscle contraction and therefore voluntary movement.

Functional areas of the cerebral cortex
(Fig. 7.20)

The main functional areas of the cerebral cortex have been identified but it is unlikely that any area is associated exclusively with only one function. Except where specially mentioned, the different areas are active in both hemispheres; however, there is some variation between individuals. There are different types of functional area:

- motor, which direct skeletal (voluntary) muscle movements
- sensory, which receive and decode sensory impulses enabling sensory perception
- association, which are concerned with integration and processing of complex mental functions such as intelligence, memory, reasoning, judgement and emotions.

In general, areas of the cortex lying anterior to the central sulcus are associated with motor functions,

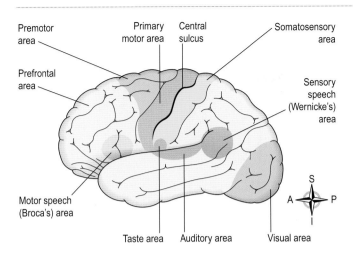

Figure 7.20 The cerebrum showing the main functional areas. Viewed from the left side.

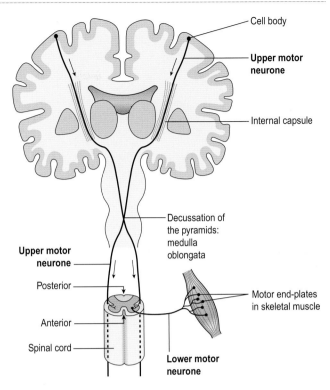

Figure 7.21 The motor nerve pathways: upper and lower motor neurones.

and those lying posterior to it are associated with sensory functions.

Motor areas of the cerebral cortex

The primary motor area. This lies in the frontal lobe immediately anterior to the central sulcus. The cell bodies are pyramid shaped (Betz's cells) and they control skeletal muscle activity. Two neurones involved in the pathway to skeletal muscle. The first, the *upper motor neurone,* descends from the motor cortex through the internal capsule to the medulla oblongata. Here it crosses to the opposite side and descends in the spinal cord. At the appropriate level in the spinal cord it synapses with a second neurone (the *lower motor neurone*), which leaves the spinal cord and travels to the target muscle. It terminates at the motor end plate of a muscle fibre (Fig. 7.21). This means that the motor area of the right hemisphere of the cerebrum controls voluntary muscle movement on the left side of the body and vice versa. Damage to either of these neurones may result in paralysis.

In the motor area of the cerebrum the body is represented upside down, i.e. the uppermost cells control the feet and those in the lowest part control the head, neck, face and fingers (Fig. 7.22A). The sizes of the areas of cortex representing different parts of the body are proportional to the complexity of movement of the body part, not to its size. Figure 7.22A shows that – in comparison with the trunk – the hand, foot, tongue and lips are represented by large cortical areas reflecting the greater degree of motor control associated with these areas.

Motor speech (Broca's) area. This is situated in the frontal lobe just above the lateral sulcus and controls the muscle movements needed for speech. It is dominant in the left hemisphere in right-handed people and vice versa.

Sensory areas of the cerebral cortex

The somatosensory area. This is the area immediately behind the central sulcus. Here sensations of pain, temperature, pressure and touch, awareness of muscular movement and the position of joints (proprioception) are perceived. The somatosensory area of the right hemisphere receives impulses from the left side of the body and vice versa. The size of the cortical areas representing different parts of the body (Fig. 7.22B) is proportional to the extent of sensory innervation, e.g. the large area for the face is consistent with the extensive sensory nerve supply by the three branches of the trigeminal nerves (5th cranial nerves).

The auditory (hearing) area. This lies immediately below the lateral sulcus within the temporal lobe. The nerve cells receive and interpret impulses transmitted from the inner ear by the cochlear (auditory) part of the vestibulocochlear nerves (8th cranial nerves).

The olfactory (smell) area. This lies deep within the temporal lobe where impulses from the nose, transmitted via the olfactory nerves (1st cranial nerves), are received and interpreted.

The taste area. This lies just above the lateral sulcus in the deep layers of the somatosensory area. Here, impulses from sensory receptors in taste buds are received and perceived as taste.

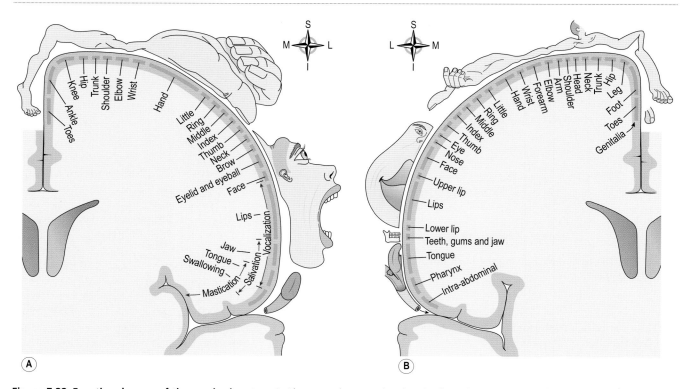

Figure 7.22 Functional areas of the cerebral cortex. A. The motor homunculus showing how the body is represented in the motor area of the cerebrum. **B.** The sensory homunculus showing how the body is represented in the sensory area of the cerebrum

The visual area. This lies behind the parieto-occipital sulcus and includes the greater part of the occipital lobe. The optic nerves (2nd cranial nerves) pass from the eye to this area, which receives and interprets the impulses as visual impressions.

Association areas

These are connected to each other and other areas of the cerebral cortex by association tracts and some are outlined below. They receive, coordinate and interpret impulses from the sensory and motor cortices permitting higher cognitive abilities and, although Figure 7.23 depicts some of the areas involved, their functions are much more complex.

The premotor area. This lies in the frontal lobe immediately anterior to the motor area. The neurones here coordinate movement initiated by the primary motor cortex, ensuring that learned patterns of movement can be repeated. For example, in tying a shoelace or writing, many muscles contract but the movements must be coordinated and carried out in a particular sequence. Such a pattern of movement, when established, is described as *manual dexterity*.

The prefrontal area. This extends anteriorly from the premotor area to include the remainder of the frontal lobe. It is a large area and is more highly developed in humans than in other animals. Intellectual functions controlled here include perception and comprehension of the

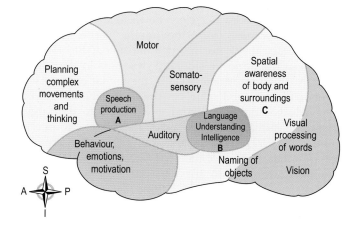

Figure 7.23 Areas of the cerebral cortex involved in higher mental functions. A. Motor speech (Broca's) area. **B.** Sensory speech (Wernicke's) area. **C.** Parieto-occipital area.

passage of time, the ability to anticipate consequences of events and the normal management of emotions.

Sensory speech (Wernicke's) area. This is situated in the temporal lobe adjacent to the parieto-occipitotemporal area. It is here that the spoken word is perceived, and comprehension and intelligence are based. Understanding language is central to higher mental functions as they are language based. This area is dominant in the left hemisphere in right-handed people and vice versa.

The parieto-occipitotemporal area This lies behind the somatosensory area and includes most of the parietal lobe. Its functions are thought to include spatial awareness, interpreting written language and the ability to name objects (Fig. 7.23). It has been suggested that objects can be recognised by touch alone because of the knowledge from past experience (memory) retained in this area.

Diencephalon (see Fig. 7.17)

This connects the cerebrum and the midbrain. It consists of several structures situated around the third ventricle, the main ones being the thalamus and hypothalamus, which are considered here. The pineal gland (p. 228) and the optic chiasma (p. 199) are situated there.

Thalamus

This consists of two masses of grey and white matter situated within the cerebral hemispheres just below the corpus callosum, one on each side of the third ventricle (Fig. 7.19). Sensory receptors in the skin and viscera send information about touch, pain and temperature, and input from the special sense organs travels to the thalamus where there is recognition, although only in a basic form, as refined perception also involves other parts of the brain. It is thought to be involved in the processing of some emotions and complex reflexes. The thalamus relays and redistributes impulses from most parts of the brain to the cerebral cortex.

Hypothalamus

The hypothalamus is a small but important structure which weighs around 7 g and consists of a number of nuclei. It is situated below and in front of the thalamus, immediately above the *pituitary gland*. The hypothalamus is linked to the posterior lobe of the pituitary gland by nerve fibres and to the anterior lobe by a complex system of blood vessels. Through these connections, the hypothalamus controls the output of hormones from both lobes of the pituitary gland (see p. 217).

Other functions of the hypothalamus include control of:

- the autonomic nervous system (p. 173)
- appetite and satiety
- thirst and water balance
- body temperature (p. 365)
- emotional reactions, e.g. pleasure, fear, rage
- sexual behaviour and child rearing
- sleeping and waking cycles.

Brain stem (Fig. 7.17)

Midbrain

The midbrain is the area of the brain situated around the cerebral aqueduct (see Fig. 7.15) between the cerebrum above and the *pons* below. It consists of nuclei and nerve fibres (tracts), which connect the cerebrum with lower parts of the brain and with the spinal cord. The nuclei act as relay stations for the ascending and descending nerve fibres and have important roles in auditory and visual reflexes.

Pons

The pons is situated in front of the cerebellum, below the midbrain and above the medulla oblongata. It consists mainly of nerve fibres (white matter) that form a bridge between the two hemispheres of the cerebellum, and of fibres passing between the higher levels of the brain and the spinal cord. There are nuclei within the pons that act as relay stations and some of these are associated with the cranial nerves. Others form the *pneumotaxic* and *apnoustic centres* that operate in conjunction with the respiratory centre in the medulla oblongata to control respiration (Ch. 10).

The anatomical structure of the pons differs from that of the cerebrum in that the cell bodies (grey matter) lie deeply and the nerve fibres are on the surface.

Medulla oblongata

The medulla oblongata, or simply the medulla, is the most interior region of the brain stem (see Fig. 7.24). Extending from the pons above, it is continuous with the spinal cord below (see Fig. 7.24). It is about 2.5 cm long and lies just within the cranium above the foramen magnum. Its anterior and posterior surfaces are marked by central fissures. The outer aspect is composed of white matter, which passes between the brain and the spinal cord, and grey matter, which lies centrally. Some cells constitute relay stations for sensory nerves passing from the spinal cord to the cerebrum.

The *vital centres*, consisting of groups of cell bodies (nuclei) associated with autonomic reflex activity, lie in its deeper structure. These are the:

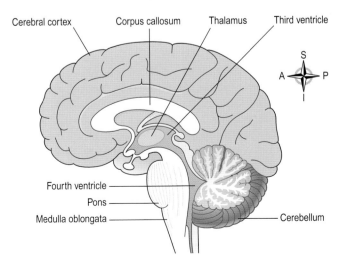

Figure 7.24 The cerebellum and associated structures.

159

- cardiovascular centre
- respiratory centre
- reflex centres of vomiting, coughing, sneezing and swallowing.

The medulla oblongata has several special features.

Decussation (crossing) of the pyramids. In the medulla, motor nerves descending from the motor area in the cerebrum to the spinal cord in the pyramidal (corticospinal) tracts cross from one side to the other. This means that the left hemisphere of the cerebrum controls the right half of the body, and vice versa. These tracts are the main pathway to skeletal (voluntary) muscles.

Sensory decussation. Some of the sensory nerves ascending to the cerebrum from the spinal cord cross from one side to the other in the medulla. Others decussate lower down in the spinal cord.

The cardiovascular centre (CVC). This area controls the rate and force of cardiac contraction (p. 97). It also controls blood pressure (p. 97). Within the CVC, other groups of nerve cells forming the *vasomotor centre* (p. 84) control the diameter of the blood vessels, especially the small arteries and arterioles. The vasomotor centre is stimulated by the arterial baroreceptors, body temperature and emotions such as sexual excitement and anger. Pain usually causes vasoconstriction although severe pain may cause vasodilation, a fall in blood pressure and fainting.

The respiratory centre. This area controls the rate and depth of respiration. From here, nerve impulses pass to the phrenic and intercostal nerves which stimulate contraction of the diaphragm and intercostal muscles, thus initiating inspiration. It functions in close association with the pnuemotaxic and apneustic centres in the pons (see p. 260).

Reflex centres. Irritants present in the stomach or respiratory tract stimulate the medulla oblongata, activating the reflex centres. Vomiting, coughing and sneezing are protective reflexes that attempt to expel irritants.

Reticular formation

The reticular formation is a collection of neurones in the core of the brain stem, surrounded by neural pathways that conduct ascending and descending nerve impulses between the brain and the spinal cord. It has a vast number of synaptic links with other parts of the brain and is therefore constantly receiving 'information' being transmitted in ascending and descending tracts.

Functions
The reticular formation is involved in:

- coordination of skeletal muscle activity associated with voluntary motor movement and the maintenance of balance

- coordination of activity controlled by the autonomic nervous system, e.g. cardiovascular, respiratory and gastrointestinal activity (p. 173)
- selective awareness that functions through the *reticular activating system* (RAS), which selectively blocks or passes sensory information to the cerebral cortex, e.g. the slight sound made by a sick child moving in bed may arouse the mother but the noise of regularly passing trains does not disturb her.

Cerebellum

The cerebellum (Fig. 7.24) is situated behind the pons and immediately below the posterior portion of the cerebrum occupying the posterior cranial fossa. It is ovoid in shape and has two hemispheres, separated by a narrow median strip called the *vermis*. Grey matter forms the surface of the cerebellum, and the white matter lies deeply.

Functions
The cerebellum is concerned with the coordination of voluntary muscular movement, posture and balance. Cerebellar activity is not under voluntary control. The cerebellum controls and coordinates the movements of various groups of muscles ensuring smooth, even, precise actions. It coordinates activities associated with the *maintenance of posture, balance* and *equilibrium*. The sensory input for these functions is derived from the muscles and joints, the eyes and the ears. *Proprioceptor impulses* from the muscles and joints indicate their position in relation to the body as a whole; impulses from the eyes and the semicircular canals in the ears provide information about the position of the head in space. The cerebellum integrates this information to regulate skeletal muscle activity so that balance and posture are maintained.

The cerebellum may also have a role in learning and language processing.

Damage to the cerebellum results in clumsy uncoordinated muscular movement, staggering gait and inability to carry out smooth, steady, precise movements.

Spinal cord

Learning outcomes

After studying this section, you should be able to:

- describe the gross structure of the spinal cord

- state the functions of the sensory (afferent) and motor (efferent) nerve tracts in the spinal cord

- explain the events of a simple reflex arc.

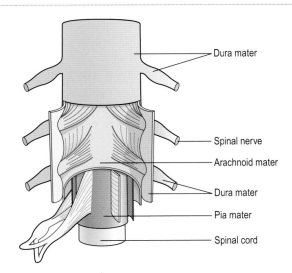

Figure 7.25 The meninges covering the spinal cord. Each cut away to show the underlying layers.

The spinal cord is the elongated, almost cylindrical part of the central nervous system, which is suspended in the vertebral canal surrounded by the meninges and cerebrospinal fluid (Fig. 7.25). The meninges are described on page 152. The spinal cord is continuous above with the medulla oblongata and extends from the upper border of the atlas (first cervical vertebra) to the lower border of the 1st lumbar vertebra (Fig. 7.26). It is approximately 45 cm long in adult males, and is about the thickness of the little finger. A specimen of cerebrospinal fluid can be taken using a procedure called *lumbar puncture* (p. 153).

Except for the cranial nerves, the spinal cord is the nervous tissue link between the brain and the rest of the body (Fig. 7.27). Nerves conveying impulses from the brain to the various organs and tissues descend through the spinal cord. At the appropriate level they leave the cord and pass to the structure they supply. Similarly, sensory nerves from organs and tissues enter and pass upwards in the spinal cord to the brain.

Some activities of the spinal cord are independent of the brain and are controlled at the level of the spinal cord by *spinal reflexes*. To facilitate these, there are extensive neurone connections between sensory and motor neurones at the same or different levels in the cord.

The spinal cord is incompletely divided into two equal parts, anteriorly by a short, shallow *median fissure* and posteriorly by a deep narrow septum, the *posterior median septum*.

A cross-section of the spinal cord shows that it is composed of grey matter in the centre surrounded by white matter supported by neuroglia. Figure 7.28 shows the parts of the spinal cord and the nerve roots on one side. The other side is the same. ▉▉ **7.8**

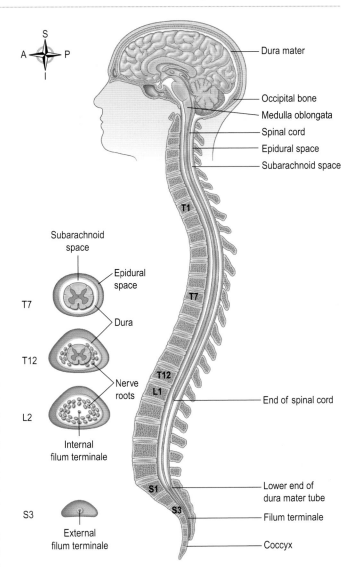

Figure 7.26 Sections of the vertebral canal showing the epidural space.

Grey matter

The arrangement of grey matter in the spinal cord resembles the shape of the letter H, having *two posterior, two anterior* and *two lateral columns*. The area of grey matter lying transversely is the *transverse commissure* and it is pierced by the central canal, an extension from the fourth ventricle, containing cerebrospinal fluid. The nerve cell bodies may belong to:

- *sensory neurones*, which receive impulses from the periphery of the body
- *lower motor neurones*, which transmit impulses to the skeletal muscles
- *connector neurones*, also known as interneurones linking sensory and motor neurones, at the same or different levels, which form spinal reflex arcs.

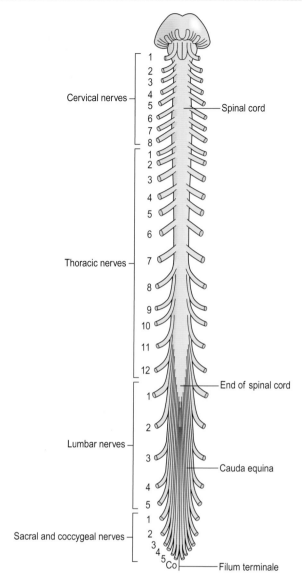

Cervical nerves
1
2
3
4
5
6
7
8

Spinal cord

Thoracic nerves
1
2
3
4
5
6
7
8
9
10
11
12

End of spinal cord

Lumbar nerves
1
2
3
4
5

Cauda equina

Sacral and coccygeal nerves
1
2
3
4
5
Co

Filum terminale

Figure 7.27 The spinal cord and spinal nerves.

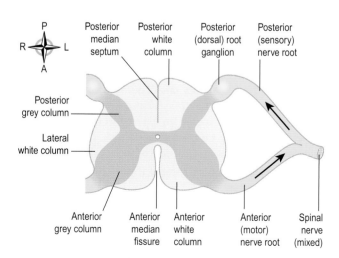

P
R — L
A

Posterior median septum
Posterior white column
Posterior (dorsal) root ganglion
Posterior (sensory) nerve root

Posterior grey column

Lateral white column

Anterior grey column
Anterior median fissure
Anterior white column
Anterior (motor) nerve root
Spinal nerve (mixed)

Figure 7.28 A transverse section of the spinal cord showing nerve roots on one side.

At each point where nerve impulses are transmitted from one neurone to another, there is a synapse (p. 147).

Posterior columns of grey matter

These are composed of cell bodies that are stimulated by sensory impulses from the periphery of the body. The nerve fibres of these cells contribute to the white matter of the cord and transmit the sensory impulses upwards to the brain.

Anterior columns of grey matter

These are composed of the cell bodies of the lower motor neurones that are stimulated by the upper motor neurones or the connector neurones linking the anterior and posterior columns to form reflex arcs.

The *posterior root* (*spinal*) *ganglia* are formed by the cell bodies of the sensory nerves.

White matter

The white matter of the spinal cord is arranged in three *columns* or *tracts*; anterior, posterior and lateral. These tracts are formed by sensory nerve fibres ascending to the brain, motor nerve fibres descending from the brain and fibres of connector neurones.

Tracts are often named according to their points of origin and destination, e.g. spinothalamic, corticospinal.

Sensory nerve tracts in the spinal cord

Neurones that transmit impulses towards the brain are called sensory (afferent, ascending). There are two main sources of sensation transmitted to the brain via the spinal cord.

1. *The skin.* Sensory receptors (nerve endings) in the skin are stimulated by pain, heat, cold and touch, including pressure (see Ch. 14). The nerve impulses generated are conducted by three neurones to the sensory area in the *opposite hemisphere of the cerebrum* where the sensation and its location are perceived (Fig. 7.29). Crossing to the other side, or decussation, occurs either at the level of entry into the cord or in the medulla.
2. *The tendons, muscles and joints.* Sensory receptors are specialised nerve endings in these structures, called *proprioceptors*, and they are stimulated by stretch. Together with impulses from the eyes and the ears, they are associated with the maintenance of balance and posture, and with perception of the position of the body in space. These nerve impulses have two destinations:
   - by a three-neurone system, the impulses reach the sensory area of the *opposite hemisphere of the cerebrum*
   - by a two-neurone system, the nerve impulses reach the *cerebellar hemisphere on the same side*.

Table 7.1 summarises the main sensory pathways.

Motor nerve tracts in the spinal cord

Neurones that transmit nerve impulses away from the brain are motor (efferent or descending) neurones. Stimulation of the motor neurones results in:

- contraction of skeletal (voluntary) muscle, or
- contraction of smooth (involuntary) muscle, cardiac muscle and the secretion by glands controlled by nerves of the autonomic nervous system (p. 173).

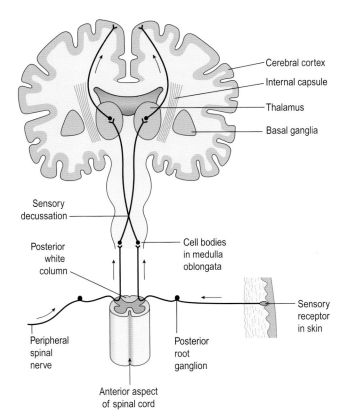

Figure 7.29 A sensory nerve pathway from the skin to the cerebrum.

Voluntary muscle movement

The contraction of muscles that move the joints is, in the main, under conscious (voluntary) control, which means that the stimulus to contract originates at the level of consciousness in the cerebrum. However, skeletal muscle activity is regulated by output from the midbrain, brain stem and cerebellum. This involuntary activity is associated with coordination of muscle activity, e.g. when very fine movement is required and in the maintenance of posture and balance.

Efferent nerve impulses are transmitted from the brain to other parts of the body via bundles of nerve fibres (tracts) in the spinal cord. The *motor pathways* from the brain to the muscles are made up of two neurones (see Fig. 7.21). These pathways, or tracts, are either:

- pyramidal (corticospinal), or
- extrapyramidal (p. 156).

The upper motor neurone. This has its cell body (Betz's cell) in the primary motor area of the cerebrum. The axons pass through the internal capsule, pons and medulla. In the spinal cord they form the lateral corticospinal tracts of white matter and the fibres synapse with the cell bodies of the lower motor neurones in the anterior columns of grey matter. The axons of the upper motor neurones make up the pyramidal tracts and decussate in the medulla oblongata, forming the pyramids.

The lower motor neurone. This has its cell body in the anterior horn of grey matter in the spinal cord. Its axon emerges from the spinal cord by the anterior root, joins with the incoming sensory fibres and forms the mixed spinal nerve that passes through the intervertebral foramen. Near its termination in skeletal muscle the axon branches into many tiny fibres, each of which is in close association with a sensitive area on the muscle fibre membrane known as a *motor end plate* (Figs 16.56 and 16.57, p. 422). The motor end plates of each nerve and the

---

Table 7.1 Sensory nerve impulses: origins, routes, destinations

Receptor	Route	Destination
Pain, touch, temperature	Neurone 1 – to spinal cord by posterior root Neurone 2 – decussation on entering spinal cord then in anterolateral spinothalamic tract to thalamus Neurone 3 –	to parietal lobe of cerebrum
Touch, proprioceptors	Neurone 1 – to medulla in posterior spinothalamic tract Neurone 2 – decussation in medulla, transmission to thalamus Neurone 3 –	to parietal lobe of cerebrum
Proprioceptors	Neurone 1 – to spinal cord Neurone 2 –	no decussation, to cerebellum in posterior spinocerebellar tract

muscle fibres they supply form a *motor unit*. The neurotransmitter that transmits the nerve impulse across the neuromuscular junction (synapse) to stimulate a skeletal muscle fibre is *acetylcholine*. Motor units contract as a whole and the strength of the muscle contraction depends on the number of motor units in action at any time.

The lower motor neurone is the *final common pathway* for the transmission of nerve impulses to skeletal muscles. The cell body of this neurone is influenced by a number of upper motor neurones originating from various sites in the brain and by some neurones which begin and end in the spinal cord. Some of these neurones stimulate the cell bodies of the lower motor neurone while others have an inhibiting effect. The outcome of these influences is smooth, coordinated muscle movement, some of which is voluntary and some involuntary.

Involuntary muscle movement

Upper motor neurones. These have their cell bodies in the brain at a level *below* the cerebrum, i.e. in the midbrain, brain stem, cerebellum or spinal cord. They influence muscle activity that maintains posture and balance, coordinates skeletal muscle movement and controls muscle tone.

Table 7.2 shows details of the area of origin of these neurones and the tracts which their axons form before reaching the cell body of the lower motor neurone in the spinal cord.

Spinal reflexes. These consist of three elements:

- sensory neurones
- connector neurones (or interneurones) in the spinal cord
- lower motor neurones. 7.9

In the simplest *reflex arc* there is only one of each type of the neurones above (Fig. 7.30). A *reflex action* is an involuntary and immediate motor response to a sensory stimulus. Many connector and motor neurones may be stimulated by afferent impulses from a small area of skin. For example, the pain impulses initiated by touching a very hot surface with the finger are transmitted to the spinal cord by sensory fibres in mixed nerves. These stimulate many connector and lower motor neurones in the spinal cord, which results in the contraction of many skeletal muscles of the hand, arm and shoulder, and the removal of the finger. Reflex action happens very quickly; in fact, the motor response may occur simultaneously with the perception of the pain in the cerebrum. Reflexes of this type are invariably protective but they can occasionally be inhibited. For example, if a precious plate is very hot when lifted every effort will be made to overcome the pain to prevent dropping it!

Stretch reflexes. Only two neurones are involved. The cell body of the lower motor neurone is stimulated directly by the sensory neurone, with no connector neurone in between (Fig. 7.30). The *knee jerk* is one example, but this type of reflex can be demonstrated at any point where a stretched tendon crosses a joint. By tapping the tendon just below the knee when it is bent, the sensory nerve endings in the tendon and in the thigh muscles are stretched. This initiates a nerve impulse that passes into the spinal cord to the cell body of the lower motor neurone in the anterior column of grey matter on the same side. As a result the thigh muscles suddenly contract and the foot kicks forward. This is used as a test of the integrity of the reflex arc. This type of reflex also has a protective function – it prevents excessive joint movement that may damage tendons, ligaments and muscles.

Autonomic reflexes. These include the pupillary light reflex when the pupil immediately constricts, in response to bright light, preventing retinal damage.

Table 7.2 Extrapyramidal upper motor neurones: origins and tracts

Origin	Name of tract	Site in spinal cord	Functions
Midbrain and pons	Rubrospinal tract decussates in brain stem	Lateral column	Control of skilled muscle movement
Reticular formation	Reticulospinal tract does not decussate	Lateral column	Coordination of muscle movement
Midbrain and pons	Tectospinal tract decussates in midbrain	Anterior colum	Maintenance of posture and balance
Midbrain and pons	Vestibulospinal tract, some fibres decussate in the cord	Anterior column	

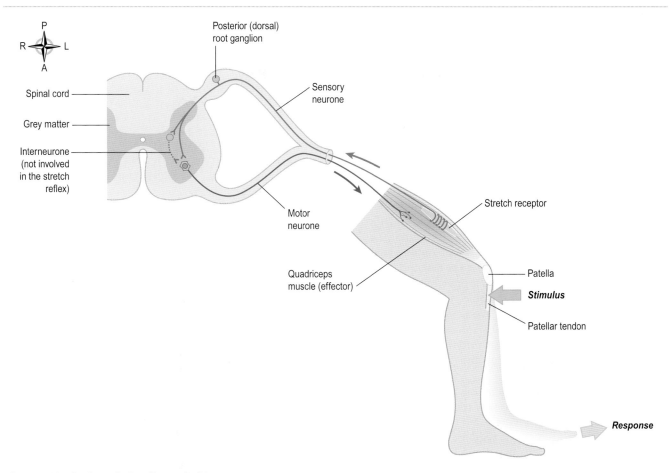

Figure 7.30 The knee jerk reflex. Left side.

Peripheral nervous system

Learning outcomes

After studying this section, you should be able to:

- outline the function of a nerve plexus

- list the spinal nerves entering each plexus and the main nerves emerging from it

- describe the areas innervated by the thoracic nerves

- outline the functions of the 12 cranial nerves

- compare and contrast the structures and neurotransmitters of the divisions of the autonomic nervous system

- compare and contrast the effects of stimulation of the divisions of the autonomic nervous system on body function.

This part of the nervous system consists of:

- 31 pairs of spinal nerves that originate from the spinal cord

- 12 pairs of cranial nerves, which originate from the brain
- the autonomic nervous system.

Most of the nerves of the peripheral nervous system are composed of sensory fibres that transmit afferent impulses from sensory organs to the brain, or motor nerve fibres that transmit efferent impulses from the brain to the effector organs, e.g. skeletal muscles, smooth muscle and glands.

Spinal nerves

Thirty-one pairs of spinal nerves leave the vertebral canal by passing through the intervertebral foramina formed by adjacent vertebrae. They are named and grouped according to the vertebrae with which they are associated (see Fig. 7.27):

- 8 cervical
- 12 thoracic
- 5 lumbar
- 5 sacral
- 1 coccygeal.

Although there are only seven cervical vertebrae, there are eight nerves because the first pair leaves the vertebral canal between the occipital bone and the atlas (first cervical vertebra) and the eighth pair leaves below the last cervical vertebra. Thereafter the nerves are given the name and number of the vertebra immediately *above*.

The lumbar, sacral and coccygeal nerves leave the spinal cord near its termination, at the level of the 1st lumbar vertebra, and extend downwards inside the vertebral canal in the subarachnoid space, forming a sheaf of nerves which resembles a horse's tail, the *cauda equina* (see Fig. 7.27). These nerves leave the vertebral canal at the appropriate lumbar, sacral or coccygeal level, depending on their destination.

Nerve roots (Fig. 7.31)

The spinal nerves arise from both sides of the spinal cord and emerge through the intervertebral foramina (see Fig 16.26, p. 404). Each nerve is formed by the union of a *motor* (anterior) and a *sensory* (posterior) *nerve root* and is, therefore, a *mixed nerve*. Thoracic and upper lumbar (L1 and L2) spinal nerves have a contribution from the sympathetic part of the autonomic nervous system in the form of a *preganglionic fibre* (neurone).

Chapter 16 describes the bones and muscles mentioned in the following sections. Bones and joints are supplied by adjacent nerves.

The *anterior nerve root* consists of motor nerve fibres, which are the axons of the lower motor neurones from the anterior column of grey matter in the spinal cord and, in the thoracic and lumbar regions, *sympathetic nerve fibres*, which are the axons of cells in the lateral columns of grey matter.

The *posterior nerve root* consists of sensory nerve fibres. Just outside the spinal cord there is a *spinal ganglion* (posterior, or dorsal, root ganglion), consisting of a little cluster of cell bodies. Sensory nerve fibres pass through these ganglia before entering the spinal cord. The area of skin whose sensory receptors contribute to each nerve is called a *dermatome* (see Figs 7.36 and 7.39).

For a very short distance after leaving the spinal cord the nerve roots have a covering of *dura* and *arachnoid maters*. These terminate before the two roots join to form the mixed spinal nerve. The nerve roots have no covering of pia mater.

Branches

Immediately after emerging from the intervertebral foramen, spinal nerves divide into branches, or *rami*: a ramus communicans, a posterior ramus and an anterior ramus.

The *rami communicante* are part of preganglionic sympathetic neurones of the autonomic nervous system (p. 173).

The *posterior rami* pass backwards and divide into smaller medial and lateral branches to supply skin and muscles of relatively small areas of the posterior aspect of the head, neck and trunk.

The *anterior rami* supply the anterior and lateral aspects of the neck, trunk and the upper and lower limbs.

Plexuses

In the cervical, lumbar and sacral regions the anterior rami unite near their origins to form large masses of nerves, or *plexuses*, where nerve fibres are regrouped and rearranged before proceeding to supply skin, bones, muscles and joints of a particular area (Fig. 7.32). This means that these structures have a nerve supply from more than one spinal nerve and therefore damage to one spinal nerve does not cause loss of function of a region. Moreover, they lie deep within the body, often under large muscles, and are therefore well protected from injury.

In the thoracic region the anterior rami do not form plexuses.

There are five large plexuses of mixed nerves formed on each side of the vertebral column. They are the:

- cervical plexuses
- brachial plexuses
- lumbar plexuses
- sacral plexuses
- coccygeal plexuses.

Cervical plexus (Fig. 7.33)

This is formed by the anterior rami of the first four cervical nerves. It lies deep within the neck opposite the 1st, 2nd, 3rd and 4th cervical vertebrae under the protection of the sternocleidomastoid muscle.

The superficial branches supply the structures at the back and side of the head and the skin of the front of the neck to the level of the sternum.

The deep branches supply muscles of the neck, e.g. the sternocleidomastoid and the trapezius.

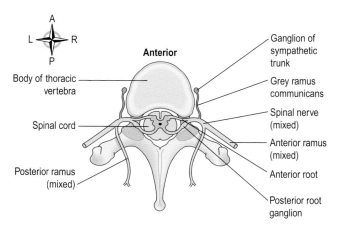

Figure 7.31 The relationship between sympathetic and mixed spinal nerves. Sympathetic nerves in green.

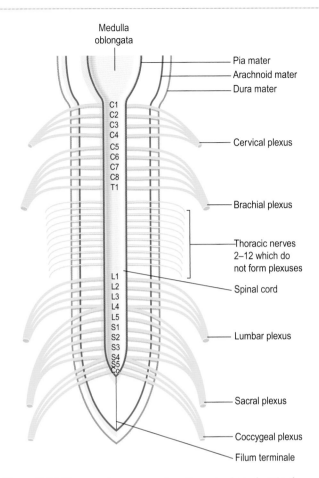

Figure 7.32 The meninges covering the spinal cord, spinal nerves and the plexuses they form.

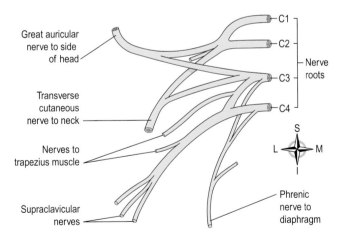

Figure 7.33 The cervical plexus. Anterior view.

The phrenic nerve originates from cervical nerve roots 3, 4 and 5 and passes downwards through the thoracic cavity in front of the root of the lung to supply the diaphragm, initiating inspiration. Disease or spinal cord injury at this level will result in death due to apnoea without assisted ventilation as spontaneous respiration is not possible.

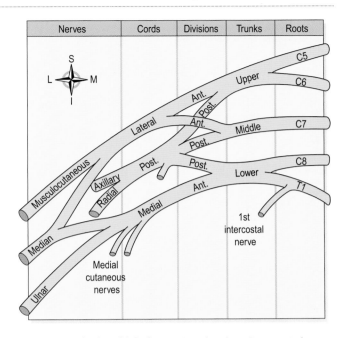

Figure 7.34 The brachial plexus. Anterior view. Ant = anterior, Post = posterior.

Brachial plexus

The anterior rami of the lower four cervical nerves and a large part of the 1st thoracic nerve form the brachial plexus. Figure 7.34 shows its formation and the nerves that emerge from it. The plexus is situated deeply within the neck and shoulder above and behind the subclavian vessels and in the axilla.

The branches of the brachial plexus supply the skin and muscles of the upper limbs and some of the chest muscles. Five large nerves and a number of smaller ones emerge from this plexus, each with a contribution from more than one nerve root, containing sensory, motor and autonomic fibres:

- axillary (circumflex) nerve: C5, 6
- radial nerve: C5, 6, 7, 8, T1
- musculocutaneous nerve: C5, 6, 7
- median nerve: C5, 6, 7, 8, T1
- ulnar nerve: C7, 8, T1
- medial cutaneous nerve: C8, T1.

The axillary (circumflex) nerve winds round the humerus at the level of the surgical neck. It then divides into minute branches to supply the deltoid muscle, shoulder joint and overlying skin.

The radial nerve is the largest branch of the brachial plexus. It supplies the triceps muscle behind the humerus, crosses in front of the elbow joint then winds round to the back of the forearm to supply extensor muscles of the wrist and finger joints. It continues into the back of the hand to supply the skin of the posterior aspect of the thumb, first two fingers and the lateral half of the third finger.

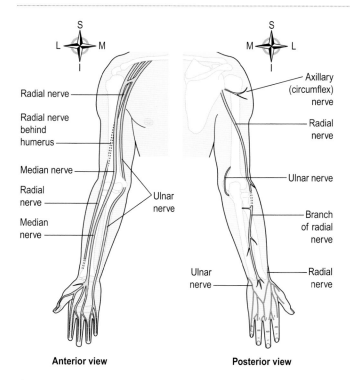

Figure 7.35 The main nerves of the arm.

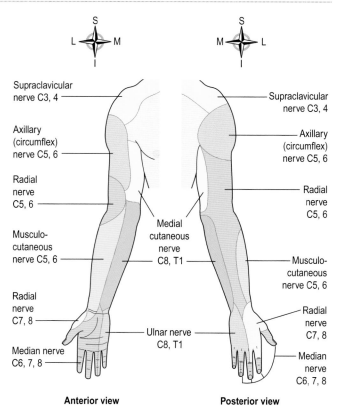

Figure 7.36 The distribution and origins of the cutaneous nerves of the arm. Colour distinguishes the dermatomes.

The musculocutaneous nerve passes downwards to the lateral aspect of the forearm. It supplies the muscles of the upper arm and the skin of the forearm.

The *median nerve* passes down the midline of the arm in close association with the brachial artery. It passes in front of the elbow joint then down to supply the muscles of the front of the forearm. It continues into the hand where it supplies small muscles and the skin of the front (palmar aspect) of the thumb, first two fingers and the lateral half of the third finger. It gives off no branches above the elbow.

The ulnar nerve descends through the upper arm lying medial to the brachial artery. It passes behind the medial epicondyle of the humerus to supply the muscles on the ulnar aspect of the forearm. It continues downwards to supply the muscles in the palm of the hand and the skin of the whole of the little finger and the medial half of the third finger. It gives off no branches above the elbow.

The main nerves of the arm are shown in Figure 7.35. The distribution and origins of the cutaneous sensory nerves of the arm, i.e. the dermatomes, are shown in Figure 7.36.

Lumbar plexus (Figs 7.37–7.39)

The lumbar plexus is formed by the anterior rami of the first three and part of the 4th lumbar nerves. The plexus is situated in front of the transverse processes of the lumbar vertebrae and behind the psoas muscle. The main branches and their nerve roots are:

- iliohypogastric nerve: L1
- ilioinguinal nerve: L1
- genitofemoral: L1, 2
- lateral cutaneous nerve of thigh: L2, 3
- femoral nerve: L2, 3, 4
- obturator nerve: L2, 3, 4
- lumbosacral trunk: L4, (5).

The iliohypogastric, ilioinguinal and *genitofemoral nerves* supply muscles and the skin in the area of the lower abdomen, upper and medial aspects of the thigh and the inguinal region.

The lateral cutaneous nerve of the thigh supplies the skin of the lateral aspect of the thigh including part of the anterior and posterior surfaces.

The femoral nerve is one of the larger branches. It passes behind the inguinal ligament to enter the thigh in close association with the femoral artery. It divides into cutaneous and muscular branches to supply the skin and the muscles of the front of the thigh. One branch, the *saphenous nerve*, supplies the medial aspect of the leg, ankle and foot.

The obturator nerve supplies the adductor muscles of the thigh and skin of the medial aspect of the thigh. It ends just above the level of the knee joint.

The lumbosacral trunk descends into the pelvis and makes a contribution to the sacral plexus.

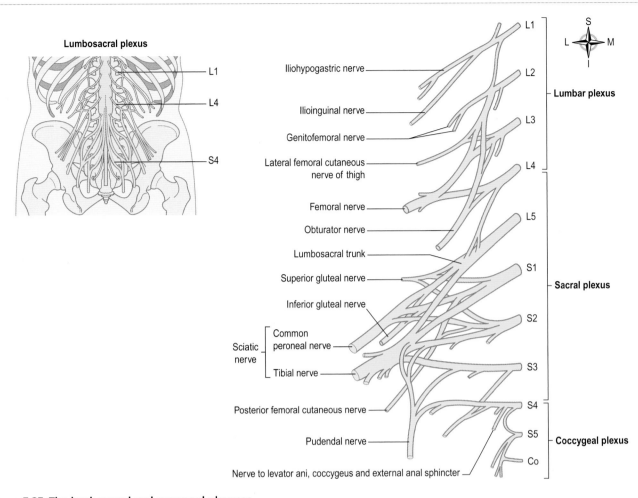

Lumbosacral plexus

L1
L4
S4

L1
L2
Lumbar plexus
L3
L4
L5
S1
Sacral plexus
S2
S3
S4
S5
Coccygeal plexus
Co

Iliohypogastric nerve
Ilioinguinal nerve
Genitofemoral nerve
Lateral femoral cutaneous nerve of thigh
Femoral nerve
Obturator nerve
Lumbosacral trunk
Superior gluteal nerve
Inferior gluteal nerve
Sciatic nerve
Common peroneal nerve
Tibial nerve
Posterior femoral cutaneous nerve
Pudendal nerve
Nerve to levator ani, coccygeus and external anal sphincter

Figure 7.37 The lumbosacral and coccygeal plexuses.

Sacral plexus (Figs 7.37–7.39)

The sacral plexus is formed by the anterior rami of the lumbosacral trunk and the 1st, 2nd and 3rd sacral nerves. The lumbosacral trunk is formed by the 5th and part of the 4th lumbar nerves. It lies in the posterior wall of the pelvic cavity.

The sacral plexus divides into a number of branches, supplying the muscles and skin of the pelvic floor, muscles around the hip joint and the pelvic organs. In addition to these it provides the sciatic nerve, which contains fibres from L4 and 5 and S1–3.

The *sciatic nerve* is the largest nerve in the body. It is about 2 cm wide at its origin. It passes through the greater sciatic foramen into the buttock then descends through the posterior aspect of the thigh supplying the hamstring muscles. At the level of the middle of the femur it divides to form the *tibial* and the *common peroneal nerves*.

The *tibial nerve* descends through the popliteal fossa to the posterior aspect of the leg where it supplies muscles and skin. It passes under the medial malleolus to supply muscles and skin of the sole of the foot and toes.

One of the main branches is the *sural nerve*, which supplies the tissues in the area of the heel, the lateral aspect of the ankle and a part of the dorsum of the foot.

The *common peroneal nerve* descends obliquely along the lateral aspect of the popliteal fossa, winds round the neck of the fibula into the front of the leg where it divides into the *deep peroneal* (anterior tibial) and the *superficial peroneal* (musculocutaneous) *nerves*. These nerves supply the skin and muscles of the anterior aspect of the leg and the dorsum of the foot and toes.

The *pudendal nerve* (S2, 3, 4) – the perineal branch supplies the external anal sphincter, the external urethral sphincter and adjacent skin. Figures 7.38 and 7.39 show the main nerves of the leg, the dermatomes and the origins of the main nerves.

Coccygeal plexus (Fig. 7.37)

The coccygeal plexus is a very small plexus formed by part of the 4th and 5th sacral and the coccygeal nerves. The nerves from this plexus supply the skin around the coccyx and anal area.

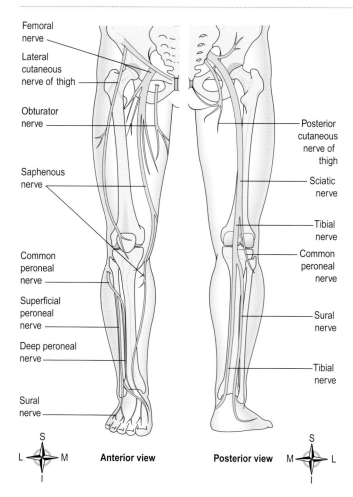

Femoral
nerve

Lateral
cutaneous
nerve of thigh

Obturator
nerve

Saphenous
nerve

Common
peroneal
nerve

Superficial
peroneal
nerve

Deep peroneal
nerve

Sural
nerve

Posterior
cutaneous
nerve of
thigh

Sciatic
nerve

Tibial
nerve

Common
peroneal
nerve

Sural
nerve

Tibial
nerve

Anterior view   **Posterior view**

Figure 7.38 The main nerves of the leg.

Thoracic nerves

The thoracic nerves *do not* intermingle to form plexuses. There are 12 pairs and the first 11 are the *intercostal nerves*. They pass between the ribs supplying them, the intercostal muscles and overlying skin. The 12th pair comprises the *subcostal nerves*. The 7th–12th thoracic nerves also supply the muscles and the skin of the posterior and anterior abdominal walls.

Cranial nerves (Fig. 7.40) ▮ 7.10

There are 12 pairs of cranial nerves originating from nuclei in the inferior surface of the brain, some sensory, some motor and some mixed. Their names suggest their distribution or function, which, in the main, is generally related to the head and neck. They are numbered using Roman numerals according to the order they connect to the brain, starting anteriorly. They are:

   I. Olfactory: sensory
  II. Optic: sensory
 III. Oculomotor: motor
 IV. Trochlear: motor

   V. Trigeminal: mixed
  VI. Abducens: motor
 VII. Facial: mixed
VIII. Vestibulocochlear (auditory): sensory
 IX. Glossopharyngeal: mixed
  X. Vagus: mixed
 XI. Accessory: motor
 XII. Hypoglossal: motor.

I. Olfactory nerves (sensory)

These are the nerves of the *sense of smell*. Their sensory receptors and nerve fibres originate in the upper part of the mucous membrane of the nasal cavity, pass upwards through the cribriform plate of the ethmoid bone and then pass to the *olfactory bulb* (see Fig. 8.23, p. 206). The nerves then proceed backwards as the olfactory tract, to the area for the perception of smell in the temporal lobe of the cerebrum (Ch. 8).

II. Optic nerves (sensory)

These are the nerves of the *sense of sight*. Their fibres originate in the retinae of the eyes and they combine to form the optic nerves (see Fig. 8.13, p. 199). They are directed backwards and medially through the posterior part of the orbital cavity. They then pass through the *optic foramina* of the sphenoid bone into the cranial cavity and join at the *optic chiasma*. The nerves proceed backwards as the *optic tracts* to the *lateral geniculate bodies* of the thalamus. Impulses pass from there to the visual areas in the occipital lobes of the cerebrum and to the cerebellum. In the occipital lobe sight is perceived, and in the cerebellum the impulses from the eyes contribute to the maintenance of balance, posture and orientation of the head in space.

III. Oculomotor nerves (motor)

These nerves arise from nuclei near the cerebral aqueduct. They supply:

- four of the six extrinsic muscles, which move the eyeball, i.e. the *superior*, *medial* and *inferior recti* and the *inferior oblique muscle* (see Table 8.1, p. 204)
- the intrinsic (intraocular) muscles:
  - *ciliary muscles*, which alter the shape of the lens, changing its refractive power
  - *circular muscles* of the iris, which constrict the pupil
- the *levator palpebrae muscles*, which raise the upper eyelids.

IV. Trochlear nerves (motor)

These nerves arise from nuclei near the cerebral aqueduct. They supply the *superior oblique muscles* of the eyes.

V. Trigeminal nerves (mixed)

These nerves contain motor and sensory fibres and are among the largest of the cranial nerves. They are the

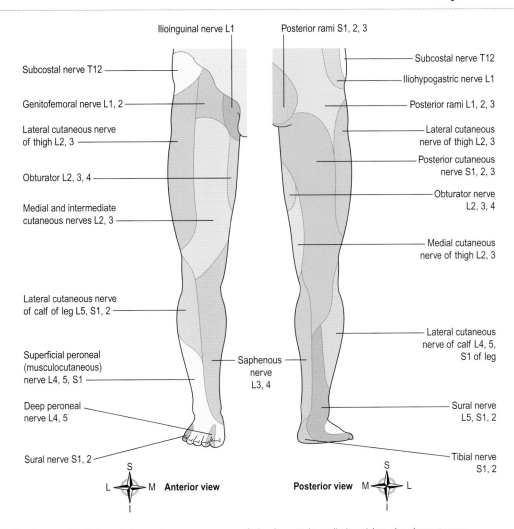

Figure 7.39 Distribution and origins of the cutaneous nerves of the leg. Colour distinguishes the dermatomes.

chief sensory nerves for the face and head (including the oral and nasal cavities and teeth), transmitting sensory impulses, e.g. for pain, temperature and touch. The motor fibres stimulate the muscles for chewing (mastication).

As the name suggests, there are three main branches of the trigeminal nerves. The dermatomes innervated by the sensory fibres on the right side are shown in Figure 7.41.

The ophthalmic nerves are sensory only and supply the lacrimal glands, conjunctiva of the eyes, forehead, eyelids, anterior aspect of the scalp and mucous membrane of the nose.

The maxillary nerves are sensory only and supply the cheeks, upper gums, upper teeth and lower eyelids.

The mandibular nerves contain both sensory and motor fibres. These are the largest of the three divisions and they supply the teeth and gums of the lower jaw, pinnae of the ears, lower lip and tongue. The motor fibres supply the muscles for chewing.

VI. Abducens nerves (motor)

These nerves arise from nuclei lying under the floor of the fourth ventricle. They supply the *lateral rectus muscles* of the eyeballs causing abduction, as the name suggests.

VII. Facial nerves (mixed)

These nerves are composed of both motor and sensory nerve fibres, arising from nuclei in the lower part of the pons. The motor fibres supply the muscles of facial expression. The sensory fibres convey impulses from the taste buds in the anterior two-thirds of the tongue to the taste perception area in the cerebral cortex (see Fig. 7.20).

VIII. Vestibulocochlear (auditory) nerves (sensory)

These nerves are composed of two divisions, the vestibular nerves and cochlear nerves.

The vestibular nerves arise from the semicircular canals of the inner ear and convey impulses to the cerebellum. They are associated with the maintenance of posture and balance.

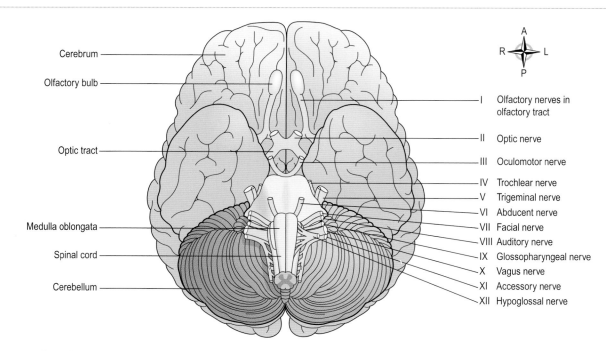

Figure 7.40 **The inferior surface of the brain showing the cranial nerves and associated structures.**

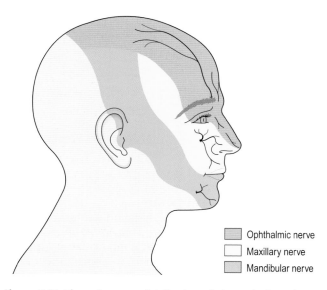

Figure 7.41 **The cutaneous distribution of the main branches of the right trigeminal nerve.**

The cochlear nerves originate in the spiral organ (of Corti) in the inner ear and convey impulses to the hearing areas in the cerebral cortex where sound is perceived.

IX. Glossopharyngeal nerves (mixed)

The motor fibres arise from nuclei in the medulla oblongata and stimulate the muscles of the tongue and pharynx and the secretory cells of the parotid (salivary) glands.

The sensory fibres convey impulses to the cerebral cortex from the posterior third of the tongue, the tonsils and pharynx and from taste buds in the tongue and pharynx. These nerves are essential for the swallowing and gag reflexes. Some fibres conduct impulses from the carotid sinus, which plays an important role in the control of blood pressure (p. 97).

X. Vagus nerves (mixed) (Fig. 7.42)

These nerves have the most extensive distribution of the cranial nerves; their name aptly means 'wanderer'. They pass downwards through the neck into the thorax and the abdomen. These nerves form an important part of the parasympathetic nervous system (see Fig. 7.44).

The motor fibres arise from nuclei in the medulla and supply the smooth muscle and secretory glands of the pharynx, larynx, trachea, bronchi, heart, carotid body, oesophagus, stomach, intestines, exocrine pancreas, gall bladder, bile ducts, spleen, kidneys, ureter and blood vessels in the thoracic and abdominal cavities.

The sensory fibres convey impulses from the membranes lining the same structures to the brain.

XI. Accessory nerves (motor)

These nerves arise from nuclei in the medulla oblongata and in the spinal cord. The fibres supply the *sternocleido-mastoid* and *trapezius muscles*. Branches join the vagus nerves and supply the *pharyngeal* and *laryngeal muscles* in the neck.

XII. Hypoglossal nerves (motor)

These nerves arise from nuclei in the medulla oblongata. They supply the muscles of the tongue and muscles surrounding the hyoid bone and contribute to swallowing and speech.

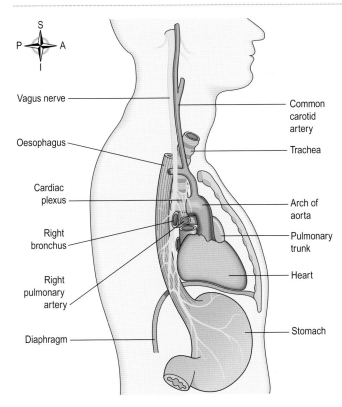

Figure 7.42 The position of the vagus nerve in the thorax viewed from the right side.

Autonomic nervous system 7.11, 7.12, 7.13

The autonomic or involuntary part of the nervous system (Fig. 7.1) controls involuntary body functions. Although stimulation does not occur voluntarily, the individual can sometimes be conscious of its effects, e.g. an increase in their heart rate.

The autonomic nervous system is separated into two divisions:

- *sympathetic* (thoracolumbar outflow)
- *parasympathetic* (craniosacral outflow).

The two divisions work in an integrated and complementary manner to maintain involuntary functions and homeostasis. Such activities include coordination and control of breathing, blood pressure, water balance, digestion and metabolic rate. Sympathetic activity predominates in stressful situations as it equips the body to respond when exertion and exercise is required. Parasympathetic activity is increased (and sympathetic activity is normally lessened) when digestion and restorative body activities predominate. There are similarities and differences between the two divisions. Some similarities are outlined in this section before the descriptions of the two divisions below.

As with other parts of the nervous system, the effects of autonomic activity are rapid. The effector organs are:

- *smooth muscle*, which controls the diameter of smaller airways and blood vessels
- *cardiac muscle*, which controls the rate and force of cardiac contraction
- *glands* that control the volumes of gastrointestinal secretions.

The *efferent (motor) nerves* of the autonomic nervous system arise from the brain and emerge at various levels between the midbrain and the sacral region of the spinal cord. Many of them travel within the same nerve sheath as peripheral nerves to reach the organs they innervate.

Each division has two efferent neurones between the central nervous system and effector organs. These are:

- *the preganglionic neurone*
- *the postganglionic neurone.*

The cell body of the preganglionic neurone is in the brain or spinal cord. Its axon terminals synapse with the cell body of the postganglionic neurone in an *autonomic ganglion* outside the CNS. The postganglionic neurone conducts impulses to the effector organ.

Sympathetic nervous system

Since the preganglionic neurones originate in the spinal cord at the thoracic and lumbar levels, the alternative name of 'thoracolumbar outflow' is apt (Fig. 7.43).

The preganglionic neurone. This has its cell body in the *lateral column of grey matter* in the spinal cord between the levels of the 1st thoracic and 2nd or 3rd lumbar vertebrae. The nerve fibre of this cell leaves the cord by the anterior root and terminates at a synapse in one of the ganglia either in the *lateral chain of sympathetic ganglia* or passes through it to one of the *prevertebral ganglia* (see below). Acetylcholine is the neurotransmitter at sympathetic ganglia.

The postganglionic neurone. This has its cell body in a ganglion and terminates in the organ or tissue supplied. Noradrenaline (norepinephrine) is usually the neurotransmitter at sympathetic effector organs. The major exception is that there is no parasympathetic supply to the sweat glands, the skin and blood vessels of skeletal muscles. These structures are supplied by only sympathetic postganglionic neurones, which are known as *sympathetic cholinergic nerves* and usually have acetylcholine as their neurotransmitter (see Fig. 7.8).

Sympathetic ganglia

The lateral chains of sympathetic ganglia. These chains extend from the upper cervical level to the sacrum, one chain lying on each side of the vertebral bodies. The ganglia are attached to each other by nerve fibres. Preganglionic neurones that emerge from the cord may synapse with the cell body of the postganglionic neurone at the

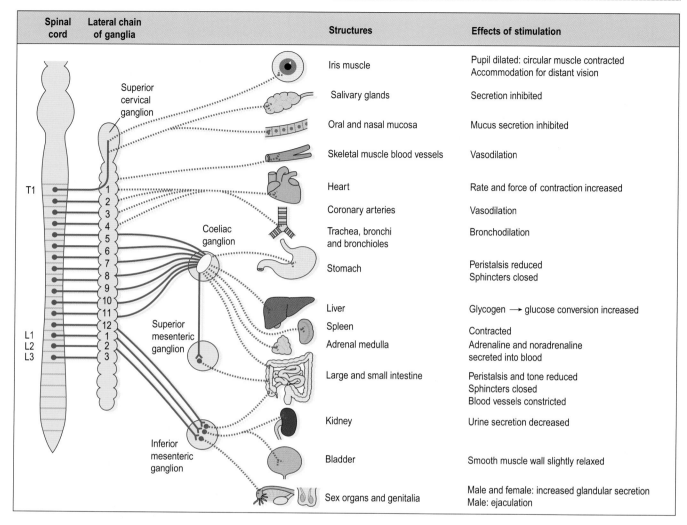

Spinal cord	Lateral chain of ganglia		Structures	Effects of stimulation
	Superior cervical ganglion		Iris muscle	Pupil dilated: circular muscle contracted Accommodation for distant vision
			Salivary glands	Secretion inhibited
			Oral and nasal mucosa	Mucus secretion inhibited
			Skeletal muscle blood vessels	Vasodilation
T1	1		Heart	Rate and force of contraction increased
	2 3		Coronary arteries	Vasodilation
	4 5	Coeliac ganglion	Trachea, bronchi and bronchioles	Bronchodilation
	6 7		Stomach	Peristalsis reduced Sphincters closed
	8 9 10			
	11		Liver	Glycogen → glucose conversion increased
	12	Superior mesenteric ganglion	Spleen	Contracted
L1 L2 L3	1 2 3		Adrenal medulla	Adrenaline and noradrenaline secreted into blood
			Large and small intestine	Peristalsis and tone reduced Sphincters closed Blood vessels constricted
			Kidney	Urine secretion decreased
		Inferior mesenteric ganglion	Bladder	Smooth muscle wall slightly relaxed
			Sex organs and genitalia	Male and female: increased glandular secretion Male: ejaculation

Figure 7.43 The sympathetic outflow, the main structures supplied and the effects of stimulation. Solid red lines – preganglionic fibres; broken lines – postganglionic fibres. There are right and left lateral chains of ganglia.

same level or they may pass up or down the chain through one or more ganglia before synapsing. For example, the nerve that dilates the pupil of the eye leaves the cord at the level of the 1st thoracic vertebra and passes up the chain to the superior cervical ganglion before it synapses with the cell body of the postsynaptic neurone. The postganglionic neurones then pass to the eyes.

The arrangement of the ganglia allows excitation of nerves at multiple levels very quickly, providing a rapid and widespread sympathetic response.

Prevertebral ganglia. There are three prevertebral ganglia situated in the abdominal cavity close to the origins of arteries of the same names:

- coeliac ganglion
- superior mesenteric ganglion
- inferior mesenteric ganglion.

The ganglia consist of nerve cell bodies rather diffusely distributed among a network of nerve fibres that form

plexuses. Preganglionic sympathetic fibres pass through the lateral chain to reach these ganglia.

Parasympathetic nervous system

Like the sympathetic nervous system, two neurones (preganglionic and postganglionic) are involved in the transmission of impulses to the effector organs (Fig. 7.44). The neurotransmitter at both synapses is acetylcholine.

The preganglionic neurone. This is usually long in comparison to its counterpart in the sympathetic nervous system and has its cell body either in the brain or in the spinal cord. Those originating in the brain form the *cranial outflow* and are the cranial nerves III, VII, IX and X, arising from nuclei in the midbrain and brain stem. The cell bodies of the *sacral outflow* are in the lateral columns of grey matter at the distal end of the spinal cord. Their fibres leave the cord in sacral segments 2, 3 and 4. The nerve fibres of parasympathetic preganglionic neurones

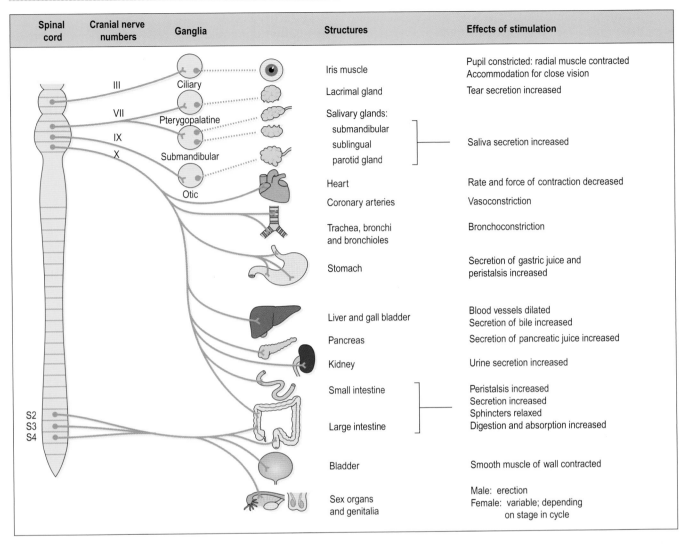

Spinal cord	Cranial nerve numbers	Ganglia	Structures	Effects of stimulation

Figure 7.44 The parasympathetic outflow, the main structures supplied and the effects of stimulation. Solid blue lines – preganglionic fibres; broken lines – postganglionic fibres. Where there are no broken lines, the postganglionic neurone is in the wall of the structure.

usually synapse with their postganglionic counterparts at or near the effector organs.

The postganglionic neurone. This is usually very short and has its cell body either in a ganglion or, more often, in the wall of the organ supplied.

Functions of the autonomic nervous system

The autonomic nervous system is involved in many complex involuntary reflex activities which, like the reflexes described in earlier sections, depend not only on sensory input to the brain or spinal cord but also on motor output. In this case the reflex action is rapid contraction, or inhibition of contraction, of involuntary (smooth and cardiac) muscle or glandular secretion. These activities are coordinated subconsciously. Sometimes sensory input does reach consciousness and may result in temporary

inhibition of the reflex action, e.g. reflex micturition can be inhibited temporarily.

The majority of the body organs are supplied by both sympathetic and parasympathetic nerves, which have complementary, and sometimes opposite effects that are finely balanced to ensure optimum functioning meets body needs at any moment.

Sympathetic stimulation prepares the body to deal with exciting and stressful situations, e.g. strengthening its defences in times of danger and in extremes of environmental temperature. A range of emotional states, e.g. fear, embarrassment and anger, also cause sympathetic stimulation. Sympathetic stimulation causes the adrenal glands to secrete the hormones adrenaline (epinephrine) and noradrenaline (norepinephrine) into the bloodstream. These hormones act as neurotransmitters when they reach target organs of the sympathetic nervous system. Through this effect, they potentiate and sustain the effects of sympathetic stimulation. It is said that sympathetic stimulation mobilises the body for 'fight or flight'. The effects of stimulation on the heart, blood vessels and lungs (see below) enable the body to respond by preparing it for exercise. Additional effects are an increase in the metabolic rate and increased conversion of glycogen to glucose. During exercise, e.g. fighting or running away, when oxygen and energy requirements of skeletal muscles are greatly increased, these changes enable the body to respond quickly to meet the increased energy demand. ▨ 7.14

Parasympathetic stimulation has a tendency to slow down cardiac and respiratory activity but it stimulates digestion and absorption of food and the functions of the genitourinary systems. Its general effect is that of a 'peace maker', allowing digestion and restorative processes to occur quietly and peacefully. ▨ 7.15

Normally the two systems function together, maintaining a regular heartbeat, normal temperature and an internal environment compatible with both physiological needs and the immediate external surroundings.

Effects of autonomic stimulation

Cardiovascular system
Sympathetic stimulation

- Accelerates firing of the sinoatrial node in the heart, increasing the rate and force of the heartbeat.
- Dilates the coronary arteries, increasing the blood supply to cardiac muscle increasing the supply of oxygen and nutritional materials and the removal of metabolic waste products, thus increasing the capacity of the muscle to work.
- Dilates the blood vessels supplying skeletal muscle, with the same effects as those on cardiac muscle above.
- Raises peripheral resistance and blood pressure by constricting the small arteries and arterioles in the skin. In this way an increased blood supply is available for highly active tissue, such as skeletal muscle, heart and brain.
- Constricts the blood vessels in the secretory glands of the digestive system. This raises the volume of blood available for circulation in dilated blood vessels, e.g. cardiac muscle, skeletal muscles.
- Accelerates blood coagulation because of vasoconstriction.

Parasympathetic stimulation

- Decreases the rate and force of the heartbeat.
- Constricts the coronary arteries, reducing the blood supply to cardiac muscle.
- Blood vessels to skeletal muscles – no effect.

The parasympathetic nervous system exerts little or no effect on blood vessels except the coronary arteries.

Respiratory system
Sympathetic stimulation. This causes smooth muscle relaxation and therefore dilation of the airways (*bronchodilation*), especially the bronchioles, allowing a greater amount of air to enter the lungs at each inspiration, and increases the respiratory rate. In conjunction with the increased heart rate, the oxygen intake and carbon dioxide output of the body are increased to deal with 'fight or flight' situations.

Parasympathetic stimulation. This causes contraction of the smooth muscle in the airway walls, leading to *bronchoconstriction*.

Digestive and urinary systems
Sympathetic stimulation

- *The liver* increases conversion of glycogen to glucose, making more carbohydrate immediately available to provide energy.
- *The stomach* and *small intestine*. Smooth muscle contraction (peristalsis) and secretion of digestive juices are inhibited, delaying digestion, onward movement and absorption of food, and the tone of sphincter muscles is increased.
- *The adrenal (suprarenal) glands* are stimulated to secrete adrenaline (epinephrine) and noradrenaline (norepinephrine) which potentiate and sustain the effects of sympathetic stimulation throughout the body.
- *Urethral* and *anal sphincters*. The muscle tone of the sphincters is increased, inhibiting micturition and defecation.
- *The bladder* wall relaxes.
- *The metabolic rate* is greatly increased.

Parasympathetic stimulation

- *The liver*. The secretion of bile is increased.
- *The stomach* and *small intestine*. Motility and secretion are increased, together with the rate of digestion and absorption of food.
- *The pancreas*. The secretion of pancreatic juice is increased.
- *Urethral* and *anal sphincters*. Relaxation of the internal urethral sphincter is accompanied by contraction of the muscle of the bladder wall, and micturition occurs. Similar relaxation of the internal anal sphincter is accompanied by contraction of the muscle of the rectum, and defecation occurs. In both cases there is voluntary relaxation of the external sphincters.
- *The adrenal glands*. No effect.
- *The metabolic rate*. No effect.

Eye
Sympathetic stimulation. This causes contraction of the radiating muscle fibres of the iris, dilating the pupil. Retraction of the levator palpebrae muscles occurs, opening the eyes wide and giving the appearance of

alertness and excitement. The ciliary muscle that adjusts the thickness of the lens is slightly relaxed, facilitating distant vision.

Parasympathetic stimulation. This contracts the circular muscle fibres of the iris, constricting the pupil. The eyelids tend to close, giving the appearance of sleepiness. The ciliary muscle contracts, facilitating near vision.

Skin

Sympathetic stimulation

- Increases sweat secretion, leading to more loss of heat generated by increased skeletal muscle activity.
- Contracts the arrector pili (the muscles in the hair follicles of the skin), giving the appearance of 'goose flesh'.
- Constricts the peripheral blood vessels, increasing blood supply available to active organs, e.g. the heart and skeletal muscle.

There is no parasympathetic nerve supply to the skin. Some sympathetic fibres are adrenergic, causing vasoconstriction, and some are cholinergic, causing vasodilation (see Fig. 7.8, p. 149).

Afferent impulses from viscera

Sensory fibres from the viscera travel with autonomic fibres and are sometimes called *autonomic afferents*. The impulses they transmit are associated with:

- visceral reflexes, usually at an unconscious level, e.g. cough, blood pressure (baroreceptors)
- sensation of, e.g., hunger, thirst, nausea, sexual sensation, rectal and bladder distension
- visceral pain.

Visceral pain

Normally the viscera are insensitive to cutting, burning and crushing. However, a sensation of dull, poorly located pain is experienced when:

- visceral nerves are stretched
- a large number of fibres are stimulated
- there is ischaemia and local accumulation of metabolites
- the sensitivity of nerve endings to painful stimuli is increased, e.g. during inflammation.

If the cause of the pain, e.g. inflammation, affects the parietal layer of a serous membrane (pleura, peritoneum, see p. 45) the pain is acute and easily located over the site of inflammation. This is because the peripheral spinal (somatic) nerves that innervate the superficial tissues also innervate the parietal layer of serous membranes. They transmit the impulses to the cerebral cortex where somatic pain is perceived and accurately located. Appendicitis is an example of this type of

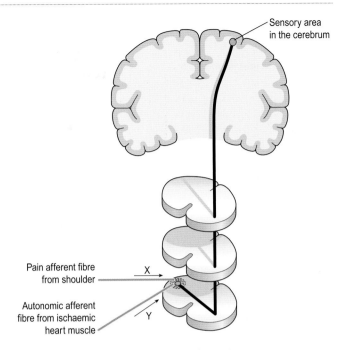

Figure 7.45 Referred pain. Ischaemic heart tissue generates impulses in nerve Y that then stimulate nerve X and pain is perceived in the shoulder.

pain. Initially it is dull and vaguely located around the midline of the abdomen. As the condition progresses the parietal peritoneum becomes involved and acute pain is clearly located in the right iliac fossa, i.e. over the appendix.

Referred pain (Fig. 7.45)

In some cases of visceral disease, pain may be felt in superficial tissues remote from its site of origin, i.e. referred pain. This occurs when sensory fibres from the affected organ enter the same segment of the spinal cord as somatic nerves, i.e. those from the superficial tissues. It is believed that the sensory nerve from the damaged organ stimulates the closely associated nerve in the spinal cord and it transmits the impulses to the sensory area in the cerebral cortex where the pain is perceived as originating in the area supplied by the somatic nerve. Examples of referred pain are given in Table 7.3.

Effect of ageing on the nervous system

Learning outcome

After studying this section, you should be able to:

■ Describe the effects of ageing on the nervous system.

Table 7.3 Referred pain

Tissue of origin of pain	Site of referred pain
Heart	Left shoulder
Liver Biliary tract	Right shoulder
Kidney Ureter	Loin and groin
Uterus	Low back
Male genitalia	Low abdomen
Prolapsed intervertebral disc	Leg

As neurones are not replaced after birth a natural decrease in numbers occurs with ageing; however, a considerable reserve means that cognitive function is not necessarily impaired. The brain of older adults is generally reduced in size and weighs less; the gyri become narrower and sulci wider. In older adults, *plaques,* accumulations of protein material, are often found around CNS neurones and *neurofibrillary tangles* may develop inside them, although their significance is unknown.

Decreased blood flow may develop in the arteries that supply the brain over a long period (*atheroma* and *arteriosclerosis,* Ch. 4) making their walls more prone to rupture. Should this occur, damage to the surrounding brain tissue causes the signs and symptoms of a *stroke* (p. 181).

Motor control of precise movement diminishes meaning that older adults take longer to carry out motor actions than younger adults and become more prone to falls. The conduction rate of nerve impulses becomes slower, and this may contribute to less effective control of, for example, vasodilation, vasoconstriction and the baroreceptor reflex (see Ch. 5).

Memory of the recent past typically becomes more difficult to access although long-term memories, including problem-solving skills, remain intact and generally remain retrievable. For unknown reasons, some older adults are much more incapacitated by progressive CNS changes than others, e.g. *dementia* (p. 183).

Effects of ageing on the special senses are almost universal and considered in Chapter 8. Thermoregulation is discussed in Chapter 14.

Disorders of the brain

Learning outcomes

After studying this section, you should be able to:

- list three causes of raised intracranial pressure (ICP)

- relate the effects of raised ICP to the functions of the brain and changes in vital signs

- outline how the brain is damaged during different types of head injury

- describe four complications of head injury

- explain the effects of cerebral hypoxia and stroke

- outline the causes and effects of dementia

- relate the pathology of Parkinson disease to its effects on body function.

Increased intracranial pressure

This is a serious complication of many conditions that affect the brain. The cranium forms a rigid cavity enclosing the brain, the cerebral blood vessels and cerebrospinal fluid (CSF). An increase in volume of any one of these will lead to raised intracranial pressure (ICP).

Sometimes its effects are more serious than the condition causing it, e.g. by disrupting the blood supply or distorting the shape of the brain, especially if the ICP rises rapidly. A slow rise in ICP allows time for compensatory adjustment to be made, i.e. a slight reduction in the volume of circulating blood and of CSF. The slower the rise in ICP, the more effective is the compensation.

Rising ICP is accompanied by bradycardia and hypertension. As it reaches its limit, a further small increase in pressure is followed by a sudden and usually serious reduction in the cerebral blood flow as autoregulation fails. The result is hypoxia and a rise in carbon dioxide levels, causing arteriolar dilation, which further increases ICP. This leads to rapid and progressive loss of functioning neurones, which exacerbates bradycardia and hypertension. Further cerebral hypoxia causes *vasomotor paralysis* and death.

The causes of increased ICP are described on the following pages and include:

- cerebral oedema
- hydrocephalus, the accumulation of excess CSF
- expanding lesions inside the skull, also known as space-occupying lesions e.g.:
  - haemorrhage or haematoma (traumatic or spontaneous)
  - tumours (primary or secondary).

Expanding lesions may occur in the brain or in the meninges and they can damage the brain in various ways (Fig. 7.46).

Effects of increased ICP

Displacement of the brain

Lesions causing displacement are usually one sided but may affect both sides. Such lesions may cause:

- *herniation* (displacement of part of the brain from its usual compartment) of the cerebral hemisphere between the corpus callosum and the free border of the falx cerebri on the same side
- herniation of the midbrain between the pons and the free border of the tentorium cerebelli on the same side
- compression of the subarachnoid space and flattening of the cerebral convolutions
- distortion of the shape of the ventricles and their ducts
- herniation of the cerebellum through the foramen magnum

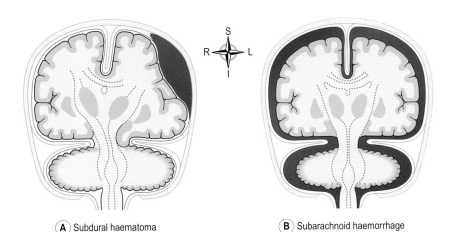
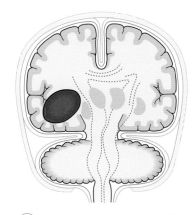

(A) Subdural haematoma (B) Subarachnoid haemorrhage (C) Tumour or intracerebral haemorrhage

Figure 7.46 Effects of different types of expanding lesions inside the skull: A. Subdural haematoma. **B.** Subarachnoid haemorrhage. **C.** Tumour or intracerebral haemorrhage.

- protrusion of the medulla oblongata through the foramen magnum ('*coning*').

Obstruction of the flow of cerebrospinal fluid

The ventricles or their ducts may be displaced or a duct obstructed. The effects depend on the position of the lesion, e.g. compression of the cerebral aqueduct causes dilation of the lateral ventricles and the third ventricle, further increasing the ICP.

Vascular damage

Blood vessels may be stretched or compressed, causing:

- haemorrhage when stretched blood vessels rupture
- ischaemia and infarction due to compression of blood vessels
- *papilloedema* (oedema round the optic disc) due to compression of the retinal vein in the optic nerve sheath where it crosses the subarachnoid space.

Neural damage

The vital centres in the medulla oblongata may be damaged when the increased ICP causes '*coning*'. Stretching may damage cranial nerves, especially the oculomotor (III) and the abducens (VI), causing disturbances of eye movement and accommodation. Dilation of a pupil and loss of the light reflex (failure of the pupil to constrict in response to bright light) is caused by compression of the oculomotor nerve.

Bone changes

Prolonged increase of ICP causes bony changes, e.g.:

- erosion, especially of the sphenoid bone
- stretching and thinning in children before ossification is complete.

Cerebral oedema

Oedema (p. 125) occurs when there is excess fluid in tissue cells and/or interstitial spaces. In the brain, this is known as cerebral oedema and increases intracranial pressure. It is associated with:

- traumatic head injury
- haemorrhage
- infections, abscesses
- hypoxia, local ischaemia or infarcts
- tumours
- inflammation of the brain or meninges
- hypoglycaemia (p. 237).

Hydrocephalus

In this condition the volume of CSF is abnormally high and is usually accompanied by increased ICP. An obstruction to CSF flow is the most common cause. It is described as *communicating* when there is free flow of CSF from the ventricular system to the subarachnoid space and *non-communicating* when there is not, i.e. there is obstruction in the system of ventricles, foramina or ducts (see Fig. 7.15).

Enlargement of the head occurs in children when ossification of the cranial bones is incomplete but, in spite of this, the ventricles dilate and cause stretching and thinning of the brain. After ossification is complete, hydrocephalus leads to a marked increase in ICP and destruction of nervous tissue.

Head injuries

Damage to the brain may be serious even when there is no outward sign of injury. At the site of injury there may be:

- a scalp wound, with haemorrhage between scalp and skull bones
- damage to the underlying meninges and/or brain with local haemorrhage inside the skull
- a depressed skull fracture, causing local damage to the underlying meninges and brain tissue
- temporal bone fracture, creating an opening between the middle ear and the meninges
- fracture involving the air sinuses of the sphenoid, ethmoid or frontal bones, making an opening between the nose and the meninges.

Acceleration–deceleration injuries

Because the brain floats relatively freely in 'a cushion' of CSF, sudden acceleration or deceleration has an inertia effect. For example, when a vehicle stops suddenly passengers are thrown forward: the head then moves forwards or backwards relative to the rest of the body causing injury to the brain at the site of impact if it moves within the skull. In '*contre coup*' injuries, brain damage is more severe on the side opposite to the site of impact. Other injuries include:

- nerve cell damage, usually to the frontal and parietal lobes, due to movement of the brain over the rough surface of bones of the base of the skull
- nerve fibre damage due to stretching, especially following rotational movement
- haemorrhage due to rupture of blood vessels in the subarachnoid space on the side opposite to the impact or many diffuse small haemorrhages, following rotational movement.

Complications of head injury

If the individual survives the immediate effects, complications may develop hours or days later. Sometimes they are the first indication of serious damage caused by a seemingly trivial injury. Their effects may increase

ICP, damage brain tissue or provide a route of entry for infection.

Traumatic intracranial haemorrhage

Haemorrhage may occur causing secondary brain damage at the site of injury, on the opposite side of the brain or diffusely throughout the brain. If bleeding continues, the expanding haematoma increases the ICP, compressing the brain. ▓ **7.16**

Extradural haemorrhage. This may follow a direct blow that may or may not cause a fracture. The individual may recover quickly and indications of increased ICP typically appear only several hours later as the haematoma grows and the outer layer of dura mater (periosteum) is stripped off the bone. The haematoma grows rapidly when arterial blood vessels are damaged. In children fractures are rare because the skull bones are still soft and the joints (sutures) have not fused. The haematoma usually remains localised.

Acute subdural haemorrhage. This is due to haemorrhage from either small veins in the dura mater or larger veins between the layers of dura mater before they enter the venous sinuses. The blood may spread in the subdural space over one or both cerebral hemispheres (Fig. 7.46A). There may be concurrent subarachnoid haemorrhage (Fig. 7.46B), especially when there are extensive brain contusions and lacerations.

Chronic subdural haemorrhage. This may occur weeks or months after minor injuries and sometimes there is no history of injury. It occurs most commonly in people in whom there is some cerebral atrophy, e.g. older adults and in alcohol misuse. Evidence of increased ICP may be delayed when brain volume is reduced. The haematoma gradually increases in size owing to repeated small haemorrhages and causes mild chronic inflammation and accumulation of inflammatory exudate. In time it is isolated by a wall of fibrous tissue.

Intracerebral haemorrhage and cerebral oedema. These occur following contusions, lacerations and shearing injuries associated with acceleration and deceleration, especially rotational movements.

Cerebral oedema (p. 180) is a common complication of contusions of the brain, leading to increased ICP, hypoxia and further brain damage.

Meningitis

(see p. 184).

Post-traumatic epilepsy

This is characterised by seizures (fits) and may develop in the first week or several months after injury. Early development is most common after severe injuries, although in children the injury itself may have appeared trivial. After depressed fractures or large haematomas, epilepsy tends to develop later.

Vegetative states

This condition is a consequence of severe cortical brain damage. The individual appears awake and is observed to undergo sleep–wake cycles; however, there are no signs of awareness or responses to the external environment. As the brain stem remains intact, the vital centres continue to function i.e. breathing and blood pressure are maintained. It is considered permanent if there is no recovery 12 months after trauma or longer than 6 months after any other cause.

Cerebral hypoxia

Hypoxia may be due to disturbances in the autoregulation of blood supply to the brain or conditions affecting cerebral blood vessels.

When the mean blood pressure falls below about 60 mmHg, the autoregulating mechanisms that control the blood flow to the brain by adjusting the diameter of the arterioles fail. The consequent rapid decrease in the cerebral blood supply leads to hypoxia and lack of glucose. If severe hypoxia is sustained for more than a few minutes there is irreversible brain damage. Neurones are affected first, then the neuroglial cells and later the meninges and blood vessels. Conditions in which autoregulation breaks down include:

- cardiorespiratory arrest
- sudden severe hypotension
- carbon monoxide poisoning
- hypercapnia (excess blood carbon dioxide)
- drug overdosage with, e.g., opioid analgesics, hypnotics.

Conditions affecting cerebral blood vessels that may lead to hypoxia include:

- occlusion of a cerebral artery by, e.g., a rapidly expanding intracranial lesion, atheroma, thrombosis or embolism (Ch. 5)
- arterial stenosis that occurs in arteritis, e.g. polyarteritis nodosa, syphilis, diabetes mellitus, degenerative changes in older adults.

If the individual survives the initial episode of ischaemia, then infarction, necrosis and loss of function of the affected area of brain may occur.

Stroke

Cerebrovascular disease is the underlying cause of most strokes and transient ischaemic attacks. Predisposing factors include:

- hypertension
- atheroma
- diabetes mellitus
- cigarette smoking.

Stroke is a very common cause of death and disability in older adults. The incidence is greater in Asian and black African populations, and increases steeply with age. Effects appear in a few minutes and include paralysis of a limb or one side of the body (*hemiparesis*) often accompanied by disturbances of speech and vision. The nature and extent of damage depend on the location of the affected blood vessels. By definition, signs and symptoms of a stroke last for longer than 24 hours. The vast majority are caused by cerebral infarction (about 85%) with spontaneous intracranial haemorrhage accounting for most of the remainder.

In contrast to a stroke, a *transient ischaemic attack* (TIA) is a brief period of reversible cerebral deficit. Typically there is a short period (minutes or hours) where there is weakness of a limb, loss of speech and/or vision followed by complete recovery. A TIA may precede a stroke (about 30% in 5 years) or, less commonly, myocardial infarction (see Ch. 5). The arbitrary definition of a TIA lasting under 24 hours is no longer used.

Around 80% of patients survive for at least a month following an acute stroke; gradual improvement of limb movement follows in about 50% of cases, which is sometimes accompanied by improved speech. Recurrence is common.

Cerebral infarction ▓ 7.17

This occurs when blood flow to the brain is suddenly interrupted resulting in cerebral hypoxia. The main cause is atheroma affecting the carotid artery or aortic arch, which is complicated by thrombosis (p. 119) although a blocked artery supplying the brain can also arise from an embolus originating in the heart, e.g. infective endocarditis (p. 128).

Spontaneous intracranial haemorrhage

The haemorrhage may be into the subarachnoid space or intracerebral (Fig. 7.47). It is commonly associated with an aneurysm or hypertension. In each case the escaped blood may cause arterial spasm, leading to ischaemia, infarction, fibrosis (gliosis) and hypoxic brain damage. A severe haemorrhage may be instantly fatal while repeated small haemorrhages have a cumulative effect in extending brain damage (*multi-infarct dementia*).

Intracerebral haemorrhage. Prolonged hypertension leads to the formation of multiple microaneurysms in the walls of very small arteries in the brain. Rupture of one or more of these, due to continuing rise in blood pressure, is usually the cause of intracerebral haemorrhage. The most common sites are branches of the middle cerebral

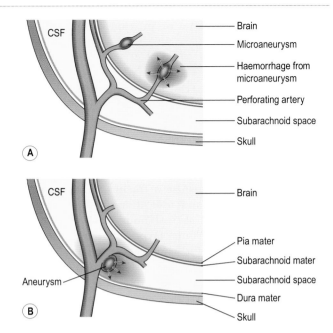

Figure 7.47 Types of haemorrhage causing stroke:
A. Intracerebral. **B.** Subarachnoid.

artery in the region of the internal capsule and the basal ganglia.

Severe haemorrhage causes compression and destruction of tissue, a sudden increase in ICP and distortion and herniation of the brain. Death follows when the vital centres in the medulla oblongata are damaged by haemorrhage or if there is coning due to increased ICP.

Less severe haemorrhage causes paralysis and loss of sensation of varying severity, affecting the side of the body opposite the haemorrhage. If the bleeding stops and does not recur, a fluid-filled cyst develops, i.e. the haematoma is walled off by gliosis, the blood clot is gradually absorbed and the cavity becomes filled with tissue exudate. When the ICP returns to normal, some function may be restored, e.g. speech and movement of limbs.

Subarachnoid haemorrhage. This accounts for a small number of strokes and is usually due to rupture of a berry aneurysm on one of the major cerebral arteries, or less often bleeding from a congenitally malformed blood vessel (Fig. 7.47B). The blood may remain localised but usually spreads in the subarachnoid space round the brain and spinal cord, causing a general increase in ICP without distortion of the brain (Fig. 7.46B). The irritant effect of the blood may cause arterial spasm, leading to ischaemia, infarction, gliosis and the effects of localised brain damage. It occurs most commonly in middle life, but occasionally in young people owing to rupture of a malformed blood vessel. This condition is often fatal or results in permanent disability.

Dementia

Dementia is caused by progressive, irreversible degeneration of the cerebral cortex and results in mental deterioration, usually over several years. There is gradual impairment of memory (especially short term), intellect and reasoning but consciousness is not affected. Emotional lability and personality change may also occur.

Alzheimer disease

This condition is the commonest form of dementia in developed countries. The aetiology is unknown although genetic factors may be involved. Females are affected twice as often as males and it usually affects those over 60 years, the incidence increasing with age. It commonly affects people with Down syndrome by the age of 40 years. There is progressive atrophy of the cerebral cortex accompanied by deteriorating mental functioning. Death usually occurs between 2 and 8 years after onset.

Huntington disease

This usually manifests itself between the ages of 30 and 50 years. It is inherited as an autosomal dominant disorder (see p. 443) associated with deficient production of the neurotransmitter gamma aminobutyric acid (GABA). By the time of onset, the individual may have already passed the genetic abnormality on to their children. Extrapyramidal changes cause chorea, rapid uncoordinated jerking movements of the limbs and involuntary twitching of the facial muscles. As the disease progresses, cortical atrophy causes personality changes and dementia.

Secondary dementias

Dementia may occur in association with other conditions:

- vascular dementia, also known as *multi-infarct dementia,* which may accompany cerebrovascular disease
- toxic – e.g. alcohol and solvent misuse and, less often, vitamin B deficiencies
- tumours – usually metastases but sometimes primary intracranial tumours
- metabolic (e.g. uraemia, liver failure) and endocrine (e.g. hypothyroidism)
- infections, although these are less common e.g. syphilis, human immunodeficiency virus (HIV) and Creutzfeldt–Jakob Disease (CJD).

Parkinson disease ▮ 7.18

In this disease there is gradual and progressive degeneration of dopamine releasing neurones in the

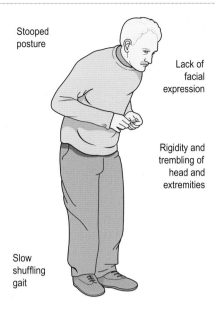

Figure 7.48 Typical posture of Parkinson disease.

Labels: Stooped posture; Lack of facial expression; Rigidity and trembling of head and extremities; Slow shuffling gait.

extrapyramidal system especially at the basal ganglia. This leads to lack of control and coordination of muscle movement resulting in:

- slowness of movement (bradykinesia) and difficulty initiating movements
- fixed muscle tone causing expressionless facial features, rigidity of voluntary muscles causing the slow and characteristic stiff shuffling gait and stooping posture
- muscle tremor of extremities that usually begins in one hand, e.g. 'pill rolling' movement of the fingers
- speech problems, excessive salivation and, in advanced disease, dysphagia.

Onset is usually between 45 and 60 years; with more men than women affected. The cause is usually unknown but some cases are associated with repeated trauma as in, e.g., 'punch drunk' boxers; tumours causing midbrain compression; drugs, e.g. phenothiazines; heavy metal poisoning. There is progressive physical disability but the intellect is not impaired (Fig. 7.48).

Effects of poisons on the brain

Many chemicals, including drugs, environmental toxins, microbial products and metabolic wastes can damage nervous tissue. This may range from short-term reversible neurological disturbance, e.g. depression of cognitive and motor functions after drinking alcohol, through to long-term permanent damage, for example heavy metal poisoning (e.g. lead) or hepatic encephalopathy (p. 334).

Infections of the central nervous system

Learning outcome

After studying this section, you should be able to:

■ describe common infections of the nervous system and their effects on body function.

The brain and spinal cord are relatively well protected from microbial infection by the blood–brain barrier.

CNS infections are usually bacterial or viral but may also be protozoal or fungal. Infections may originate in the meninges (*meningitis*) or in the brain (*encephalitis*), then spread from one site to the other.

Bacterial infections

Entry of bacteria into the CNS may be:

- direct – through a compound skull fracture or through the skull bones from, e.g., middle ear or paranasal sinus infections, mastoiditis
- blood-borne – from infection elsewhere in the body, e.g. septicaemia, bacterial endocarditis (p. 128)
- iatrogenic – introduced during an invasive procedure, e.g. lumbar puncture.

Bacterial meningitis

The term 'meningitis' usually refers to inflammation of the subarachnoid space and is most commonly transmitted through contact with an infected individual. Bacterial meningitis is usually preceded by a mild upper respiratory tract infection during which a few bacteria enter the bloodstream and are carried to the meninges. Common microbes include:

- *Haemophilus influenzae* in children between the ages of 2 and 5 years
- *Neisseria meningitidis* in those between 5 and 30 years, the most common type
- *Streptococcus pneumoniae* in people over 30 years.

Other pathogenic bacteria can also cause meningitis, e.g. those causing tuberculosis (p. 268) and syphilis.

Meningitis can also affect the dura mater, especially when spread is direct through a compound skull fracture as leakage of CSF and blood from the site also provides a route of entry for microbes. CSF and blood may escape through the:

- skin, in compound skull fractures
- middle ear, in fractures of the temporal bone (*CSF otorrhoea*)
- nose, in fractures of the sphenoid, ethmoid or frontal bones when air sinuses are involved (*CSF rhinorrhoea*).

It may also arise from nearby infections, e.g., of the ear. If an extradural or subdural abscess forms, the infection may spread further locally should it rupture.

The onset is usually sudden with severe headache, neck stiffness, photophobia (intolerance of bright light) and fever. This is sometimes accompanied by a petechial rash. CSF appears cloudy owing to the presence of many bacteria and neutrophils. Mortality and morbidity rates are considerable.

Viral infections

Entry of viruses into the CNS is usually blood-borne from viral infection elsewhere in the body and, less commonly, through the nervous system. In the latter situation, *neurotropic viruses*, i.e. those with an affinity for nervous tissue, travel along peripheral nerve from a site elsewhere, e.g. poliovirus. They enter the body via:

- the alimentary tract, e.g. poliomyelitis
- the respiratory tract, e.g. shingles
- skin abrasions, e.g. rabies.

The effects of viral infections vary according to the site and the amount of tissue destroyed. Viruses may damage neurones by multiplying within them or stimulating an immune reaction which may explain why signs of some infections do not appear until there is a high antibody titre, 1–2 weeks after infection.

Viral meningitis

This is the most common form of meningitis, which is usually relatively mild and followed by complete recovery.

Viral encephalitis

Viral encephalitis is rare and usually associated with a recent viral infection. Most cases are mild and recovery is usually complete. More serious cases are usually associated with rabies or *Herpes simplex* viruses. Many different sites can be affected and, as neurones cannot be replaced, loss of function reflects the extent of damage. In severe infections neurones and neuroglia may be affected, followed by necrosis and gliosis. If the individual survives the initial acute phase there may be residual dysfunction, e.g. cognitive impairment and epilepsy. If vital centres in the medulla are involved the condition can be fatal.

Herpes zoster (shingles)

Herpes zoster viruses cause chickenpox (varicella), mainly in children, and shingles (zoster) in adults. Susceptible children may contract chickenpox from a person with shingles but not the reverse. Infected adults may show no immediate signs of disease. The viruses may remain dormant in posterior root ganglia of the spinal nerves then become active years later, causing shingles. Reactivation may be either spontaneous or associated with intercurrent illness or depression of the immune system, e.g. by drugs, old age, AIDS.

The posterior root ganglion becomes acutely inflamed. From there the viruses travel along the sensory nerve to the surface tissues supplied, e.g. skin, cornea. The infection is usually unilateral and the most common sites are:

- nerves supplying the trunk, sometimes two or three adjacent dermatomes
- the ophthalmic division of the trigeminal nerve (Fig. 7.41), causing *trigeminal neuralgia*, and, if vesicles form on the cornea, there may be ulceration, scarring and residual interference with vision.

Affected tissues become inflamed and vesicles, containing serous fluid and viruses, develop along the course of the nerve. This is accompanied by persistent pain and hypersensitivity to touch (*hyperaesthesia*). Recovery is usually slow and there may be some loss of sensation, depending on the severity of the disease.

Poliomyelitis

This disease is usually caused by *polioviruses* and, occasionally, by other *enteroviruses*. The infection is spread by food contaminated by infected faecal matter and, initially, viral multiplication occurs in the alimentary tract. The viruses are then blood-borne to the nervous system and invade anterior horn cells in the spinal cord. Usually there is a mild febrile illness with no indication of nerve damage. In mild cases there is complete recovery but there is permanent disability in many others. Irreversible damage to lower motor neurones (p. 163) causes muscle paralysis which, in the limbs, may lead to deformity because of the unopposed tonal contraction of antagonistic muscles. Death may occur owing to respiratory paralysis if the intercostal muscles are affected. Vaccination programmes have now almost eradicated this disease in developed countries.

Rabies

All warm-blooded animals are susceptible to the rabies virus, which is endemic in many countries but not in the UK. The main reservoirs of this virus are wild animals, some of which may be carriers. When these infect domestic pets they then become the source of human infection. The viruses multiply in the salivary glands and are present in large numbers in saliva. They enter the body through skin abrasions and are believed to travel to the brain along peripheral nerves. The incubation period varies from about 2 weeks to several months, possibly reflecting the distance viruses travel between the site of entry and the brain. There is acute encephalomyelitis with extensive damage to the basal ganglia, midbrain and medulla oblongata. Involvement of the posterior root ganglia of the peripheral nerves causes meningeal irritation, extreme hyperaesthesia, muscle spasm and convulsions. *Hydrophobia* (hatred of water) and overflow of

saliva from the mouth are due to painful spasm of the throat muscles that inhibits swallowing. In the advanced stages muscle spasm may alternate with flaccid paralysis and death is usually due to respiratory muscle spasm or paralysis.

Not all people exposed to the virus contract rabies, but in those who do, the mortality rate is high.

Human immunodeficiency virus (HIV)

The brain is often affected in individuals with AIDS (p. 386) resulting in opportunistic infection (e.g. meningitis) and dementia.

Creutzfeldt–Jakob disease

This infective condition may be caused by a 'slow' virus, the nature and transmission of which is poorly understood. It is thought to be via a heat-resistant transmissible particle known as a *prion protein*. It is a rapidly progressive form of dementia (p. 183) for which there is no known treatment so the condition is always fatal.

Myalgic encephalitis (ME)

This condition is also known as post-viral syndrome or chronic fatigue syndrome. It affects mostly teenagers and young adults and the aetiology is unknown. Sometimes the condition follows a viral illness. The effects include malaise, severe fatigue, poor concentration and myalgia. Recovery is usually spontaneous but sometimes results in chronic disability.

Demyelinating diseases

Learning outcome

After studying this section, you should be able to:

- explain how the signs and symptoms of demyelinating disease are related to pathological changes in the nervous system.

These diseases are caused either by injury to axons or by disorders of cells that secrete myelin, i.e. oligodendrocytes and Schwann cells.

Multiple sclerosis (MS)

In this disease areas of demyelinated white matter, called plaques, replace myelin. They are irregularly distributed throughout the brain and spinal cord. Grey matter in the brain and spinal cord may also be affected because of the arrangement of satellite oligodendrocytes round cell bodies. In the early stages there may be little damage to axons.

It usually develops between the ages of 20 and 40 years and affects twice as many women as men. The actual cause(s) of MS are not known but several factors seem to be involved. It appears to be an autoimmune disorder, possibly triggered by a viral infection, e.g. measles.

Environment before adolescence is implicated because the disease is most prevalent in people who spend their pre-adolescent years in temperate climates, and those who move to other climates after that age retain their susceptibility to MS. People from equatorial areas moving into a temperate climate during adolescence or later life appear not to be susceptible.

Genetic factors are implicated too as there is an increased incidence of MS among siblings, especially identical twins, and parents of patients.

Effects of multiple sclerosis

Symptoms depend on the size and location of the developing plaques and include:

- weakness of skeletal muscles and sometimes paralysis
- loss of coordination and movement
- disturbed sensation, e.g. burning or pins and needles
- incontinence of urine
- visual disturbances, especially blurring and double vision. The optic nerves are commonly affected early in the disease.

The disease pattern is usually one of relapses and remissions of widely varying duration. Each relapse causes further loss of nervous tissue and progressive dysfunction. In some cases there may be chronic progression without remission, or acute disease rapidly leading to death.

Acute disseminated encephalomyelitis

This is a rare but serious condition that may occur as a complication of a viral infection, e.g. measles, chickenpox, or rarely following primary immunisation against viral diseases, mainly in older children and adults.

The cause of the acute diffuse demyelination is not known. It has been suggested that an autoimmune effect on myelin is triggered either by viruses during viral infection such as measles, or by an immune response to vaccines. The effects vary considerably, according to the distribution and degree of demyelination and are similar to those of MS. The early febrile state may progress to paralysis and coma. Most patients survive the initial phase and recover completely but some have severe neurological impairment.

Diseases of the spinal cord

Learning outcome

After studying this section, you should be able to:

- explain how disorders of the spinal cord cause abnormal function.

Because space in the neural canal and intervertebral foramina is limited, any condition that distorts their shape or reduces the space may damage the spinal cord or peripheral nerve roots, or compress blood vessels causing ischaemia. Such conditions include:

- fracture and/or dislocation of vertebrae
- tumours of the meninges or vertebrae
- prolapsed intervertebral disc.

The effects of disease or injury depend on the severity of the damage, the type and position of the neurones involved.

Motor neurones

Table 7.4 gives a summary of the effects of damage to the motor neurones. The parts of the body affected depend on which neurones have been damaged and their site in the brain, spinal cord or peripheral nerve.

Upper motor neurone (UMN) lesions

Lesions of the UMNs above the level of the decussation of the pyramids affect the opposite side of the body, e.g. haemorrhage or infarction in the internal capsule of one hemisphere causes paralysis of the opposite side of the body. Lesions below the decussation affect the same side of the body. The lower motor neurones are released from cortical control and muscle tone is increased (Table 7.4).

Lower motor neurone (LMN) lesions

The cell bodies of LMNs are in the spinal cord and the axons are part of peripheral nerves. Lesions of LMNs lead to weakness or paralysis and atrophy of the effector muscles they supply.

Motor neurone disease

This is a chronic progressive degeneration of upper and lower motor neurones, occurring more commonly in men over 50 years of age. The cause is seldom known, although a few cases are inherited as an autosomal dominant disorder (p. 443). Motor neurones in the cerebral cortex, brain stem and anterior horns of the spinal cord are

Table 7.4 Summary of effects of damage to motor neurones

Upper motor neurone	Lower motor neurone
Muscle weakness and spastic paralysis	Muscle weakness and flaccid paralysis
Exaggerated tendon reflexes	Absence of tendon reflexes
Muscle twitching	Muscle wasting Contracture of muscles Impaired circulation

destroyed and replaced by gliosis. Early effects are usually weakness and twitching of the small muscles of the hand, and muscles of the arm and shoulder girdle. The legs are affected later. Death occurs within 3–5 years and is usually due to respiratory difficulties or complications of immobility.

Mixed motor and sensory conditions

Subacute combined degeneration of the spinal cord

This condition most commonly occurs as a complication of pernicious anaemia (p. 74). Vitamin B_{12} is needed for the formation and maintenance of myelin by Schwann cells and oligodendrocytes. Although degeneration of the spinal cord may be apparent before the anaemia, it is arrested by treatment with vitamin B_{12}.

The degeneration of myelin occurs in the posterior and lateral columns of white matter in the spinal cord, especially in the upper thoracic and lower cervical regions. Less frequently the changes occur in the posterior root ganglia and peripheral nerves. Demyelination of proprioceptor fibres (sensory) leads to ataxia and involvement of upper motor neurones leads to increased muscle tone and spastic paralysis. Without treatment, death may occur within 5 years.

Compression of the spinal cord and nerve roots

The causes include:

- prolapsed intervertebral disc
- syringomyelia
- tumours: metastatic, meningeal or nerve sheath
- fractures with displacement of bone fragments.

Prolapsed intervertebral disc (Fig. 7.49)

This is the most common cause of compression of the spinal cord and/or nerve roots. The vertebral bodies are separated by the intervertebral discs, each consisting of an outer rim of cartilage, the *annulus fibrosus*, and a central core of soft gelatinous material, the *nucleus pulposus*.

Prolapse of a disc is herniation of the nucleus pulposus, causing the annulus fibrosus and the posterior longitudinal ligament to protrude into the neural canal. It is most common in the lumbar region, usually below the level of the spinal cord, i.e. below L2, and therefore affects nerve roots only. If it occurs in the cervical region, the cord may also be compressed. Herniation may occur suddenly, typically in young adults during strenuous exercise or exertion, or progressively in older people when there is bone disease or degeneration of the disc, which leads to rupture during minimal exercise. The hernia may be:

- one sided, causing pressure damage to a nerve root
- midline, compressing the spinal cord, the anterior spinal artery and possibly bilateral nerve roots.

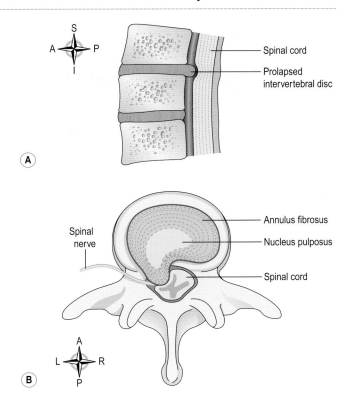

Figure 7.49 Prolapsed intervertebral disc. A. Viewed from the side. **B.** Viewed from above.

The outcome depends upon the size of the hernia and the length of time the pressure is applied. Small herniations cause local pain due to pressure on the nerve endings in the posterior longitudinal ligament. Large herniations may cause:

- unilateral or bilateral paralysis
- acute or chronic pain perceived to originate from the area supplied by the compressed sensory nerve, e.g. in the leg or foot
- compression of the anterior spinal artery, causing ischaemia and possibly necrosis of the spinal cord
- local muscle spasm due to pressure on motor nerves.

Syringomyelia

This dilation (syrinx) of the central canal of the spinal cord occurs most commonly in the cervical region and is associated with congenital abnormality of the distal end of the fourth ventricle. As the central canal dilates, pressure causes progressive damage to sensory and motor neurones.

Early effects include *dissociated anaesthesia*, i.e. insensibility to heat and pain, due to compression of the sensory fibres that cross the cord immediately they enter. In the long term there is destruction of motor and sensory tracts, leading to spastic paralysis and loss of sensation and reflexes.

187

Diseases of peripheral nerves

Learning outcomes

After studying this section, you should be able to:

■ compare and contrast the causes and effects of polyneuropathies and mononeuropathies

■ describe the effects of Guillain–Barré syndrome and Bell's palsy.

Peripheral neuropathy

This is a group of diseases of peripheral nerves not associated with inflammation. They are classified as:

• polyneuropathy: several nerves are affected

• mononeuropathy: a single nerve is usually affected.

Polyneuropathy

Damage to a number of nerves and their myelin sheaths occurs in association with other disorders, e.g.:

• vitamin deficiencies, e.g. vitamins B_1, B_6, B_{12}

• metabolic disorders, e.g. diabetes mellitus, uraemia (in renal failure), hepatic failure, malignancy

• toxic reactions to, e.g., alcohol, lead, mercury, aniline dyes and some drugs, such as phenytoin, isoniazid.

Long nerves are usually affected first, e.g. those supplying the feet and legs. The outcome depends upon the cause of the neuropathy and the extent of the damage.

Mononeuropathy

Usually only one nerve is damaged and the most common cause is ischaemia due to pressure. The resultant dysfunction depends on the site and extent of the injury. Examples include:

• pressure applied to cranial nerves in cranial bone foramina due to distortion of the brain by increased ICP

• compression of a nerve in a confined space caused by surrounding inflammation and oedema, e.g. the median nerve in carpal tunnel syndrome (see p. 435)

• external pressure on a nerve, e.g. an unconscious person lying with an arm hanging over the side of a bed or trolley

• compression of the axillary (circumflex) nerve by ill-fitting crutches

• trapping of a nerve between the broken ends of a bone

• ischaemia due to thrombosis of blood vessels supplying a nerve.

Guillain–Barré syndrome

Also known as acute inflammatory polyneuropathy, this is sudden, acute, progressive, bilateral ascending muscular weakness or paralysis. It begins in the lower limbs and spreads to the arms, trunk and cranial nerves. It usually occurs 1–3 weeks after an upper respiratory tract infection. There is widespread inflammation accompanied by some demyelination of spinal, peripheral and cranial nerves and the spinal ganglia. Paralysis may affect all the limbs and the respiratory muscles. Patients who survive the acute phase usually recover completely in weeks or months.

Bell's palsy

Compression of a facial nerve in the temporal bone foramen causes paralysis of facial muscles with drooping and loss of facial expression on the affected side. The immediate cause is inflammation and oedema of the nerve. The underlying cause is thought to be viral. The onset may be sudden or develop over several hours. Distortion of the features is due to muscle tone on the unaffected side, the affected side being expressionless. Recovery is usually complete within 3–8 weeks although the condition is sometimes permanent.

Developmental abnormalities of the nervous system

Learning outcomes

After studying this section, you should be able to:

■ describe developmental abnormalities of the nervous system

■ relate their effects to abnormal body function.

Spina bifida

This is a congenital malformation of the embryonic neural tube and spinal cord (Fig. 7.50). The vertebral (neural) arches are absent and the dura mater is abnormal, most commonly in the lumbosacral region. The causes are not known, although the condition is associated with dietary deficiency of folic acid at the time of conception. These neural tube defects may be of genetic origin or due to environmental factors, e.g. irradiation, or maternal infection (rubella) at a critical stage in development of the fetal vertebrae and spinal cord. The effects depend on the extent of the abnormality.

Occult spina bifida

In this 'hidden' condition the skin over the defect is intact and excessive growth of hair over the site may be the only sign of abnormality. This is sometimes associated with minor nerve defects that commonly affect the bladder.

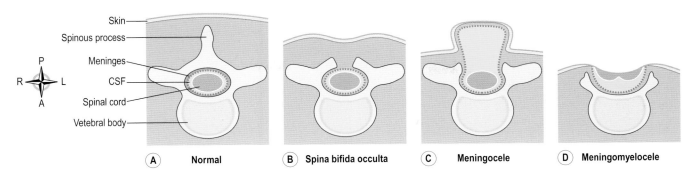

Figure 7.50 **Spina bifida.** Vertebrae viewed from above.

Meningocele

The skin over the defect is very thin and may rupture after birth. There is dilation of the subarachnoid space posteriorly. The spinal cord is correctly positioned.

Meningomyelocele

The meninges and spinal cord are grossly abnormal. The skin may be absent or rupture. In either case there is leakage of CSF, and the meninges may become infected. Serious nerve defects result in paraplegia and lack of sphincter control causing incontinence of urine and faeces. There may also be mental impairment.

Hydrocephalus

(see p. 180.)

Tumours of the nervous system

Learning outcome

After studying this section, you should be able to:

■ outline the effects of tumours of the nervous system.

Some 50% of brain tumours are metastases from the other primary sites, often the bronchus, breast, stomach or prostate (see below).

Primary tumours of the nervous system usually arise from the neuroglia, meninges or blood vessels. Neurones are rarely involved because they do not normally multiply. Nervous tissue tumours rarely metastise. Because of this, the rate of growth of an intracranial tumour is more important than the likelihood of spread outside the nervous system. In this context, 'benign' means slow growing and 'malignant' rapid growing. Early signs typically include headache, vomiting, visual disturbances and *papilloedema* (swelling of the optic disc seen by ophthalmoscopy). Signs of raised ICP appear after the limits of compensation have been reached (see p. 179).

Within the confined space of the skull, haemorrhage within a tumour exacerbates the increased ICP caused by the tumour.

Slow-growing tumours

These allow time for compensation for increasing intracranial pressure, so the tumour may be quite large before its effects are evident. Compensation involves gradual reduction in the volume of cerebrospinal fluid and circulating blood.

Rapidly growing tumours

These do not allow time for adjustment to compensate for the rapidly increasing ICP, so the effects quickly become apparent (Fig. 7.46C). Complications include:

- neurological impairment, depending on tumour site and size
- effects of increased ICP (p. 179)
- necrosis of the tumour, causing haemorrhage and oedema.

Specific tumours

Brain tumours typically arise from different cells in adults and children, and may range from benign to highly malignant. The most common tumours in adults are *glioblastomas* and *meningiomas*, which are usually benign and originate from arachnoid granulations. *Astrocytomas* and *medulloblastomas* account for most brain tumours in children.

Metastases in the brain

The prognosis of this condition is poor and the effects depend on the site(s) and rate of growth of metastases. There are two forms: discrete multiple tumours, mainly in the cerebrum, and diffuse tumours in the arachnoid mater.

For a range of self-assessment exercises on the topics in this chapter, visit Evolve online resources: https://evolve.elsevier.com/Waugh/anatomy/

The special senses

ANIMATIONS

The special senses of hearing, sight, smell and taste all have specialised sensory receptors that collect and transmit information to specific areas of the brain. Incoming nerve impulses from sensory receptors in the ears, eyes, nose and mouth are integrated and coordinated within the brain allowing perception of this sensory information. Up to 80% of what we perceive comes from external sensory stimuli. The first sections of this chapter explore the special senses, while the later ones consider the effect of ageing and problems that arise when disorders occur in the structures involved in hearing and vision.

Hearing and the ear

Learning outcomes

After studying this section, you should be able to:

- describe the structure of the outer, middle and inner parts of the ear
- explain the physiology of hearing.

The ear is the organ of hearing and is also involved in balance. It is supplied by the 8th cranial nerve, i.e. the *cochlear part* of the *vestibulocochlear nerve*, which is stimulated by vibrations caused by sound waves.

With the exception of the auricle (pinna), the structures that form the ear are encased within the petrous portion of the temporal bone.

Structure

The ear is divided into three distinct parts (Fig. 8.1): the outer ear, middle ear (tympanic cavity) and inner ear.

The outer ear collects the sound waves and directs them to the middle ear, which in turn transfers them to the inner ear, where they are converted into nerve impulses and transmitted to the hearing area in the cerebral cortex.

Outer ear

The outer ear consists of the auricle (pinna) and the external acoustic meatus (auditory canal).

The auricle (pinna)

The auricle is the visible part of the ear that projects from the side of the head. It is composed of fibroelastic cartilage covered with skin. It is deeply grooved and ridged; the most prominent outer ridge is the *helix*.

The *lobule* (earlobe) is the soft pliable part at the lower extremity, composed of fibrous and adipose tissue richly supplied with blood.

External acoustic meatus (auditory canal)

This is a slightly 'S'-shaped tube about 2.5 cm long extending from the auricle to the *tympanic membrane* (eardrum). The lateral third is embedded in cartilage and the remainder lies within the temporal bone. The meatus is lined with skin continuous with that of the auricle. There are numerous *ceruminous glands* and hair follicles, with associated *sebaceous glands*, in the skin of the lateral third. Ceruminous glands are modified sweat glands that secrete *cerumen* (earwax), a sticky material containing protective substances including the bacteriocidal enzyme lysozyme and immunoglobulins. Foreign materials, e.g. dust, insects and microbes, are prevented from reaching the tympanic membrane by wax, hairs and the curvature of the meatus. Movements of the temporomandibular

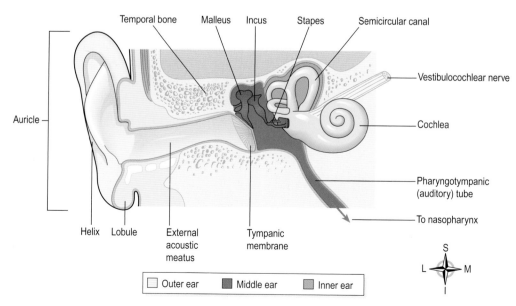

Figure 8.1 The parts of the ear.

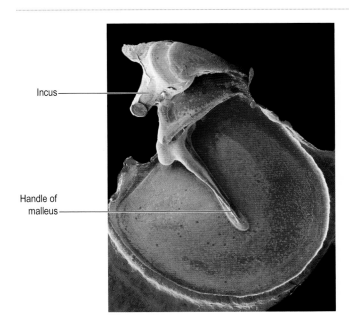

Figure 8.2 The tympanic membrane. Coloured scanning electron micrograph showing the malleus and the incus.

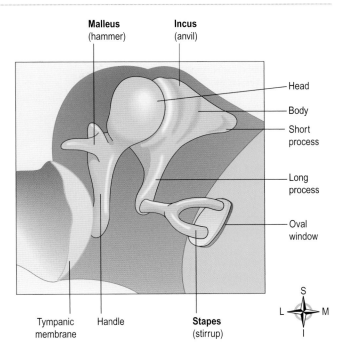

Figure 8.3 The auditory ossicles.

joint during chewing and speaking 'massage' the cartilaginous meatus, moving the wax towards the exterior.

The tympanic membrane (eardrum) (Fig. 8.2) completely separates the external acoustic meatus from the middle ear. It is oval-shaped with the slightly broader edge upwards and is formed by three types of tissue: the outer covering of hairless skin, the middle layer of fibrous tissue and the inner lining of mucous membrane continuous with that of the middle ear.

Middle ear (tympanic cavity)

This is an irregular-shaped air-filled cavity within the petrous portion of the temporal bone (Figs 8.1 and 8.3). The cavity, its contents and the air sacs which open out of it are lined with either simple squamous or cuboidal epithelium.

The *lateral wall* of the middle ear is formed by the tympanic membrane.

The *roof and floor* are formed by the temporal bone.

The *posterior wall* is formed by the temporal bone with openings leading to the mastoid antrum through which air passes to the air cells within the mastoid process.

The *medial wall* is a thin layer of temporal bone in which there are two openings:

- oval window
- round window (see Fig. 8.6).

The oval window is occluded by part of a small bone called the *stapes* and the round window, by a fine sheet of fibrous tissue.

Air reaches the cavity through the *pharyngotympanic* (*auditory* or *Eustachian*) *tube*, which links the nasopharynx

and middle ear. It is about 4 cm long and lined with ciliated columnar epithelium. The presence of air at atmospheric pressure on both sides of the tympanic membrane is maintained by the pharyngotympanic tube and enables the membrane to vibrate when sound waves strike it. The pharyngotympanic tube is normally closed but when there is unequal pressure across the tympanic membrane, e.g. at high altitude, it is opened by swallowing or yawning and the ears 'pop', equalising the pressure again.

Auditory ossicles (Fig. 8.3)

These are three very small bones only a few millimetres in size that extends across the middle ear from the tympanic membrane to the oval window (Fig. 8.1). They form a series of movable joints with each other and with the medial wall of the cavity at the oval window. The ossicles are held in place by fine ligaments and are named according to their shapes.

The malleus. This is the lateral hammer-shaped bone. The handle is in contact with the tympanic membrane and the head forms a movable joint with the incus.

The incus. This is the middle anvil-shaped bone. Its body articulates with the malleus, the long process with the stapes, and it is stabilised by the short process, fixed by fibrous tissue to the posterior wall of the tympanic cavity.

The stapes. This is the medial stirrup-shaped bone. Its head articulates with the incus and its footplate fits into the oval window.

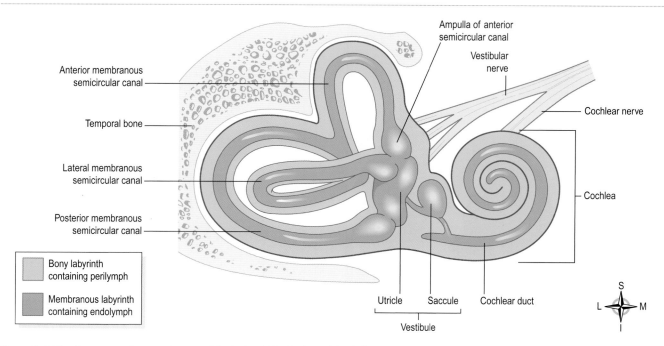

Figure 8.4 The inner ear. The membranous labyrinth within the bony labyrinth.

Inner ear (Fig. 8.4)

The inner ear or labyrinth (meaning 'maze') contains the organs of hearing and balance. It is described in two parts, the *bony labyrinth* and the *membranous labyrinth* and is divided into three main regions:

- the vestibule, containing the utricle and saccule
- three semicircular canals
- the cochlea.

The inner ear is formed from a network of channels and cavities in the temporal bone (the *bony labyrinth*). Within the bony labyrinth, like a tube within a tube, is the *membranous labyrinth*, a network of fluid-filled membranes that lines and fills the bony labyrinth (Fig. 8.4).

The bony labyrinth. This is lined with periosteum. Within the bony labyrinth, the membranous labyrinth is suspended in a watery fluid called *perilymph*.

The membranous labyrinth. This is filled with *endolymph*.

The vestibule

This is the expanded part nearest the middle ear. The oval and round windows are located in its lateral wall. It contains two membranous sacs, the utricle and the saccule, which are important in balance (p. 196).

The semicircular canals

These are three tubes arranged so that one is situated in each of the three planes of space. They are continuous with the vestibule and are also important in balance (p. 196).

The cochlea

This resembles a snail's shell. It has a broad base where it is continuous with the vestibule and a narrow apex, and it spirals round a central bony column.

A cross-section of the cochlea (Fig. 8.5) contains three compartments:

- the scala vestibuli
- the scala media, or *cochlear duct*
- the scala tympani.

In cross-section the bony cochlea has two compartments containing perilymph: the scala vestibuli, which originates at the oval window, and the scala tympani, which ends at the round window. The two compartments are continuous with each other and Figure 8.6 shows the relationship between these structures. The cochlear duct is part of the membranous labyrinth and is triangular in shape. On the *basilar membrane*, or base of the triangle, are *supporting cells* and specialised *cochlear hair cells* containing auditory receptors. These cells form the *spiral organ* (of Corti), the sensory organ that responds to vibration by initiating nerve impulses that are then perceived as hearing within the brain. The *auditory receptors* are dendrites of efferent (sensory) nerves that combine forming the cochlear (auditory) part of the vestibulocochlear nerve (8th cranial nerve), which passes through a foramen in the temporal bone to reach the hearing area in the temporal lobe of the cerebrum (see Fig. 7.20, p. 157).

Physiology of hearing ▪ 8.1

Every sound produces sound waves or vibrations in the air, which travel at about 332 metres per second. The

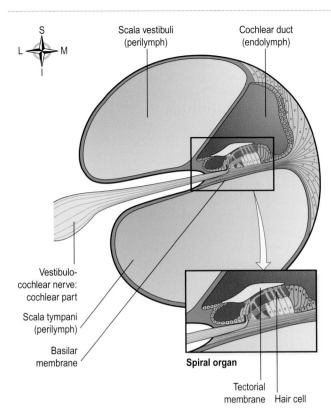

Figure 8.5 A cross-section of the cochlea showing the spiral organ (of Corti).

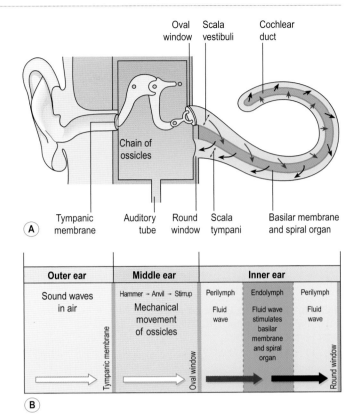

Figure 8.6 Passage of sound waves: A. The ear with cochlea uncoiled. **B.** Summary of transmission.

auricle, because of its shape, collects and concentrates the waves and directs them along the auditory canal causing the tympanic membrane to vibrate. Tympanic membrane vibrations are transmitted and amplified through the middle ear by movement of the ossicles (Fig. 8.6). At their medial end the footplate of the stapes rocks to and fro in the oval window, setting up fluid waves in the perilymph of the scala vestibuli. Some of the force of these waves is transmitted along the length of the scala vestibuli and scala tympani, but most of the pressure is transmitted into the cochlear duct. This causes a corresponding wave motion in the endolymph, resulting in vibration of the basilar membrane and stimulation of the auditory receptors in the hair cells of the spiral organ. The nerve impulses generated pass to the brain in the cochlear (auditory) portion of the vestibulocochlear nerve (8th cranial nerve). The fluid wave is finally expended into the middle ear by vibration of the membrane of the round window. The vestibulocochlear nerve transmits the impulses to the auditory nuclei in the medulla, where they synapse before they are conducted to the auditory area in the temporal lobe of the cerebrum (see Fig. 7.20, p. 157). Because some fibres cross over in the medulla and others remain on the same side, the left and right auditory areas of the cerebrum receive impulses from both ears.

Sound waves have the properties of *pitch* and *volume*, or intensity (Fig. 8.7). Pitch is determined by the frequency of the sound waves and is measured in Hertz (Hz). Sounds of different frequencies stimulate the basilar membrane (Fig. 8.6A) at different places along its length, allowing discrimination of pitch.

The volume depends on the magnitude of the sound waves and is measured in decibels (dB). The greater the amplitude of the wave created in the endolymph, the greater is the stimulation of the auditory receptors in the hair cells in the spiral organ, enabling perception of volume. Long-term exposure to excessive noise causes hearing loss because it damages the sensitive hair cells of the spiral organ.

Balance and the ear

Learning outcome

After studying this section, you should be able to:

■ describe the physiology of balance.

The semicircular canals and vestibule (Fig. 8.4)

The semicircular canals have no auditory function although they are closely associated with the cochlea.

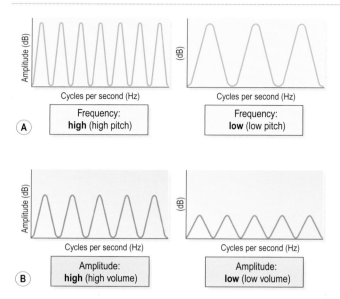

Figure 8.7 Behaviour of sound waves. A. Difference in frequency but of the same amplitude. **B.** Difference in amplitude but of the same frequency.

Instead they provide information about the position of the head in space, contributing to maintenance of posture and balance.

There are three semicircular canals, one lying in each of the three planes of space. They are situated above, beside and behind the vestibule of the inner ear and open into it.

The semicircular canals, like the cochlea, are composed of an outer bony wall and inner membranous tubes or *ducts*. The membranous ducts contain endolymph and are separated from the bony wall by perilymph.

The utricle is a membranous sac which is part of the vestibule and the three membranous ducts open into it at their dilated ends, the *ampullae*. The saccule is a part of the vestibule and communicates with the utricle and the cochlea.

In the walls of the utricle, saccule and ampullae are fine, specialised epithelial cells with minute projections, called *hair cells*. Amongst the hair cells there are receptors on sensory nerve endings, which combine forming the vestibulocochlear nerve.

Physiology of balance

The semicircular canals and the vestibule (utricle and saccule) are concerned with balance, or *equilibrium*. The arrangement of the three semicircular canals, one in each plane, not only allows perception of the position of the head in space but also the direction and rate of any movement. Any change of position of the head causes movement in the perilymph and endolymph, which bends the hair cells and stimulates the sensory receptors in the

utricle, saccule and ampullae. The resultant nerve impulses are transmitted by the vestibular nerve, which joins the cochlear nerve to form the vestibulocochlear nerve. The vestibular branch passes first to the *vestibular nucleus*, then to the cerebellum.

The cerebellum also receives nerve impulses from the eyes and proprioceptors (sensory receptors) in the skeletal muscles and joints. The cerebellum coordinates incoming impulses from the vestibular nerve, the eyes and proprioceptors. Thereafter, impulses are transmitted to the cerebrum and skeletal muscles enabling perception of body position and any adjustments needed to maintain posture and balance. This maintains upright posture and fixing of the eyes on the same point, independently of head movements.

Sight and the eye

Learning outcomes

After studying this section, you should be able to:

- describe the gross structure of the eye

- describe the route taken by nerve impulses from the retina to the cerebrum

- explain how light entering the eye is focused on the retina

- state the functions of the extraocular eye muscles

- explain the functions of the accessory organs of the eye.

The eye is the organ of sight. It is situated in the orbital cavity and supplied by the *optic nerve* (2nd cranial nerve).

It is almost spherical in shape and about 2.5 cm in diameter. The space between the eye and the orbital cavity is occupied by adipose tissue. The bony walls of the orbit and the fat protect the eye from injury.

Structurally the two eyes are separate but, unlike the ears, some of their activities are coordinated so that they normally function as a pair. It is possible to see with only one eye (monocular vision), but three-dimensional vision is impaired when only one eye is used, especially in relation to the judgement of speed and distance.

Structure (Fig. 8.8)

There are three layers of tissue in the walls of the eye:

- the outer fibrous layer: *sclera* and *cornea*
- the middle vascular layer or *uveal tract*: consisting of the choroid, ciliary body and iris
- the inner nervous tissue layer: the *retina*.

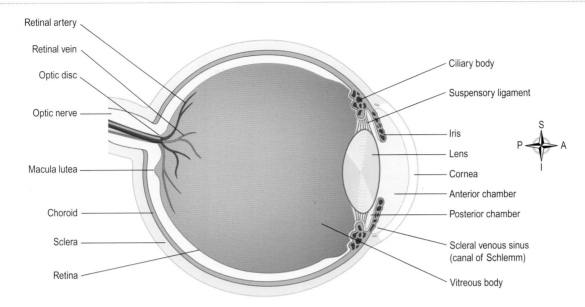

Figure 8.8 Section of the eye.

Structures inside the eyeball include the lens, aqueous fluid and vitreous body.

Sclera and cornea

The sclera, or white of the eye, forms the outermost layer of the posterior and lateral aspects of the eyeball and is continuous anteriorly with the cornea. It consists of a firm fibrous membrane that maintains the shape of the eye and gives attachment to the *extrinsic muscles* of the eye (see Table 8.1, p. 204).

Anteriorly the sclera continues as a clear transparent epithelial membrane, the cornea. Light rays pass through the cornea to reach the retina. The cornea is convex anteriorly and is involved in refracting (bending) light rays to focus them on the retina.

Choroid (Figs 8.8 and 8.9)

The choroid lines the posterior five-sixths of the inner surface of the sclera. It is very rich in blood vessels and is deep chocolate brown in colour. Light enters the eye through the pupil, stimulates the sensory receptors in the retina (p. 198) and is then absorbed by the choroid.

Ciliary body

The ciliary body is the anterior continuation of the choroid consisting of *ciliary muscle* (smooth muscle fibres) and secretory epithelial cells. As many of the smooth muscle fibres are circular, the ciliary muscle acts like a sphincter. The lens is attached to the ciliary body by radiating *suspensory ligaments*, like the spokes of a wheel (see Fig. 8.10). Contraction and relaxation of the ciliary muscle fibres, which are attached to these ligaments, control the size

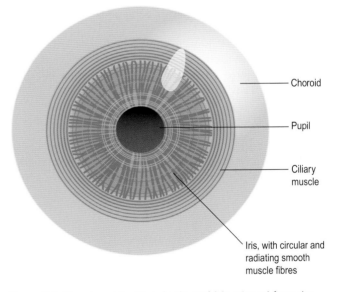

Figure 8.9 The choroid, ciliary body and iris. Viewed from the front.

and thickness of the lens. The epithelial cells secrete *aqueous fluid* into the anterior segment of the eye, i.e. the space between the lens and the cornea (anterior and posterior chambers) (Fig. 8.8). The ciliary body is supplied by parasympathetic branches of the oculomotor nerve (3rd cranial nerve). Stimulation causes contraction of the ciliary muscle and accommodation of the eye (p. 202).

Iris

The iris is the visible coloured ring at the front of the eye and extends anteriorly from the ciliary body, lying behind the cornea and in front of the lens. It divides the *anterior segment* of the eye into anterior and posterior chambers which contain aqueous fluid secreted by the ciliary body. It is a circular body composed of pigment cells and two layers of smooth muscle fibres, one circular and the other radiating (Fig. 8.9). In the centre is an aperture called the *pupil*.

The iris is supplied by parasympathetic and sympathetic nerves. Parasympathetic stimulation constricts the pupil and sympathetic stimulation dilates it (see Figs 7.44 and 7.43, respectively, pp. 174 and 175).

The colour of the iris is genetically determined and depends on the number of pigment cells present. Albinos have no pigment cells and people with blue eyes have fewer than those with brown eyes.

Lens (Fig. 8.10)

The lens is a highly elastic circular biconvex body, lying immediately behind the pupil. It consists of fibres enclosed within a capsule and is suspended from the ciliary body by the suspensory ligament. Its thickness is controlled by the ciliary muscle through the suspensory ligament. The lens bends (refracts) light rays reflected by objects in front of the eye. It is the only structure in the eye that can vary its refractory power, which is achieved by changing its thickness.

When the ciliary muscle contracts, it moves forward, releasing its pull on the lens, increasing its thickness. The nearer is the object being viewed, the thicker the lens becomes to allow focusing (see Fig. 8.18).

Retina

The retina is the innermost lining of the eye (Fig. 8.8). It is an extremely delicate structure and well adapted for stimulation by light rays. It is composed of several layers of nerve cell bodies and their axons, lying on a pigmented layer of epithelial cells. The light-sensitive layer consists of sensory receptor cells, *rods* and *cones*, which contain photosensitive pigments that convert light rays into nerve impulses.

The retina lines about three-quarters of the eyeball and is thickest at the back. It thins out anteriorly to end just behind the ciliary body. Near the centre of the posterior part is the *macula lutea*, or yellow spot (Figs 8.11A and 8.12). In the centre of the yellow spot is a little depression called the *fovea centralis*, consisting of only cones. Towards the anterior part of the retina there are fewer cones than rods.

About 0.5 cm to the nasal side of the macula lutea all the nerve fibres of the retina converge to form the optic nerve. The small area of retina where the optic nerve

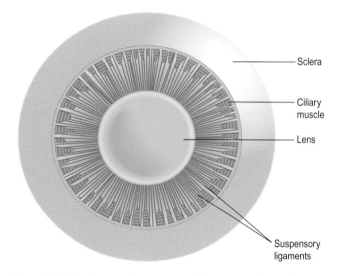

Figure 8.10 The lens and suspensory ligaments viewed from the front. The iris has been removed.

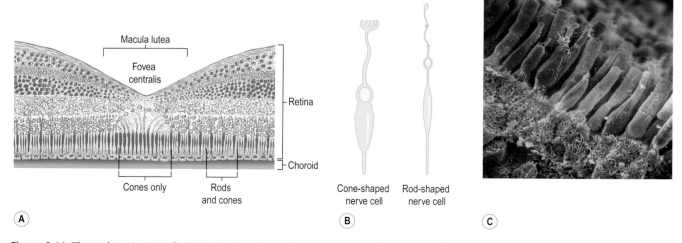

Figure 8.11 The retina. A. Magnified section. **B.** Light-sensitive nerve cells: rods and cones. **C.** Coloured scanning electron micrograph of rods (green) and cones (blue).

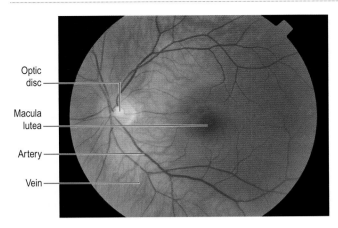

Optic disc
Macula lutea
Artery
Vein

Figure 8.12 The retina as seen through the pupil with an ophthalmoscope.

leaves the eye is the *optic disc* or *blind spot*. It has no light-sensitive cells.

Blood supply to the eye

The eye is supplied with arterial blood by the *ciliary arteries* and the *central retinal artery*. These are branches of the ophthalmic artery, a branch of the internal carotid artery.

Venous drainage is by a number of veins, including the *central retinal vein*, which eventually empty into a deep venous sinus.

The central retinal artery and vein are encased in the optic nerve, which enters the eye at the optic disc (Fig. 8.8).

Interior of the eye

The anterior segment of the eye, i.e. the space between the cornea and the lens, is incompletely divided into anterior and posterior chambers by the iris (Fig. 8.8). Both chambers contain a clear aqueous fluid secreted into the posterior chamber by the ciliary glands. It circulates in front of the lens, through the pupil into the anterior chamber and returns to the venous circulation through the *scleral venous sinus* (canal of Schlemm) in the angle between the iris and cornea (Fig. 8.8). The intraocular pressure remains fairly constant between 1.3 and 2.6 kPa (10 to 20 mmHg) as production and drainage rates of aqueous fluid are equal. An increase in this pressure causes *glaucoma* (p. 211). Aqueous fluid supplies nutrients and removes wastes from the transparent structures in the front of the eye that have no blood supply, i.e. the cornea, lens and lens capsule.

Behind the lens and filling the posterior segment (cavity) of the eyeball is the *vitreous body*. This is a soft, colourless, transparent, jelly-like substance composed of 99% water, some salts and mucoprotein. It maintains sufficient intraocular pressure to support the retina against the choroid and prevent the eyeball from collapsing.

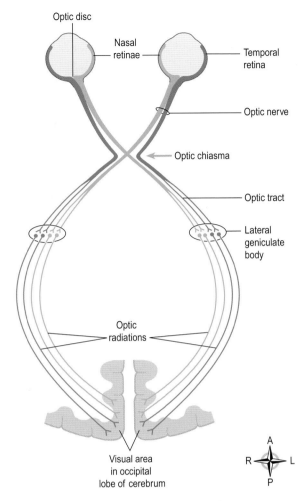

Figure 8.13 The optic nerves and their pathways.

The eye keeps its shape because of the intraocular pressure exerted by the vitreous body and the aqueous fluid. It remains fairly constant throughout life.

Optic nerves (second cranial nerves) (Fig. 8.13)

The fibres of the optic nerve originate in the retina and they converge to form the optic nerve about 0.5 cm to the nasal side of the macula lutea at the optic disc. The nerve pierces the choroid and sclera to pass backwards and medially through the orbital cavity. It then passes through the optic foramen of the sphenoid bone, backwards and medially to meet the nerve from the other eye at the *optic chiasma*.

Optic chiasma

This is situated immediately in front of and above the pituitary gland, which is in the hypophyseal fossa of the sphenoid bone (see Fig. 9.2, p. 217). In the optic chiasma the nerve fibres of the optic nerve from the nasal side of each retina cross over to the opposite side. The fibres from the temporal side do not cross but continue backwards

199

on the same side. This crossing over provides both cere-bral hemispheres with sensory input from each eye.

Optic tracts

These are the pathways of the optic nerves, posterior to the optic chiasma (Fig. 8.13). Each tract consists of the nasal fibres from the retina of one eye and the temporal fibres from the retina of the other. The optic tracts pass backwards to synapse with nerve cells of the *lateral genic-ulate bodies* of the thalamus. From there the nerve fibres proceed backwards and medially as the *optic radiations* to terminate in the *visual area* of the cerebral cortex in the occipital lobes of the cerebrum (see Fig. 7.20, p. 157). Other neurones originating in the lateral geniculate bodies transmit impulses from the eyes to the cerebellum where, together with impulses from the semicircular canals of the inner ears and from the skeletal muscles and joints, they contribute to the maintenance of posture and balance.

Physiology of sight 8.2

Light waves travel at a speed of 300 000 kilometres (186 000 miles) per second. Light is reflected into the eyes by objects within the field of vision. White light is a combina-tion of all the colours of the visual spectrum (rainbow), i.e. red, orange, yellow, green, blue, indigo and violet. This is demonstrated by passing white light through a glass prism which bends the rays of the different colours to a greater or lesser extent, depending on their wave-lengths (Fig. 8.14). Red light has the longest wavelength and violet the shortest.

This range of colour is the *spectrum of visible light*. In a rainbow, white light from the sun is broken up by rain-drops, which act as prisms and reflectors.

The electromagnetic spectrum

The electromagnetic spectrum is broad, but only a small part is visible to the human eye (Fig. 8.15). Beyond the long end are infrared waves (heat), microwaves and radio waves. Beyond the short end are ultraviolet (UV), X-rays and gamma rays. UV light is not normally visible because it is absorbed by a yellow pigment in the lens. Following

removal of the lens (cataract extraction), it is usually replaced with an artificial one to prevent long term damage to the retina from UV light rays.

A specific colour is perceived when only one wave-length is reflected by the object and all the others are absorbed, e.g. an object appears red when it only reflects red light. Objects appear white when all wavelengths are reflected, and black when they are all absorbed.

In order to achieve clear vision, light reflected from objects within the visual field is focused on to the retina of each eye. The processes involved in producing a clear image are *refraction of the light rays*, changing the *size of the pupils* and *accommodation* (adjustment of the lens for near vision, see p. 202).

Although these may be considered as separate pro-cesses, effective vision is dependent upon their coordination.

Refraction of the light rays

When light rays pass from a medium of one density to a medium of a different density they are bent; for example, a glass prism (Fig. 8.14). In the eye, the biconvex lens bends and focuses light rays (Fig. 8.16). This principle is

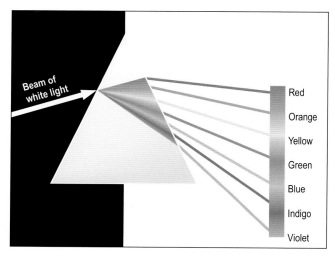

Figure 8.14 Refraction: white light broken into the colours of the visible spectrum when it passes through a glass prism.

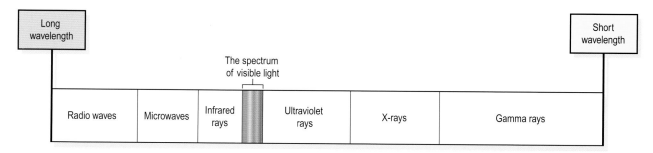

Figure 8.15 The electromagnetic spectrum.

used to focus light on the retina. Before reaching the retina, light rays pass successively through the conjunctiva, cornea, aqueous fluid, lens and vitreous body. They are all denser than air and, with the exception of the lens, they have a constant refractory power, similar to that of water.

Focusing of an image on the retina

Light rays reflected from an object are bent (refracted) by the lens when they enter the eye in the same way as shown in Figure 8.16, although the image on the retina is actually upside down (Fig. 8.17). The brain adapts to this early in life so that objects are perceived 'the right way up'.

Abnormal refraction within the eye is corrected using biconvex or biconcave lenses, which are shown on page 212.

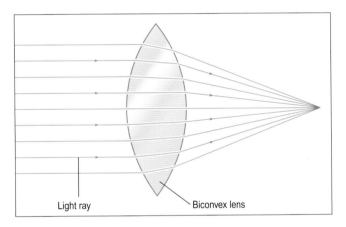

Figure 8.16 Refraction of light rays passing through a biconvex lens.

Lens

The lens is a biconvex elastic transparent body suspended behind the iris from the ciliary body by the suspensory ligament (Fig. 8.10). It is the only structure in the eye able to change its refractive power. Light rays entering the eye need to be refracted to focus them on the retina. Light from distant objects needs least refraction and, as the object comes closer, the amount of refraction needed increases. To focus light rays from near objects on the retina, the refractory power of the lens must be increased – by accommodation. To do this, the ciliary muscle (a sphincter) contracts moving the ciliary body inwards towards the lens. This lessens the pull on the suspensory ligaments and allows the lens to bulge, increasing its convexity and focusing light rays on the retina (see Fig. 8.18B).

To focus light rays from distant objects on the retina, the ciliary muscle relaxes, increasing its pull on the suspensory ligaments. This makes the lens thinner and focuses light rays from distant objects on the retina (see Fig. 8.18A).

Size of the pupils

Pupil size contributes to clear vision by controlling the amount of light entering the eye. In bright light the pupils are constricted. In dim light they are dilated.

If the pupils were dilated in bright light, too much light would enter the eye and damage the sensitive retina. In dim light, if the pupils were constricted, insufficient light would enter the eye to activate the light-sensitive pigments in the rods and cones, which stimulate the nerve endings in the retina enabling vision.

The iris consists of one layer of circular and one of radiating smooth muscle fibres. Contraction of the

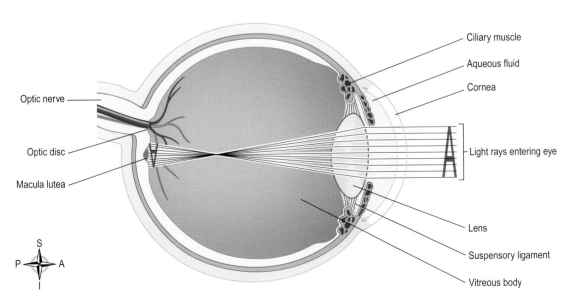

Figure 8.17 Section of the eye showing the focusing of light rays on the retina.

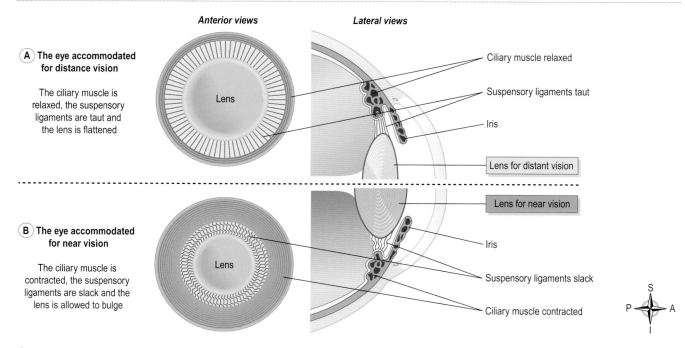

Anterior views   *Lateral views*

A The eye accommodated for distance vision

The ciliary muscle is relaxed, the suspensory ligaments are taut and the lens is flattened

Lens

Ciliary muscle relaxed

Suspensory ligaments taut

Iris

Lens for distant vision

Lens for near vision

B The eye accommodated for near vision

The ciliary muscle is contracted, the suspensory ligaments are slack and the lens is allowed to bulge

Lens

Iris

Suspensory ligaments slack

Ciliary muscle contracted

Figure 8.18 Accommodation: action of the ciliary muscle on the shape of the lens. A. Distant vision. **B.** Near vision.

circular fibres constricts the pupil, and contraction of the radiating fibres dilates it. The size of the pupil is controlled by the autonomic nervous system; sympathetic stimulation dilates the pupils and parasympathetic stimulation constricts them.

Accommodation

Near vision

In order to focus on near objects, i.e. within about 6 metres, accommodation is required and the eye must make the following adjustments:

- constriction of the pupils
- convergence
- changing the refractory power of the lens.

Constriction of the pupils. This assists accommodation by reducing the width of the beam of light entering the eye so that it passes through the central curved part of the lens (Fig. 8.17).

Convergence (movement of the eyeballs). Light rays from nearby objects enter the two eyes at different angles and for clear vision they must stimulate corresponding areas of the two retinae. Extrinsic muscles move the eyes and to obtain a clear image they rotate the eyes so that they converge on the object viewed. This coordinated muscle activity is under autonomic control. When there is voluntary movement of the eyes, both eyes move and convergence is maintained. The nearer an object is to the eyes the greater the eye rotation needed to achieve convergence, e.g. focusing near the tip of one's nose gives the

appearance of being 'cross-eyed'. If convergence is not complete, the eyes are focused on different objects or on different points of the same object. There are then two images sent to the brain and this can lead to double vision, *diplopia*. If convergence is not possible, the brain tends to ignore the impulses received from the divergent eye (see Squint, p. 211).

Changing the refractory power of the lens. Changes in the thickness of the lens are made to focus light on the retina. The amount of adjustment depends on the distance of the object from the eyes, i.e. the lens is thicker for near vision and at its thinnest when focusing on objects more than 6 metres away (Fig. 8.18). Looking at near objects 'tires' the eyes more quickly, owing to the continuous use of the ciliary muscle. The lens loses its elasticity and stiffens with age, a condition known as *presbyopia* (p. 208).

Distant vision

Objects more than 6 metres away from the eyes are focused on the retina without adjustment of the lens or convergence of the eyes.

Functions of the retina

The retina is the light-sensitive (photosensitive) part of the eye. The light-sensitive nerve cells are the rods and cones and their distribution in the retina is shown in Figure 8.11A. Light rays cause chemical changes in light-sensitive pigments in these cells and they generate nerve impulses which are conducted to the occipital lobes of the cerebrum via the optic nerves (Fig. 8.13).

The *rods* are much more light sensitive than the cones (see Fig. 8.11), so they are used when light levels are low. Stimulation of rods leads to monochromic (black and white) vision. Rods outnumber cones in the retina by about 16:1 and are more numerous towards the periphery of the retina. *Visual purple* (*rhodopsin*) is a light-sensitive pigment present only in the rods. It is bleached (degraded) by bright light and is quickly regenerated, provided an adequate supply of vitamin A is available.

The *cones* are sensitive to light and colour; bright light is required to activate them and give sharp, clear colour vision. The different wavelengths of visible light light-sensitive pigments in the cones, resulting in the perception of different colours.

Colour blindness. This is a common condition that affects more men than women. Although affected individuals see colours, they cannot always differentiate between them as the light-sensitive pigments (to red, green or blue) in cones are abnormal. There are different forms but the most common is red–green colour blindness which is transmitted a by sex-linked recessive gene (see Fig. 17.11, p. 445) where greens, oranges, pale reds and browns all appear to be the same colour and can only be distinguished by their intensity.

Dark adaptation. When exposed to bright light, the rhodopsin within the sensitive rods is completely degraded. This does not affect vision in good light, when there is enough light to activate the cones. However, moving into a darkened area where the light intensity is insufficient to stimulate the cones causes temporary visual impairment whilst the rhodopsin is being regenerated within the rods, 'dark adaptation'. When regeneration of rhodopsin has occurred, normal sight returns.

It is easier to see a dim star in the sky at night if the head is turned slightly away from it because light of low intensity is then focused on an area of the retina where there is a greater concentration of rods. If looked at directly, the light intensity of a dim star is not sufficient to stimulate the less sensitive cones in the area of the macula lutea. In dim evening light, colours cannot be distinguished because the light intensity is insufficient to stimulate colour-sensitive pigments in cones.

Breakdown and regeneration of the visual pigments in cones is similar to that of rods.

Binocular vision ▮8.3

Binocular or stereoscopic vision enables three-dimensional views although each eye 'sees' a scene from a slightly different angle (Fig. 8.19). The visual fields overlap in the middle but the left eye sees more on the left than can be seen by the other eye and vice versa. The images from the two eyes are fused in the cerebrum so that only one image is perceived.

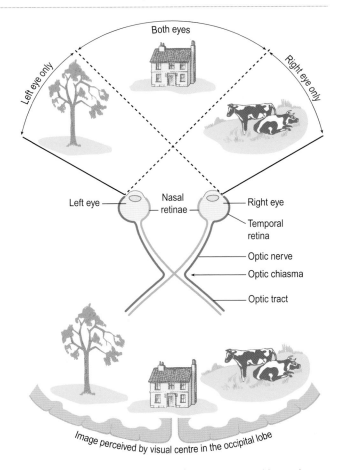

Figure 8.19 Parts of the visual field: monocular and binocular.

Binocular vision provides a much more accurate assessment of one object relative to another, e.g. its distance, depth, height and width. People with monocular vision may find it difficult, for example, to judge the speed and distance of an approaching vehicle.

Extraocular muscles of the eye

These include the muscles of the eyelids and those that move the eyeballs. The eyeball is moved by six *extrinsic muscles*, attached at one end to the eyeball and at the other to the walls of the orbital cavity. There are four *straight* (rectus) muscles and two *oblique* muscles (Fig. 8.20).

Moving the eyes to look in a particular direction is under voluntary control, but coordination of movement, needed for convergence and accommodation to near or distant vision, is under autonomic (involuntary) control. Movements of the eyes resulting from the action of these muscles are shown in Table 8.1.

Nerve supply to the muscles of the eye

Table 8.1 shows the nerves that supply the extrinsic muscles. The *oculomotor nerves* supply the *intrinsic eye muscles* of the iris and ciliary body.

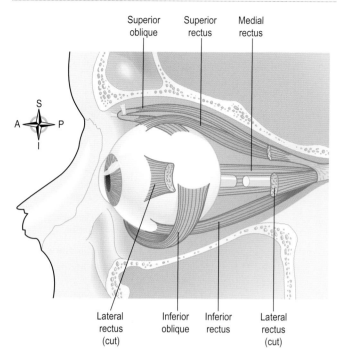

Figure 8.20 The extrinsic muscles of the eye.

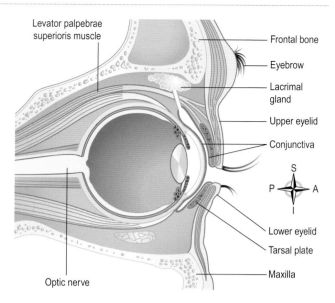

Figure 8.21 Section of the eye and its accessory structures.

Table 8.1 Extrinsic muscles of the eye: their actions and cranial nerve supply		
Name	**Action**	**Cranial nerve supply**
Medial rectus	Rotates eyeball inwards	Oculomotor nerve (3rd cranial nerve)
Lateral rectus	Rotates eyeball outwards	Abducent nerve (6th cranial nerve)
Superior rectus	Rotates eyeball upwards	Oculomotor nerve (3rd cranial nerve)
Inferior rectus	Rotates eyeball downwards	Oculomotor nerve (3rd cranial nerve)
Superior oblique	Rotates eyeball downwards and outwards	Trochlear nerve (4th cranial nerve)
Inferior oblique	Rotates eyeball upwards and outwards	Oculomotor nerve (3rd cranial nerve)

Accessory organs of the eye

The eye is a delicate organ which is protected by several structures (Fig. 8.21):

- eyebrows
- eyelids and eyelashes
- lacrimal apparatus.

Eyebrows

These are two arched ridges of the supraorbital margins of the frontal bone. Numerous hairs (eyebrows) project obliquely from the surface of the skin. They protect the eyeball from sweat, dust and other foreign bodies.

Eyelids (palpebrae)

The eyelids are two movable folds of tissue situated above and below the front of each eye. On their free edges are short curved hairs, the *eyelashes*. The layers of tissue forming the eyelids are:

- a thin covering of skin
- a thin sheet of subcutaneous connective (loose areolar) tissue
- two muscles – the *orbicularis oculi* and *levator palpebrae superioris*
- a thin sheet of dense connective tissue, the *tarsal plate*, larger in the upper than the lower eyelid, which supports the other structures
- a membranous lining, the *conjunctiva*.

Conjunctiva

This is a fine transparent membrane that lines the eyelids and the front of the eyeball (Fig. 8.21). Where it lines the eyelids it consists of highly vascular columnar epithelium. Corneal conjunctiva consists of avascular stratified epithelium, i.e. epithelium without blood vessels. When the eyelids are closed the conjunctiva becomes a closed sac. It protects the delicate cornea and the front of the eye. When eyedrops are administered they are placed in the lower conjunctival sac. The medial and lateral angles of the eye where the upper and lower lids come together are called respectively the *medial canthus* and the *lateral canthus*.

Eyelid margins

Along the edges of the lids are numerous *sebaceous glands*, some with ducts opening into the hair follicles of the eyelashes and some on to the eyelid margins between the hairs. *Tarsal glands* are modified sebaceous glands embedded in the tarsal plates with ducts that open on to the inside of the free margins of the eyelids. They secrete an oily material, spread over the conjunctiva by blinking, which delays evaporation of tears.

Functions

The eyelids and eyelashes protect the eye from injury:

- reflex closure of the lids occurs when the conjunctiva or eyelashes are touched, when an object comes close to the eye or when a bright light shines into the eye – this is called the *corneal reflex*
- blinking at about 3- to 7-second intervals spreads tears and oily secretions over the cornea, preventing drying.

When the orbicularis oculi contract, the eyes close. When the levator palpebrae contract, the eyelids open (see Fig. 16.58, p. 424).

Lacrimal apparatus (Fig. 8.22)

For each eye this consists of the structures that secrete tears and drain them from the front of the eyeball:

- 1 lacrimal gland and its ducts
- 2 lacrimal canaliculi
- 1 lacrimal sac
- 1 nasolacrimal duct.

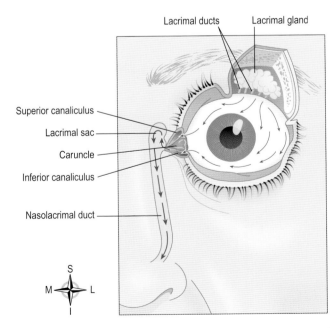

Lacrimal ducts   Lacrimal gland

Superior canaliculus

Lacrimal sac

Caruncle

Inferior canaliculus

Nasolacrimal duct

S
M — L
I

Figure 8.22 The lacrimal apparatus. Arrows show the direction of the flow of tears.

The lacrimal glands are exocrine glands situated in recesses in the frontal bones on the lateral aspect of each eye just behind the supraorbital margin. Each gland is approximately the size and shape of an almond, and is composed of secretory epithelial cells. The glands secrete *tears* composed of water, mineral salts, antibodies (immunoglobulins, see Ch. 15) and *lysozyme*, a bactericidal enzyme.

The tears leave the lacrimal gland by several small ducts and pass over the front of the eye under the lids towards the medial canthus where they drain into the *two lacrimal canaliculi*; the opening of each is called the *punctum*. The two canaliculi lie one above the other, separated by a small red body, the *caruncle*. The tears then drain into the *lacrimal sac*, which is the upper expanded end of the *nasolacrimal duct*. This is a membranous canal approximately 2 cm long, extending from the lower part of the lacrimal sac to the nasal cavity, opening at the level of the inferior concha. Normally the rate of secretion of tears keeps pace with the rate of drainage. When a foreign body or other irritant enters the eye the secretion of tears is greatly increased and the conjunctival blood vessels dilate. Secretion of tears is also increased in emotional states, e.g. crying, laughing.

Functions

The fluid that fills the conjunctival sac is a mixture of tears and the oily secretion of tarsal glands, which is spread over the cornea by blinking. The functions of this fluid include:

- provision of oxygen and nutrients to the avascular corneal conjunctiva and drainage of wastes
- washing away irritating materials, e.g. dust, grit
- the bactericidal enzyme *lysozyme* prevents microbial infection
- its oiliness delays evaporation and prevents friction or drying of the conjunctiva.

Sense of smell

Learning outcome

After studying this section, you should be able to:

- describe the physiology of smell.

The sense of smell, or *olfaction*, originates in the nasal cavity, which also acts as a passageway for respiration (see Ch. 10).

Olfactory nerves (first cranial nerves)

These are the sensory nerves of smell. They originate as *chemoreceptors* (specialised olfactory nerve endings) in the mucous membrane of the roof of the nasal cavity above the superior nasal conchae (Fig. 8.23). On each side of the nasal septum nerve fibres pass through the cribriform plate of the ethmoid bone to the *olfactory bulb* where interconnections and synapses occur (Fig. 8.24). From the bulb, bundles of nerve fibres form the *olfactory tract*, which passes backwards to the olfactory area in the temporal lobe of the cerebral cortex in each hemisphere where the impulses are interpreted and odour perceived (see Fig. 7.20, p. 157). 8.4

Physiology of smell

The human sense of smell is less acute than in other animals. Many animals secrete odorous chemicals called *pheromones*, which play an important part in chemical communication in, for example, territorial behaviour, mating and the bonding of mothers and their newborn. The role of pheromones in human communication is unknown.

All odorous materials give off volatile molecules, which are carried into the nose with inhaled air and even very low concentrations, when dissolved in mucus, stimulate the olfactory chemoreceptors.

The air entering the nose is warmed, and convection currents carry eddies of inspired air to the roof of the nasal cavity. 'Sniffing' concentrates volatile molecules in the roof of the nose. This increases the number of olfactory receptors stimulated and thus perception of the smell. The sense of smell and the sense of taste are closely related; the sense of smell may affect the appetite. If the odours are pleasant the appetite may improve and vice versa. When accompanied by the sight of food, an appetising smell increases salivation and stimulates the digestive system (see Ch. 12). The sense of smell and the sense of taste are closely related; the sense of smell may create powerful and long-lasting memories, especially for distinctive odours, e.g. hospital smells, favourite or least-liked foods.

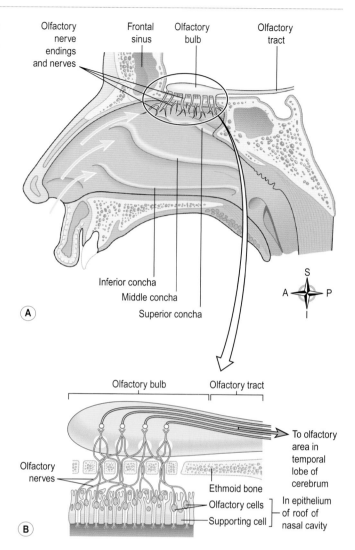

Figure 8.23 The sense of smell. A. The olfactory structures. **B.** An enlarged section of the olfactory apparatus in the nose and on the inferior surface of the cerebrum.

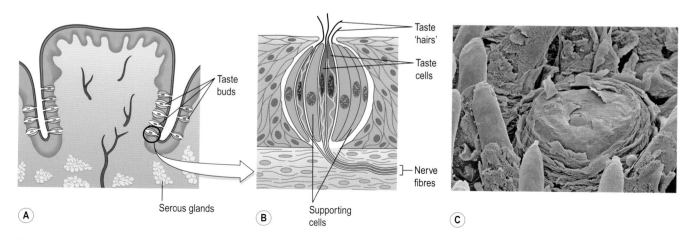

Figure 8.24 Structure of taste buds. A. A section of a papilla. **B.** A taste bud – greatly magnified. **C.** Coloured scanning electron micrograph of a taste bud (centre) on the tongue.

Inflammation of the nasal mucosa prevents odorous substances from reaching the olfactory area of the nose, causing loss of the sense of smell (*anosmia*). The usual cause is a cold.

Adaptation. When an individual is continuously exposed to an odour, perception of the odour decreases and ceases within a few minutes. This loss of perception affects only that specific odour.

Sense of taste

Learning outcome

After studying this section, you should be able to:

■ describe the physiology of taste.

The sense of taste, or *gustation*, is closely linked to the sense of smell and, like smell, also involves stimulation of chemoreceptors by dissolved chemicals.

Taste buds contain chemoreceptors (sensory receptors) that are found in the papillae of the tongue and widely distributed in the epithelia of the tongue. They consist of small sensory nerve endings of the glossopharyngeal, facial and vagus nerves (cranial nerves VII, IX and X). Some of the cells have hair-like cilia on their free border, projecting towards tiny pores in the epithelium (Fig. 8.24). The sensory receptors are highly sensitive and stimulated by very small amounts of chemicals that enter the pores dissolved in saliva. Nerve impulses are generated and conducted along the glossopharyngeal, facial and vagus nerves before synapsing in the medulla and thalamus. Their final destination is the *taste area* in the parietal lobe of the cerebral cortex where taste is perceived (see Fig. 7.20, p. 157).

Physiology of taste

Four fundamental sensations of taste have been described – sweet, sour, bitter and salt; however, others have also been suggested, including metallic and umami (a Japanese 'savoury' taste). However, perception varies widely and many 'tastes' cannot be easily classified. It is thought that all taste buds are stimulated by all 'tastes'. Taste is impaired when the mouth is dry, because substances can only be 'tasted' when in solution.

The sense of taste is closely linked to the sense of smell. For example when one has a cold, it is common for food to taste bland and unappealing. In addition, taste triggers salivation and the secretion of gastric juice (see Ch. 12). The sense of taste also has a protective function, e.g. when foul-tasting food is eaten, reflex gagging or vomiting may be induced.

The effect of ageing on the special senses

Learning outcome

After studying this section, you should be able to:

■ describe the impact of ageing on the special senses.

Changes in hearing and vision that occur as part of normal ageing are almost universal and often accompanied by diminished senses of taste and smell. The number of olfactory receptors reduces around the age of 50, diminishing the sense of taste; older adults may complain of their food being bland while children can find the same food too spicy. In a similar way, older adults may not smell (perceive) weak odours. The effect of changes associated with ageing on hearing and vision are considered below.

Presbycusis

This form of hearing impairment accompanies the ageing process and is therefore common in older adults. Degenerative changes in the sensory cells of the spiral organ result in sensorineural hearing loss (p. 209). Perception of high-frequency sound is impaired first and later low-frequency sound may also be affected. Difficulty in discrimination develops, e.g. following a conversation, especially in the presence of background noise.

Vision

Presbyopia and cataracts are common consequences of normal ageing.

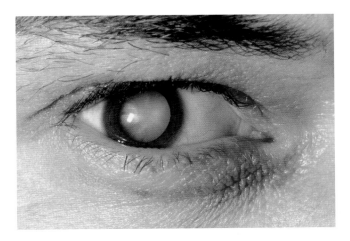

Figure 8.25 Cataract.

Presbyopia

Age-related changes in the lens lead to loss of accommodation as the lens loses its elasticity and becomes firmer. This prevents focusing of light on the retina, giving blurred vision. Correction is achieved using glasses with convex lenses for near vision, e.g. reading (see Fig. 8.27).

Cataracts

Cataracts arise when there is opacity of the lens (Fig. 8.25). Weak light rays cannot easily pass through a less transparent or cloudy lens and is the reason why many older adults use brighter light for reading and may also experience difficulty with night vision. It is most commonly age-related occurring as a result of exposure to predisposing factors which include UV light, X-rays and cigarette smoke. There are also other important causes of cataracts (p. 211).

Disorders of the ear

Learning outcomes

After studying this section, you should be able to:

■ compare and contrast the features of conductive and sensorineural hearing loss

■ describe the causes and effects of diseases of the ear.

Hearing loss

Hearing impairment can be classified in two main categories: *conductive* and *sensorineural*. Hearing impairment can also be mixed when there is a combination of conductive and sensorineural hearing loss in one ear.

Conductive hearing impairment

This occurs when an abnormality of the outer or middle ear impairs conduction of sound waves to the oval window; common examples are listed in Box 8.1.

Otosclerosis. This is a common cause of progressive conductive hearing loss in young adults that may affect one ear but is more commonly bilateral. It is usually hereditary, more common in females than males and often worsens during pregnancy. Abnormal bone develops around the footplate of the stapes, fusing it to the oval window, reducing the ability to transmit sound waves across the tympanic cavity.

Serous otitis media. Also known as *'glue ear'*, or secretory otitis media, this is a collection of fluid (*effusion*) in the middle ear cavity. Causes include:

• obstruction of the auditory tube by, for example, pharyngeal swelling, enlarged adenoids or tumour

• barotrauma (usually caused by descent in an aeroplane when suffering from a cold)

• untreated acute otitis media.

The air already present in the middle ear is absorbed and a negative pressure develops causing retraction of the tympanic membrane. Thereafter fluid is drawn into the low-pressure cavity from surrounding blood vessels causing conductive hearing loss.

Adults experience hearing loss and, usually painless, blockage of the ear. However, this is a common cause of hearing impairment in preverbal children which may manifest as delayed speech and/or achievement of developmental milestones. Secondary infection can complicate this condition in both adults and children.

Sensorineural hearing impairment

This is the more prevalent form of hearing impairment and is the result of a disorder of the nerves of the inner ear or the central nervous system, e.g. the cochlea, cochlear branch of the vestibular nerve or the auditory area of the cerebrum. Noise-induced hearing loss is one cause of sensorineural hearing impairment which may arise as a consequence of:

• employment e.g. construction work, manufacturing or the music industry

• social activities e.g. listening to loud music on personal equipment or at nightclubs.

Other causes are listed in Box 8.1.

Risk factors for congenital sensorineural hearing impairment include family history, exposure to intrauterine viruses, e.g. maternal rubella and acute hypoxia at birth.

Ménière's disease. In this condition there is accumulation of endolymph causing distension and increased pressure within the membranous labyrinth with destruction of the sensory cells in the ampulla and cochlea. It is usually unilateral at first but both ears may be affected later. The cause is not known. Ménière's disease is associated with recurrent episodes of incapacitating dizziness (*vertigo*), nausea and vomiting, lasting for several hours. Periods of remission vary from days to months. During and between attacks there may be continuous ringing in the affected ear (*tinnitus*). Loss of hearing is experienced during episodes, which may gradually become permanent over a period of years as the spiral organ is destroyed.

Presbycusis. (see p. 207).

Ear infections

External otitis

Infection by *Staphylococcus aureus* is the usual cause of localised inflammation (boils) in the auditory canal. More

---

Box 8.1 Common causes of hearing loss

Conductive	Sensorineural
Acute otitis media	Impacted earwax or foreign body
Serous otitis media	Presbycusis
Chronic otitis media	Long-term exposure to excessive noise
Barotrauma	Congenital
Otosclerosis	Ménière's disease
External otitis	Ototoxic drugs, e.g. aminoglycoside antibiotics, diuretics, chemotherapy
Injury of the tympanic membrane	Infections, e.g. mumps, herpes zoster, meningitis, syphilis

generalised inflammation may be caused by prolonged exposure to bacteria or fungi or by an allergic reaction to, e.g., dandruff, soaps, hair sprays, hair dyes.

Acute otitis media

This is inflammation of the middle ear cavity, usually caused by upward spread of microbes from an upper respiratory tract infection via the auditory tube. It is very common in children and is accompanied by severe earache. Occasionally it spreads inwards from the outer ear through a perforation in the tympanic membrane.

Bacterial infection leads to the accumulation of pus and the outward bulging of the tympanic membrane. Sometimes the tympanic membrane ruptures and pus discharges from the middle ear (*otorrhoea*). The spread of infection may cause *mastoiditis* and *labyrinthitis* (see below). As the petrous portion of the temporal bone is very thin, the infection may spread through the bone and cause meningitis (p. 184) and brain abscess.

Chronic otitis media

In this condition there is permanent perforation of the tympanic membrane following acute otitis media (especially when recurrent, persistent or untreated) and mechanical or blast injuries. During the healing process stratified epithelium from the outer ear sometimes grows into the middle ear, forming a *cholesteatoma*. This is a collection of desquamated epithelial cells and purulent material. Continued development of cholesteatoma may lead to:

- destruction of the ossicles and conductive hearing loss
- erosion of the roof of the middle ear and meningitis
- spread of infection to the inner ear that may cause labyrinthitis (see below).

Labyrinthitis

This complication of middle ear infection may be caused by development of a fistula from a cholesteatoma (see above). It is accompanied by vertigo, nausea and vomiting, and nystagmus. In some cases the spiral organ is destroyed, causing sudden profound sensorineural hearing loss in the affected ear.

Motion sickness

This occurs when the brain receives conflicting sensory information; the visual information received from the eye does not match the information from the semicircular canals of the inner ear about one's position in relation to the environment. It causes nausea and vomiting in some people, and is usually associated with travel, e.g. by car, train or aeroplane.

Disorders of the eye

Learning outcome

After studying this section, you should be able to:

- describe the pathological changes and effects of diseases of the eye.

Inflammatory conditions

Stye

Also known as hordeolum, this is an acute and painful bacterial infection of sebaceous or tarsal glands of the eyelid margin. The most common cause is *Staphylococcus aureus*. A 'crop' of styes may occur due to localised spread to adjacent glands. Infection of tarsal glands may block their ducts, leading to cyst formation (*chalazion*), which may damage the cornea.

Blepharitis

This is chronic inflammation of the eyelid margins, usually caused by bacterial infection or allergy, e.g. staphylococcal infection or *seborrhoea* (excessive sebaceous gland secretion). If ulceration occurs, healing by fibrosis may distort the eyelid margins, preventing complete closure of the eye. This may lead to drying of the eye, conjunctivitis and possibly corneal ulceration.

Conjunctivitis

Inflammation of the conjunctiva may be caused by irritants, such as smoke, dust, wind, cold or dry air, microbes or antigens and may be acute or chronic (Fig. 8.26). Corneal ulceration (see below) is a rare complication.

Infection. This is highly contagious and in adults is usually caused by strains of staphylococci, streptococci or haemophilus.

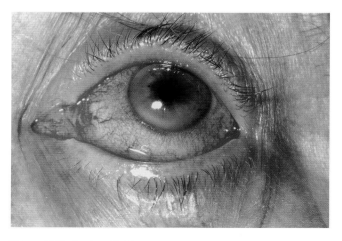

Figure 8.26 Conjunctivitis.

Neonatal conjunctivitis. Sexually transmitted disease in the mother, including gonorrhoea, chlamydia and genital herpes, can infect the newborn infant's eyes as the baby passes through the birth canal.

Allergic conjunctivitis. This may be a complication of hay fever, or be caused by a wide variety of airborne antigens, e.g. dust, pollen, fungus spores, animal dander, cosmetics, hair sprays, soaps. The condition sometimes becomes chronic.

Trachoma

This chronic inflammatory condition is caused by *Chlamydia trachomatis* and is a common cause of sight loss in developing countries. Deposition of fibrous tissue in the conjunctiva and cornea leads to eyelid deformity and corneal scarring as the eyelashes rub against the surface of the eye. The microbes are spread by poor hygiene, e.g. communal use of contaminated washing water, cross-infection between mother and child, or contaminated towels and clothing.

Corneal ulcer

This is local necrosis of corneal tissue, usually associated with corneal infection (*keratitis*) following trauma (e.g. abrasion), or infection spread from the conjunctiva or eyelids. Causative organisms include staphylococci, streptococci and herpes viruses. Acute pain, *injection* (redness of the cornea), photophobia and lacrimation interfere with sight during the acute phase. In severe cases extensive ulceration or perforation and healing by fibrosis can cause opacity of the cornea requiring corneal transplantation.

Glaucoma

This is a group of conditions in which intraocular pressure rises due to impaired drainage of aqueous fluid through the scleral venous sinus (canal of Schlemm) in the angle between the iris and cornea in the anterior chamber (Fig. 8.8). Persistently raised intraocular pressure may damage the optic nerve by mechanical compression or compression of its blood supply causing ischaemia.

Damage to the optic nerve impairs vision; the extent of which varies from some visual impairment to complete loss of sight.

In addition to the primary glaucomas below, it is occasionally congenital or secondary to other causes, e.g. anterior uveitis or a tumour.

Primary glaucomas

Primary open-angle glaucoma (POAG). There is a gradual painless rise in intraocular pressure with progressive loss of vision. Peripheral vision is lost first but may not be noticed until only central (*tunnel*) vision remains. As the condition progresses, atrophy of the optic disc occurs leading to irreversible loss of vision. It is commonly bilateral and occurs mostly in people over 40 years of age. The cause is not known but there is a familial tendency.

Acute closed-angle glaucoma. This is most common in people over 40 years of age and usually affects one eye. During life the lens gradually increases in size, pushing the iris forward. In dim light when the pupil dilates, the lax iris bulges still further forward, and may come into contact with the cornea, blocking the scleral venous sinus (canal of Schlemm) suddenly raising the intraocular pressure. Sudden severe pain, photophobia, headache, nausea and blurred vision accompany an acute attack. It may resolve spontaneously if the iris responds to bright light, constricting the pupil and releasing the pressure on the scleral venous sinus. After repeated attacks spontaneous recovery may be incomplete and vision is progressively impaired.

Chronic closed-angle glaucoma. The intraocular pressure rises gradually without symptoms. Later, peripheral vision deteriorates followed by atrophy of the optic disc and loss of sight.

Strabismus (squint, cross-eye)

In normal binocular vision, the eyes are aligned so that each eye sees the same image, meaning that both eyes send the same image to the brain. In strabismus only one eye is directed at the observed object and the other diverges (is directed elsewhere). The result is that two different images are sent to the brain, one from each eye, instead of one. It is caused by one-sided extrinsic muscle weakness or impairment of the cranial nerve (III, IV or VI) supply to the extrinsic muscles. In most cases the image from the squinting eye is suppressed by the brain, otherwise there is double vision (*diplopia*).

Presbyopia

(see p. 208).

Cataract

This is opacity of the lens which impairs vision especially in poor light and darkness when weak light rays can no longer pass through the cloudy lens to the retina (Fig. 8.25). Although most commonly age-related (p. 208) this condition also be congenital or secondary to other conditions e.g. ocular trauma, uveitis, diabetes mellitus.

The most common cause of visual impairment worldwide, cataracts can affect one or both eyes. The extent of visual impairment depends on the location and extent of the opacity.

Congenital cataract may be idiopathic, or due to genetic abnormality or maternal infection in early pregnancy, e.g. rubella. Early treatment is required to prevent permanent loss of sight.

Retinopathies

Vascular retinopathies

Occlusion of the central retinal artery or vein causes sudden painless unilateral loss of vision. *Arterial occlusion* is usually due to embolism from, e.g., atheromatous plaques, endocarditis. *Venous occlusion* is usually associated with increased intraocular pressure in, for example, glaucoma, diabetes mellitus, hypertension, increased blood viscosity. The retinal veins become distended and retinal haemorrhages occur.

Diabetic retinopathy

This occurs in type I and type II diabetes mellitus (p. 236) and is the commonest cause of blindness in adults aged between 30 and 65 years in developed countries. Changes in retinal blood vessels increase with the severity and duration of hyperglycaemia. Capillary microaneurysms develop and later there may be proliferation of blood vessels. Haemorrhages, fibrosis and secondary retinal detachment may follow and, over time, there may be severe retinal degeneration and loss of vision.

Retinopathy of prematurity (ROP)

This condition affects premature babies. Known risk factors include: birth before 32 weeks' gestation, birth weight less than 1500 g, requirement for oxygen therapy and serious illness. There is abnormal development of retinal blood vessels and formation of fibrovascular tissue in the vitreous body causing varying degrees of interference with light transmission. The prognosis depends on the severity and many cases resolve spontaneously. In severe cases there may also be haemorrhage in the vitreous body, retinal detachment and loss of vision.

Retinal detachment

This painless condition occurs when a tear or hole in the retina allows fluid to accumulate between the layers of retinal cells or between the retina and choroid. It is usually localised at first but as fluid collects the detachment spreads. There are visual disturbances, often spots before the eyes or flashes of light due to abnormal stimulation of sensory receptors, and progressive loss of vision, sometimes described as a 'shadow' or 'curtain'. In many cases the cause is unknown but it may be associated with trauma to the eye or head, tumours, haemorrhage, cataract surgery when intraocular pressure is reduced or diabetic retinopathy.

Retinitis pigmentosa

This is a group of hereditary diseases in which there is degeneration of the retina, mainly affecting the rods. Progressive impairment of peripheral vision, especially in dim light, usually becomes apparent in early childhood. Over time this leads to tunnel vision and, eventually, loss of sight.

Tumours

Choroidal malignant melanoma

This is the most common ocular malignancy in adults, occurring between 40 and 70 years of age. Vision is not normally affected until the tumour causes retinal detachment or secondary glaucoma, usually when well advanced. The tumour spreads locally in the choroid, and blood-borne metastases usually develop in the liver.

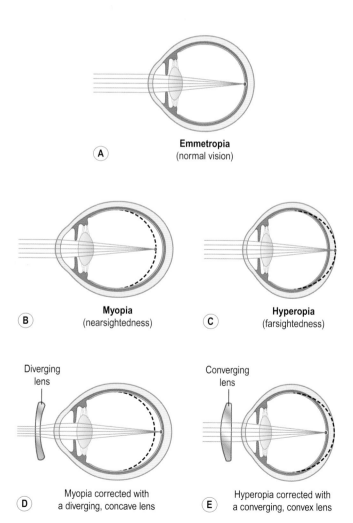

Figure 8.27 Common refractive errors of the eye and corrective lenses. A. Normal eye. **B.** Nearsightedness. **C.** Farsightedness. **D.** Correction of nearsightedness. **E.** Correction of farsightedness.

Retinoblastoma

This is the most common malignant tumour in children. A small number of cases are familial. It is usually evident before the age of 4 years and usually affects one side. The condition presents with a squint and enlargement of the eye. As the tumour grows visual impairment develops and the pupil looks pale. It spreads locally to the vitreous body and may grow along the optic nerve, invading the brain.

Refractive errors of the eye

Learning outcome

After studying this section, you should be able to:

■ explain how corrective lenses overcome refractive errors of the eye.

In the *emetropic* or normal eye, light from near and distant objects is focused on the retina (Fig. 8.27).

In *myopia*, or nearsightedness, the eyeball is too long and distant objects are focused in front of the retina (Fig. 8.27B). Close objects are focused normally, but distant vision is blurred. Correction is achieved using a biconcave lens (Fig. 8.27D).

In *hyperopia*, or farsightedness, a near image is focused behind the retina because the eyeball is too short (Fig. 8.27C). Distant objects are focused normally, but close vision is blurred. A convex lens corrects this (Fig. 8.27E).

Astigmatism is the abnormal curvature of part of the cornea or lens. This interferes with the light path though the eye and prevents focusing of light on the retina, causing blurred vision. Correction requires cylindrical lenses. It may coexist with hypermetropia, myopia or presbyopia.

For a range of self-assessment exercises on the topics in this chapter, visit Evolve online resources: https://evolve.elsevier.com/Waugh/anatomy/

The endocrine system

ANIMATIONS

The endocrine system consists of glands widely separated from each other with no physical connections (Fig. 9.1). Endocrine glands are groups of secretory cells surrounded by an extensive network of capillaries that facilitates diffusion of *hormones* (chemical messengers) from the secretory cells into the bloodstream. They are also referred to as *ductless glands* because hormones diffuse directly into the bloodstream. Hormones are then carried in the bloodstream to *target tissues* and *organs* that may be quite distant, where they influence cell growth and metabolism.

Homeostasis of the internal environment is maintained partly by the autonomic nervous system and partly by the endocrine system. The autonomic nervous system is concerned with rapid changes, while endocrine control is mainly involved in slower and more precise adjustments.

Although the hypothalamus is classified as a part of the brain rather than an endocrine gland, it controls the pituitary gland and indirectly influences many others.

The ovaries and the testes secrete hormones associated with the reproductive system after puberty; their functions are described in Chapter 18. The placenta that develops to nourish the developing fetus during pregnancy also has an endocrine function, which is outlined in Chapter 5. In addition to the main endocrine glands

shown in Figure 9.1 many other organs and tissues also secrete hormones as a secondary function e.g. adipose tissue produces leptin (p. 284), involved in the regulation of appetite; the heart secretes atrial natriuretic peptide (ANP, p. 99) that acts on the kidneys. Other hormones do not travel to remote organs but act locally e.g. prostaglandins.

The endocrine glands are explored in the early sections of the chapter. Some local hormones are considered briefly on page 229. Changes in endocrine functions that accompany ageing are explored. Problems that arise when abnormalities occur are usually caused by the over- or under-activity of endocrine glands and are explained in the final sections of this chapter.

Overview of hormone action

When a hormone arrives at its target cell, it binds to a specific *receptor*, where it acts as a switch influencing chemical or metabolic reactions inside the cell. Receptors for peptide hormones are situated on the cell membrane and those for lipid-based hormones are located inside cells. Examples are shown in Box 9.1. ▮ 9.1

The level of a hormone in the blood is variable and self-regulating within its normal range. A hormone is released in response to a specific stimulus and usually its action reverses or negates the stimulus through a *negative*

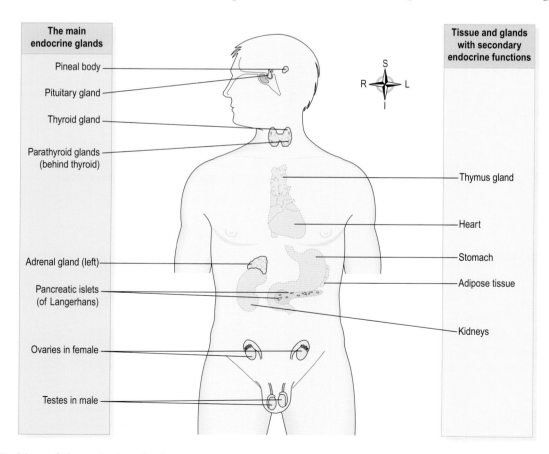

The main endocrine glands	Tissue and glands with secondary endocrine functions
Pineal body	
Pituitary gland	
Thyroid gland	
Parathyroid glands (behind thyroid)	
	Thymus gland
	Heart
Adrenal gland (left)	Stomach
Pancreatic islets (of Langerhans)	Adipose tissue
	Kidneys
Ovaries in female	
Testes in male	

Figure 9.1 Positions of the endocrine glands.

Box 9.1 Examples of lipid-based and peptide hormones

Lipid-based hormones	Peptide hormones
Steroids e.g. glucocorticoids, mineralocorticoids	Adrenaline (epinephrine), noradrenaline (norepinephrine)
Thyroid hormones	Insulin
	Glucagon

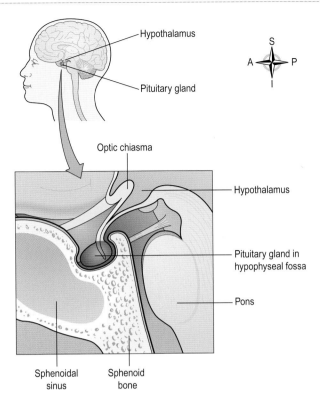

Figure 9.2 **Median section showing the position of the pituitary gland and its associated structures.**

feedback mechanism (see p. 6). This may be controlled either indirectly through the release of hormones by the hypothalamus and the anterior pituitary gland, e.g. steroid and thyroid hormones, or directly by blood levels of the stimulus, e.g. insulin and glucagon and determined by plasma glucose levels.

The effect of a *positive feedback mechanism* is amplification of the stimulus and increasing release of the hormone until a particular process is complete and the stimulus ceases, e.g. release of oxytocin during labour (p. 7).

Pituitary gland and hypothalamus

Learning outcomes

After studying this section, you should be able to:

- describe the structure of the hypothalamus and the pituitary gland

- explain the influence of the hypothalamus on the lobes of the pituitary gland

- outline the actions of the hormones secreted by the anterior and posterior lobes of the pituitary gland.

The pituitary gland and the hypothalamus act as a unit, regulating the activity of most of the other endocrine glands. The pituitary gland lies in the hypophyseal fossa of the sphenoid bone below the hypothalamus, to which it is attached by a *stalk* (Fig. 9.2). It is the size of a pea, weighs about 500 mg and consists of two main parts that originate from different types of cells. The *anterior pituitary* (adenohypophysis) is an upgrowth of glandular epithelium from the pharynx and the *posterior pituitary* (neurohypophysis) a downgrowth of nervous tissue from the brain. There is a network of nerve fibres between the hypothalamus and the posterior pituitary.

Blood supply

Arterial blood. This is from branches of the internal carotid artery. The anterior lobe is supplied indirectly

by blood that has already passed through a capillary bed in the hypothalamus but the posterior lobe is supplied directly.

Venous drainage. Containing hormones from both lobes, venous blood leaves the gland in short veins that enter the venous sinuses between the layers of dura mater.

The influence of the hypothalamus on the pituitary gland

The hypothalamus controls release of hormones from both the anterior and posterior pituitary but in different ways (see below).

Anterior pituitary

The anterior pituitary is supplied indirectly with arterial blood that has already passed through a capillary bed in the hypothalamus (Fig. 9.3A). This network of blood vessels forms part of the *pituitary portal system*, which transports blood from the hypothalamus to the anterior pituitary where it enters thin-walled sinusoids that are in close contact with the secretory cells. As well as providing oxygen and nutrients, this blood transports *releasing* and *inhibiting hormones* secreted by the hypothalamus.

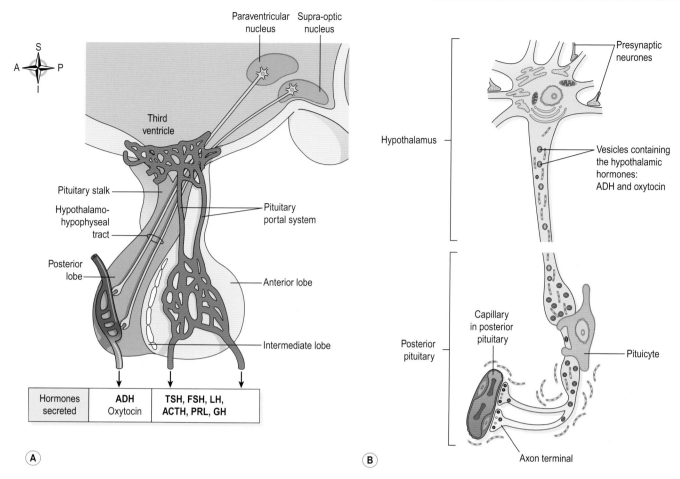

Figure 9.3 The pituitary gland. A. The lobes of the pituitary gland and their relationship with the hypothalamus. **B.** Synthesis and storage of antidiuretic hormone and oxytocin.

These hormones specifically influence secretion and release of other hormones formed in the anterior pituitary (Table 9.1).

Some of the hormones secreted by the anterior lobe stimulate or inhibit secretion by other endocrine glands (target glands) while others have a direct effect on target tissues. Table 9.1 summarises the main relationships between the hormones of the hypothalamus, the anterior pituitary and target glands or tissues.

Secretion of an anterior pituitary hormone follows stimulation of the gland by a specific *releasing hormone* produced by the hypothalamus and carried to the gland through the pituitary portal system (see above). The whole system is controlled by a *negative feedback mechanism* (Ch. 1). That is, when the level of a hormone in the blood supplying the hypothalamus is low it produces the appropriate releasing hormone that stimulates release of a *trophic hormone* by the anterior pituitary. This in turn stimulates the target gland to produce and release its hormone. As a result the blood level of that hormone rises and inhibits secretion of its releasing factor by the hypothalamus (Fig. 9.4).

Growth hormone (GH)

This is the most abundant hormone synthesised by the anterior pituitary. It stimulates growth and division of most body cells but especially those in the bones and skeletal muscles. Body growth in response to the secretion of GH is evident during childhood and adolescence, and thereafter secretion of GH maintains the mass of bones and skeletal muscles. It also regulates aspects of metabolism in many organs, e.g. liver, intestines and pancreas; stimulates protein synthesis, especially tissue growth and repair; promotes breakdown of fats and increases blood glucose levels (see Ch. 12).

Its release is stimulated by *growth hormone releasing hormone* (GHRH) and suppressed by *growth hormone release inhibiting hormone* (GHRIH), also known as *somatostatin*, both of which are secreted by the hypothalamus. Secretion of GH is greater at night during sleep and is also stimulated by hypoglycaemia (low blood sugar), exercise and anxiety. Secretion peaks in adolescence and then declines with age.

GH secretion is controlled by a negative feedback system; it is inhibited when the blood level rises and also

Table 9.1 Hormones of the hypothalamus, anterior pituitary and their target tissues

Hypothalamus	Anterior pituitary	Target gland or tissue
GHRH	GH	Most tissues Many organs
GHRIH	GH inhibition TSH inhibition	Thyroid gland Pancreatic islets Most tissues
TRH	TSH	Thyroid gland
CRH	ACTH	Adrenal cortex
PRH	PRL	Breast
PIH	PRL inhibition	Breast
LHRH or	FSH	Ovaries and testes
GnRH	LH	Ovaries and testes

GHRH = growth hormone releasing hormone
GH = growth hormone (somatotrophin)
GHRIH = growth hormone release inhibiting hormone
      (somatostatin)
TRH = thyrotrophin releasing hormone
TSH = thyroid stimulating hormone
CRH = corticotrophin releasing hormone
ACTH = adrenocorticotrophic hormone
PRH = prolactin releasing hormone
PRL = prolactin (lactogenic hormone)
PIH = prolactin inhibiting hormone (dopamine)
LHRH = luteinising hormone releasing hormone
GnRH = gonadotrophin releasing hormone
FSH = follicle stimulating hormone
LH = luteinising hormone

when GHRIH is released by the hypothalamus. GHRIH also suppresses secretion of TSH and gastrointestinal secretions, e.g. gastric juice, gastrin and cholecystokinin (see Ch. 12).

Thyroid stimulating hormone (TSH)

The release of this hormone is stimulated by *thyrotrophin releasing hormone* (TRH) from the hypothalamus. It stimulates growth and activity of the thyroid gland, which secretes the hormones *thyroxine* (T_4) and *tri-iodothyronine* (T_3). Release is lowest in the early evening and highest during the night. Secretion is regulated by a negative feedback mechanism, i.e. when the blood level of thyroid hormones is high, secretion of TSH is reduced, and vice versa (Fig. 9.4).

Adrenocorticotrophic hormone (ACTH, corticotrophin)

Corticotrophin releasing hormone (CRH) from the hypothalamus promotes the synthesis and release of ACTH by the anterior pituitary. This increases the concentration of

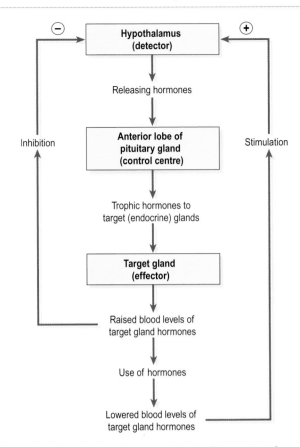

Figure 9.4 Negative feedback regulation of secretion of hormones by the anterior lobe of the pituitary gland.

cholesterol and steroids within the adrenal cortex and the output of steroid hormones, especially *cortisol*.

ACTH levels are highest at about 8 a.m. and fall to their lowest about midnight, although high levels sometimes occur at midday and 6 p.m. This circadian rhythm is maintained throughout life. It is associated with the sleep pattern and adjustment to changes takes several days, e.g. following changing work shifts, travelling to a different time zone (jet lag).

Secretion is also regulated by a negative feedback mechanism, being suppressed when the blood level of ACTH rises (Fig. 9.4). Other factors that stimulate secretion include hypoglycaemia, exercise and other stressors, e.g. emotional states and fever.

Prolactin

This hormone is secreted during pregnancy to prepare the breasts for *lactation* (milk production) after childbirth. The blood level of prolactin is stimulated by *prolactin releasing hormone* (PRH) released from the hypothalamus and it is lowered by *prolactin inhibiting hormone* (PIH, *dopamine*) and by an increased blood level of prolactin. Immediately after birth, suckling stimulates prolactin secretion and lactation. The resultant high blood level is a factor in reducing the incidence of conception during lactation.

Prolactin, together with oestrogens, corticosteroids, insulin and thyroxine, is involved in initiating and maintaining lactation. Prolactin secretion is related to sleep, rising during any period of sleep, night or day.

Gonadotrophins

Just before puberty two gonadotrophins (sex hormones) are secreted in gradually increasing amounts by the anterior pituitary in response to *luteinising hormone releasing hormone* (LHRH), also known as *gonadotrophin releasing hormone* (GnRH). Rising levels of these hormones at puberty promotes mature functioning of the reproductive organs. In both males and females the hormones responsible are:

- follicle stimulating hormone (FSH)
- luteinising hormone (LH).

In both sexes. FSH stimulates production of gametes (ova or spermatozoa) by the gonads.

In females. LH and FSH are involved in secretion of the hormones *oestrogen* and *progesterone* during the menstrual cycle (see Figs 18.9 and 18.10, pp. 456 and 457). As the levels of oestrogen and progesterone rise, secretion of LH and FSH is suppressed.

In males. LH, also called interstitial cell stimulating hormone (ICSH) stimulates the interstitial cells of the testes to secrete the hormone *testosterone* (see Ch. 18).

Table 9.2 summarises the hormonal secretions of the anterior pituitary.

Posterior pituitary

The posterior pituitary is formed from nervous tissue and consists of nerve cells surrounded by supporting glial cells called *pituicytes*. These neurones have their cell bodies in the supraoptic and paraventricular nuclei of the hypothalamus and their axons form a bundle known as the *hypothalamohypophyseal tract* (Fig. 9.3A). Posterior pituitary hormones are synthesised in the nerve cell bodies, transported along the axons and stored in vesicles within the axon terminals in the posterior pituitary (Fig. 9.3B).

Nerve impulses from the hypothalamus trigger exocytosis of the vesicles, releasing their hormones into the bloodstream.

The structure of the posterior pituitary gland and its relationship with the hypothalamus is explained on page 217. *Oxytocin* and *antidiuretic hormone* (ADH, *vasopressin*) are the hormones released from axon terminals within the posterior pituitary (Fig. 9.3B). These hormones act directly on non-endocrine tissue.

Oxytocin

Oxytocin stimulates two target tissues during and after childbirth (parturition): uterine smooth muscle and the muscle cells of the lactating breast.

During childbirth increasing amounts of oxytocin are released from the posterior pituitary into the bloodstream in response to increasing stimulation of sensory stretch receptors in the uterine cervix as the baby's head progressively dilates it. Sensory impulses are generated and travel to the control centre in the hypothalamus, stimulating the posterior pituitary to release more oxytocin. In turn this stimulates more forceful uterine contractions and greater stretching of the uterine cervix as the baby's head is forced further downwards. This is an example of a *positive feedback mechanism* which stops soon after the baby is delivered when distension of the uterine cervix is greatly reduced (Fig. 9.5).

The process of milk ejection also involves a positive feedback mechanism. Suckling generates sensory impulses that are transmitted from the breast to the hypothalamus. The impulses trigger release of oxytocin from the posterior pituitary. On reaching the lactating breast, oxytocin stimulates contraction of the milk ducts

Table 9.2 Summary of the hormones secreted by the anterior pituitary gland and their functions

Hormone	Function
Growth hormone (GH)	Regulates metabolism, promotes tissue growth especially of bones and muscles
Thyroid stimulating hormone (TSH)	Stimulates growth and activity of thyroid gland and secretion of T_3 and T_4
Adrenocorticotrophic hormone (ACTH)	Stimulates the adrenal cortex to secrete glucocorticoids
Prolactin (PRL)	Stimulates growth of breast tissue and milk production
Follicle stimulating hormone (FSH)	Stimulates production of sperm in the testes, stimulates secretion of oestrogen by the ovaries, maturation of ovarian follicles, ovulation
Luteinising hormone (LH)	Stimulates secretion of testosterone by the testes, stimulates secretion of progesterone by the corpus luteum

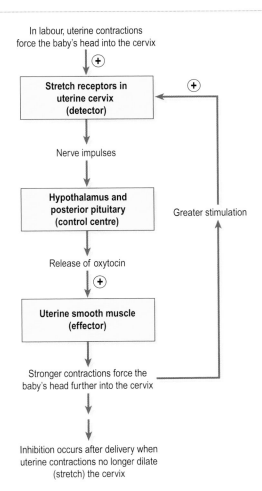

Figure 9.5 Regulation of secretion of oxytocin through a positive feedback mechanism.

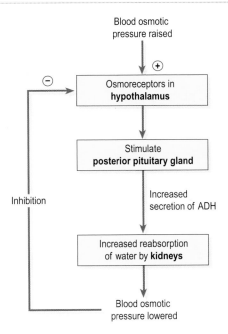

Figure 9.6 Negative feedback regulation of secretion of antidiuretic hormone (ADH).

and myoepithelial cells around the glandular cells, ejecting milk. Suckling also inhibits the release of *prolactin inhibiting hormone* (PIH), prolonging prolactin secretion and lactation.

Oxytocin levels rise during sexual arousal in both males and females. This increases smooth muscle contraction which is associated with glandular secretion and ejaculation in males. In females, contraction of smooth muscle in the vagina and uterus promotes movement of sperm towards the uterine tubes. It is believed that the smell of oxytocin may be involved in social recognition and bonding (between mother and newborn baby).

Antidiuretic hormone (ADH, vasopressin)

The main effect of antidiuretic hormone is to reduce urine output (diuresis is the production of a large volume of urine). ADH acts on the distal convoluted tubules and collecting ducts of the nephrons of the kidneys (Ch. 13). It increases their permeability to water and more of the glomerular filtrate is reabsorbed. ADH secretion is determined by the osmotic pressure of the blood circulating to the *osmoreceptors* in the hypothalamus.

As osmotic pressure rises, for example as a result of dehydration, secretion of ADH increases. More water is therefore reabsorbed and the urine output is reduced. This means that the body retains more water and the rise in osmotic pressure is reversed. Conversely, when the osmotic pressure of the blood is low, for example after a large fluid intake, secretion of ADH is reduced, less water is reabsorbed and more urine is produced (Fig. 9.6).

At high concentrations, for example after severe blood loss, ADH causes smooth muscle contraction, especially vasoconstriction in small arteries. This has a *pressor effect*, raising systemic blood pressure; the alternative name of this hormone, vasopressin, reflects this effect.

Thyroid gland (Fig. 9.7)

Learning outcomes

After studying this section, you should be able to:

- describe the position of the thyroid gland and its related structures

- describe the microscopic structure of the thyroid gland

- outline the actions of the thyroid hormones

- explain how blood levels of the thyroid hormones T₃ and T₄ are regulated.

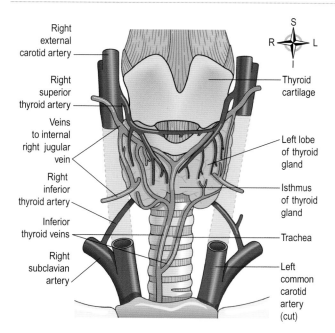

Figure 9.7 The position of the thyroid gland and its associated structures. Anterior view.

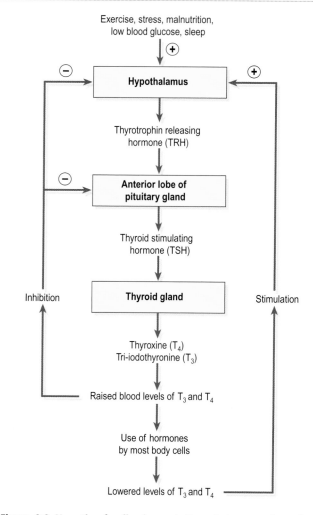

Figure 9.8 Negative feedback regulation of the secretion of thyroxine (T₄) and tri-iodothyronine (T₃).

The thyroid gland is situated in the neck in front of the larynx and trachea at the level of the 5th, 6th and 7th cervical and 1st thoracic vertebrae. It is a highly vascular gland that weighs about 25 g and is surrounded by a fibrous capsule. It resembles a butterfly in shape, consisting of two lobes, one on either side of the thyroid cartilage and upper cartilaginous rings of the trachea. The lobes are joined by a narrow *isthmus*, lying in front of the trachea.

The lobes are roughly cone shaped, about 5 cm long and 3 cm wide.

The *arterial blood supply* to the gland is through the superior and inferior thyroid arteries. The superior thyroid artery is a branch of the external carotid artery and the inferior thyroid artery is a branch of the subclavian artery.

The *venous return* is by the thyroid veins, which drain into the internal jugular veins.

The recurrent laryngeal nerves pass upwards close to the lobes of the gland and, especially on the right side, lie near the inferior thyroid artery (see Fig. 9.10).

The gland is composed of largely spherical follicles formed from cuboidal epithelium (Fig. 9.9). These secrete and store *colloid*, a thick sticky protein material. Between the follicles are other cells found singly or in small groups: *parafollicular cells*, also called C-cells, which secrete the hormone *calcitonin*.

Thyroxine and tri-iodothyronine

Iodine is essential for the formation of the thyroid hormones, thyroxine (T₄) and tri-iodothyronine (T₃), so numbered as these molecules contain four and three atoms of the element iodine respectively. The main dietary sources of iodine are seafood, vegetables grown in iodine-rich soil and iodinated table salt. The thyroid gland selectively takes up iodine from the blood, a process called *iodine trapping*.

Thyroid hormones are synthesised as large precursor molecules called *thyroglobulin*, the major constituent of colloid. The release of T₃ and T₄ into the blood is stimulated by *thyroid stimulating hormone* (TSH) from the anterior pituitary.

Secretion of TSH is stimulated by *thyrotrophin releasing hormone* (TRH) from the hypothalamus and secretion of TRH is stimulated by exercise, stress, malnutrition, low plasma glucose levels and sleep. TSH secretion depends on the plasma levels of T₃ and T₄ because it is these hormones that control the sensitivity of the anterior pituitary to TRH. Through the negative feedback mechanism, increased levels of T₃ and T₄ decrease TSH secretion and vice versa (Fig. 9.8). Dietary iodine deficiency greatly increases TSH secretion causing proliferation of thyroid

Table 9.3 Common effects of abnormal secretion of thyroid hormones

Hyperthyroidism: increased T$_3$ and T$_4$ secretion	Hypothyroidism: decreased T$_3$ and T$_4$ secretion
Increased basal metabolic rate	Decreased basal metabolic rate
Weight loss, good appetite	Weight gain, anorexia
Anxiety, physical restlessness, mental excitability	Depression, psychosis, mental slowness, lethargy
Hair loss	Dry skin, brittle hair
Tachycardia, palpitations, atrial fibrillation	Bradycardia
Warm sweaty skin, heat intolerance	Dry cold skin, prone to hypothermia
Diarrhoea	Constipation
Exophthalmos in Graves' disease (see Fig. 9.17)	

gland cells and enlargement of the gland (goitre, see Fig. 9.16). Secretion of T$_3$ and T$_4$ begins about the third month of fetal life and increases at puberty and in women during the reproductive years, especially during pregnancy. Otherwise, it remains fairly constant throughout life. Of the two thyroid hormones, T$_4$ is much more abundant. However it is less potent than T$_3$, which is more physiologically important. Most T$_4$ is converted into T$_3$ inside target cells. 9.2

Thyroid hormones enter the cell nucleus and regulate gene expression, i.e. they increase or decrease protein synthesis (see Ch. 17). They enhance the effects of other hormones, e.g. adrenaline (epinephrine) and noradrenaline (norepinephrine). T$_3$ and T$_4$ affect most cells of the body by:

- increasing the basal metabolic rate and heat production
- regulating metabolism of carbohydrates, proteins and fats.

T$_3$ and T$_4$ are essential for normal growth and development, especially of the skeleton and nervous system. Most other organs and systems are also influenced by thyroid hormones. Physiological effects of T$_3$ and T$_4$ on the heart, skeletal muscles, skin, digestive and reproductive systems are more evident when there is underactivity or overactivity of the thyroid gland and can be profound in childhood (Table 9.3).

Calcitonin

This hormone is secreted by the parafollicular or C-cells in the thyroid gland (Fig. 9.9). Calcitonin lowers raised blood calcium (Ca^{2+}) levels. It does this by acting on:

- bone cells promoting their storage of calcium
- kidney tubules inhibiting the reabsorption of calcium.

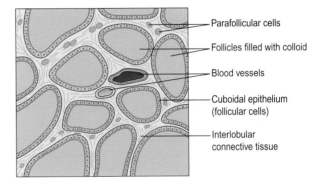

Parafollicular cells

Follicles filled with colloid

Blood vessels

Cuboidal epithelium (follicular cells)

Interlobular connective tissue

Figure 9.9 The microscopic structure of the thyroid gland.

Its effect is opposite to that of parathyroid hormone, the hormone secreted by the parathyroid glands. Release of calcitonin is stimulated by increased blood calcium levels.

This hormone is important during childhood when bones undergo considerable changes in size and shape.

Parathyroid glands

Learning outcomes

After studying this section, you should be able to:

- describe the position and gross structure of the parathyroid glands

- outline the functions of parathyroid hormone and calcitonin

- explain how blood levels of parathyroid hormone and calcitonin are regulated.

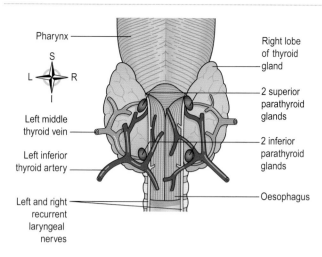

Figure 9.10 The positions of the parathyroid glands and their related structures, viewed from behind.

There are four small parathyroid glands, each weighing around 50 g, two embedded in the posterior surface of each lobe of the thyroid gland (Fig. 9.10). They are surrounded by fine connective tissue capsules that contain spherical cells arranged in columns with sinusoids containing blood in between them.

Function

These glands secrete *parathyroid hormone* (PTH, parathormone). Secretion is regulated by blood calcium levels. When they fall, secretion of PTH is increased and vice versa.

The main function of PTH is to increase blood calcium levels. This is achieved by increasing the calcium absorption from the small intestine and reabsorption from the renal tubules. If these sources provide inadequate supplies then PTH stimulates osteoclasts (bone-destroying cells) and calcium is released from bones into the blood.

Parathormone and calcitonin from the thyroid gland act in a complementary manner to maintain blood calcium levels within the normal range. This is needed for:

- muscle contraction
- transmission of nerve impulses
- blood clotting
- normal action of many enzymes.

Learning outcomes

After studying this section, you should be able to:

- describe the structure of the adrenal glands
- describe the actions of each of the three groups of adrenocorticoid hormones
- explain how blood levels of glucocorticoids are regulated
- describe the actions of adrenaline (epinephrine) and noradrenaline (norepinephrine)
- outline how the adrenal glands respond to stress.

The two adrenal (suprarenal) glands are situated on the upper pole of each kidney enclosed within the renal fascia (Fig. 9.1). They are about 4 cm long and 3 cm thick.

The *arterial blood supply* is by branches from the abdominal aorta and renal arteries.

The *venous return* is by suprarenal veins. The right gland drains into the inferior vena cava and the left into the left renal vein.

The glands are composed of two parts which have different structures and functions. The outer part is the *cortex* and the inner part the *medulla*. The adrenal cortex is essential to life but the medulla is not.

Adrenal cortex

The adrenal cortex produces three groups of steroid hormones from cholesterol. They are collectively called *adrenocorticoids* (corticosteroids).The groups are:

- glucocorticoids
- mineralocorticoids
- sex hormones (androgens).

The hormones in each group have different characteristic actions but as they are structurally similar their actions may overlap.

Glucocorticoids

Cortisol (hydrocortisone) is the main glucocorticoid but small amounts of *corticosterone* and *cortisone* are also produced. Commonly these are collectively known as 'steroids'; they are essential for life, regulating metabolism and responses to stress (see Fig. 9.13). Secretion is controlled through a negative feedback system involving the hypothalamus and anterior pituitary. It is stimulated by ACTH from the anterior pituitary and by stress (Fig. 9.11). Cortisol secretion shows marked circadian variation peaking between 4 a.m. and 8 a.m. and being lowest between midnight and 3 a.m. When the sleeping waking

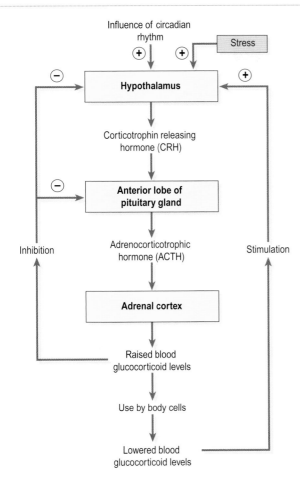

Figure 9.11 Negative feedback regulation of glucocorticoid secretion.

pattern is changed, e.g. night shift working, it takes several days for ACTH/cortisol secretion to readjust (p. 219). Glucocorticoid secretion increases in response to stress (Fig. 9.11), including infection and surgery.

Glucocorticoids have widespread metabolic effects generally concerned with catabolism (breakdown) of protein and fat that makes glucose and other substances available for use. These include:

- hyperglycaemia (raised blood glucose levels) caused by breakdown of glycogen and *gluconeogenesis* (formation of new sugar from, for example, protein)
- *lipolysis* (breakdown of triglycerides into fatty acids and glycerol for energy production) raising circulating levels of free fatty acids
- stimulating breakdown of protein, releasing amino acids, and increasing blood levels. Amino acids are then used for synthesis of other proteins, e.g. enzymes, or for energy production (Ch. 12)
- promoting absorption of sodium and water from renal tubules (a weak mineralocorticoid effect).

In pathological and pharmacological quantities glucocorticoids also have other effects including:

- anti-inflammatory actions
- suppression of immune responses
- delayed wound healing.

When corticosteroids are administered in the treatment of common disorders, e.g. asthma, the high circulating levels exert a negative feedback effect on the hypothalamus and pituitary and can completely suppress natural secretion of CRH and ACTH respectively.

Mineralocorticoids (aldosterone)

Aldosterone is the main mineralocorticoid. It is involved in maintaining water and electrolyte balance. Through a negative feedback system it stimulates the reabsorption of sodium (Na^+) by the renal tubules and excretion of potassium (K^+) in the urine. Sodium reabsorption is also accompanied by retention of water and therefore aldosterone is involved in the regulation of blood volume and blood pressure too.

Blood potassium levels regulate aldosterone secretion by the adrenal cortex. When blood potassium levels rise, more aldosterone is secreted (Fig. 9.12). Low blood potassium has the opposite effect. *Angiotensin* (see below) also stimulates the release of aldosterone.

Renin–angiotensin–aldosterone system. When renal blood flow is reduced or blood sodium levels fall, the enzyme *renin* is secreted by kidney cells. Renin converts the plasma protein *angiotensinogen*, produced by the liver, to *angiotensin 1*. *Angiotensin converting enzyme* (ACE), formed in small quantities in the lungs, proximal kidney tubules and other tissues, converts angiotensin 1 to *angiotensin 2*, which stimulates secretion of aldosterone. Angiotensin 2 causes vasoconstriction and increases blood pressure closing the negative feedback loop (Fig. 9.12).

Sex hormones

Sex hormones secreted by the adrenal cortex are mainly *androgens* (male sex hormones) although the amounts produced are insignificant compared with those secreted by the testes and ovaries in late puberty and adulthood (see Ch. 18).

Adrenal medulla 9.3

The medulla is completely surrounded by the adrenal cortex. It develops from nervous tissue in the embryo and is part of the sympathetic nervous system (Ch. 7). When stimulated by extensive sympathetic nerve supply, the glands release the hormones *adrenaline* (epinephrine, 80%) and *noradrenaline* (norepinephrine, 20%).

Adrenaline (epinephrine) and noradrenaline (norepinephrine)

Noradrenaline is the postganglionic neurotransmitter of the sympathetic division of the autonomic nervous system (see Fig. 7.43, p. 174). Adrenaline and some noradrenaline

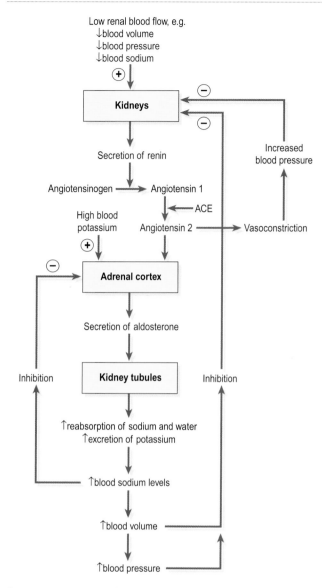

Figure 9.12 Negative feedback regulation of aldosterone secretion.

are released into the blood from the adrenal medulla during stimulation of the sympathetic nervous system (see Fig. 7.44, p. 175). The action of these hormones prolongs and augments stimulation of the sympathetic nervous system. Structurally they are very similar, which explains their similar effects. Together they potentiate the fight or flight response by:

- increasing heart rate
- increasing blood pressure
- diverting blood to essential organs, including the heart, brain and skeletal muscles, by dilating their blood vessels and constricting those of less essential organs, such as the skin
- increasing metabolic rate
- dilating the pupils.

Adrenaline has a greater effect on the heart and metabolic processes whereas noradrenaline has more influence on blood vessel diameter.

Response to stress

When the body is under stress homeostasis is disturbed. To restore it and, in some cases, to maintain life there are immediate and, if necessary, longer-term responses. Stressors include exercise, fasting, fright, temperature changes, infection, disease and emotional situations.

The *immediate response* is sometimes described as preparing for 'fight or flight' (p. 176). This is mediated by the sympathetic nervous system and the principal effects are shown in Figure 9.13.

In the *longer term*, ACTH from the anterior pituitary stimulates the release of glucocorticoids and mineralocorticoids from the adrenal cortex providing a more prolonged response to stress (Fig. 9.13).

Pancreatic islets

Learning outcomes

After studying this section, you should be able to:

- list the hormones secreted by the endocrine pancreas
- describe the actions of insulin and glucagon
- explain how blood glucose levels are regulated.

The gross structure of the pancreas is described in Chapter 12. The endocrine pancreas consists of clusters of cells, known as the pancreatic islets (islets of Langerhans), scattered throughout the gland. Pancreatic hormones are secreted directly into the bloodstream and circulate throughout the body. This is in contrast to the exocrine pancreas and its associated ducts (p. 308).

There are three main types of cells in the pancreatic islets:

- α (alpha) cells, which secrete *glucagon*
- β (beta) cells, which are the most numerous, secrete *insulin*
- δ (delta) cells, which secrete *somatostatin* (GHRIH, pp. 218 and 228).

The normal blood glucose level is between 3.5 and 8 mmol/litre (63 to 144 mg/100 mL). Blood glucose levels are controlled mainly by the opposing actions of insulin and glucagon:

- glucagon increases blood glucose levels
- insulin reduces blood glucose levels.

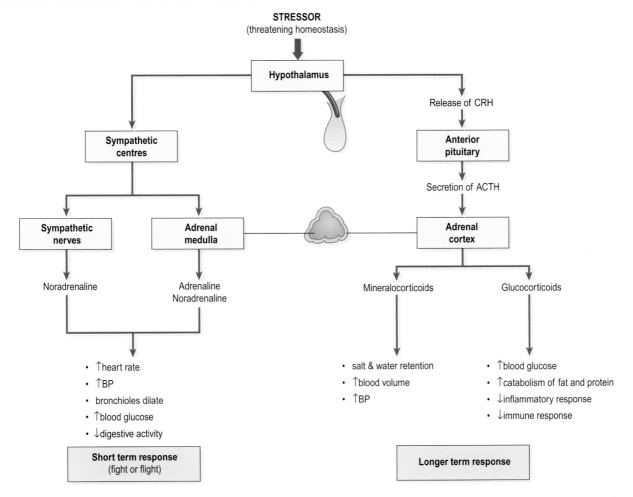

Figure 9.13 Responses to stressors that threaten homeostasis. CRH = corticotrophin releasing hormone. ACTH = adrenocorticotrophic hormone.

Insulin

Insulin is a polypeptide consisting of about 50 amino acids. Its main function is to lower raised blood nutrient levels, not only glucose but also amino acids and fatty acids. These effects are described as anabolic, i.e. they promote storage of nutrients. When nutrients, especially glucose, are in excess of immediate needs insulin promotes their storage by:

- acting on cell membranes and stimulating uptake and use of glucose by muscle and connective tissue cells
- increasing conversion of glucose to glycogen (*glycogenesis*), especially in the liver and skeletal muscles
- accelerating uptake of amino acids by cells, and the synthesis of protein
- promoting synthesis of fatty acids and storage of fat in adipose tissue (*lipogenesis*)
- decreasing *glycogenolysis* (breakdown of glycogen into glucose)

- preventing the breakdown of protein and fat, and *gluconeogenesis* (formation of new sugar from, e.g., protein).

Secretion of insulin is stimulated by increased blood glucose levels, for example after eating a meal, and to a lesser extent by parasympathetic stimulation, raised blood amino acid and fatty acid levels, and gastrointestinal hormones, e.g. gastrin, secretin and cholecystokinin. Secretion is decreased by sympathetic stimulation, glucagon, adrenaline, cortisol and somatostatin (GHRIH), which is secreted by the hypothalamus and pancreatic islets.

Glucagon

Glucagon increases blood glucose levels by stimulating:

- conversion of glycogen to glucose in the liver and skeletal muscles (glycogenolysis)
- gluconeogenesis.

Secretion of glucagon is stimulated by low blood glucose levels and exercise, and decreased by somatostatin and insulin.

Somatostatin (GHRIH)

This hormone, also produced by the hypothalamus, inhibits the secretion of both insulin and glucagon in addition to inhibiting the secretion of GH from the anterior pituitary (p. 218).

Pineal gland

Learning outcomes

After studying this section, you should be able to:

■ state the position of the pineal gland

■ outline the actions of melatonin.

The pineal gland is a small body attached to the roof of the third ventricle and is connected to it by a short stalk containing nerves, many of which terminate in the hypothalamus. The pineal gland is about 10 mm long, reddish brown in colour and surrounded by a capsule. The gland tends to atrophy after puberty and may become calcified in later life.

Melatonin

This is the main hormone secreted by the pineal gland. Secretion is controlled by daylight and darkness; levels fluctuate during each 24-hour period, the being highest at night and the lowest around midday. Secretion is also influenced by the number of daylight hours, i.e. there may be seasonal variations. Although its functions are not fully understood, melatonin is believed to be associated with:

• coordination of the circadian and diurnal rhythms of many tissues, possibly by influencing the hypothalamus

• inhibition of growth and development of the sex organs before puberty, possibly by preventing synthesis or release of gonadotrophins.

Organs with secondary endocrine functions

Learning outcome

After studying this section, you should be able to:

■ Outline the functions of some other hormones.

In addition to the glands with primary endocrine functions described above, many other organs and tissues secrete hormones as a secondary function (see Fig. 9.1). Examples of such organs and the hormones they secrete are shown in Table 9.4.

Table 9.4 Organs with secondary endocrine functions

Organ	Hormone	Site of action	Function
Kidney	Erythropoietin	Red bone marrow	Stimulation of red blood cell production (Ch. 4)
Gastrointestinal tract			
Gastric mucosa	Gastrin	Gastric glands	Stimulates secretion of gastric juice (Ch. 12)
Intestinal mucosa	Secretin	Stomach and pancreas	Stimulates secretion of pancreatic juice, slows emptying of the stomach (Ch. 12)
Intestinal mucosa	Cholecystokinin (CCK)	Gallbladder and pancreas	Stimulates release of bile and pancreatic juice (Ch. 12)
Adipose tissue	Leptin	Hypothalamus and other tissues	Provides a feeling of fullness ('satiety') after eating (Ch. 11); needed for GnRH and gonadotrophin synthesis (Ch. 18)
Ovary and testis	Inhibin	Anterior pituitary	Inhibits secretion of FSH
Heart (atria)	Atrial natriuretic peptide (ANP)	Kidney tubules	Decreases reabsorption of sodium and water in renal tubules (Ch. 13)
Placenta	hCG	Ovary	Stimulates secretion of oestrogen and progesterone during pregnancy (Ch. 5)
Thymus	Thymosin	White blood cells (T-lymphocytes)	Development of T-lymphocytes (Ch. 15)

Local hormones

A number of body tissues not normally described as endocrine glands secrete substances that act in tissues nearby (locally). Some of these are described below.

Histamine

This is synthesised and stored by mast cells in the tissues and basophils in blood. It is released as part of the inflammatory responses, especially when caused by allergy (p. 386), increasing capillary permeability and causing vasodilation. It also acts as a neurotransmitter, causes contraction of smooth muscle of the bronchi and alimentary tract, and stimulates the secretion of gastric juice.

Serotonin (5-hydroxytryptamine, 5-HT)

This is present in platelets, in the brain and in the intestinal wall. It causes intestinal secretion and contraction of smooth muscle and its role in haemostasis (blood clotting) is outlined in Chapter 4. It is a neurotransmitter in the CNS and is known to influence mood.

Prostaglandins (PGs)

These are lipid substances found in most tissues. They act on neighbouring cells but their actions are short-lived as they are quickly metabolized. Prostaglandins have potent and wide-ranging physiological effects in:

- the inflammatory response
- potentiating pain
- fever
- regulating blood pressure
- blood clotting
- uterine contractions during labour.

Other chemically similar compounds include *leukotrienes*, which are involved in inflammatory responses, and *thromboxanes*, e.g. thromboxane A_2, which is a potent aggregator of platelets. All of these active substances are found in only small amounts, as they are rapidly degraded.

The effects of ageing on endocrine function

Adrenal cortex

Osteoporosis caused by oestrogen deficiency in postmenopausal women is reviewed in Chapter 16. Reduced secretion of androgens in women after the menopause may be accompanied by changing hair patterns, e.g. increased facial hair and thinning of hair on the scalp.

Pancreatic islets

In the pancreatic islets, β-cell function declines with age. Especially when associated with weight gain in middle life and older age, this predisposes to type 2 diabetes mellitus (p. 236).

Endocrine disorders are commonly caused by tumours or autoimmune diseases and their effects are usually the result of:

- hypersecretion (overproduction) of hormones, or
- hyposecretion (underproduction) of hormones.

The effects of many conditions explained in this section can therefore be readily linked to the underlying abnormality.

Disorders of the pituitary gland

Learning outcomes

After studying this section, you should be able to:

- list the causes of diseases in this section

- relate the features of conditions affecting the anterior pituitary to the actions of the hormones involved

- relate the features of diabetes insipidus to abnormal secretion of antidiuretic hormone.

Hypersecretion of anterior pituitary hormones

Gigantism and acromegaly

The most common cause is prolonged hypersecretion of growth hormone (GH), usually by a hormone-secreting pituitary tumour. The conditions are occasionally due to excess growth hormone releasing hormone (GHRH) secreted by the hypothalamus. As the tumour increases in size, compression of nearby structures may lead to hyposecretion of other pituitary hormones (from both lobes) and damage to the optic nerves, causing visual disturbances. The effects of excess GH include:

- excessive growth of bones
- enlargement of internal organs
- formation of excess connective tissue
- enlargement of the heart and raised blood pressure
- reduced glucose tolerance and a predisposition to diabetes mellitus.

Gigantism. This occurs in children when there is excess GH while epiphyseal cartilages of long bones are still growing, i.e. before ossification of bones is complete. It is evident mainly in the bones of the limbs, and affected individuals may grow to heights of 2.1 to 2.4 m, although body proportions remain normal (Fig. 9.14).

Acromegaly. This means 'large extremities' and occurs in adults when there is excess GH after ossification is complete. The bones become abnormally thick and there is also thickening of the soft tissues. These changes are most noticeable as coarse facial features (especially

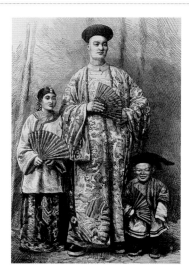

Figure 9.14 Historical artwork showing effects of normal and abnormal growth hormone secretion. From left to right: normal stature, gigantism (2.3 m tall) and dwarfism (0.9 m tall).

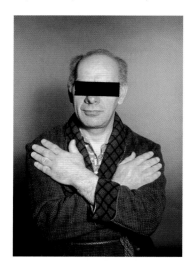

Figure 9.15 Facial features and large hands in acromegaly.

excessive growth of the lower jaw), an enlarged tongue and excessively large hands and feet (Fig. 9.15).

Hyperprolactinaemia

This is caused by a tumour that secretes large amounts of prolactin. It causes *galactorrhoea* (inappropriate milk secretion), *amenorrhoea* (cessation of menstruation) and sterility in women and impotence in men.

Hyposecretion of anterior pituitary hormones

The number of hormones involved and the extent of hyposecretion varies. *Panhypopituitarism* is the absence of all anterior pituitary hormones. Causes of hyposecretion include:

- tumours of the hypothalamus or pituitary
- trauma, usually caused by fractured base of skull, or surgery

- pressure caused by a tumour adjacent to the pituitary gland, e.g. glioma, meningioma
- infection, e.g. meningitis, encephalitis, syphilis
- ischaemic necrosis
- ionising radiation or cytotoxic drugs.

Ischaemic necrosis

Simmond's disease is hypofunction of the anterior pituitary gland, which only rarely affects the posterior lobe. The arrangement of the blood supply makes the gland unusually susceptible to a fall in systemic BP. Severe hypotensive shock may cause ischaemic necrosis. The effects include deficient stimulation of target glands and hypofunction of all or some of the thyroid, adrenal cortex and gonads. The outcome depends on the extent of pituitary necrosis and hormone deficiency. In severe cases, glucocorticoid deficiency may be life threatening or fatal. When this condition is associated with severe haemorrhage during or after childbirth it is known as *postpartum necrosis* (Sheehan's syndrome*)*, and in this situation the other effects are preceded by failure of lactation.

Pituitary dwarfism (Lorain–Lévi syndrome)

This is caused by severe deficiency of GH, and possibly of other hormones, in childhood. The individual is of small stature but is normally proportioned and cognitive development is not affected. Puberty is delayed and there may be episodes of hypoglycaemia. The condition may be due to genetic abnormality or a tumour.

Fröhlich's syndrome

In this condition there is panhypopituitarism but the main features are associated with deficiency of GH, FSH and LH. In children the effects are diminished growth, lack of sexual development, obesity with female distribution of fat and learning disabilities. Obesity and sterility are the main features in a similar condition in adults. It may arise from a tumour of the anterior pituitary and/or the hypothalamus but in most cases the cause is unknown.

Disorders of the posterior pituitary

Diabetes insipidus

This is a relatively rare condition usually caused by hyposecretion of ADH due to damage to the hypothalamus by, for example, trauma, tumour or encephalitis. Occasionally it occurs when the renal tubules fail to respond to ADH. Water reabsorption by the renal tubules is impaired, leading to excretion of excessive amounts of dilute urine, often more than 10 litres daily, causing dehydration and extreme thirst (polydipsia). Water balance is disturbed unless fluid intake is greatly increased to compensate for excess losses.

Disorders of the thyroid gland

Learning outcome

After studying this section, you should be able to:

■ compare and contrast the effects of hyperthyroidism and hypothyroidism, relating them to the actions of T_3 and T_4.

These fall into three main categories:

- abnormal secretion of thyroid hormones (T3 and T4) causing hyperthyroidism or hypothyroidism
- goitre – enlargement of the thyroid gland
- tumours.

Abnormal thyroid function may arise not only from thyroid disease but also from disorders of the pituitary or hypothalamus; in addition, insufficient dietary iodine impairs thyroid hormone production. The main effects are caused by an abnormally high or low basal metabolic rate.

Hyperthyroidism

This syndrome, also known as *thyrotoxicosis*, arises as the body tissues are exposed to excessive levels of T_3 and T_4. The main effects are due to increased basal metabolic rate (see Table 9.3).

In older adults, cardiac failure is another common consequence as the ageing heart must work harder to deliver more blood and nutrients to the hyperactive body cells. The main causes are:

- Graves' disease
- toxic nodular goitre
- adenoma (a benign tumour, p. 232).

Graves' disease

Sometimes called *Graves' thyroiditis*, this condition accounts for 75% of cases of hyperthyroidism. It affects more women than men and may occur at any age, being most common between the ages of 30 and 50 years. It is an autoimmune disorder in which an antibody that mimics the effects of TSH is produced, causing:

- increased release of T_3 and T_4 and signs of hyperthyroidism (see Table 9.3)
- goitre (visible enlargement of the gland, Fig. 9.16) as the antibody stimulates thyroid growth
- exophthalmos in many cases.

Exophthalmos. This is protrusion of the eyeballs that gives the appearance of staring, which is due to the deposition of excess fat and fibrous tissue behind the eyes (Fig. 9.17); it is often present in Graves' disease. Effective treatment of hyperthyroidism does not completely reverse

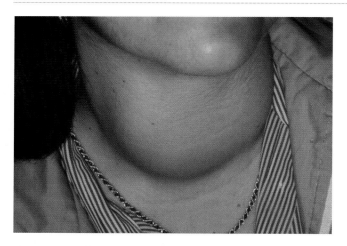

Figure 9.16 Enlarged thyroid gland in goitre.

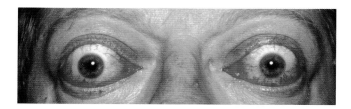

Figure 9.17 Abnormally bulging eyes in exophthalmos.

exophthalmos, although it may lessen after 2–3 years. In severe cases the eyelids become retracted and may not completely cover the eyes during blinking and sleep, leading to drying of the conjunctiva and predisposing to infection. It does not occur in other forms of hyperthyroidism.

Toxic nodular goitre

In this condition one or two nodules of a gland that is already affected by goitre (see Fig. 9.16) become active and secrete excess T_3 and T_4 causing the effects of hyperthyroidism (Table 9.3). It is more common in women than men and after middle age. As this condition affects an older age group than Graves' disease, arrhythmias and cardiac failure are more common. Exophthalmos does not occur in this condition.

Hypothyroidism

This condition is prevalent in older adults and is five times more common in females than males. Deficiency of T_3 and T_4 in adults results in an abnormally low metabolic rate and other effects shown in Table 9.3. There may be accumulation of mucopolysaccharides in the subcutaneous tissues causing swelling (non-pitting oedema), especially of the face, hands, feet and eyelids (myxoedema). The commonest causes are autoimmune thyroiditis, severe iodine deficiency (see goitre) and healthcare

interventions, e.g. antithyroid drugs, surgical removal of thyroid tissue or ionising radiation.

Autoimmune thyroiditis. The most common cause of acquired hypothyroidism is *Hashimoto's disease*. It is more common in women than men and, like Graves' disease, an organ-specific autoimmune condition. Autoantibodies that react with thyroglobulin and thyroid gland cells develop and prevent synthesis and release of thyroid hormones causing hypothyroidism. Goitre is sometimes present.

Congenital hypothyroidism. This is a profound deficiency or absence of thyroid hormones that becomes evident a few weeks or months after birth. Hypothyroidism is endemic in parts of the world where the diet is severely deficient in iodine and contains insufficient for synthesis of T_3 and T_4. Absence of thyroid hormones results in profound impairment of growth and cognitive development. Unless treatment begins early in life, cognitive impairment is permanent and the individual typically has disproportionately short limbs, a large protruding tongue, coarse dry skin, poor abdominal muscle tone and, often, an umbilical hernia.

Simple goitre ▦9.4

This is enlargement of the thyroid gland without signs of hyperthyroidism. It is caused by a relative lack of T_3 and T_4 and the low levels stimulate secretion of TSH resulting in hyperplasia of the thyroid gland (Fig. 9.16). Sometimes the extra thyroid tissue is able to maintain normal hormone levels but if not, hypothyroidism develops. Causes are:

- persistent iodine deficiency. In parts of the world where there is dietary iodine deficiency, this is a common condition known as *endemic goitre*
- genetic abnormality affecting synthesis of T_3 and T_4
- iatrogenic, e.g. antithyroid drugs, surgical removal of excess thyroid tissue.

The enlarged gland may cause pressure damage to adjacent tissues, especially if it lies in an abnormally low position, i.e. behind the sternum. The structures most commonly affected are the oesophagus, causing dysphagia; the trachea, causing dyspnoea; and the recurrent laryngeal nerve, causing hoarseness.

Tumours of the thyroid gland

Malignant tumours are rare.

Benign tumours

Single adenomas are fairly common and may become cystic. Sometimes the adenoma secretes hormones and hyperthyroidism may develop. The tumours may become malignant, especially in older adults.

Disorders of the parathyroid glands

Learning outcome

After studying this section, you should be able to:

■ explain how the diseases in this section are related to abnormal secretion of parathyroid hormone.

Hyperparathyroidism

This condition is characterised by high blood calcium levels (hypercalcaemia) and is usually caused by a benign parathyroid tumour which secretes high levels of parathormone (PTH). This results in release of calcium from bones, raising blood calcium levels. The effects may include:

- polyuria and polydipsia
- formation of renal calculi
- anorexia and constipation
- muscle weakness
- general fatigue.

Hypoparathyroidism

Parathyroid hormone (PTH) deficiency causes hypocalcaemia, i.e. abnormally low blood calcium levels, and is much rarer than hyperparathyroidism. There is reduced absorption of calcium from the small intestine and less reabsorption from bones and glomerular filtrate. Low blood calcium causes:

- *tetany* (Fig. 9.18)
- anxiety
- paraesthesia
- grand mal seizures
- in some cases, cataracts (opacity of the lens, Fig. 8.25, p. 207) and brittle nails.

Causes of hypoparathyroidism include damage to or removal of the glands during thyroidectomy, ionising radiation, development of autoantibodies to PTH and parathyroid cells, and congenital abnormalities.

Tetany

This is caused by hypocalcaemia because low blood calcium levels increase excitability of peripheral nerves. There are very strong painful spasms of skeletal muscles, causing characteristic bending inwards of the hands, forearms and feet (Fig. 9.18). In children there may also be laryngeal spasm and seizures.

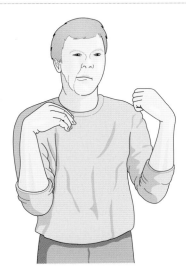

Figure 9.18 Characteristic positions adopted during tetanic spasms.

Hypocalcaemia

In addition to hyperthyroidism, this may be associated with:

- chronic renal failure when there is excessive excretion of excess calcium in the urine
- deficiency of vitamin D or dietary deficiency of calcium
- alkalosis; metabolic or respiratory
- acute pancreatitis.

Disorders of the adrenal cortex

Learning outcomes

After studying this section, you should be able to:

■ relate the features of Cushing's syndrome to the physiological actions of adrenocorticoids

■ relate the features of Addison's disease to the physiological actions of adrenocorticoids.

Hypersecretion of glucocorticoids (Cushing's syndrome)

Cortisol is the main glucocorticoid hormone secreted by the adrenal cortex. Causes of hypersecretion include:

- hormone-secreting adrenal tumours
- hypersecretion of adrenocorticotrophic hormone (ACTH) by the anterior pituitary
- abnormal secretion of ACTH by a non-pituitary tumour, e.g. bronchial or pancreatic tumour.

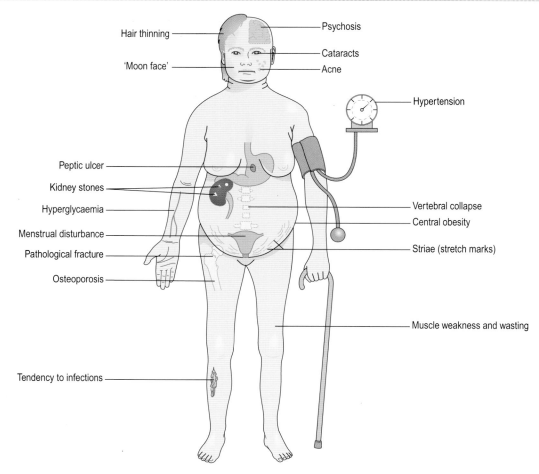

Hair thinning

Psychosis

Cataracts

'Moon face'

Acne

Hypertension

Peptic ulcer

Kidney stones

Hyperglycaemia

Menstrual disturbance

Pathological fracture

Osteoporosis

Vertebral collapse

Central obesity

Striae (stretch marks)

Muscle weakness and wasting

Tendency to infections

Figure 9.19 The systemic features of Cushing's syndrome.

Prolonged therapeutic use of systemic ACTH or glucocorticoids is another cause of Cushing's syndrome where high blood levels arise from drug therapy. Any of the features shown in Figure 9.19 may occur as side effects of this treatment.

Hypersecretion of cortisol exaggerates its physiological effects (Fig. 9.19). These include:

- adiposity of the face (*moon face*), neck and abdomen
- excessive tissue protein breakdown, causing thinning of subcutaneous tissue and muscle wasting, especially of the limbs
- diminished protein synthesis
- suppression of growth hormone secretion preventing normal growth in children
- osteoporosis (p. 431), and kyphosis if vertebral bodies are involved
- pathological fractures caused by calcium loss from bones
- excessive gluconeogenesis resulting in hyperglycaemia and glycosuria which can precipitate diabetes mellitus (p. 236)
- atrophy of lymphoid tissue and depression of the immune response

- susceptibility to infection due to reduced febrile response, depressed immune and inflammatory responses
- impaired collagen production, leading to capillary fragility, cataract and striae
- insomnia, excitability, euphoria, depression or psychosis
- hypertension due to salt and water retention
- menstrual disturbances
- formation of renal calculi
- peptic ulceration.

Hyposecretion of glucocorticoids

Inadequate cortisol secretion causes diminished gluconeogenesis, low blood glucose levels, muscle weakness and pallor. This may be primary, i.e. due to disease of the adrenal cortex, or secondary due to deficiency of ACTH from the anterior pituitary. In primary deficiency there is also hyposecretion of aldosterone (see below) but in secondary deficiency, aldosterone secretion is not usually affected because aldosterone release is controlled by the renin–angiotensin–aldosterone system (p. 225).

Hypersecretion of mineralocorticoids

Excess aldosterone affects kidney function, with consequences elsewhere:

- excessive reabsorption of sodium chloride and water, causing increased blood volume and hypertension
- excessive excretion of potassium, causing *hypokalaemia*, which leads to cardiac arrhythmias, alkalosis, syncope and muscle weakness.

Primary hyperaldosteronism is due to excessive secretion of mineralocorticoids, independent of the renin–angiotensin–aldosterone system. It is usually caused by a tumour affecting only one adrenal gland.
Secondary hyperaldosteronism is caused by overstimulation of normal glands by the excessively high blood levels of renin and angiotensin that result from low renal perfusion or low blood sodium.

Hyposecretion of mineralocorticoids

Hypoaldosteronism results in failure of the kidneys to regulate sodium, potassium and water excretion, leading to:

- blood sodium deficiency (hyponatraemia) and potassium excess (hyperkalaemia)
- dehydration, low blood volume and low blood pressure.

There is usually hyposecretion of other adrenal cortical hormones, as in Addison's disease.

Chronic adrenocortical insufficiency (Addison's disease)

This is due to destruction of the adrenal cortex that results in hyposecretion of glucocorticoid and mineralocorticoid hormones. The most common causes are development of autoantibodies to cortical cells, metastasis (secondary tumours) and infections. Autoimmune disease of other glands can be associated with Addison's disease, e.g. diabetes mellitus, thyrotoxicosis and hypoparathyroidism. The most important effects are:

- muscle weakness and wasting
- gastrointestinal disturbances, e.g. vomiting, diarrhoea, anorexia
- increased skin pigmentation, especially of exposed areas
- listlessness and tiredness
- hypoglycaemia
- confusion
- menstrual disturbances and loss of body hair in women

- electrolyte imbalance, including hyponatraemia, low blood chloride levels and hyperkalaemia
- chronic dehydration, low blood volume and hypotension.

The adrenal glands have a considerable tissue reserve and Addison's disease is not usually severely debilitating unless more than 90% of cortical tissue is destroyed, but this condition is fatal without treatment.

Acute adrenocortical insufficiency (Addisonian crisis)

This is characterised by sudden severe nausea, vomiting, diarrhoea, hypotension, electrolyte imbalance (hyponatraemia and hyperkalaemia) and, in severe cases, circulatory collapse. It is precipitated when an individual with chronic adrenocortical insufficiency is subjected to stress, e.g. an acute infection.

Disorders of the adrenal medulla

Learning outcome

After studying this section, you should be able to:

- explain how the features of the diseases in this section are related to excessive secretion of adrenaline (epinephrine) and noradrenaline (norepinephrine).

Tumours

Hormone-secreting tumours are the most common problem. The effects of excess adrenaline (epinephrine) and noradrenaline (norepinephrine) include:

- hypertension
- weight loss
- nervousness and anxiety
- headache
- excessive sweating and alternate flushing and blanching of the skin
- hyperglycaemia and glycosuria
- constipation.

Phaeochromocytoma

This is usually a *benign tumour*, occurring in one or both glands. Hormone secretion may be constantly elevated or in intermittent bursts, often precipitated by raised intra-abdominal pressure, e.g. coughing or defaecation.

Neuroblastoma

This is a rare and *malignant tumour*, occurring in infants and children. Tumours that develop early tend to be highly malignant but there may be spontaneous regression.

Disorders of the pancreatic islets

Learning outcomes

After studying this section, you should be able to:

■ compare and contrast the onset and features of types 1 and 2 diabetes mellitus

■ relate the signs and symptoms of diabetes mellitus to deficiency of insulin

■ explain how the causes and effects of the following conditions occur: diabetic ketoacidosis and hypoglycaemic coma

■ describe the long-term complications of diabetes mellitus.

Diabetes mellitus (DM)

This is the most common endocrine disorder; the primary sign is hyperglycaemia which is accompanied by varying degrees of disruption of carbohydrate and fat metabolism. DM is caused by complete absence of, relative deficiency of or resistance to the hormone insulin. Box 9.2 shows the classification of diabetes. *Primary DM* is categorised as type 1 or type 2. In *secondary DM*, the disorder arises as a result of other conditions, and *gestational diabetes* develops in pregnancy. The incidence of types 1 and 2 DM, especially type 2, is rapidly increasing worldwide. Table 9.5 shows some distinguishing features of types 1 and 2 DM.

Type 1 diabetes mellitus

Previously known as insulin-dependent diabetes mellitus (IDDM), this occurs mainly in children and young adults;

Box 9.2 Classification of diabetes mellitus

Primary
Type 1 diabetes mellitus
Type 2 diabetes mellitus

Secondary
Due to other situations, e.g.:

• acute or chronic pancreatitis (p. 331)
• some drug therapy, e.g. corticosteroids
• other endocrine disorders involving hormones that increase plasma glucose levels, e.g. growth hormone, thyroid hormones, cortisol (Cushing's syndrome, p. 233)

Gestational diabetes

This develops during pregnancy and may disappear after delivery but often recurs in later life. It is associated with birth of heavier than normal and stillborn babies, and deaths shortly after birth.

---

the onset is usually sudden and can be life threatening. There is severe deficiency or absence of insulin secretion due to destruction of β-islet cells of the pancreas. Treatment with injections of insulin is required. There is usually evidence of an autoimmune mechanism that destroys the β-islet cells. Genetic predisposition and environmental factors, including viral infections, are also implicated.

Type 2 diabetes mellitus

Previously known as non-insulin-dependent diabetes mellitus (NIDDM), this is the most common form of diabetes, accounting for about 90% of cases. The causes are multifactorial and predisposing factors include:

• obesity
• sedentary lifestyle
• increasing age: predominantly affecting middle-aged and older adults
• genetic factors.

Its onset is gradual, often over many years, and it frequently goes undetected until signs are found on routine investigation or a complication occurs. Insulin secretion may be below or above normal. Deficiency of glucose inside body cells occurs despite hyperglycaemia and a high insulin level. This may be due to insulin resistance, i.e. changes in cell membranes that block the insulin-assisted movement of glucose into cells. Treatment involves diet and/or drugs, although sometimes insulin injections are required. ▧ **9.5**

Pathophysiology of DM

Raised plasma glucose level

After eating a carbohydrate-rich meal the plasma glucose level remains high because:

Table 9.5 Features of type1 and type 2 diabetes mellitus		
	Type 1 DM	**Type 2 DM**
Age of onset	Usually childhood	Adulthood and later life
Body weight at onset	Normal or low	Obese
Onset of symptoms	Weeks	Months/years
Main cause(s)	Autoimmune	Obesity, lack of exercise
Insulin requirement	100% of cases	Up to 20% of cases
Ketonuria	Yes	No
Complications at diagnosis	No	Up to 25%
Family history	Rare	Common

- cells are unable to take up and use glucose from the bloodstream, despite high plasma levels
- conversion of glucose to glycogen in the liver and muscles is diminished
- there is gluconeogenesis from protein, in response to deficiency of intracellular glucose.

Glycosuria and polyuria

The concentration of glucose in the glomerular filtrate is the same as in the blood and, although diabetes raises the renal threshold for glucose, it is not all reabsorbed by the tubules. The glucose remaining in the filtrate raises its osmotic pressure, water reabsorption is reduced and the volume of urine is increased (*polyuria*). This results in electrolyte imbalance and excretion of urine of high specific gravity. Polyuria leads to dehydration, extreme thirst (*polydipsia*) and increased fluid intake.

Weight loss

The cells are essentially starved of glucose because, in the absence of insulin, they are unable to extract it from the bloodstream, leading to derangement of energy metabolism as cells must use alternative pathways to produce the energy they need. This results in weight loss due to:

- gluconeogenesis from amino acids and body protein, causing muscle wasting, tissue breakdown and further increases in blood glucose
- catabolism of body fat, releasing some of its energy and excess production of ketone bodies.

This is very common in type 1 DM and sometimes occurs in type 2 DM.

Ketosis and ketoacidosis

This nearly always affects people with type 1 DM.

In the absence of insulin to promote normal intracellular glucose metabolism, alternative energy sources must be used instead and increased breakdown of fat occurs (see Fig. 12.43, p. 317). This leads to excessive production of weakly acidic ketone bodies, which can be used for metabolism by the liver. Normal buffering systems maintain pH balance so long as the levels of ketone bodies are not excessive. *Ketosis* (see p. 318) develops as ketone bodies accumulate. Excretion of ketones is via the urine (ketonuria) and/or the lungs giving the breath a characteristic smell of acetone or 'pear drops'.

Ketoacidosis develops owing to increased insulin requirement or increased resistance to insulin due to some added stress, such as pregnancy, infection, infarction, or cerebrovascular accident. It may occur when insufficient insulin is administered during times of increased requirement. Severe and dangerous ketoacidosis may occur without loss of consciousness. When worsening ketosis swamps the compensatory buffer systems, control of acid–base balance is lost; the blood pH falls and *ketoacidosis* occurs. The consequences if untreated are:

- increasing acidosis (↓ blood pH) due to accumulation of ketoacids
- increasing hyperglycaemia
- hyperventilation as the lungs excrete excess hydrogen ions as CO_2
- acidification of urine – the result of kidney buffering
- polyuria as the renal threshold for glucose is exceeded
- dehydration and hypovolaemia (↓ BP and ↑ pulse) – caused by polyuria
- disturbances of electrolyte balance accompanying fluid loss, hyponatraemia (↓ plasma sodium) and hypokalaemia (↓ plasma potassium)
- confusion, coma and death.

Acute complications of diabetes mellitus

Diabetic ketoacidosis

The effects and consequences of diabetic ketoacidosis are outlined above.

Hypoglycaemic coma

This occurs when insulin administered is in excess of that needed to balance the food intake and expenditure of energy. Hypoglycaemia is of sudden onset and may be the result of:

- accidental overdose of insulin
- delay in eating after insulin administration
- drinking alcohol on an empty stomach
- strenuous exercise.

It may also arise from an insulin-secreting tumour, especially if it produces irregular bursts of secretion. Because neurones are more dependent on glucose for their energy needs than are other cells, glucose deprivation causes disturbed neurological function, leading to coma and, if prolonged, irreversible damage.

Common signs and symptoms of hypoglycaemia include drowsiness, confusion, speech difficulty, sweating, trembling, anxiety and a rapid pulse. This can progress rapidly to coma without treatment, which usually enables rapid recovery. Most people can readily recognize the symptoms of hypoglycaemia and can take appropriate action.

Long-term complications of diabetes mellitus

These increase with the severity and duration of hyperglycaemia and represent significant causes of morbidity (poor health) and mortality (death) in people with both type 1 and type 2 diabetes.

Cardiovascular disturbances

Diabetes mellitus is a significant risk factor for cardiovascular disorders. Blood vessel abnormalities (angiopathies) may still occur even when the disease is well controlled.

Diabetic macroangiopathy. The most common lesions are atheroma and calcification of the tunica media of the large arteries. In type 1 diabetes these changes may occur at a relatively early age. The most common consequences are serious and often fatal:

- ischaemic heart disease, i.e. angina and myocardial infarction (p. 127)
- stroke (p. 181)
- peripheral vascular disease.

Diabetic microangiopathy. This affects small blood vessels and there is thickening of the epithelial basement membrane of arterioles, capillaries and, sometimes, venules. These changes may lead to:

- peripheral vascular disease, progressing to gangrene and 'diabetic foot'
- diabetic retinopathy and visual impairment (see p. 212)
- diabetic nephropathy and chronic renal failure (p. 352)
- peripheral neuropathy causing sensory deficits and motor weakness (p. 188), especially when myelination is affected.

Infection

DM predisposes to infection, especially by bacteria and fungi, possibly because phagocyte activity is depressed by insufficient intracellular glucose. Infection may cause:

- boils and carbuncles
- vaginal candidiasis (thrush, p. 466)
- pyelonephritis (p. 352)
- diabetic foot.

Renal failure

This is due to diabetic nephropathy (p. 352) and is a common cause of death.

Visual impairment and blindness

Diabetic retinopathy (p. 212) is the commonest cause of blindness in adults between 30 and 65 years in

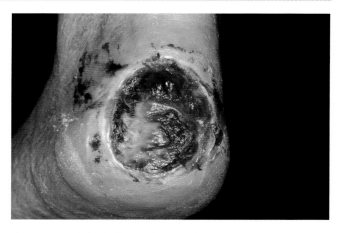

Figure 9.20 Diabetic foot: a large heel ulcer.

developed countries. Diabetes also increases the risk of early development of cataracts (p. 211) and other visual disorders.

Diabetic foot

Many factors commonly present in DM contribute to the development of this serious situation. Disease of large and small blood vessels impairs blood supply to and around the extremities. If peripheral neuropathy is present, sensation is reduced. A small injury to the foot may go unnoticed, especially when there is visual impairment. In DM healing is slower and injuries easily worsen if aggravated, e.g. by chafing shoes, and often become infected. An ulcer may form (Fig. 9.20) and the healing process is lengthy, if at all. In severe cases the injured area ulcerates and enlarges, and may become gangrenous, sometimes to the extent that amputation is required.

For a range of self-assessment exercises on the topics in this chapter, visit Evolve online resources: https://evolve.elsevier.com/Waugh/anatomy/

Intake of raw materials and elimination of waste

The respiratory system

This chapter describes the structure and functions of the respiratory system.

The cells of the body need energy for all their metabolic activities. Most of this energy is derived from chemical reactions, which can only take place in the presence of oxygen (O_2). The main waste product of these reactions is carbon dioxide (CO_2). The respiratory system provides the route by which the supply of oxygen present in the atmospheric air enters the body, and it provides the route of excretion for carbon dioxide.

The condition of the atmospheric air entering the body varies considerably according to the external environment, e.g. it may be dry or moist, warm or cold, and carry varying quantities of pollutants, dust or dirt. As the air breathed in moves through the air passages to reach the lungs, it is warmed or cooled to body temperature, saturated with water vapour and 'cleaned' as particles of dust stick to the mucus which coats the lining

membrane. Blood provides the transport system for O_2 and CO_2 between the lungs and the cells of the body. Exchange of gases between the blood and the lungs is called *external respiration* and that between the blood and the cells *internal respiration*. The organs of the respiratory system are:

- nose
- pharynx
- larynx
- trachea
- two bronchi (one bronchus to each lung)
- bronchioles and smaller air passages
- two lungs and their coverings, the pleura
- muscles of breathing – the intercostal muscles and the diaphragm.

Figure 10.1 shows the organs of the respiratory system and associated structures. 🎬 **10.1, 10.2**

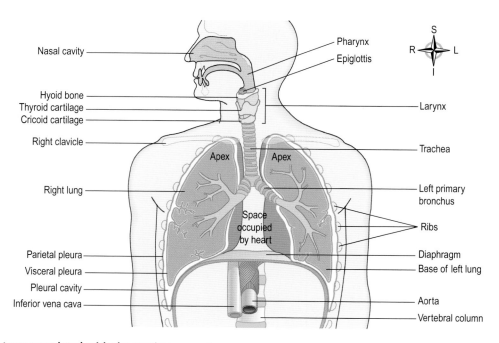

Figure 10.1 Structures associated with the respiratory system.

The effects of ageing on respiratory function are described on p. 261, and important respiratory disorders on p. 262.

Nose and nasal cavity

Learning outcomes

After studying this section, you should be able to:

- describe the location of the nasal cavities

- relate the structure of the nasal cavities to their function in respiration

- outline the physiology of smell.

Position and structure

The nasal cavity is the main route of air entry, and consists of a large irregular cavity divided into two equal passages by a *septum*. The posterior bony part of the septum is formed by the perpendicular plate of the ethmoid bone and the vomer. Anteriorly, it consists of hyaline cartilage (Fig. 10.2).

The roof is formed by the cribriform plate of the ethmoid bone and the sphenoid bone, frontal bone and nasal bones.

The floor is formed by the roof of the mouth and consists of the hard palate in front and the soft palate behind. The hard palate is composed of the maxilla and palatine bones and the soft palate consists of involuntary muscle.

The medial wall is formed by the septum.

The lateral walls are formed by the maxilla, the ethmoid bone and the inferior conchae (Fig. 10.3).

The posterior wall is formed by the posterior wall of the pharynx.

Lining of the nasal cavity 10.3

The nasal cavity is lined with very vascular *ciliated columnar epithelium* (ciliated mucous membrane, see Fig. 10.12, respiratory mucosa) which contains mucus-secreting goblet cells (p. 249). At the anterior nares this blends with the skin and posteriorly it extends into the nasal part of the pharynx (the nasopharynx).

Openings into the nasal cavity

The anterior nares, or nostrils, are the openings from the exterior into the nasal cavity. Nasal hairs are found here, coated in sticky mucus.

The posterior nares are the openings from the nasal cavity into the pharynx.

The paranasal sinuses are cavities in the bones of the face and the cranium, containing air. There are tiny openings between the paranasal sinuses and the nasal cavity. They

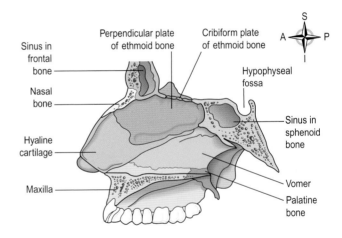

Figure 10.2 Structures forming the nasal septum.

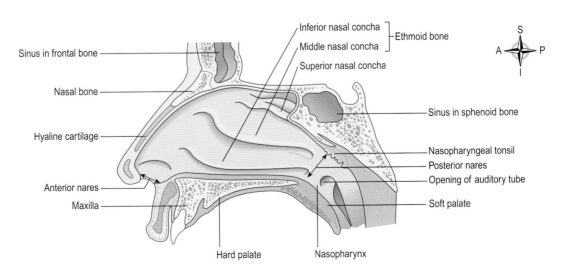

Figure 10.3 Lateral wall of right nasal cavity.

are lined with mucous membrane, continuous with that of the nasal cavity. The main sinuses are:

- maxillary sinuses in the lateral walls
- frontal and sphenoidal sinuses in the roof (Fig. 10.3)
- ethmoidal sinuses in the upper part of the lateral walls.

The sinuses are involved in speech (p. 248) and also lighten the skull. *The nasolacrimal ducts* extend from the lateral walls of the nose to the conjunctival sacs of the eye (p. 204). They drain tears from the eyes.

Respiratory function of the nose

The nose is the first of the respiratory passages through which the inspired air passes. In the nasal cavity, air is warmed, moistened and filtered. The three projecting *conchae* (Figs 10.3 and 10.4) increase the surface area and cause turbulence, spreading inspired air over the whole nasal surface. The large surface area maximises warming, humidification and filtering.

Warming. The immense vascularity of the mucosa permits rapid warming as the air flows past. This also explains the large blood loss when a nosebleed (epistaxis) occurs.

Filtering and cleaning. Hairs at the anterior nares trap larger particles. Smaller particles such as dust and bacteria settle and adhere to the mucus. Mucus protects the underlying epithelium from irritation and prevents

drying. Synchronous beating of the cilia wafts the mucus towards the throat where it is swallowed or coughed up (expectorated).

Humidification. As air travels over the moist mucosa, it becomes saturated with water vapour. Irritation of the nasal mucosa results in *sneezing*, a reflex action that forcibly expels an irritant.

The sense of smell

The nose is the organ of the sense of smell (*olfaction*). Specialised receptors that detect smell are located in the roof of the nose in the area of the cribriform plate of the ethmoid bones and the superior conchae (Figs 10.4 and 8.23A). These receptors are stimulated by airborne odours. The resultant nerve signals are carried by the *olfactory nerves* to the brain where the sensation of smell is perceived (p. 206).

Pharynx

Learning outcomes

After studying this section, you should be able to:

- describe the location of the pharynx
- relate the structure of the pharynx to its function.

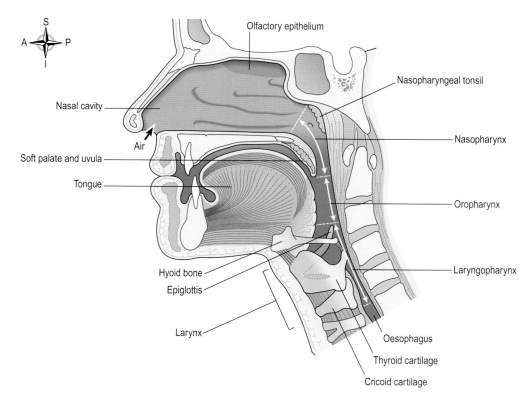

Figure 10.4 The pathway of air from the nose to the larynx.

Position

The pharynx (throat) is a passageway about 12–14 cm long. It extends from the posterior nares, and runs behind the mouth and the larynx to the level of the 6th thoracic vertebra, where it becomes the oesophagus.

Structures associated with the pharynx

Superiorly – the inferior surface of the base of the skull
Inferiorly – it is continuous with the oesophagus
Anteriorly – the wall is incomplete because of the openings into the nose, mouth and larynx
Posteriorly – areolar tissue, involuntary muscle and the bodies of the first six cervical vertebrae.

For descriptive purposes the pharynx is divided into three parts: *nasopharynx, oropharynx* and *laryngopharynx*.

The nasopharynx

The nasal part of the pharynx lies behind the nose above the level of the soft palate. On its lateral walls are the two openings of the *auditory tubes* (p. 193), one leading to each middle ear. On the posterior wall are the *pharyngeal tonsils* (adenoids), consisting of lymphoid tissue. They are most prominent in children up to approximately 7 years of age. Thereafter they gradually atrophy.

The oropharynx

The oral part of the pharynx lies behind the mouth, extending from below the level of the soft palate to the level of the upper part of the body of the 3rd cervical vertebra. The lateral walls of the pharynx blend with the soft palate to form two folds on each side. Between each pair of folds is a collection of lymphoid tissue called the *palatine tonsil.*

When swallowing, the soft palate and uvula are pushed upwards, sealing off the nasal cavity and preventing the entry of food and fluids.

The laryngopharynx

The laryngeal part of the pharynx extends from the oropharynx above and continues as the oesophagus below, with the larynx lying anteriorly.

Structure

The walls of the pharynx contain several types of tissue.

Mucous membrane lining

The mucosa varies slightly in the different regions. In the nasopharynx it is continuous with the lining of the nose and consists of ciliated columnar epithelium; in the oropharynx and laryngopharynx it is formed by tougher stratified squamous epithelium, which is continuous with the lining of the mouth and oesophagus. This lining protects underlying tissues from the abrasive action of foodstuffs passing through during swallowing.

Submucosa

The layer of tissue below the epithelium (the submucosa) is rich in mucosa-associated lymphoid tissue (MALT, p. 139), involved in protection against infection. Tonsils are masses of MALT that bulge through the epithelium. Some glandular tissue is also found here.

Smooth muscle

The pharyngeal muscles help to keep the pharynx permanently open so that breathing is not interfered with. Sometimes in sleep, and particularly if sedative drugs or alcohol have been taken, the tone of these muscles is reduced and the opening through the pharynx can become partially or totally obstructed. This contributes to snoring and periodic wakenings, which disturb sleep.

Constrictor muscles close the pharynx during swallowing, pushing food and fluid into the oesophagus.

Blood and nerve supply

Blood is supplied to the pharynx by several branches of the facial artery. The venous return is into the facial and internal jugular veins.

The nerve supply is from the pharyngeal plexus, and includes both parasympathetic and sympathetic nerves. Parasympathetic supply is by the *vagus* and *glossopharyngeal* nerves. Sympathetic supply is by nerves from the *superior cervical ganglia* (p. 174).

Functions

Passageway for air and food

The pharynx is involved in both the respiratory and the digestive systems: air passes through the nasal and oral sections, and food through the oral and laryngeal sections.

Warming and humidifying

By the same methods as in the nose, the air is further warmed and moistened as it passes towards the lungs.

Hearing

The auditory tube, extending from the nasopharynx to each middle ear, allows air to enter the middle ear. This leads to air in the middle ear being at the same pressure as the outer ear, protecting the tympanic membrane (eardrum, p. 193) from any changes in atmospheric pressure.

Protection

The lymphatic tissue of the pharyngeal and laryngeal tonsils produces antibodies in response to swallowed or inhaled antigens (Ch. 15). The tonsils are larger in children and tend to atrophy in adults.

Speech

The pharynx functions in speech; by acting as a resonating chamber for sound ascending from the larynx, it helps (together with the sinuses) to give the voice its individual characteristics.

Larynx

Learning outcomes

After studying this section, you should be able to:

■ describe the structure and function of the larynx

■ outline the physiology of speech generation.

Position

The larynx or 'voice box' links the laryngopharynx and the trachea (Figs 10.1 and 10.4). It lies in front of the laryngopharynx and the 3rd, 4th, 5th and 6th cervical vertebrae. Until puberty there is little difference in the size of the larynx between the sexes. Thereafter, it grows larger in the male, which explains the prominence of the 'Adam's apple' and the generally deeper voice.

Structures associated with the larynx

Superiorly – the hyoid bone and the root of the tongue
Inferiorly – it is continuous with the trachea
Anteriorly – the muscles attached to the hyoid bone and the muscles of the neck
Posteriorly – the laryngopharynx and 3rd–6th cervical vertebrae
Laterally – the lobes of the thyroid gland.

Structure

Cartilages

The larynx is composed of several irregularly shaped cartilages attached to each other by ligaments and membranes. The main cartilages are:

- 1 thyroid cartilage ⎫
- 1 cricoid cartilage ⎬ hyaline cartilage
- 2 arytenoid cartilages ⎭
- 1 epiglottis   elastic fibrocartilage.

Several ligaments attach the cartilages to each other and to the hyoid bone (Figs 10.5, 10.6 and 10.8).

The thyroid cartilage (Figs 10.5 and 10.6). This is the most prominent of the laryngeal cartilages. Made of hyaline cartilage, it lies to the front of the neck. Its anterior wall projects into the soft tissues of the front of the throat, forming the *laryngeal prominence* or Adam's apple, which is easily felt and often visible in adult males. The anterior wall is partially divided by the *thyroid notch*. The cartilage is incomplete posteriorly, and is bound with ligaments to the hyoid bone above and the cricoid cartilage below.

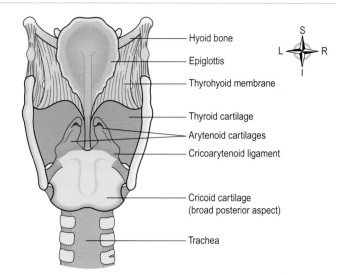

Figure 10.5 Larynx. Viewed from behind.

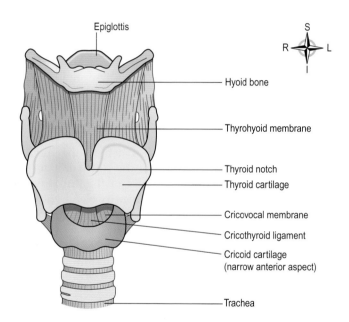

Figure 10.6 Larynx. Viewed from the front.

The upper part of the thyroid cartilage is lined with stratified squamous epithelium like the larynx, and the lower part with ciliated columnar epithelium like the trachea. There are many muscles attached to its outer surface.

The thyroid cartilage forms most of the anterior and lateral walls of the larynx.

The cricoid cartilage (Fig. 10.7). This lies below the thyroid cartilage and is also composed of hyaline cartilage. It is shaped like a signet ring, completely encircling the larynx with the narrow part anteriorly and the broad part posteriorly. The broad posterior part articulates with the arytenoid cartilages and with the thyroid cartilage. It is lined with ciliated columnar epithelium and there are

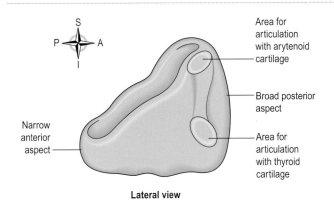

Figure 10.7 The cricoid cartilage.

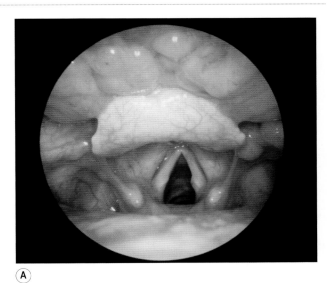

A

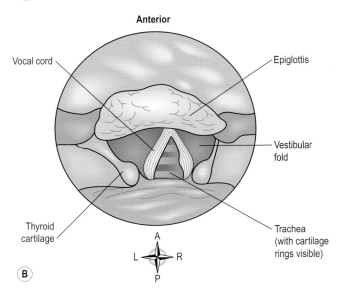

B

Figure 10.8 **Vocal cords. A.** Bronchoscopic image of the open (abducted) vocal cords. **B.** Diagram of the vocal cords showing the principal structures.

muscles and ligaments attached to its outer surface (Fig. 10.7). The lower border of the cricoid cartilage marks the end of the upper respiratory tract.

The arytenoid cartilages. These are two roughly pyramid-shaped hyaline cartilages situated on top of the broad part of the cricoid cartilage forming part of the posterior wall of the larynx (Fig. 10.5). They give attachment to the vocal cords and to muscles and are lined with ciliated columnar epithelium.

The epiglottis (Figs 10.4–10.6 and 10.8). This is a leaf-shaped fibroelastic cartilage attached on a flexible stalk of cartilage to the inner surface of the anterior wall of the thyroid cartilage immediately below the thyroid notch. It rises obliquely upwards behind the tongue and the body of the hyoid bone. It is covered with stratified squamous epithelium. If the larynx is likened to a box then the epiglottis acts as the lid; it closes off the larynx during swallowing, protecting the lungs from accidental inhalation of foreign objects.

Blood and nerve supply

Blood is supplied to the larynx by the superior and inferior laryngeal arteries and drained by the thyroid veins, which join the internal jugular vein.

The parasympathetic nerve supply is from the superior laryngeal and recurrent laryngeal nerves, which are branches of the vagus nerves. The sympathetic nerves are from the superior cervical ganglia, one on each side. These provide the motor nerve supply to the muscles of the larynx and sensory fibres to the lining membrane.

Interior of the larynx (Fig. 10.8)

The *vocal cords* are two pale folds of mucous membrane with cord-like free edges, stretched across the laryngeal opening. They extend from the inner wall of the thyroid prominence anteriorly to the arytenoid cartilages posteriorly.

When the muscles controlling the vocal cords are relaxed, the vocal cords open and the passageway for air coming up through the larynx is clear; the vocal cords are said to be *abducted* (open, Fig. 10.9A). Vibrating the vocal cords in this position produces low-pitched sounds. When the muscles controlling the vocal cords contract, the vocal cords are stretched out tightly across the larynx (Fig. 10.9B), and are said to be *adducted* (closed). When the vocal cords are stretched to this extent, and are vibrated by air passing through from the lungs, the sound produced is high pitched. The pitch of the voice is therefore determined by the tension applied to the vocal cords by the appropriate sets of muscles. When not in use, the vocal cords are adducted. The space between the vocal cords is called the *glottis*.

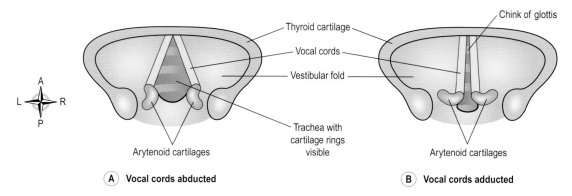

Figure 10.9 The extreme positions of the vocal cords. A. Abducted (open). **B.** Adducted (closed).

Functions

Production of sound. Sound has the properties of *pitch*, *volume* and *resonance*.

- Pitch of the voice depends upon the *length* and *tightness* of the cords. Shorter cords produce higher pitched sounds. At puberty, the male vocal cords begin to grow longer, hence the lower pitch of the adult male voice.
- Volume of the voice depends upon the *force* with which the cords vibrate. The greater the force of expired air, the more strongly the cords vibrate and the louder the sound emitted.
- Resonance, or tone, is dependent upon the shape of the mouth, the position of the tongue and the lips, the facial muscles and the air in the paranasal sinuses.

Speech. This is produced when the sounds produced by the vocal cords are amplified and manipulated by the tongue, cheeks and lips.

Protection of the lower respiratory tract. During swallowing (p. 297) the larynx moves upwards, blocking the opening into it from the pharynx. In addition, the hinged epiglottis closes over the larynx. This ensures that food passes into the oesophagus and not into the trachea.

Passageway for air. The larynx links the pharynx above with the trachea below.

Humidifying, filtering and warming. These processes continue as inspired air travels through the larynx.

Trachea

Learning outcomes

After studying this section, you should be able to:

- describe the location of the trachea
- outline the structure of the trachea
- explain the functions of the trachea in respiration.

Position

The trachea or windpipe is a continuation of the larynx and extends downwards to about the level of the 5th thoracic vertebra where it divides at the *carina* into the right and left primary bronchi, one bronchus going to each lung. It is approximately 10–11 cm long and lies mainly in the median plane in front of the oesophagus (Fig. 10.10).

Structures associated with the trachea

(Fig. 10.10)

Superiorly – the larynx
Inferiorly – the right and left bronchi
Anteriorly – upper part: the isthmus of the thyroid gland; lower part: the arch of the aorta and the sternum
Posteriorly – the oesophagus separates the trachea from the vertebral column
Laterally – the lungs and the lobes of the thyroid gland.

Structure

The tracheal wall is composed of three layers of tissue, and is held open by between 16 and 20 incomplete (C-shaped) rings of hyaline cartilage lying one above the other. The rings are incomplete posteriorly where the trachea lies against the oesophagus (Fig. 10.11). The cartilages are embedded in a sleeve of smooth muscle and connective tissue, which also forms the posterior wall where the rings are incomplete.

Three layers of tissue 'clothe' the cartilages of the trachea.

- The outer layer contains fibrous and elastic tissue and encloses the cartilages.
- The middle layer consists of cartilages and bands of smooth muscle that wind round the trachea in a helical arrangement. There is some areolar tissue, containing blood and lymph vessels and autonomic nerves. The free ends of the

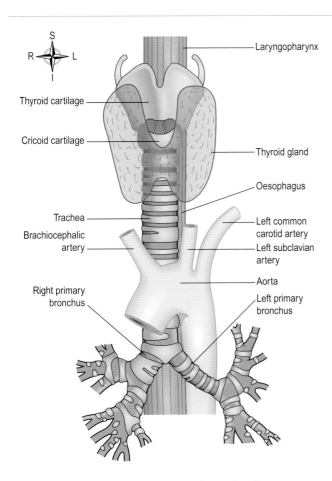

Figure 10.10 The trachea and some of its related structures.

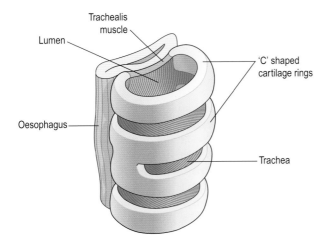

Figure 10.11 The relationship of the trachea to the oesophagus.

incomplete cartilages are connected by the trachealis muscle, which allows for adjustment of tracheal diameter.

- The lining is ciliated columnar epithelium, containing mucus-secreting goblet cells (Fig. 10.12).

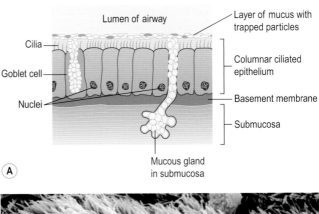

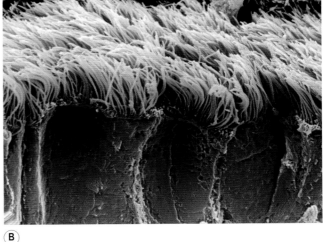

Figure 10.12 Cells lining the trachea. A. Ciliated mucous membrane. **B.** Coloured scanning electron micrograph of bronchial cilia.

Blood and nerve supply, lymph drainage

Arterial blood supply is mainly by the inferior thyroid and bronchial arteries and venous return is by the inferior thyroid veins into the brachiocephalic veins.

Parasympathetic nerve supply is by the recurrent laryngeal nerves and other branches of the vagi. Sympathetic supply is by nerves from the sympathetic ganglia. Parasympathetic stimulation constricts the trachea, and sympathetic stimulation dilates it.

Lymph from the respiratory passages drains through lymph nodes situated round the trachea and in the carina, the area where it divides into two bronchi.

Functions

Support and patency. Tracheal cartilages hold the trachea permanently open (patent), but the soft tissue bands in between the cartilages allow flexibility so that the head and neck can move freely without obstructing or kinking the trachea. The absence of cartilage posteriorly permits the oesophagus to expand comfortably during swallowing. Contraction or relaxation of the trachealis muscle, which links the free ends of the

C-shaped cartilages, helps to regulate the diameter of the trachea.

Mucociliary escalator. This is the synchronous and regular beating of the cilia of the mucous membrane lining that wafts mucus with adherent particles upwards towards the larynx where it is either swallowed or coughed up (Fig. 10.12B).

Cough reflex. Nerve endings in the larynx, trachea and bronchi are sensitive to irritation, which generates nerve impulses conducted by the vagus nerves to the respiratory centre in the brain stem (p. 160). The reflex motor response is deep inspiration followed by closure of the glottis, i.e. closure of the vocal cords. The abdominal and respiratory muscles then contract causing a sudden and rapid increase of pressure in the lungs. Then the glottis opens, expelling air through the mouth, taking mucus and/or foreign material with it.

Warming, humidifying and filtering. These continue as in the nose, although air is normally saturated and at body temperature when it reaches the trachea.

Lungs

Learning outcomes

After studying this section, you should be able to:

- name the air passage of the bronchial tree in descending order of size
- describe the structure and changing functions of the different levels of airway
- describe the location and gross anatomy of the lungs
- identify the functions of the pleura
- describe the pulmonary blood supply.

Position and gross structure (Fig. 10.13)

There are two lungs, one lying on each side of the midline in the thoracic cavity. They are cone-shaped and have an *apex*, a *base*, a *tip*, *costal surface* and *medial surface.*

The apex This is rounded and rises into the root of the neck, about 25 mm above the level of the middle third of the clavicle. It lies close to the first rib and the blood vessels and nerves in the root of the neck.

The base This is concave and semilunar in shape, and lies on the upper (thoracic) surface of the diaphragm.

The costal surface This is the broad outer surface of the lung that lies directly against the costal cartilages, the ribs and the intercostal muscles.

The medial surface The medial surface of each lung faces the other directly across the space between the lungs, the *mediastinum.* Each is concave and has a roughly triangular-shaped area, called the *hilum*, at the level of the 5th, 6th and 7th thoracic vertebrae. The primary bronchus, the pulmonary artery supplying the lung and the two pulmonary veins draining it, the bronchial artery and veins, and the lymphatic and nerve supply enter and leave the lung at the hilum (Fig. 10.14).

The mediastinum contains the heart, great vessels, trachea, right and left bronchi, oesophagus, lymph nodes, lymph vessels and nerves.

The right lung is divided into three distinct lobes: superior, middle and inferior. The left lung is smaller because the heart occupies space left of the midline. It is divided into only two lobes: superior and inferior. The divisions between the lobes are called *fissures.*

Pleura and pleural cavity

The pleura consists of a closed sac of serous membrane (one for each lung) which contains a small amount of serous fluid. The lung is pushed into this sac so that it forms two layers: one adheres to the lung and the other to the wall of the thoracic cavity (Figs 10.1 and 10.15).

The visceral pleura
This is adherent to the lung, covering each lobe and passing into the fissures that separate them.

The parietal pleura
This is adherent to the inside of the chest wall and the thoracic surface of the diaphragm. It is not attached to other structures in the mediastinum and is continuous with the visceral pleura round the edges of the hilum.

The pleural cavity
This is only a potential space and contains no air, so the pressure within is negative relative to atmospheric pressure. In health, the two layers of pleura are separated by a thin film of serous fluid (pleural fluid), which allows them to glide over each other, preventing friction between them during breathing. The pleural fluid is secreted by the epithelial cells of the membrane. The double membrane arrangement of the pleura is similar to the serous pericardium of the heart (p. 87).

The two layers of pleura, with pleural fluid between them, behave in the same way as two pieces of glass separated by a thin film of water. They glide over each other easily but can be pulled apart only with difficulty, because of the surface tension between the membranes and the fluid. This is essential for keeping the lung inflated against the inside of the chest wall. The airways and the alveoli of the lungs are embedded in elastic tissue, which constantly pull the lung tissues towards the hilum, but

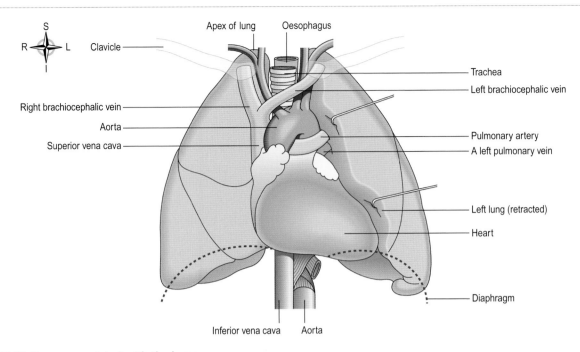

Figure 10.13 **Organs associated with the lungs.**

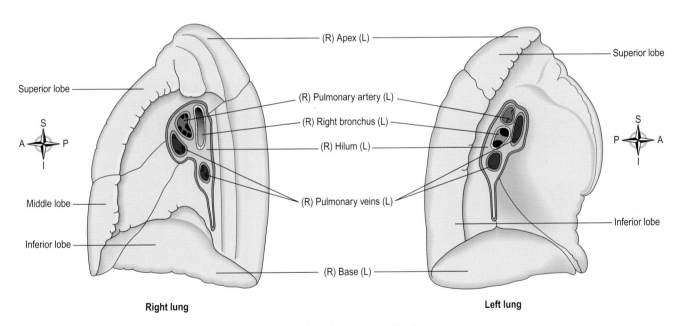

Figure 10.14 **The lobes of the lungs and vessels/airways of each hilum.** Medial views.

because pleural fluid holds the two pleura together, the lung remains expanded. If either layer of pleura is punctured, air is sucked into the pleural space and part or all of the entire underlying lung collapses.

Interior of the lungs

The lungs are composed of the bronchi and smaller air passages, alveoli, connective tissue, blood vessels, lymph vessels and nerves, all embedded in an elastic connective tissue matrix. Each lobe is made up of a large number of *lobules*.

Pulmonary blood supply (Fig. 10.16)

The *pulmonary trunk* divides into the right and left pulmonary arteries, carrying deoxygenated blood to each lung. Within the lungs each pulmonary artery divides into many branches, which eventually end in a dense capillary network around the alveoli (see Fig. 10.18). The walls of

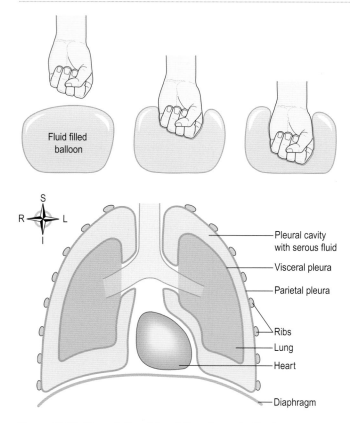

Figure 10.15 The relationship of the pleura to the lungs.

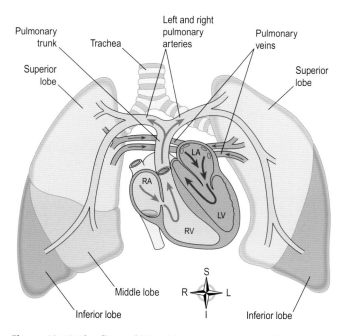

Figure 10.16 The flow of blood between heart and lungs.

the alveoli and the capillaries each consist of only one layer of flattened epithelial cells. The exchange of gases between air in the alveoli and blood in the capillaries takes place across these two very fine membranes (together called the *respiratory membrane*). The pulmonary capillaries

merge into a network of pulmonary venules, which in turn form two pulmonary veins carrying oxygenated blood from each lung back to the left atrium of the heart.

The blood supply to the respiratory passages, lymphatic drainage and nerve supply is described later (p. 253).

Bronchi and bronchioles

The two primary bronchi are formed when the trachea divides, at about the level of the 5th thoracic vertebra (Fig. 10.17).

The right bronchus. This is wider, shorter and more vertical than the left bronchus and is therefore more likely to become obstructed by an inhaled foreign body. It is approximately 2.5 cm long. After entering the right lung at the hilum it divides into three branches, one to each lobe. Each branch then subdivides into numerous smaller branches.

The left bronchus. This is about 5 cm long and is narrower than the right. After entering the lung at the hilum it divides into two branches, one to each lobe. Each branch then subdivides into progressively smaller airways within the lung substance.

Structure 10.4

The bronchial walls contain the same three layers of tissue as the trachea, and are lined with ciliated columnar epithelium. The bronchi progressively subdivide into bronchioles (Fig. 10.17), terminal bronchioles, respiratory bronchioles, alveolar ducts and finally, alveoli. The wider passages are called *conducting airways* because their function is to bring air into the lungs, and their walls are too thick to permit gas exchange.

Structural changes in the bronchial passages
As the bronchi divide and become progressively smaller, their structure changes to match their function.

Cartilage. Since rigid cartilage would interfere with expansion of lung tissue and the exchange of gases, it is present for support in the larger airways only. The bronchi contain cartilage rings like the trachea, but as the airways divide, these rings become much smaller plates, and at the bronchiolar level there is no cartilage present in the airway walls at all.

Smooth muscle. As the cartilage disappears from airway walls, it is replaced by smooth muscle. This allows the diameter of the airways to be increased or decreased through the influence of the autonomic nervous system, regulating airflow within each lung.

Epithelial lining. The ciliated epithelium is gradually replaced with non-ciliated epithelium, and goblet cells disappear.

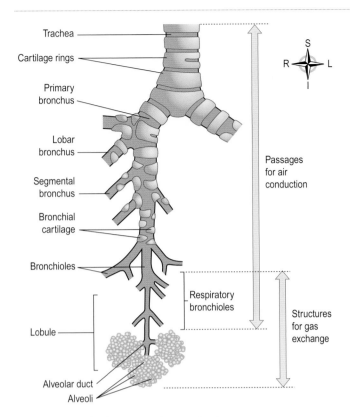

Trachea

Cartilage rings

Primary bronchus

Lobar bronchus

Segmental bronchus

Bronchial cartilage

Bronchioles

Lobule

Alveolar duct

Alveoli

S
R — L
I

Passages for air conduction

Respiratory bronchioles

Structures for gas exchange

Figure 10.17 The lower respiratory tract.

Blood and nerve supply, lymph drainage

The arterial supply to the walls of the bronchi and smaller air passages is through branches of the right and left bronchial arteries and the venous return is mainly through the bronchial veins. On the right side they empty into the azygos vein and on the left into the superior intercostal vein (see Fig. 5.29, p. 104).

The vagus nerves (parasympathetic) stimulate contraction of smooth muscle in the bronchial tree, causing bronchoconstriction, and sympathetic stimulation causes bronchodilation (see below).

Lymph is drained from the walls of the air passages in a network of lymph vessels. It passes through lymph nodes situated around the trachea and bronchial tree then into the thoracic duct on the left side and right lymphatic duct on the other.

Functions

Control of air entry. The diameter of the respiratory passages is altered by contraction or relaxation of the smooth muscle in their walls, regulating the speed and volume of airflow into and within the lungs. These changes are controlled by the autonomic nerve supply: parasympathetic stimulation causes constriction and sympathetic stimulation causes dilation (p. 176).

The following functions continue as in the upper airways:

- warming and humidifying
- support and patency
- removal of particulate matter
- cough reflex.

Respiratory bronchioles and alveoli 10.5

Structure

Within each lobe, the lung tissue is further divided by fine sheets of connective tissue into *lobules*. Each lobule is supplied with air by a terminal bronchiole, which further subdivides into respiratory bronchioles, alveolar ducts and large numbers of alveoli (air sacs). There are about 150 million alveoli in the adult lung. It is in these structures that the process of gas exchange occurs. As airways progressively divide and become smaller and smaller, their walls gradually become thinner until muscle and connective tissue disappear, leaving a single layer of simple squamous epithelial cells in the alveolar ducts and alveoli. These distal respiratory passages are supported by a loose network of elastic connective tissue in which macrophages, fibroblasts, nerves and blood and lymph vessels are embedded. The alveoli are surrounded by a dense network of capillaries (Fig. 10.18). Exchange of gases in the lung (external respiration) takes place across a membrane made up of the alveolar wall and the capillary wall fused firmly together. This is called the *respiratory membrane*.

On microscopic examination, the extensive air spaces are clearly seen and healthy lung tissue has a honeycomb appearance (Fig. 10.19). **10.6**

Lying between the squamous cells are *septal* cells that secrete *surfactant*, a phospholipid fluid which prevents the alveoli from drying out and reduces surface tension preventing alveolar collapse during expiration. Secretion of surfactant into the distal air passages and alveoli begins about the 35th week of fetal life. Its presence in newborn babies permits expansion of the lungs and the establishment of respiration immediately after birth. It may not be present in sufficient amounts in the immature lungs of premature babies, causing serious breathing problems.

Nerve supply to bronchioles

Parasympathetic stimulation, from the vagus nerve, causes bronchoconstriction. The absence of supporting cartilage means that small airways may be completely closed off by constriction of their smooth muscle. Sympathetic stimulation relaxes bronchiolar smooth muscle (bronchodilation).

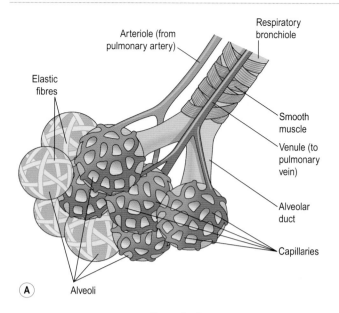

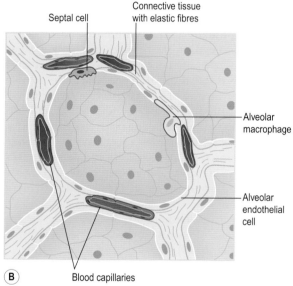

Figure 10.18 **The alveoli and their capillary network.**
A. A group of intact alveoli. **B.** Section through an alveolus.

Functions

External respiration. (See p. 259.)

Defence against infection. At this level, ciliated epithelium, goblet cells and mucus are no longer present, because their presence would impede gas exchange and encourage infection. By the time inspired air reaches the alveoli, it is usually clean. Defence relies on protective cells present within the lung tissue. These include lymphocytes and plasma cells, which produce antibodies, and phagocytes, including alveolar macrophages. These cells are most active in the distal air passages where ciliated epithelium has been replaced by squamous (flattened) cells.

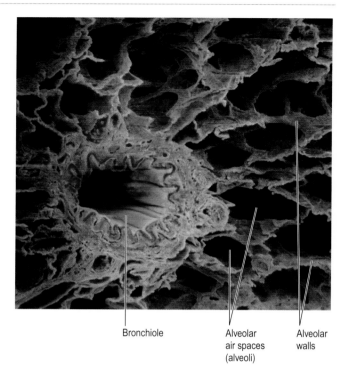

Figure 10.19 **Coloured scanning electron micrograph of lung alveoli and a bronchiole.**

Warming and humidifying. These continue as in the upper airways. Inhalation of dry or inadequately humidified air over a period of time irritates the mucosa and encourages infection.

Respiration

Learning outcomes

After studying this section, you should be able to:

- describe the actions of the main muscles involved in breathing

- compare and contrast the mechanical events occurring in inspiration and expiration

- define the terms compliance, elasticity and airflow resistance

- describe the principal lung volumes and capacities

- compare the processes of internal and external respiration, using the concept of diffusion of gases

- describe O_2 and CO_2 transport in the blood

- explain the main mechanisms by which respiration is controlled.

The term respiration means the exchange of gases between body cells and the environment. This involves two main processes.

Breathing (pulmonary ventilation). This is movement of air into and out of the lungs.

Exchange of gases. This takes place:

- in the lungs: external respiration
- in the tissues: internal respiration.

Each of these will be considered later in this section.

Breathing

Breathing supplies oxygen to the alveoli, and eliminates carbon dioxide.

Muscles of breathing

Expansion of the chest during inspiration occurs as a result of muscular activity, partly voluntary and partly involuntary. The main muscles used in normal quiet breathing are the *external intercostal muscles* and the *diaphragm*.

Intercostal muscles

There are 11 pairs of intercostal muscles occupying the spaces between the 12 pairs of ribs. They are arranged in two layers, the external and internal intercostal muscles (Fig. 10.20).

The external intercostal muscles These extend downwards and forwards from the lower border of the rib above to the upper border of the rib below. They are involved in inspiration.

The internal intercostal muscles These extend downwards and backwards from the lower border of the rib above to the upper border of the rib below, crossing the external intercostal muscle fibres at right angles. The internal intercostals are used when expiration becomes active, as in exercise.

The first rib is fixed. Therefore, when the external intercostal muscles contract they pull all the other ribs towards the first rib. The ribcage moves as a unit, upwards and outwards, enlarging the thoracic cavity. The intercostal muscles are stimulated to contract by the *intercostal nerves*.

Diaphragm 10.7

The diaphragm is a dome-shaped muscular structure separating the thoracic and abdominal cavities. It forms the floor of the thoracic cavity and the roof of the abdominal cavity and consists of a central tendon from which muscle fibres radiate to be attached to the lower ribs and sternum and to the vertebral column by two crura. When the diaphragm is relaxed, the central tendon is at the level of the 8th thoracic vertebra (Fig. 10.21). When it contracts, its muscle fibres shorten and the central tendon is pulled downwards to the level of the 9th thoracic vertebra, lengthening the thoracic cavity. This decreases pressure in the thoracic cavity and increases it in the abdominal and pelvic cavities. The diaphragm is supplied by the *phrenic nerves*.

Quiet, restful breathing is sometimes called *diaphragmatic breathing* because 75% of the work is done by the diaphragm.

During inspiration, the external intercostal muscles and the diaphragm contract simultaneously, enlarging the thoracic cavity in all directions, that is from back to front, side to side and top to bottom (Fig. 10.22).

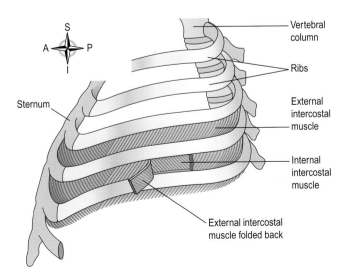

Figure 10.20 The intercostal muscles and the bones of the thorax.

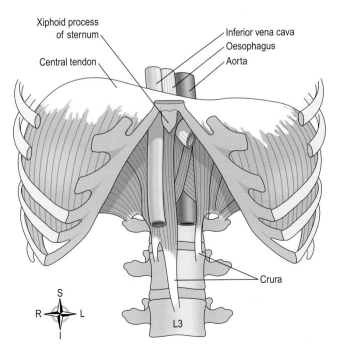

Figure 10.21 The diaphragm.

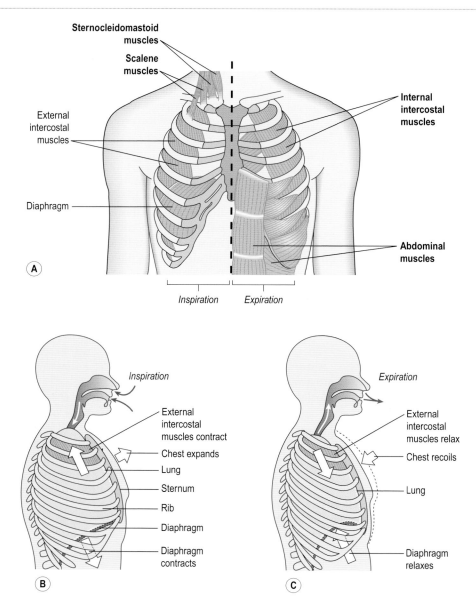

Figure 10.22 Changes in chest size during inspiration. A. Muscles involved in respiration (accessory muscles labelled in bold). **B, C.** Changes in chest volume.

Accessory muscles of respiration (Fig. 10.22A)

When extra respiratory effort is required, additional muscles are used. Forced inspiration is assisted by the *sternocleidomastoid* muscles (p. 425) and the *scalene* muscles, which link the cervical vertebrae to the first two ribs, and increase ribcage expansion. Forced expiration is helped by the activity of the internal intercostal muscles and sometimes the abdominal muscles, which increase the pressure in the thorax by squeezing the abdominal contents.

Cycle of breathing ▮ 10.8

The average respiratory rate is 12–15 breaths per minute. Each breath consists of three phases: inspiration, expiration and pause.

The visceral pleura is adherent to the lungs and the parietal pleura to the inner wall of the thorax and to the diaphragm. Between them is a thin film of pleural fluid (p. 250).

Breathing depends upon changes in pressure and volume in the thoracic cavity. It follows the underlying physical principle that increasing the volume of a container decreases the pressure inside it, and that decreasing the volume of a container increases the pressure inside it. Since air flows from an area of high pressure to an area of low pressure, changing the pressure inside the lungs determines the direction of airflow.

Inspiration

Simultaneous contraction of the external intercostal muscles and the diaphragm expands the thorax. As the parietal pleura is firmly adhered to the diaphragm and the inside of the ribcage, it is pulled outward along with them. This pulls the visceral pleura outwards too, since the two pleura are held together by the thin film of pleural fluid. Because the visceral pleura is firmly adherent to the lung, the lung tissue is, therefore, also pulled up and out with the ribs, and downwards with the diaphragm. This expands the lungs, and the pressure within the alveoli and in the air passages falls, drawing air into the lungs in an attempt to equalise atmospheric and alveolar air pressures.

The process of inspiration is *active*, as it needs energy for muscle contraction. The negative pressure created in the thoracic cavity aids venous return to the heart and is known as the *respiratory pump*.

At rest, inspiration lasts about 2 seconds.

Expiration

Relaxation of the external intercostal muscles and the diaphragm results in downward and inward movement of the ribcage (Fig. 10.22) and elastic recoil of the lungs. As this occurs, pressure inside the lungs rises and expels air from the respiratory tract. At the end of expiration, the lungs still contain some air, and are pre-vented from complete collapse by the intact pleura. This process is *passive* as it does not require the expenditure of energy.

At rest, expiration lasts about 3 seconds, and after expiration there is a pause before the next cycle begins.

Physiological variables affecting breathing

Elasticity. Elasticity is the ability of the lung to return to its normal shape after each breath. Loss of elasticity, e.g. in emphysema (p. 263), of the connective tissue in the lungs necessitates forced expiration and increased effort on inspiration.

Compliance. This is the stretchability of the lungs, i.e. the effort required to inflate the alveoli. The healthy lung is very compliant, and inflates with very little effort. When compliance is low the effort needed to inflate the lungs is greater than normal, e.g. when insufficient surfactant is present. Note that compliance and elasticity are opposing forces.

Airway resistance. When this is increased, e.g. in bron-choconstriction, more respiratory effort is required to inflate the lungs.

Lung volumes and capacities (Fig. 10.23)

In normal quiet breathing there are about 15 complete respiratory cycles per minute. The lungs and the air passages are never empty and, as the exchange of gases takes place only across the walls of the alveolar ducts and alveoli, the remaining capacity of the respiratory passages is called the *anatomical dead space* (about 150 mL).

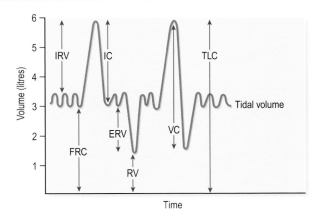

Figure 10.23 Lung volumes and capacities. IRV: inspiratory reserve volume; IC: inspiratory capacity; FRC: functional residual capacity; ERV: expiratory reserve volume; RV: residual volume; VC: vital capacity; TLC: total lung capacity.

Tidal volume (TV). This is the amount of air passing into and out of the lungs during each cycle of breathing (about 500 mL at rest).

Inspiratory reserve volume (IRV). This is the extra volume of air that can be inhaled into the lungs during maximal inspiration, i.e. over and above normal TV.

Inspiratory capacity (IC). This is the amount of air that can be inspired with maximum effort. It consists of the tidal volume (500 ml) plus the inspiratory reserve volume.

Functional residual capacity (FRC). This is the amount of air remaining in the air passages and alveoli at the end of quiet expiration. Tidal air mixes with this air, causing relatively small changes in the composition of alveolar air. As blood flows continuously through the pulmonary capillaries, this means that exchange of gases is not inter-rupted between breaths, preventing moment-to-moment changes in the concentration of blood gases. The func-tional residual volume also prevents collapse of the alveoli on expiration.

Expiratory reserve volume (ERV). This is the largest volume of air which can be expelled from the lungs during maximal expiration.

Residual volume (RV). This cannot be directly measured but is the volume of air remaining in the lungs after forced expiration.

Vital capacity (VC). This is the maximum volume of air which can be moved into and out of the lungs:

$$VC = \text{Tidal volume} + IRV + ERV$$

Total lung capacity (TLC). This is the maximum amount of air the lungs can hold. In an adult of average build, it is normally around 6 litres. Total lung capacity represents the sum of the vital capacity and the residual volume. It cannot be directly measured in clinical tests because even after forced expiration, the residual volume of air still remains in the lungs.

Alveolar ventilation. This is the volume of air that moves into and out of the alveoli per minute. It is equal to the tidal volume minus the anatomical dead space, multiplied by the respiratory rate:

$$\text{Alveolar ventilation} = \text{TV} - \text{anatomical dead space} \times$$
$$\text{respiratory rate}$$
$$= (500 - 150)\ \text{mL} \times 15\ \text{per minute}$$
$$= 5.25\ \text{litres per minute}$$

Lung function tests are carried out to determine respiratory function and are based on the parameters outlined above. Results of these tests can help in diagnosis and monitoring of respiratory disorders.

Exchange of gases

Although breathing involves the alternating processes of inspiration and expiration, gas exchange at the respiratory membrane and in the tissues is a continuous and ongoing process. Diffusion of oxygen and carbon dioxide depends on pressure differences, e.g. between atmospheric air and the blood, or blood and the tissues.

Composition of air

Atmospheric pressure at sea level is 101.3 kilopascals (kPa) or 760 mmHg. With increasing height above sea level, atmospheric pressure is progressively reduced and at 5500 m, about two-thirds the height of Mount Everest (8850 m), it is about half that at sea level. Under water, pressure increases by approximately 1 atmosphere per 10 m below sea level.

Air is a mixture of gases: nitrogen, oxygen, carbon dioxide, water vapour and small quantities of inert gases. The percentage of each in inspired and expired air is listed in Table 10.1. Each gas in the mixture exerts a part of the total pressure proportional to its concentration, i.e. the *partial pressure* (Table 10.2). This is denoted as, e.g. PO_2, PCO_2.

Alveolar air

The composition of alveolar air remains fairly constant and is different from atmospheric air. It is saturated with water vapour, and contains more carbon dioxide and less oxygen. Saturation with water vapour provides 6.3 kPa (47 mmHg) thus reducing the partial pressure of all the other gases present. Gaseous exchange between the alveoli and the bloodstream (*external respiration*) is a continuous process, as the alveoli are never empty, so it is independent of the respiratory cycle. During each inspiration only some of the alveolar gases are exchanged.

Diffusion of gases

Exchange of gases occurs when a difference in partial pressure exists across a semipermeable membrane. Gases move by diffusion from the higher concentration to the lower until equilibrium is established (p. 29). Atmospheric nitrogen is not used by the body so its partial pressure remains unchanged and is the same in inspired and expired air, alveolar air and in the blood.

These principles govern the diffusion of gases in and out of the alveoli across the respiratory membrane

Table 10.1 The composition of inspired and expired air

	Inspired air %	Expired air %
Oxygen	21	16
Carbon dioxide	0.04	4
Nitrogen	78	78
Water vapour	Variable	Saturated

Table 10.2 Partial pressures of gases

Gas	Alveolar air		Deoxygenated blood		Oxygenated blood	
	kPa	mmHg	kPa	mmHg	kPa	mmHg
Oxygen	13.3	100	5.3	40	13.3	100
Carbon dioxide	5.3	40	5.8	44	5.3	40
Nitrogen	76.4	573	76.4	573	76.4	573
Water vapour	6.3	47				
Total	101.3	760				

(*external respiration*) and across capillary membranes in the tissues (*internal respiration*).

External respiration (Fig. 10.24A) 🎞 **10.9**

This is exchange of gases by diffusion between the alveoli and the blood in the alveolar capillaries, across the respiratory membrane. Each alveolar wall is one cell thick and is surrounded by a network of tiny capillaries (the walls of which are also only one cell thick). The total area of respiratory membrane for gas exchange in the lungs is about equivalent to the area of a tennis court. Venous blood arriving at the lungs in the pulmonary artery has travelled from all the tissues of the body, and contains high levels of CO_2 and low levels of O_2. Carbon dioxide diffuses from venous blood down its concentration gradient into the alveoli until equilibrium with alveolar air is

reached. By the same process, oxygen diffuses from the alveoli into the blood. The relatively slow flow of blood through the capillaries increases the time available for gas exchange to occur. When blood leaves the alveolar capillaries, the oxygen and carbon dioxide concentrations are in equilibrium with those of alveolar air (Fig. 10.24A).

Internal respiration (Fig. 10.24B) 🎞 **10.10**

This is exchange of gases by diffusion between blood in the capillaries and the body cells. Gas exchange does not occur across the walls of the arteries carrying blood from the heart to the tissues, because their walls are too thick. PO_2 of blood arriving at the capillary bed is therefore the same as blood leaving the lungs. Blood arriving at the tissues has been cleansed of its CO_2 and saturated with O_2 during its passage through the lungs, and therefore has a higher PO_2 and a lower PCO_2 than the tissues. This creates concentration gradients between capillary blood and the tissues, and gas exchange therefore occurs (Fig. 10.24B). O_2 diffuses from the bloodstream through the capillary wall into the tissues. CO_2 diffuses from the cells into the extracellular fluid, then into the bloodstream towards the venous end of the capillary.

Figure 10.25 summarises the processes of internal and external respiration. 🎞 **10.11**

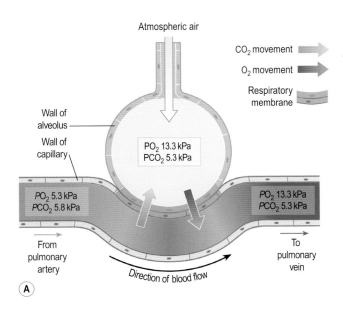

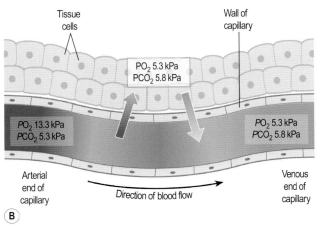

Figure 10.24 Respiration. A. External respiration. **B.** Internal respiration.

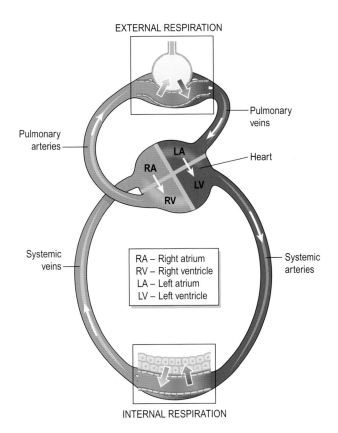

Figure 10.25 Summary of external and internal respiration.

Transport of gases in the bloodstream

Oxygen and carbon dioxide are carried in the blood in different ways.

Oxygen

Oxygen is carried in the blood in:

- chemical combination with haemoglobin (see Fig. 4.6, p. 66) as *oxyhaemoglobin* (98.5%)
- solution in plasma water (1.5%).

Oxyhaemoglobin is unstable, and under certain conditions readily dissociates releasing oxygen. Factors that increase dissociation include low O_2 levels, low pH and raised temperature (see Ch. 4). In active tissues there is increased production of carbon dioxide and heat, which leads to increased release of oxygen. In this way oxygen is available to tissues in greatest need. Whereas oxyhaemoglobin is bright red, deoxygenated blood is bluish-purple in colour.

Carbon dioxide

Carbon dioxide is one of the waste products of metabolism. It is excreted by the lungs and is transported by three mechanisms:

- as bicarbonate ions (HCO_3^-) in the plasma (70%)
- some is carried in erythrocytes, loosely combined with haemoglobin as *carbaminohaemoglobin* (23%)
- some is dissolved in the plasma (7%).

Carbon dioxide levels must be finely managed, as either an excess or a deficiency leads to significant disruption of acid-base balance. Sufficient CO_2 is essential for the bicarbonate buffering system that protects against a fall in body pH. Excess CO_2 on the other hand reduces blood pH, because it dissolves in body water to form carbonic acid.

Regulation of air and blood flow in the lung

During quiet breathing, only a small portion of the lung's total capacity is ventilated with each breath. This means that only a fraction of the total alveolar numbers are being ventilated, usually in the upper lobes, and much of the remaining lung is temporarily collapsed. Airways supplying alveoli that are not being used are constricted, directing airflow into functioning alveoli. In addition, the pulmonary arterioles bringing blood into the ventilated alveoli are dilated, to maximise gas exchange, and blood flow (perfusion) past the non-functioning alveoli is reduced.

When respiratory requirements are increased, e.g. in exercise, the increased tidal volume expands additional alveoli, and the blood flow is redistributed to perfuse these too. In this way, air flow (ventilation) and blood flow (perfusion) are matched to maximise the opportunity for gas exchange.

Control of respiration

Effective control of respiration enables the body to regulate blood gas levels over a wide range of physiological, environmental and pathological conditions, and is normally involuntary. Voluntary control is exerted during activities such as speaking and singing but is overridden if blood CO_2 rises (hypercapnia).

The respiratory centre

This is formed by groups of nerves in the medulla, the *respiratory rhythmicity centre*, which control the respiratory pattern, i.e. the rate and depth of breathing (Fig. 10.26). Regular discharge of *inspiratory neurones* within this centre set the rate and depth of breathing. Activity of the respiratory rhythmicity centre is adjusted by nerves in the pons (the *pneumotaxic centre* and the *apneustic centre*), in response to input from other parts of the brain.

Motor impulses leaving the respiratory centre pass in the *phrenic* and *intercostal nerves* to the diaphragm and intercostal muscles respectively to stimulate respiration.

Chemoreceptors

These are receptors that respond to changes in the partial pressures of oxygen and carbon dioxide in the blood and cerebrospinal fluid. They are located centrally and peripherally.

Central chemoreceptors. These are located on the surface of the medulla oblongata and are bathed in cerebrospinal fluid. When arterial PCO_2 rises (hypercapnia), even slightly, the central chemoreceptors respond by stimulating the respiratory centre, increasing ventilation of the lungs and reducing arterial PCO_2. The sensitivity of the central chemoreceptors to raised arterial PCO_2 is the most important factor in controlling normal blood gas levels. A small reduction in PO_2 (hypoxaemia) has the same, but less pronounced effect, but a substantial reduction depresses breathing.

Peripheral chemoreceptors. These are situated in the arch of the aorta and in the carotid bodies (Fig. 10.26). They respond to changes in blood CO_2 and O_2 levels, but are much more sensitive to carbon dioxide than oxygen. Even a slight rise in CO_2 levels activates these receptors, triggering nerve impulses to the respiratory centre via the glossopharyngeal and vagus nerves. This stimulates an immediate rise in the rate and depth of respiration. An increase in blood acidity (decreased pH or raised $[H^+]$) also stimulates the peripheral chemoreceptors, resulting in increased ventilation, increased CO_2 excretion and increased blood pH. These chemoreceptors also help to regulate blood pressure (p. 97).

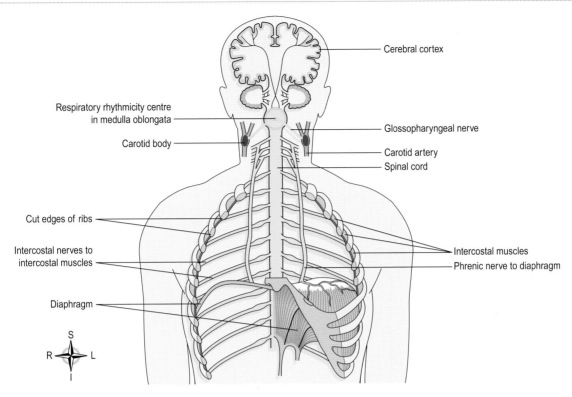

Figure 10.26 Some of the structures involved in control of respiration.

Exercise and respiration

Physical exercise increases both the rate and depth of respiration to supply the increased oxygen requirements of the exercising muscles. Exercising muscles produces higher quantities of CO_2, which stimulates central and peripheral chemoreceptors. The increased respiratory effort persists even after exercise stops, in order to supply enough oxygen to repay the 'oxygen debt'. This represents mainly the oxygen needed to get rid of wastes, including lactic acid.

Other factors that influence respiration

Breathing may be modified by the higher centres in the brain by:

- speech, singing
- emotional displays, e.g. crying, laughing, fear
- drugs, e.g. sedatives, alcohol
- sleep.

Body temperature influences breathing. In fever, respiration is increased due to increased metabolic rate, while in hypothermia respiration and metabolism are depressed. Temporary changes in respiration occur in swallowing, sneezing and coughing.

The Hering–Breuer reflex prevents overinflation of the lungs. Stretch receptors in the lung, linked to the respiratory centre by the vagus nerve, inhibit respiration when lung volume approaches maximum.

Ageing and the respiratory system

Learning outcome

After studying this section, you should be able to:

- describe the main consequences of ageing on respiratory structure and function.

Respiratory performance declines with age, beginning in the mid-20s. General loss of elastic tissue in the lungs increases the likelihood that small airways will collapse during expiration and decreases the functional lung volume. Varying degrees of emphysema (p. 263) are normal in older people, usually without symptoms. Cartilage in general becomes less flexible with age and there is an increased risk of arthritic joint changes. The ribcage therefore becomes stiffer which, along with the general age-related reduction in muscle function, reduces the respiratory minute volume.

The risk of respiratory infections rises because of age-related immune decline and loss of mucus production in the airways. The respiratory reflexes that increase respiratory effort in response to rising blood CO_2/falling blood O_2 levels become less efficient, so older people may respond less well to adverse changes in blood gases.

Age-related respiratory compromise is greatly enhanced in smokers.

Disorders of the upper respiratory tract

Learning outcome

After studying this section, you should be able to:

■ describe the common inflammatory and infectious disorders of the upper respiratory tract.

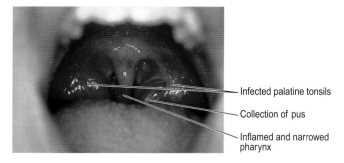

Figure 10.27 Streptococcal tonsillitis.

Labels: Infected palatine tonsils; Collection of pus; Inflamed and narrowed pharynx

Infectious and inflammatory disorders

Inflammation of the upper respiratory tract can be caused by inhaling irritants, such as cigarette smoke or air pollutants, but is commonly due to infection. Such infections are usually caused by viruses that lower the resistance of the respiratory tract to other infections. This allows bacteria to invade the tissues. Such infections are only life-threatening if they spread to the lungs or other organs, or if inflammatory swelling and exudate block the airway.

Pathogens are usually spread by droplet infection (tiny droplets containing pathogenic material suspended in the air), in dust or by contaminated equipment and dressings. If not completely resolved, acute infection may become chronic.

Viral infections cause acute inflammation of the mucous membrane, leading to tissue congestion and profuse exudate of watery fluid. Secondary bacterial infection is particularly likely in vulnerable people such as children and older adults.

Viral infections are most dangerous in infants, young children and the elderly.

Common cold and influenza

The common cold (coryza) is usually caused by the rhinoviruses and is a highly infectious, normally mild illness characterised mainly by a runny nose (rhinorrhoea), sneezing, sore throat and sometimes slight fever. Normally a cold runs its course over a few days. Influenza is caused by a different group of viruses and produces far more severe symptoms than a cold, including very high temperatures and muscle pains; complete recovery can take weeks and secondary bacterial infections are more common than with a simple cold. In healthy adults, most strains of influenza are incapacitating but rarely fatal unless infection spreads to the lungs.

Sinusitis

This is usually caused by spread of microbes from the nose and pharynx to the mucous membrane lining the paranasal sinuses. The primary viral infection is usually followed by bacterial infection. The congested mucosa may block the openings between the nose and the sinuses, preventing drainage of mucopurulent discharge. Symptoms include facial pain and headache. If there are repeated attacks or if recovery is not complete, the infection may become chronic.

Tonsillitis

Viruses and *Streptococcus pyogenes* are common causes of inflammation of the palatine tonsils, palatine arches and walls of the pharynx (Fig. 10.27). Severe infection may lead to suppuration and abscess formation (*quinsy*). Occasionally the infection spreads into the neck causing cellulitis. Following acute tonsillitis, swelling subsides and the tonsil returns to normal but repeated infection may lead to chronic inflammation, fibrosis and permanent enlargement. Endotoxins from tonsillitis caused by *Streptococcus pyogenes* are associated with the development of rheumatic fever (p. 434) and glomerulonephritis (p. 350). Repeated infection of the nasopharyngeal tonsil (adenoids, Fig. 10.3) can leave them enlarged and fibrotic, and can cause airway obstruction, especially in children.

Pharyngitis, laryngitis and tracheitis

The pharynx, larynx and trachea may become infected secondary to other upper respiratory tract infections, e.g. the common cold or tonsillitis

Laryngotracheobronchitis (croup in children) is a rare but serious complication of upper respiratory tract infections. The airway is obstructed by marked swelling around the larynx and epiglottis, accompanied by wheeze and breathlessness (dyspnoea).

Diphtheria

This is a bacterial infection of the pharynx which may extend to the nasopharynx and trachea, caused by *Corynebacterium diphtheriae*. A thick fibrous membrane forms over the area and may obstruct the airway. The microbe produces powerful exotoxins that may severely damage cardiac and skeletal muscle, the liver, kidneys and adrenal glands. Where immunisation is widespread, diphtheria is rare.

Hay fever (allergic rhinitis)

In this condition, *atopic* ('immediate') hypersensitivity (p. 385) develops to foreign proteins (antigens), e.g. pollen, mites in pillow feathers, animal dander. The acute inflammation of nasal mucosa and conjunctiva causes *rhinorrhoea* (excessive watery exudate from the nose), redness of the eyes and excessive tear production. Atopic hypersensitivity tends to run in families, but no single genetic factor has yet been identified; it is likely to involve multiple genes. Other forms of atopic hypersensitivity include childhood onset asthma (see below), eczema (p. 371) in infants and young children and food allergies.

Obstructive lung disorders

Learning outcomes

After studying this section, you should be able to:

■ compare the causes and pathology of chronic and acute bronchitis

■ discuss the pathologies of the main forms of emphysema

■ discuss the causes and disordered physiology of asthma

■ explain the main physiological abnormality in bronchiectasis

■ describe the effect of cystic fibrosis on lung function.

Obstructive lung disorders are characterised by blockage of airflow through the airways. Obstruction may be acute or chronic.

Bronchitis

Acute bronchitis

This is usually a secondary bacterial infection of the bronchi, usually preceded by a common cold or influenza, which may also complicate measles and whooping cough in children. Viral infection depresses normal defence mechanisms, allowing pathogenic bacteria already present in the respiratory tract to multiply. Downward spread of infection may lead to bronchiolitis and/or bronchopneumonia, especially in children and in debilitated or older adults.

Chronic bronchitis

This is a common disorder that becomes increasingly debilitating as it progresses. Chronic bronchitis is defined clinically when an individual has had a cough with sputum for 3 months in 2 successive years. It is a progressive inflammatory disease resulting from prolonged irritation of the bronchial epithelium, often worsened by damp or cold conditions.

It is often a consequence of cigarette smoking, but can also follow episodes of acute bronchitis (often caused by *Haemophilus influenzae* or *Streptococcus pneumoniae*) and chronic exposure to airborne irritants such as urban fog, vehicular exhaust fumes or industrial pollutants.

It develops mostly in middle-aged men who are chronic heavy smokers and may have a familial predisposition. Acute exacerbations are common, and often associated with infection. The changes occurring in the bronchi include:

Increased size and number of mucus glands. The increased volume of mucus may block small airways, and overwhelm the ciliary escalator, leading to reduced clearance, a persistent cough and infection.

Oedema and other inflammatory changes. These cause swelling of the airway wall, narrowing the passageway and obstructing airflow.

Reduction in number and function of ciliated cells. Ciliated epithelium is progressively destroyed and replaced by a different type of epithelium with no cilia. This may precede neoplastic (cancerous) change. As ciliary efficiency is reduced, the problem of mucus accumulation is worsened, further increasing the risk of infection.

Fibrosis of the airways. Inflammatory changes lead to fibrosis and stiffening of airway walls, further reducing airflow.

Breathlessness (dyspnoea). This is worse with physical exertion and increases the work of breathing.

Ventilation of the lungs becomes severely impaired, causing breathlessness, leading to hypoxia, pulmonary hypertension and right-sided heart failure. As respiratory failure develops, arterial blood PO_2 is reduced (*hypoxaemia*) and is accompanied by a rise in arterial blood PCO_2 (*hypercapnia*). When the condition becomes more severe, the respiratory centre in the medulla responds to hypoxaemia rather than to hypercapnia. In the later stages, the inflammatory changes begin to affect the smallest bronchioles and the alveoli themselves, and emphysema develops (see below). The term *chronic obstructive pulmonary disease* (COPD) is sometimes used to describe this situation.

Emphysema (Figs 10.28, 10.29)

Pulmonary emphysema

Pulmonary emphysema, generally referred to simply as emphysema, usually develops as a result of long-term inflammatory conditions or irritation of the airways, e.g. in smokers or coal miners. Occasionally, it may be due to a genetic deficiency in the lung of an antiproteolytic enzyme, α_1 anti-trypsin. These conditions lead to progressive destruction of supporting elastic tissue in the lung, and the lungs progressively expand (barrel chest) because their ability to recoil is lost. In addition, there is irreversible distension of the respiratory bronchioles, alveolar

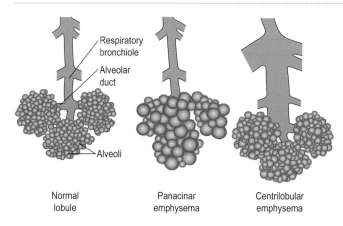

Respiratory
bronchiole

Alveolar
duct

Alveoli

Normal
lobule

Panacinar
emphysema

Centrilobular
emphysema

Figure 10.28 Emphysema.

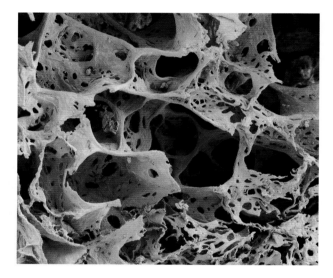

Figure 10.29 Coloured scanning electron micrograph of lung tissue with emphysema.

ducts and alveoli, reducing the surface area for the exchange of gases.

On microscopic examination, the lung tissue is full of large, irregular cavities created by the destruction of alveolar walls (Fig. 10.29, and compare with Fig. 10.19). There are two main types and both are usually present.

Panacinar emphysema

The walls between adjacent alveoli break down, the alveolar ducts dilate and interstitial elastic tissue is lost. The lungs become distended and their capacity is increased. Because the volume of air in each breath remains unchanged, it constitutes a smaller proportion of the total volume of air in the distended alveoli, reducing the partial pressure of oxygen. This reduces the concentration gradient of O_2 across the alveolar membrane, decreasing diffusion of O_2 into the blood. Merging of alveoli reduces the surface area for exchange of gases. In the early stages of the disease, normal arterial blood O_2 and CO_2 levels are maintained at rest by hyperventilation. As the disease

progresses the combined effect of these changes may lead to hypoxia, pulmonary hypertension and eventually right-sided heart failure.

Centrilobular emphysema

In this form there is irreversible dilation of the respiratory bronchioles supplying lung lobules. When inspired air reaches the dilated area the pressure falls, leading to a reduction in alveolar air pressure, reduced ventilation efficiency and reduced partial pressure of oxygen. As the disease progresses the resultant hypoxia leads to pulmonary hypertension and right-sided heart failure.

Interstitial emphysema

Interstitial emphysema means the presence of air in the thoracic interstitial tissues, and this may happen in one of the following ways:

- from the outside by injury, e.g. fractured rib, stab wound
- from the inside when an alveolus ruptures through the pleura, e.g. during an asthmatic attack, in bronchiolitis, coughing as in whooping cough.

The air in the tissues usually tracks upwards to the soft tissues of the neck where it is gradually absorbed, causing no damage. A large quantity in the mediastinum may, however, limit heart movement.

It is important to distinguish between interstitial emphysema and pneumothorax (p. 271), where the air is trapped between the pleura.

Asthma (Fig. 10.30)

Asthma is a common inflammatory disease of the airways associated with episodes of reversible over-reactivity of the airway smooth muscle. The mucous membrane and muscle layers of the bronchi become thickened and the mucous glands enlarge, reducing airflow in the lower respiratory tract. The walls swell and thicken with inflammatory exudate and an influx of inflammatory cells, especially eosinophils. During an asthmatic attack, spasmodic contraction of bronchial muscle (*bronchospasm*) constricts the airways and there is excessive secretion of thick sticky mucus, which further narrows the airway. Only partial expiration is achieved, so the lungs become hyperinflated and there is severe dyspnoea and wheezing. The duration of attacks usually varies from a few minutes to hours. In severe acute attacks the bronchi may be obstructed by mucus plugs, blocking airflow and leading to acute respiratory failure, hypoxia and possibly death.

Non-specific factors that may precipitate asthma attacks include cold air, cigarette smoking, air pollution, upper respiratory tract infection, emotional stress and strenuous exercise.

There are two clinical categories of asthma, which generally give rise to identical symptoms and are

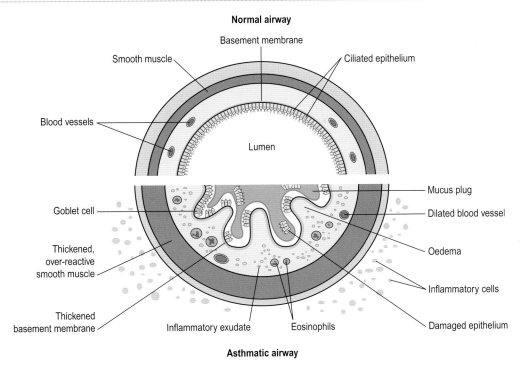

Normal airway

Basement membrane

Smooth muscle

Ciliated epithelium

Blood vessels

Lumen

Goblet cell

Mucus plug

Dilated blood vessel

Thickened, over-reactive smooth muscle

Oedema

Inflammatory cells

Thickened basement membrane

Inflammatory exudate

Eosinophils

Damaged epithelium

Asthmatic airway

Figure 10.30 Cross-section of the airway wall in asthma.

treated in the same way. Important differences include typical age of onset and the contribution of an element of allergy. Asthma, whatever the aetiology, can usually be well controlled with inhaled anti-inflammatory and bronchodilator agents, enabling people to live a normal life.

Atopic (childhood onset, extrinsic) asthma

This occurs in children and young adults who have atopic (type I) hypersensitivity (p. 385) to foreign protein, e.g. pollen, dust containing mites from carpets, feather pillows, animal dander, fungi. A history of infantile eczema or food allergies is common and there are often close family members with a history of allergy.

As in hayfever, antigens (allergens) are inhaled and absorbed by the bronchial mucosa. This stimulates the production of IgE antibodies that bind to the surface of mast cells and basophils round the bronchial blood vessels. When the allergen is encountered again, the antigen/antibody reaction results in the release of histamine and other related substances that stimulate mucus secretion and muscle contraction that narrows the airways. Attacks tend to become less frequent and less severe with age.

Non-atopic (adult onset, intrinsic) asthma

This type occurs later in adult life and there is no history of childhood allergic reactions. It can be associated with chronic inflammation of the upper respiratory tract, e.g.

chronic bronchitis, nasal polyps. Other trigger factors include exercise and occupational exposure, e.g. inhaled paint fumes. Aspirin triggers an asthmatic reaction in some people. Attacks tend to increase in severity over time and lung damage may be irreversible. Eventually, impaired lung ventilation leads to hypoxia, pulmonary hypertension and right-sided heart failure.

Bronchiectasis

This is permanent abnormal dilation of bronchi and bronchioles. It is associated with chronic bacterial infection, and sometimes with a history of childhood bronchiolitis and bronchopneumonia, cystic fibrosis, or bronchial tumour. The bronchi become obstructed by mucus, pus and inflammatory exudate and the alveoli distal to the blockage collapse as trapped air is absorbed. Interstitial elastic tissue degenerates and is replaced by fibrous adhesions that attach the bronchi to the parietal pleura. The pressure of inspired air in these damaged bronchi leads to dilation proximal to the blockage. The persistent severe coughing to remove copious purulent sputum causes intermittent increases in pressure in the blocked bronchi, leading to further dilation.

The lower lobe of the lung is usually affected. Suppuration is common. If a blood vessel is eroded, haemoptysis may occur, or pyaemia, leading to abscess formation elsewhere in the body, commonly the brain. Progressive fibrosis of the lung leads to hypoxia, pulmonary hypertension and right-sided heart failure.

Cystic fibrosis (mucoviscidosis)

This is one of the most common genetic diseases (p. 446), affecting 1 in 2500 babies. It is estimated that almost 5% of people carry the abnormal recessive gene which must be present in both parents to cause the disease.

The secretions of all exocrine glands have abnormally high viscosity, but the most severely affected are those of the lungs, pancreas, intestines, biliary tract, and the reproductive system in the male. Sweat glands secrete abnormally large amounts of salt during excessive sweating. In the pancreas, highly viscous mucus is secreted by the walls of the ducts and causes obstruction, parenchymal cell damage, the formation of cysts and defective enzyme secretion. In the newborn, intestinal obstruction may be caused by a plug of meconium (fetal faeces) and viscid mucus, leading to perforation of the alimentary canal wall and meconium peritonitis which is often fatal. In less acute cases there may be impairment of protein and fat digestion resulting in malabsorption, steatorrhoea and failure to thrive in infants. In older children, common consequences include:

- digestion of food and absorption of nutrients is impaired
- there may be obstruction of bile ducts in the liver, causing cirrhosis
- bronchitis, bronchiectasis and pneumonia may develop.

The life span of affected individuals is around 50 years; the main treatments offered are aimed at maintaining effective respiratory function and preventing infection. Chronic lung and heart disease are common complications.

Restrictive disorders

Learning outcomes

After studying this section, you should be able to:

- describe the main pneumoconioses
- outline the main causes and consequences of chemically induced lung disease.

Restrictive lung disorders are characterised by increasing stiffness (low compliance) of lung tissue, making it harder to inflate the lung and increasing the work of breathing. Chronic restrictive disease is often associated with progressive fibrosis caused by repeated and ongoing inflammation of the lungs.

Pneumoconioses

This group of lung diseases is caused by prolonged exposure to inhaled organic dusts, which triggers a generalised inflammation and progressive fibrosis of lung tissues. Inhalation of work-related pollutants was a major cause of lung disease prior to the introduction of legislation that limits workers' exposure to them. To cause disease, particles must be so small that they are carried in inspired air to the level of the respiratory bronchioles and alveoli, where they can only be cleared by phagocytosis. Larger particles are trapped by mucus higher up the respiratory tract and expelled by ciliary action and coughing. The risk increases with the duration and concentration of exposure, and in cigarette smokers.

Coal worker's pneumoconiosis

Inhalation of coal dust over a prolonged period leads to varying degrees of respiratory impairment; many miners develop little or no disease but others suffer massive progressive fibrosis that is ultimately fatal. The inhaled dust collects in the lung and is phagocytosed by macrophages, which collect around airways and trigger varying degrees of fibrosis. If the fibrosis remains restricted to these small collections of macrophages and there is no significant reduction in lung function, the disorder is referred to as *simple coal worker's pneumoconiosis*, and is unlikely to progress once exposure to dust stops. For reasons that are unclear, the fibrotic changes in the lungs progress much more aggressively in some people, with formation of large dense fibrotic nodules, destruction and cavitation of lung tissue and potentially fatal respiratory impairment.

Silicosis

This may be caused by long-term exposure to dust containing silicon compounds. High-risk industries include quarrying, mining of minerals, stone masonry, sand blasting, glass making and pottery production.

Inhaled silica particles accumulate in the alveoli and are ingested by macrophages to which silica is toxic. The inflammatory reaction triggered when the macrophages die causes significant fibrosis.

Silicosis appears to predispose to the development of tuberculosis, which rapidly progresses to tubercular bronchopneumonia and possibly miliary TB. Gradual destruction of lung tissue leads to progressive reduction in pulmonary function, pulmonary hypertension and right-sided heart failure.

Asbestosis

Asbestosis, caused by inhaling asbestos fibres, usually develops after 10–20 years' exposure, but sometimes after only 2 years. Asbestos miners and workers involved in making and using some products containing asbestos are at risk. There are different types of asbestos, but blue asbestos is associated with the most serious disease.

In spite of their large size, asbestos particles penetrate to the level of respiratory bronchioles and alveoli. Macrophages accumulate in the alveoli and ingest shorter fibres. The larger fibres form *asbestos bodies*, consisting of fibres surrounded by macrophages, protein material and iron deposits. Their presence in sputum indicates exposure to asbestos but not necessarily asbestosis. The macrophages that have engulfed fibres migrate out of the alveoli and accumulate around respiratory bronchioles and blood vessels, stimulating the formation of fibrous tissue. Lung tissue is progressively destroyed, with the development of dyspnoea, chronic hypoxia, pulmonary hypertension and right-sided heart failure. The link between inhaled asbestos and fibrosis is not clear. It may be that asbestos stimulates the macrophages to secrete enzymes that promote fibrosis or that it stimulates an immune reaction causing fibrosis. Asbestos is linked to the development of mesothelioma (p. 270).

Extrinsic allergic alveolitis

This group of conditions is caused by inhaling organic dusts, including those in Table 10.3. The contaminants act as antigens causing a type III hypersensitivity reaction in the walls of the alveoli.

Initially, the allergy causes bronchiolitis, dyspnoea, cough, accumulation of inflammatory cells and granuloma (collections of macrophages) formation. If the exposure is brief, the inflammatory response may resolve but on repeated exposures, pulmonary fibrosis develops.

Pulmonary toxins

Lung disease can be triggered by a range of toxins and drugs, including:

Paraquat. This weedkiller causes pulmonary oedema, irreversible pulmonary fibrosis and renal damage and ingestion can be fatal.

Drugs. The mechanism and severity of drug-induced pulmonary damage varies depending on the drug and the general condition of the patient. Some drugs used to treat cancer, including bleomycin and methotrexate, can trigger

progressive fibrotic changes. Other common drugs, including angiotensin converting enzyme inhibitors (used in hypertension and other cardiovascular conditions), phenytoin (an anticonvulsant) and hydralazine (used in hypertension) can also have pulmonary side-effects.

High concentration oxygen therapy. Premature babies may require oxygen treatment while their lung function matures, but the high concentrations used can cause permanent fibrotic damage to the lungs, as well as to the retina of the eye (p. 212). People of any age who require high concentration oxygen therapy may also develop pulmonary fibrosis.

Lung infections

Learning outcome

After studying this section, you should be able to:

■ describe the causes and effects of lung infection, including pneumonia, abscess and tuberculosis.

Pneumonia (Fig. 10.31)

Pneumonia means infection of the alveoli. This occurs when pulmonary defence mechanisms fail to prevent

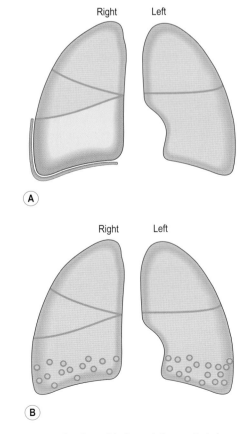

Figure 10.31 Distribution of infected tissue. A. Lobar pneumonia. **B.** Bronchopneumonia.

Table 10.3 Conditions caused by organic dusts	
Disease	**Contaminant**
Farmer's lung	Mouldy hay
Bagassosis	Mouldy sugar waste
Bird handler's lung	Moulds in bird droppings
Malt worker's lung	Mouldy barley
Byssinosis	Cotton fibres

inhaled or blood-borne microbes reaching and colonising the lungs. The following are some predisposing factors.

Impaired coughing. Coughing is an effective cleaning mechanism, but if it is impaired or lost by, e.g., damage to respiratory muscles or the nerves supplying them, or painful coughing, then respiratory secretions may accumulate and become infected.

Damage to the epithelial lining of the tract. Ciliary action may be impaired or the epithelium destroyed by, e.g., tobacco smoking, inhaling noxious gases, infection.

Impaired alveolar phagocytosis. Depressed macrophage activity may be caused by tobacco smoking, alcohol, anoxia, oxygen toxicity.

Hospitalisation. Especially when mechanically assisted ventilation is required.

Other factors. The risk of pneumonia is increased in:

- extremes of age
- leukopenia
- chronic disease, e.g. heart failure, cancer, chronic renal failure, alcoholism
- suppression of immunity caused by, e.g. ionising radiation, corticosteroid drugs
- hypothermia.

Causative organisms

A wide variety of organisms, including bacteria, viruses, mycoplasma, protozoa and fungi, can cause pneumonia under appropriate conditions. The commonest pathogen, especially in lobar pneumonia, is the bacterium *Streptococcus pneumoniae*. Others include *Staphylococcus aureus* and *Haemophilus influenzae*. *Legionella pneumophila* spreads through water distribution systems, e.g. air conditioning systems, and is transmitted via droplet inhalation. *Klebsiella pneumoniae* and *Pseudomonas aeruginosa* are common causes of hospital-acquired pneumonia.

Lobar pneumonia (Fig. 10.31A)

This is infection of one or more lobes, usually by *Streptococcus pneumoniae*, leading to production of watery inflammatory exudate in the alveoli. This accumulates and fills the lobule which then overflows into and infects adjacent lobules. It is of sudden onset and pleuritic pain accompanies inflammation of the visceral pleura. If not treated with antibiotics the disease follows its course and resolves within 2–3 weeks. This form of pneumonia is most common in previously healthy young adults.

Bronchopneumonia (Fig. 10.31B)

Infection spreads from the bronchi to terminal bronchioles and alveoli. As these become inflamed, fibrous exudate accumulates and there is an influx of leukocytes. Small foci of consolidation (fluid-filled alveoli) develop.

There is frequently incomplete resolution with fibrosis. Bronchiectasis is a common complication leading to further acute attacks, lung fibrosis and progressive destruction of lung substance. Bronchopneumonia occurs most commonly in infancy and old age, and death is fairly common, especially when the condition complicates debilitating diseases. Predisposing factors include:

- debility due to, e.g., cancer, uraemia, cerebral haemorrhage, congestive heart failure, malnutrition, hypothermia
- lung disease, e.g. bronchiectasis, cystic fibrosis or acute viral infection
- general anaesthesia, which depresses respiratory and ciliary activity
- inhalation of gastric contents (*aspiration pneumonia*) in, e.g., unconsciousness, very deep sleep, following excessive alcohol consumption, drug overdose
- inhalation of infected material from the paranasal sinuses or upper respiratory tract.

Lung abscess

This is localised suppuration and necrosis within the lung substance.

Sources of infection

The abscess may develop from local infection:

- if pneumonia is inadequately treated
- as a result of trauma, e.g. rib fracture, stab wound or surgery
- of adjacent structures, e.g. oesophagus, spine, pleural cavity, or a subphrenic abscess.

Occasionally a lung abscess develops when infected material travelling in the bloodstream, a *septic embolus*, arrives and lodges in the lung. Such material usually originates from a thrombophlebitis (p. 123) or infective endocarditis (p. 128).

Outcomes

Recovery from lung abscess may either be complete or lead to complications, e.g.:

- chronic suppuration
- septic emboli may spread to other parts of the body, e.g. the brain, causing cerebral abscess or meningitis
- subpleural abscesses may spread and cause empyema and possibly bronchopleural fistula formation
- erosion of a pulmonary blood vessel, leading to haemorrhage.

Tuberculosis (TB)

TB is a major health problem worldwide, particularly in low-income countries that cannot afford effective prevention or treatment, and in countries where HIV disease is common. It is caused by one of two similar forms of mycobacteria, the main one being *Mycobacterium tuberculosis*. Humans are the main host. The microbes are spread by inhalation, either by aerosol droplet infection from an individual with active tuberculosis, or in dust contaminated by infected sputum.

Less commonly in developed countries because of pasteurisation of milk, TB can be caused by *Mycobacterium bovis*, from cows.

Pulmonary tuberculosis

Primary tuberculosis

Initial infection usually involves the apex of the lung. Inflammatory cells, including macrophages and lymphocytes, are recruited in defence, sealing off the infected lesions in *Ghon foci*. The centres of Ghon foci are filled with a cheese-like necrotic material that may contain significant numbers of active bacteria that have survived inside macrophages. If infection spreads to the regional lymph nodes, the Ghon foci and these infected nodes together are called the *primary complex*. At this stage, the disease is likely to have caused few, if any, clinical symptoms and in the great majority of people progresses no further, although calcified primary complexes are clearly identifiable on X-ray. Exposure to the bacterium causes *sensitisation*, which leads to a strong T-cell mediated immune reaction (p. 380) if the infection becomes reactivated.

Secondary TB

This is usually due to reactivation of disease from latent bacteria surviving primary TB, and can occur decades after the initial exposure in response to factors such as stress, ageing, immunocompromise or malnutrition. The infection is now much more likely to progress than it was at the primary stage, with significant destruction and cavitation of lung tissues. Symptoms include fever, cough, malaise, haemoptysis, weight loss and night sweats. Nearly half of patients with secondary TB develop non-pulmonary involvement.

Non-pulmonary TB

Primary TB rarely affects tissues other than the lung, but non-pulmonary involvement in secondary TB is very common. Widely disseminated TB is nearly always fatal unless adequately treated.

Miliary TB

Blood-borne spread from the lungs leads to widespread dissemination of the bacilli throughout body tissues, and foci of infection can establish in any organ, including the bone marrow, liver, spleen, kidneys and CNS. Numerous tiny nodules develop in the lungs, which on X-ray look like sprinkled millet seeds (hence 'miliary'). Rapid treatment is essential to prevent further spread.

Lymph node TB

This is the second commonest site of infection after the lung. Lymph nodes in the mediastinum, neck, axilla and groin are most likely to be affected. Infection causes swelling and central necrosis of the node. It is usually painless.

Joint and bone TB

The intervertebral, hip and knee joints are most commonly affected, and in children are usually a consequence of primary TB. Infection of the intervertebral disc or synovial membrane of a synovial joint is followed by extensive destruction of cartilage and adjacent bone, which in turn can progress to tuberculous osteomyelitis.

Other affected tissues

The pericardium, skin and GI tract may all become involved. One in five people with extrapulmonary disease develop CNS infection, which requires urgent treatment and, if not fatal, can leave survivors with permanent neurological damage.

Lung tumours

Learning objective

After studying this section, you should be able to:

- describe the pathology of the common lung tumours.

Benign tumours of the lung are rare.

Bronchial carcinoma

Primary bronchial carcinoma is a very common malignancy. The vast majority of cases (up to 90%) occur in smokers or those who inhale other people's smoke (passive smokers). Other risk factors include exposure to airborne dusts and the presence of lung fibrosis. The primary tumour has usually spread by the time of diagnosis, and therefore the prognosis of this type of cancer is usually extremely poor.

The tumour usually develops in a main bronchus, forming a large friable mass projecting into the lumen, sometimes causing obstruction. Mucus then collects and predisposes to infection. As the tumour grows it may erode a blood vessel, causing haemoptysis.

Spread of bronchial carcinoma

This does not follow any particular pattern or sequence. Spread is by infiltration of local tissues and the transport of tumour fragments in blood and lymph. If blood or lymph vessels are eroded, fragments may spread while the tumour is still quite small. A metastatic tumour may, therefore, cause symptoms before the primary in the lung has been detected.

Local spread. This may be within the lung or to mediastinal structures, e.g. blood vessels, nerves, oesophagus.

Lymphatic spread. Tumour fragments spread along lymph vessels to successive lymph nodes in which they may cause metastatic tumours. Fragments may enter lymph draining from a tumour or gain access to a larger vessel if its walls have been eroded by a growing tumour.

Blood spread. Tumour cells can enter the blood if a blood vessel is eroded by a growing tumour. The most common sites of blood-borne metastases are the liver, brain, adrenal glands, bones and kidneys.

Pleural mesothelioma

The majority of cases of this malignant tumour of the pleura are linked with previous exposure to asbestos dust, e.g. asbestos workers and people living near asbestos mines and factories. Smoking multiplies the risk of mesothelioma several fold in people exposed to asbestos. Mesothelioma may develop after widely varying duration of asbestos exposure, from 3 months to 60 years, and is usually associated with crocidolite fibres (blue asbestos). The tumour involves both layers of pleura and as it grows it obliterates the pleural cavity, compressing the lung. Lymph and blood-spread metastases are commonly found in the hilar and mesenteric lymph nodes, the other lung, liver, thyroid and adrenal glands, bone, skeletal muscle and the brain. The prognosis is usually very poor.

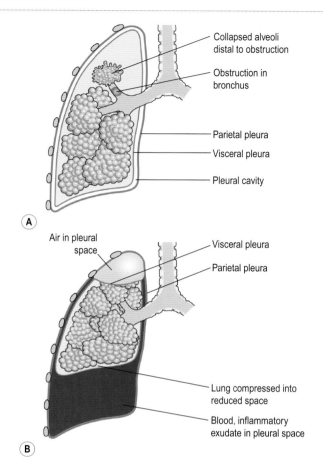

Figure 10.32 Collapse of a lung. A. Absorption collapse. **B.** Pressure collapse.

Lung collapse (Fig. 10.32)

Learning objectives

After studying this section, you should be able to:

- list the main causes of lung collapse
- describe the effects of lung collapse.

The clinical effects of collapse (*atelectasis*) of all or part of a lung depend on how much of the lung is affected. Fairly large sections of a single lung can be out of action without obvious symptoms. There are four main causes of this condition:

- obstruction of an airway (absorption collapse)
- impaired surfactant function
- pressure collapse
- alveolar hypoventilation.

Obstruction of an airway (absorption collapse, Fig. 10.32A)

The amount of lung affected depends on the size of the obstructed air passage. Distal to the obstruction air is trapped and absorbed, the lung collapses and secretions collect. These may cause infection, and sometimes abscess formation. Short-term obstruction is usually followed by reinflation of the lung without lasting ill-effects. Prolonged obstruction leads to progressive fibrosis and permanent collapse. Sudden obstruction may be due to inhalation of a foreign body (usually into the (R) primary bronchus, which is wider and more steeply angled than the left) or a mucus plug formed during an asthmatic attack or in chronic bronchitis. Gradual obstruction may be due to a bronchial tumour or pressure on a bronchus by, e.g., enlarged mediastinal lymph nodes, aortic aneurysm.

Impaired surfactant function

Premature babies, born before the 34th week, may be unable to expand their lungs by their own respiratory effort because their lungs are too immature to produce surfactant (p. 253). These babies may need to be mechanically ventilated until their lungs begin to produce surfactant. This is called *neonatal respiratory distress syndrome* (NRDS).

In *adult respiratory distress syndrome* (ARDS), dilution of surfactant by fluid collecting in the alveoli (pulmonary oedema) leads to atelectasis. These patients are nearly always gravely ill already, and collapse of substantial areas of lung contributes to the mortality rate of around one-third.

Pressure collapse

When air or fluid enters the pleural cavity the negative pressure becomes positive, preventing lung expansion. Fluids settle in the lung bases, whereas collections of air are usually found towards the lung apex (Fig. 10.32B). The collapse usually affects only one lung and may be partial or complete. There is no obstruction of the airway.

Pneumothorax

In this condition there is air in the pleural cavity. It may occur spontaneously or be the result of trauma.

Spontaneous pneumothorax. This may be either primary or secondary. *Primary spontaneous pneumothorax* is of unknown cause, often recurrent, and occurs in fit and healthy people, usually males between 20 and 40 years. *Secondary spontaneous pneumothorax* occurs when air enters the pleural cavity after the visceral pleura ruptures due to lung disease, e.g. emphysema, asthma, pulmonary tuberculosis, bronchial cancer.

Traumatic pneumothorax. This is due to a penetrating injury that breaches the pleura, e.g. compound fracture of rib, stab or gunshot wound, surgery.

Tension pneumothorax (Fig. 10.33). This occurs as a complication when a flap or one-way valve develops between the lungs and the pleural cavity. Air enters the pleural cavity during inspiration but cannot escape on expiration and steadily, sometimes rapidly, accumulates. This expansion of the affected lung pushes the mediastinum towards the unaffected side, compressing its contents, including the unaffected lung and great vessels. Without prompt treatment, severe respiratory distress precedes cardiovascular collapse.

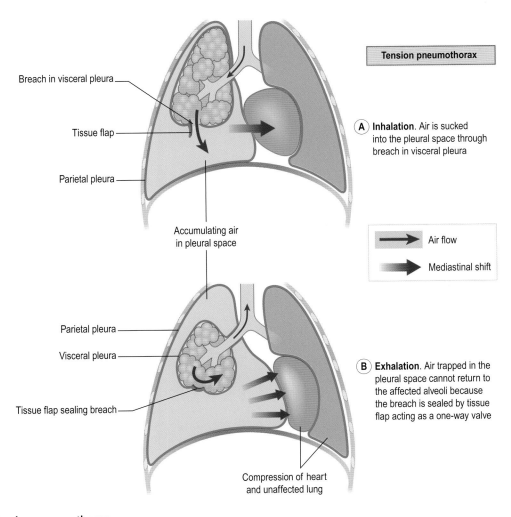

Figure 10.33 Tension pneumothorax.

Haemothorax

This is blood in the pleural cavity. It may be caused by:

- penetrating chest injury involving blood vessels
- ruptured aortic aneurysm
- erosion of a blood vessel by a malignant tumour.

Pleural effusion

This is excess fluid in the pleural cavity that may be caused by:

- increased hydrostatic pressure, e.g. heart failure (p. 126), increased blood volume
- increased capillary permeability due to local inflammation, e.g. lobar pneumonia, pulmonary tuberculosis, bronchial cancer, mesothelioma
- decreased plasma osmotic pressure, e.g. nephrotic syndrome (p. 351), liver cirrhosis (p. 334)
- impaired lymphatic drainage, e.g. malignant tumour involving the pleura.

Following haemothorax and pleural effusion, fibrous adhesions which limit reinflation may form between the layers of pleura.

Alveolar hypoventilation

In the normal individual breathing quietly at rest, there are always some collapsed lobules within the lungs because of the low tidal volume. These lobules re-expand without difficulty at the next deep inspiration. Non-physiological causes of hypoventilation collapse include post-operative collapse, particularly after chest and upper abdominal surgery, when pain restricts thoracic expansion. This predisposes to chest infections, because mucus collects in the underventilated airways and is not coughed up (expectorated).

For a range of self-assessment exercises on the topics in this chapter, visit Evolve online resources: https://evolve.elsevier.com/Waugh/anatomy/

Introduction to nutrition

Before discussing the digestive system it is necessary to understand the body's nutritional needs, i.e. the dietary constituents and their functions. Food provides nutrients, some of which are broken down to provide energy while others are needed to maintain health, e.g. for growth and cellular metabolism. These substances are:

- carbohydrates
- proteins
- fats
- vitamins
- mineral salts, trace elements and water.

Many foods contain a combination of nutrients, e.g. potatoes and bread are mainly carbohydrate, but both also contain protein and some vitamins. *Fibre*, more correctly known as *non-starch polysaccharide* (NSP), consists of indigestible material. Although it is not a nutrient as it is neither a source of energy nor essential for cellular metabolism, NSP is important in the diet as it has many beneficial effects on the body.

The *diet* is the selection of foods eaten by an individual. A *balanced diet* is essential for health and provides appropriate amounts of all nutrients in the correct proportions to meet body requirements. An *essential nutrient* is a substance that cannot be made by the body and must therefore be eaten in the diet.

The first parts of this chapter explore the balanced diet and its constituents. Nutrition and its impact on older adults is discussed.

Many health problems arise as the result of poor diet. In developed countries obesity is increasingly common, while in other countries malnutrition is widespread; the final section considers some consequences of poor nutrition.

The balanced diet

Learning outcomes

After studying this section, you should be able to:

- list the constituent food groups of a balanced diet

- calculate body mass index from an individual's weight and height.

A balanced diet contains appropriate proportions of all nutrients required for health, which is normally achieved by eating a variety of foods, with the exception of breast milk, this is because no single food contains the correct proportions of the essential nutrients. If any nutrient is eaten in excess, or is deficient, health may be adversely affected. For example, a high-energy diet can lead to obesity, and an iron-deficient one to anaemia.

Box 11.1 Body mass index: WHO classification

Calculation of BMI

$$\text{Body mass index BMI} = \frac{\text{Weight (kg)}}{\text{Height (m}^2)}$$

Interpretation of BMI

<16	Severely underweight
16–18.4	Underweight
18.5–24.9	Normal range
25–29.9	Overweight
30–39.9	Obese
>40	Severely obese

A balanced diet is important in maintaining a healthy body weight, which can be assessed by calculating body mass index (BMI) (Box 11.1).

Healthy eating, i.e. eating a balanced diet, requires some knowledge and planning. An important dietary consideration is the amount of energy required, which should meet individual requirements. Daily energy requirements depend on several factors including basal metabolic rate (p. 314), age, gender and activity levels. Dietary carbohydrates, fats and proteins are the principal energy sources and fat is the most concentrated form. Dietary energy is correctly expressed in joules or kilojoules (kJ) although the older terms calories and kilocalories (kcal or Cal) are also still used in the UK.

This section is based on the recommendations of the British Nutrition Foundation (2013). Recommendations for daily food intake sort foods of similar origins and nutritional values into food groups, and advise that from the age of two years a certain proportion from each group be eaten daily (Fig. 11.1). If this plan is followed, the resulting dietary intake is likely to be well balanced. The five food groups are:

- bread, rice, potatoes, pasta
- fruit and vegetables
- milk and dairy foods
- meat, fish, eggs, beans
- foods and drinks high in fat and/or sugar.

The first two groups above should form two-thirds of the diet with the other groups forming the remainder with only limited amounts of food and drinks high in fat and/or sugar.

Bread, rice, potatoes, pasta

The British Nutrition Foundation recommends that this group should make up one-third of the diet and that each meal should be based around one food from this group. Potatoes, yams, plantains and sweet potato are classified as 'starchy carbohydrates' and are, therefore, considered within this group rather than as fruit and vegetables. Other foods in this group include breakfast cereals, rice and

The eatwell plate

Use the eatwell plate to help you get the balance right. It shows how much of what you eat should come from each food group.

eatwell.gov.uk

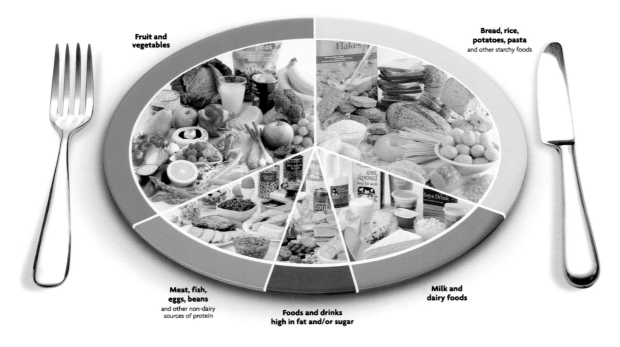

Figure 11.1 The eatwell plate. The main food groups and their recommended proportions within a balanced diet.

noodles. These foods are sources of carbohydrate and fibre that provide sustained energy release. Some also contain iron and B-group vitamins including folic acid (p. 279).

Fruit and vegetables
Foods in this group include fresh, frozen and canned products, 100% fruit or vegetable juices and pure fruit smoothies. These foods provide carbohydrate, fibre, vitamin C, folic acid and fibre. A minimum of five portions per day is recommended.

> One portion (80 g) = one piece of medium fruit, e.g. apple, orange, banana; three tablespoons of cooked vegetables, one bowl of mixed salad; 150 mL fruit juice or fruit smoothie

Milk and dairy foods
Foods in this group provide protein and minerals including calcium and zinc; some are also a source of vitamins A, B_2 and B_{12}. They include milk, cheese, fromage frais and yoghurt, and often contain considerable amounts of fat. Intake should therefore be limited to three servings per day.

> One serving = 200 mL milk, 150 g yoghurt or 30 g cheese

Meat, fish, eggs, beans
In addition to the food shown in Figure 11.1, this group includes meat products such as bacon, sausages, beef-burgers, salami and paté. Moderate amounts are recommended because many have a high fat content. It is suggested that fish, including one portion of oily fish, e.g. salmon, trout, sardines or fresh tuna, is eaten twice weekly. This food group provides protein, iron, vitamins B and D and sometimes minerals. Vegetarian alternatives include tofu, nuts, beans and pulses, e.g. lentils. Beans and pulses are also a good source of fibre.

Foods and drinks high in fat and/or sugar
These foods are illustrated in Figure 11.1 and also include oils, butter, margarine (including low-fat spreads), mayonnaise, fried food including chips, crisps, sweets, chocolate, cream, ice cream, puddings, jam, sugar and soft drinks, but not diet drinks. Fats are classified as saturated or unsaturated and the differences between these are explained on page 277. Foods in this group should only be used sparingly, if at all, as they are high in energy and have little other nutritional value.

Additional recommendations

The British Nutrition Foundation makes other specific recommendations about *salt* (p. 280) and *fluid intake* (1.5–2 L per day). This includes water, tea, coffee, squash and fruit juice. *Alcohol* intake should not exceed 3–4 units per day for men and 2–3 units per day for women.

> One unit of alcohol = 125 mL (small glass) wine; 300 mL (half pint) of standard strength beer, lager or cider; 25 mL of spirits

Groups of people with specific dietary requirements

Certain groups of people require a diet different from the principles outlined above. For example, pregnant and lactating women have higher energy requirements to support the growing baby and milk production. Menstruating women need more iron in their diet than non-menstruating women to compensate for blood loss during menstruation. Babies and growing children have higher energy requirements than adults because they have relatively higher growth and metabolic rates. In some gastrointestinal disorders there is intolerance of certain foods, which restricts dietary choices, e.g. coeliac disease (p. 331).

Digestion, absorption and use of nutrients are explained in Chapter 12. Structures of carbohydrates, proteins and fats are described in Chapter 2.

Nutrients

Learning outcomes

After studying this section, you should be able to:

■ describe the functions of dietary carbohydrate, protein and fat.

■ outline the sources and functions of fat- and water-soluble vitamins

■ outline the sources and functions of minerals, trace elements and water.

Carbohydrates

Carbohydrates are mainly sugars and starches, which are found in a wide variety of foods, e.g. sugar, jam, cereals, bread, biscuits, pasta, convenience foods, fruit and vegetables. Chemically, they consist of carbon, hydrogen and oxygen, the hydrogen and oxygen being in the same proportion as in water. Carbohydrates are classified according to the complexity of the chemical substances from which they are formed.

Monosaccharides

Carbohydrates are digested in the alimentary canal and absorbed as monosaccharides. Examples include glucose (see Fig. 2.7, p. 26), fructose and galactose. These are, chemically, the simplest form of carbohydrates.

Disaccharides

These consist of two monosaccharide molecules chemically combined, e.g. sucrose (see Fig. 2.7, p. 26), maltose and lactose.

Polysaccharides

These are complex molecules made up of large numbers of monosaccharides in chemical combination, e.g. starches, glycogen and cellulose.

Not all polysaccharides can be digested by humans; e.g. cellulose and other substances present in vegetables, fruit and some cereals pass through the alimentary canal almost unchanged (see NSP, p. 281).

Functions of digestible carbohydrates

These include:

- provision of energy and heat; the breakdown of monosaccharides, preferably in the presence of oxygen, releases heat and chemical energy for metabolic work – glucose is the main fuel molecule used by body cells
- 'protein sparing'; i.e. when there is an adequate supply of carbohydrate in the diet, protein does not need to be used to provide energy and heat, and is used for its main purpose, i.e. building new and replacement body proteins
- providing energy stores when carbohydrate is eaten in excess of the body's needs as it is converted to:
  - glycogen – as a short-term energy store in the liver and skeletal muscles (see p. 315)
  - fat, that is stored in adipose tissue, e.g. under the skin.

Proteins (nitrogenous foods)

During digestion proteins are broken down into their constituent amino acids and it is in this form that they are absorbed into the bloodstream. A constant supply of amino acids is needed to build new proteins, e.g. structural proteins, enzymes and some hormones.

Amino acids (see Fig. 2.8)

These are composed of the elements carbon, hydrogen, oxygen and nitrogen. Some contain minerals such as iron, copper, zinc, iodine, sulphur and phosphate. Amino acids are divided into two categories: *essential* and *non-essential*.

Essential amino acids cannot be synthesised in the body, therefore they must be included in the diet. *Non-essential*

Box 11.2 Essential and non-essential amino acids

Essential amino acids	Non-essential amino acids
Histidine (in infants only)	Alanine
Isoleucine	Arginine
Leucine	Asparagine
Lysine	Aspartic acid
Methionine	Cysteine
Phenylalanine	Cystine
Threonine	Glutamic acid
Tryptophan	Glutamine
Valine	Glycine
	Hydroxyproline
	Proline
	Serine
	Tyrosine

amino acids are those that can be synthesised in the body. The essential and non-essential amino acids are shown in Box 11.2.

Nitrogen balance

Excess amino acids are broken down. The amino group ($\sim NH_2$) is converted to the nitrogenous waste product urea and excreted by the kidneys. The remainder of the molecule is converted to either glucose or a ketone body (see ketosis, Ch. 12), depending on the amino acid. *Negative nitrogen balance* occurs when amino acid supply does not meet body needs. This situation may arise either when dietary protein intake is inadequate, e.g. deficiency or absence of amino acids, or protein requirement is increased, e.g. during growth spurts and following injury or surgery.

Biological value of protein

The nutritional value of a protein, its *biological value*, is measured by how well it meets the nutritional needs of the body. Protein of high biological value is usually of animal origin, easily digested and contains all essential amino acids in the proportions required by the body.

A balanced diet, containing all the amino acids required, may also be achieved by eating a range of foods containing proteins of lower biological values, provided that deficiencies in amino acid content of any one of the constituent proteins of the diet is supplied by another. A balanced vegetarian diet consists primarily of proteins with lower biological values, e.g. vegetables, cereals and pulses. When proteins from different plant sources are combined, they complement each other providing higher biological values than a single plant source. Through this complementary action the biological value of vegetarian diets can be similar to those based on animal protein.

Functions of proteins

Amino acids are used for:

- growth and repair of body cells and tissues
- synthesis of enzymes, plasma proteins, antibodies (immunoglobulins) and some hormones
- provision of energy. Normally a secondary function, this becomes important only when there is not enough carbohydrate in the diet and fat stores are depleted.

When protein is eaten in excess of the body's needs, the nitrogenous amino group is detached, i.e. it is deaminated, and excreted by the kidneys. The remainder is converted to fat for storage in the fat depots, e.g. in the fat cells of adipose tissue (p. 41).

Fats

Fats consist of carbon, hydrogen and oxygen, but they differ from carbohydrates in that the hydrogen and oxygen are not in the same proportions as in water. There are several groups of fats and lipids important in nutrition.

Fats (triglycerides)

Commonly known as 'fats', a triglyceride molecule consists of three fatty acids liked to a glycerol molecule (see Fig. 2.9, p. 27). Depending on the type and relative amounts of fatty acids they contain, fats are classified as *saturated* or *unsaturated*. In general, saturated fats are solid at room temperature and originate from animal sources, while unsaturated fats are oils, usually derived from vegetables or plants. A high intake of saturated fat can predispose to coronary heart disease (Ch. 5).

Linoleic, linolenic and arachadonic acids are *essential fatty acids*, which cannot be synthesised by the body in significant amounts, but are needed for synthesis of prostaglandins, phospholipids and leukotrienes. These fatty acids are found in oily fish.

Cholesterol

Unlike other lipids whose molecules are composed of chains of atoms, this molecule contains four rings, which give it the characteristic steroid structure. It can be synthesised by the body (around 20%) with the remainder coming from saturated fats in the diet as a constituent of full-fat dairy products, fatty meat and egg yolk. Cholesterol is needed for synthesis of steroid hormones, e.g. glucocorticoids and mineralocorticoids (Ch. 9) and is an important constituent of cell membranes.

Cholesterol is transported in the blood combined with proteins, forming *lipoproteins*. Two examples are:

- *low-density lipoprotein* (LDL): this carries cholesterol from the liver to the body cells. Excessive blood LDL levels are harmful to health as LDL can build up in arterial walls, leading to atherosclerosis. LDL is sometimes known as 'bad cholesterol'

- *high-density lipoprotein* (HDL): this carries cholesterol back from body cells to the liver, where it is either broken down or excreted. This may be referred to as 'good cholesterol' and raised HDL levels are cardioprotective.

High blood cholesterol levels are associated with an increased risk of atherosclerosis (p. 122), hypertension (high blood pressure, p. 131) and diabetes mellitus (p. 236).

Functions of fats

These include:

- provision of the most concentrated source of chemical energy and heat
- support of some organs, e.g. the kidneys, the eyes
- transport and storage of the fat-soluble vitamins: A, D, E, K
- constituent of myelin sheaths (p. 146) and of sebum (p. 365)
- formation of steroid hormones from cholesterol
- storage of energy as fat in adipose tissue under the skin and in the mesentery, especially when eaten in excess of requirements
- insulation – as a subcutaneous layer it reduces heat loss through the skin
- *satiety value* – the emptying time of the stomach is prolonged after eating food that is high in fat, postponing the return of hunger.

As the body stores excess fat, it is important not to eat too much as this will lead to weight gain and becoming over-weight or obese (p. 283).

Vitamins

Vitamins are chemicals required in very small quantities for essential metabolic processes. As most cannot be made by the body, they are an essential part of the diet and insuf-ficiency may lead to a deficiency disease. They are in found a wide range of foods and are divided into two groups:

- fat-soluble vitamins: A, D, E and K
- water-soluble vitamins: B complex and C.

Daily vitamin requirements for adults are shown on page 480.

Fat-soluble vitamins

Bile is needed for absorption of these vitamins from the small intestine. The presence of mineral oils in the intes-tine and malabsorption impair their absorption.

Vitamin A (retinol)

This vitamin is found in such foods as cream, egg yolk, liver, fish oil, milk, cheese and butter. It is absent from vegetable fats and oils but is added to margarine during manufacture. In addition, Vitamin A can be formed in the body from certain carotenes, the main dietary sources of which are green vegetables, orange-coloured fruit (e.g. mangoes, apricots) and carrots. The main roles of vitamin A in the body are:

- generation of the light-sensitive pigment rhodopsin (visual purple) in the retina of the eye (Ch. 8)
- cell growth and differentiation; this is especially important in fast-growing cells, such as the epithelial cells covering both internal and external body surfaces
- promotion of immunity and defence against infection
- promotion of growth, e.g. in bones.

The first sign of vitamin A deficiency is night blindness due to formation of abnormal retinal pigment. Other con-sequences include xerophthalmia, which is drying and thickening of the conjunctiva and, ultimately, ulceration and destruction of the conjunctiva. This is a common cause of blindness in developing countries. Atrophy and keratinisation of other epithelial tissues leads to increased incidence of infections of the ear and the respiratory, geni-tourinary and alimentary tracts. Immunity is compro-mised and bone development may be abnormal and delayed.

Vitamin D

Vitamin D is found mainly in animal fats such as eggs, butter, cheese, fish liver oils. Humans can synthesise this vitamin by the action of the ultraviolet rays in sunlight on a form of cholesterol (7-dehydrocholesterol) in the skin.

Vitamin D increases calcium and phosphate absorp-tion from the gut and stimulates their retention by the kidneys. It therefore promotes the calcification of bones and teeth.

Deficiency causes *rickets* in children and *osteomalacia* in adults (p. 431), due to impaired absorption and use of calcium and phosphate. Stores in fat and muscle are such that deficiency may not be apparent for several years.

Vitamin E

Also known as *tocopherol*, this is found in nuts, egg yolk, wheat germ, whole cereal, milk and butter.

Vitamin E is an antioxidant, which means that it pro-tects body constituents such as membrane lipids from being destroyed in oxidative reactions caused by free radicals. Recently, vitamin E has been shown to protect against coronary heart disease.

Deficiency is rare, because this vitamin is present in many foods, and is usually seen only in premature babies and in conditions associated with impaired fat absorp-tion, e.g. cystic fibrosis.

Vitamin K

The sources of vitamin K are liver, some vegetable oils and leafy green vegetables. It is also synthesised by bacteria in the large intestine and significant amounts are absorbed. A small amount is stored in the liver. Vitamin K is required by the liver for the production of prothrombin and factors VII, IX and X, all essential for blood clotting (p. 70). Deficiency therefore prevents normal blood coagulation. It may occur in adults when there is obstruction to the flow of bile, severe liver damage and in malabsorption, e.g. coeliac disease. Premature babies may be given vitamin K to prevent haemorrhagic disease of the newborn (p. 78). This is because their intestines are sterile and require several weeks to become colonised with vitamin K-producing bacteria allowing normal blood clotting.

Water-soluble vitamins

Water soluble vitamins are lost in the urine, so body stores are usually limited.

Vitamin B complex

This is a group of water-soluble vitamins that promote activity of enzymes involved in the chemical breakdown (catabolism) of nutrients to release energy.

Vitamin B$_1$ (thiamin). This is present in nuts, yeast, egg yolk, liver, legumes, meat and the germ of cereals. It is rapidly destroyed by heat. Thiamin is essential for the complete aerobic release of energy from carbohydrate. Absence or deficiency causes accumulation of lactic and pyruvic acids, which may lead to accumulation of tissue fluid (oedema) and heart failure. Thiamin is also important for nervous system function because of the dependency of these tissues on glucose for fuel.

Deficiency causes *beriberi*, which mainly occurs in countries where polished rice is the chief constituent of the diet. In beriberi there is:

- severe muscle wasting
- delayed growth in children
- polyneuritis, causing degeneration of motor, sensory and some autonomic nerves
- susceptibility to infections.

If untreated, death from cardiac failure or severe microbial infection may occur.

The main cause of thiamin deficiency in developed countries is alcoholism, where the diet is usually poor. This affects the central nervous system causing neurological symptoms, which are usually irreversible. These include memory loss, ataxia and visual disturbances known as Wernicke-Korsakoff syndrome.

Vitamin B$_2$ (riboflavin). Riboflavin is found in yeast, green vegetables, milk, liver, eggs, cheese and fish roe. Only small amounts are stored in the body and it is destroyed by light and alkalis. It is involved in carbohydrate and protein metabolism, especially in the eyes and skin. Deficiency leads to cracking of the skin, commonly around the mouth (angular stomatitis), and inflammation of the tongue (glossitis).

Vitamin B$_3$ (niacin). This is present in liver, cheese, yeast, whole cereals, eggs and dairy products; in addition, the body can synthesise it from the amino acid tryptophan. It is central to energy release from carbohydrates in cells. In fat metabolism it inhibits the production of cholesterol and assists in fat breakdown. Deficiency is rare and occurs mainly in areas where maize is the chief constituent of the diet because niacin in maize is in an unusable form. *Pellagra* develops within 6 to 8 weeks of severe deficiency. It is characterised by:

- dermatitis – sunburn-like skin sensitivity affecting areas exposed to sunlight
- delirium and dementia.

Vitamin B$_6$ (pyridoxine). This stable vitamin is found in egg yolk, peas, beans, soya beans, yeast, poultry, white fish and peanuts. Dietary deficiency is very rare. Vitamin B$_6$ is associated with amino acid metabolism, including the synthesis of non-essential amino acids and important molecules such as haem and nucleic acids.

Vitamin B$_{12}$ (cobalamin). This is a group of cobalt-containing compounds. It is found in almost all foods of animal origin, and is destroyed by heat.

Vitamin B$_{12}$ is essential for DNA synthesis, and deficiency leads to megaloblastic anaemia (p. 74), which is correctable with supplements. However, vitamin B$_{12}$ is also required for formation and maintenance of myelin, the fatty substance that surrounds and protects some nerves. Deficiency accordingly causes irreversible damage such as peripheral neuropathy and/or subacute spinal cord degeneration and usually affects older adults. The presence of intrinsic factor in the stomach is essential for vitamin B$_{12}$ absorption, and deficiency is usually associated with insufficient intrinsic factor.

Folic acid (folate). This is found in liver, leafy green vegetables, brown rice, beans, nuts and milk. It is synthesised by bacteria in the large intestine, and significant amounts derived from this source are believed to be absorbed. It is destroyed by heat and moisture. As only a small amount is stored in the body, deficiency quickly becomes evident. Like vitamin B$_{12}$, folic acid is also essential for DNA synthesis, and when lacking mitosis (cell division) is impaired. This manifests particularly in rapidly dividing tissues such as blood, and folate deficiency therefore leads to megaloblastic anaemia (p. 74), which is reversible with folate supplements. It is involved in development of the embryonic neural tube, which later becomes the spinal cord and skull. Deficiency at conception and during early pregnancy is linked to spina bifida (p. 188).

Pantothenic acid. This is found in many foods and is associated with energy-yielding carbohydrate metabolism; no deficiency diseases have been identified. It is destroyed by excessive heat and freezing.

Biotin. This is found in a wide range of foods including yeast, egg yolk, liver, kidney and tomatoes and is synthesised by microbes in the intestine. It is associated with the metabolism of carbohydrates, lipids and some amino acids; deficiency is very rare.

Vitamin C (ascorbic acid)

This is found in fresh fruit, especially blackcurrants, oranges, grapefruit and lemons, and also in rosehips and green vegetables. The vitamin is very water soluble and is easily destroyed by heat, ageing, chopping, salting and drying. These processes may predispose to the development of *scurvy* (deficiency). Deficiency becomes apparent after 4–6 months.

Vitamin C is associated with protein metabolism, especially the laying down of collagen fibres in connective tissue. Vitamin C, like vitamin E, acts as an antioxidant, protecting body molecules from damaging oxidative reactions caused by free radicals. When scurvy affects collagen production there is fragility of blood vessels, delayed wound healing and poor bone repair. Gums become swollen and spongy and the teeth loosen in their sockets. Systemic affects include fatigue, weakness and aching joints and muscles.

Minerals, trace elements and water

Minerals and trace elements

Minerals are inorganic substances needed in small amounts for normal cellular functioning. Some minerals, e.g. calcium, phosphate, sodium and potassium are needed in larger amounts than others. Those required in only tiny quantities are known as trace elements or trace minerals, e.g. iron, iodine, zinc, copper, cobalt, selenium and fluoride. The main minerals and trace elements are outlined below.

Calcium

This is found in milk, cheese, eggs, green vegetables and some fish, e.g. sardines. An adequate supply should be obtained from a normal, well-balanced diet, although requirements are higher in pregnant women and growing children. The most abundant of the minerals, 99% of calcium (about 1 kg in adults) is found in the bones and teeth, where it is an essential structural component. Calcium is also involved in blood clotting, and nerve and muscle function. Deficiency of calcium causes *rickets* in children and *osteomalacia* in adults (p. 431).

Phosphate

Sources include milk and dairy products, red meat, fish, poultry, bread and rice. If there is sufficient calcium in the diet it is unlikely that there will be phosphate deficiency.

It is associated with calcium and vitamin D in the hardening of bones and teeth; 85% of body phosphate is found in these sites. Phosphates are an essential part of nucleic acids (DNA and RNA, see Ch. 17), cell membranes and energy storage molecules such as adenosine triphosphate (ATP, Fig. 2.10, p. 28).

Sodium

Sodium is found in most foods, especially fish, meat, eggs, milk and especially in processed foods. It is also frequently added during cooking or as table salt. Intake of sodium chloride usually exceeds recommendations and excess is normally excreted in the urine. High sodium intake is associated with hypertension (p. 131), which is a risk factor for ischaemic heart disease (p. 127) and stroke (p. 181). The recommended daily salt (sodium chloride) intake for adults should not exceed 6 g. In practice, food is usually labelled with sodium content, and to convert this to salt, the sodium content is multiplied by 2.5.

It is the most common *extracellular cation* and is essential for muscle contraction and transmission of nerve impulses.

Potassium

This is found widely distributed in all foods, especially fruit and vegetables, and intake usually exceeds requirements.

It is the most common *intracellular cation* and is involved in muscle contraction and transmission of nerve impulses.

Iron

Iron, as a soluble compound, is found in liver, red meat, pulses, nuts, eggs, dried fruit, wholemeal bread and leafy green vegetables. In normal adults about 1 mg of iron is lost from the body daily. The normal daily diet contains more, i.e. 9 to 15 mg, but only 5–15% of intake is absorbed. Iron is essential for the formation of haemoglobin in red blood cells. It is also necessary for carbohydrate metabolism and the synthesis of some hormones and neurotransmitters. Menstruating and pregnant women have increased iron requirements, as do young people experiencing growth spurts.

Iron deficiency anaemia (p. 73) is relatively common and occurs when iron stores become depleted. Iron deficiency anaemia may also occur arise from chronic bleeding, e.g. peptic ulcer disease.

Iodine

Iodine is found in seafoods and vegetables grown in soil rich in iodine. In parts of the world where iodine is deficient in soil, very small quantities are added to table salt to prevent *goitre* (p. 232).

It is essential for the formation of *thyroxine* and *tri-iodothyronine*, two hormones secreted by the thyroid gland (p. 222) which regulate metabolic rate, and physical and mental development.

Water

Water is the most abundant constituent of the human body, accounting for around 60% of the body weight in an adult (see Fig. 2.14, p. 30).

A large amount of water is lost each day in urine, sweat and faeces. This is normally balanced by intake in food and fluids, to satisfy thirst. Water requirements are increased following exercise and in high environmental temperatures. Dehydration, with serious consequences, may occur if intake does not balance loss. Water balance is finely regulated by the action of hormones on the kidney tubules (Ch. 13).

Functions of water

These include:

- providing the moist internal environment required by all living cells, e.g. for metabolic reactions
- moistening food for swallowing (see saliva, p. 295)
- regulation of body temperature – as a constituent of sweat, which is secreted onto the skin, it evaporates, cooling the body surface (Ch. 14)
- being the major constituent of blood and tissue fluid, it transports substances round the body and allows exchange between the blood, tissue fluid and body cells
- dilution of waste products and toxins in the body
- providing the medium for excretion of waste products, e.g. urine and faeces.

Non-starch polysaccharide (NSP)

Learning outcome

After studying this section, you should be able to:

- describe the sources and functions of non-starch polysaccharide.

Non-starch polysaccharide (NSP) is the correct term for dietary fibre although the latter term continues to be more commonly used in the UK. It is the indigestible part of the diet and consists of bran, cellulose and other polysaccharides found in fruit, vegetables and cereals. Dietary fibre is partly digested by microbes in the large intestine and is associated with gas (flatus) formation. The recommended daily intake is at least 18 g, at least 5 portions of fruit or vegetables ('5 a day').

Functions of NSP (dietary fibre)

Dietary fibre:

- provides bulk to the diet and helps to satisfy the appetite
- stimulates peristalsis (see p. 289) ⎫
- attracts water, increasing faecal bulk ⎬ prevents constipation ⎭
- protects against some gastrointestinal disorders, e.g. colorectal cancer and diverticular disease (p. 328).

Nutrition and ageing

Learning outcome

After studying this section, you should be able to:

- describe the factors affecting diet and nutrition in older adults.

The importance of good nutrition to health and wellbeing at all stages of the lifespan is well established. The relationship between nutrition, diet and ageing is complex as many diseases arise from poor diet, e.g. atherosclerosis predisposes to coronary heart disease (p. 127). Good nutrition during early and middle life can significantly reduce the risk of problems in later life e.g. osteoporosis (p. 431) can be greatly reduced by an adequate intake of calcium, phosphate and vitamin D.

The senses of smell and taste decline with age (Ch. 8) which can reduce appetite and enjoyment of eating.

Basal metabolic rate (BMR, p. 314) gradually declines with age from the fourth or fifth decades of life. This is mainly due to a reduction in muscle mass and a corresponding increase in body fat; BMR is higher in those with more muscle as muscle is more metabolically active than adipose tissue (fat). Physical activity generally lessens with age, further reducing BMR in older adults.

UK dietary recommendations for older adults are the same as those for other adults although energy requirements gradually reduce as the BMR falls, especially when physical activity is limited. As for other age groups, it is important for older adults to eat a balanced diet with sufficient fibre and vitamins.

Nutritional disorders in older adults

Malnutrition and obesity are both prevalent in older adults as well as other conditions considered below. Malnutrition is more prevalent in those living in institutions, whereas being overweight or obese tends to be more common in people living at home.

Malnutrition

Being underweight (BMI < 18.5) predisposes to health problems e.g. development of pressure ulcers which take longer to heal in older adults. In the oldest adults, anorexia and weight loss become increasingly common and the incidence of protein-energy malnutrition (PEM, p. 283) increases. Malnutrition in healthcare settings is considered in the following section.

Obesity

It is common for body weight to increase between the ages of 40 and 65 ('middle age spread'). This is generally attributed to a reduction in physical activity and BMR rather than increased dietary energy intake. Overweight is defined as BMI above 25 and obesity when BMI is above 30 (Box 11.1). After 65 years, there is usually weight loss accompanied by a lower dietary intake, a decline in muscle mass and an increasing risk of malnutrition. Being overweight or obese at any age carries many health risks (see p. 284), for example, type 2 diabetes mellitus (p. 236). In older adults, obesity is associated with a decline in BMR (see above) and lessened secretion of and responsiveness to hormones which is often accompanied by a more sedentary lifestyle.

Vitamin deficiency

Some vitamin deficiencies become more common in older adults. Vitamin D deficiency (p. 278) is linked to older adults who live in institutions, or are Asian, black or housebound. Those who habitually cover their skin are also vulnerable due to limited exposure to sunlight. The British Nutrition Foundation (2009) recommends that vitamin D intake is maintained by eating oily fish and fortified cereals regularly and that those over 65 years take supplements (10 µg per day). Vitamin B_{12} deficiency, perhaps due to decreased absorption of intrinsic factor, is also more common in older adults and may result in pernicious anaemia (p. 74).

Constipation

Constipation becomes more common as muscle tone and peristaltic activity of the colon lessens with age. This is exacerbated by a lower fluid and/or fibre intake, taking less exercise and reduced mobility. If there is difficulty with activities related to nutrition, e.g. mobility problems which prevent shopping, impaired cognitive function or loss of the manual dexterity required to prepare and eat food and drinks, this further predisposes to constipation.

Disorders of nutrition

Learning outcome

After studying this section, you should be able to:

■ describe the main consequences of malnutrition and obesity.

The importance of nutrition is increasingly recognised as essential for health, and illness often alters nutritional requirements.

Protein-energy malnutrition (PEM)

This is the result of inadequate intake of protein, carbohydrate and fat. It occurs during periods of starvation and when dietary intake is insufficient to meet increased requirements, e.g. trauma, fever and illness. Malnutrition is relatively rare in developed countries except when there is an underlying condition, e.g. sepsis, trauma, surgery or a concurrent illness. Under-nutrition is seen where poverty is prevalent and is usually the result of a poor diet which is not adequately balanced. In the UK many older adults admitted to healthcare establishments (e.g. hospitals and care homes) have signs of undernutrition which often worsens during admission. Anorexia (loss of appetite) from any cause may lead to malnutrition. People with advanced cancer or some chronic illnesses can experience loss of appetite accompanied by profound weight loss and muscle wasting as a symptom of *cachexia* (p. 57).

If dietary intake is inadequate, it is not uncommon for vitamin deficiency to develop at the same time. Poor nutrition reduces the ability to combat other illness and infection. The degree of malnutrition can be assessed from measurement of body mass index (see Box 11.1).

Infants and young children are particularly susceptible as their nutritional requirements for normal growth and development are high. In developing countries where people experience long periods of near-total starvation the two conditions below are found in children under 5 years.

Kwashiorkor

This is malnutrition with oedema that typically occurs when breastfeeding stops and is often precipitated by infections such as measles or gastroenteritis. Severe liver damage significantly reduces the production of plasma proteins leading to ascites and oedema in the lower limbs that masks emaciation (Fig. 11.2A).

Growth stops and there is loss of weight and loss of pigmentation of skin and hair accompanied by listlessness, apathy and irritability. There is susceptibility to infection and recovery from injury and infection takes longer.

Marasmus

This malnutrition with severe muscle wasting is characterised by emaciation due to breakdown (catabolism) of

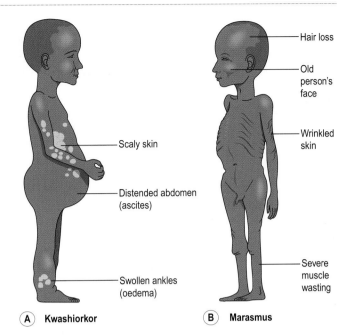

Figure 11.2 Features of protein-energy malnutrition.

muscle and fat (Fig. 11.2B). There is no oedema. Growth is retarded and the skin becomes wrinkled due to absence of subcutaneous fat; hair is lost.

Malabsorption

The causes of malabsorption vary widely, from short-term problems such as gastrointestinal infections (p. 325) to chronic conditions such as cystic fibrosis (p. 266). Malabsorption may be specific for one nutrient, e.g. vitamin B_{12} in pernicious anaemia (p. 74), or it may apply across a spectrum of nutrients, e.g. tropical sprue (p. 331).

Obesity

In developed countries, this is increasingly common although it is also prevalent in some developing countries. The WHO define obesity as a body mass index that exceeds 29.9 (Box 11.1). It occurs when energy intake exceeds energy expenditure, e.g. in inactive individuals whose food intake exceeds daily energy requirements.

Obesity (Fig. 11.3) is a growing public health challenge worldwide that affects people of all ages and predisposes to many other conditions (Box 11.3). Worldwide, around 33% of adults are obese and 10% are overweight (see definitions in Box 11.1). There are more than 40 million obese children aged under five worldwide, of whom 75% live in urban areas of developing countries (WHO, 2013). Childhood obesity is of particular concern, especially in developing countries (where malnutrition can also be widespread), because this preventable condition is likely to continue into and during adulthood with its associated health risks, especially diabetes and cardiovascular disease.

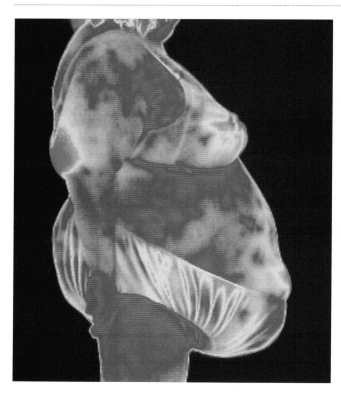

Figure 11.3 Obese woman (thermogram).

Box 11.3 Conditions with obesity as a predisposing factor

Cardiovascular diseases, e.g. hypertension (p. 131), ischaemic heart disease (p. 127)

Type 2 diabetes (p. 236)

Some cancers

Gallstones (p. 335)

Osteoarthritis (p. 434)

Varicose veins (p. 123)

Increased risk of postoperative complications

The hormone *leptin* is associated with obesity. It has several functions, one of which is control of appetite. After eating, this hormone is released by adipose tissue and acts on the hypothalamus resulting in a feeling of satiety, or fullness, which suppresses the appetite. In obesity, there are usually high blood levels of leptin and the negative feedback system, which usually suppresses the appetite, no longer operates normally.

Another function of leptin is involvement in the synthesis of GnRH and gonadotrophins at puberty (Ch. 18). Being secreted by fat tissue, levels are low in thin individuals which explains why:

- thin girls with little body fat reach puberty later than their peers of normal weight
- very thin women may have difficulty in conceiving
- menstruation stops in females with very little body fat.

Obesity predisposes to:

- cardiovascular diseases, e.g. ischaemic heart disease (p. 127), hypertension (p. 131)
- type 2 diabetes mellitus (p. 236)
- some cancers
- hernias (p. 329)
- gallstones (p. 335)
- varicose veins (p. 123)
- osteoarthritis (p. 434)
- increased incidence of postoperative complications.

Conditions with dietary implications

In addition to nutritional disorder there are many conditions where dietary modifications are needed. Some of these are listed in Box 11.4.

Box 11.4 Conditions that require dietary modification

Obesity	Phenylketonuria (p. 446)
Malnutrition	Acute renal failure (p. 352)
Diabetes mellitus (p. 236)	Chronic renal failure (p. 353)
Diverticular disease (p. 328)	Liver failure (p. 334)
Coeliac disease (p. 331)	Lactose intolerance

Further reading

British Nutrition Foundation. Nutrition science. Available online at: http://www.nutrition.org.uk/nutritionscience Accessed 31 March 2013

British Nutrition Foundation. The Eatwell plate. Available online at: http://www.food.gov.uk/multimedia/pdfs/publication/eatwellplate0210.pdf Accessed 31 March 2013

WHO 2009 Global database on body mass index. Available online at: http://www.who.int/bmi/index.jsp?introPage=intro_3.html Accessed 4 November 2013

WHO (2010) Global Strategy on Diet, Physical Activity and Health: childhood overweight and obesity. Available online at: http://www.who.int/dietphysicalactivity/childhood/en/ Accessed 31 March 2013

WHO (2013) Factsheet: Obesity and overweight. Available online at: http://www.who.int/mediacentre/factsheets/fs311/en/ Accessed 31 March 2013

 For a range of self-assessment exercises on the topics in this chapter, visit Evolve online resources: https://evolve.elsevier.com/Waugh/anatomy/

The digestive system

The digestive system describes the *alimentary canal*, its *accessory organs* and a variety of digestive processes that prepare food eaten in the diet for absorption. The alimentary canal begins at the mouth, passes through the thorax, abdomen and pelvis and ends at the anus (Fig. 12.1). It has a basic structure which is modified at different levels to provide for the processes occurring at each level (Fig. 12.2). The digestive processes gradually break down the foods eaten until they are in a form suitable for absorption. For example, meat, even when cooked, is chemically too complex to be absorbed from the alimentary canal. Digestion releases its constituents:

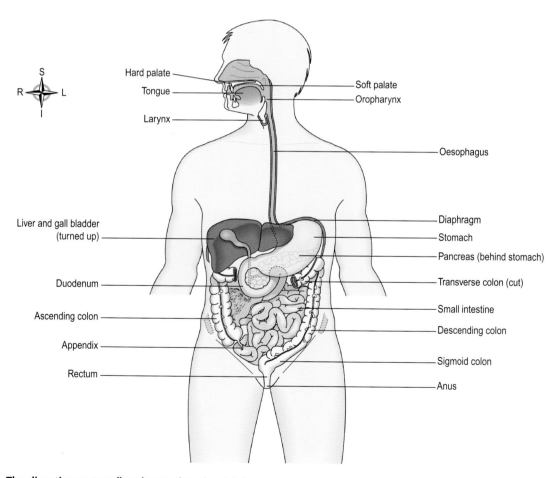

Figure 12.1 The digestive system (head turned to the right).

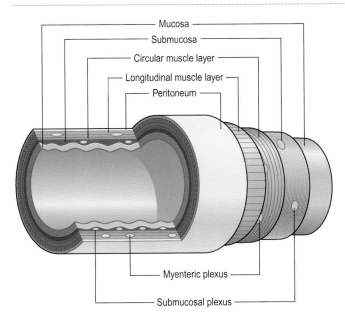

Figure 12.2 **General structure of the alimentary canal.**

the alimentary canal as *faeces* by the process of *defaecation*.

The fate of absorbed nutrients and how they are used by the body is explored and the effects of ageing on the digestive system are considered. In the final section disorders of the digestive system are explained.

Organs of the digestive system
(Fig. 12.1)

Learning outcomes

After studying this section, you should be able to:

■ identify the main organs of the alimentary canal

■ list the accessory organs of digestion.

amino acids, mineral salts, fat and vitamins. Digestive *enzymes* (p. 28) responsible for these changes are secreted into the canal by specialised glands, some of which are in the walls of the canal and some outside the canal, but with ducts leading into it. ▉ **12.1**

After absorption, nutrients provide the raw materials for the manufacture of new cells, hormones and enzymes. The energy needed for these and other processes, and for the disposal of waste materials, is generated from the products of digestion.

The activities of the digestive system can be grouped under five main headings.

Ingestion. This is the taking of food into the alimentary tract, i.e. eating and drinking.

Propulsion. This mixes and moves the contents along the alimentary tract.

Digestion. This consists of:

- *mechanical breakdown* of food by, e.g. mastication (chewing)
- *chemical digestion* of food into small molecules by enzymes present in secretions produced by glands and accessory organs of the digestive system.

Absorption. This is the process by which digested food substances pass through the walls of some organs of the alimentary canal into the blood and lymph capillaries for circulation and use by body cells.

Elimination. Food substances that have been eaten but cannot be digested and absorbed are excreted from

Alimentary canal

Also known as the gastrointestinal (GI) tract, this is essentially a long tube through which food passes. It commences at the mouth and terminates at the anus, and the various organs along its length have different functions, although structurally they are remarkably similar. The parts are:

- mouth
- pharynx
- oesophagus
- stomach
- small intestine
- large intestine
- rectum and anal canal.

Accessory organs

Various secretions are poured into the alimentary tract, some by glands in the lining membrane of the organs, e.g. gastric juice secreted by glands in the lining of the stomach, and some by glands situated outside the tract. The latter are the accessory organs of digestion and their secretions pass through ducts to enter the tract. They consist of:

- three pairs of salivary glands
- the pancreas
- the liver and biliary tract.

The organs and glands are linked physiologically as well as anatomically in that digestion and absorption occur in stages, each stage being dependent upon the previous stage or stages.

Basic structure of the alimentary canal (Fig. 12.2)

Learning outcomes

After studying this section, you should be able to:

■ describe the distribution of the peritoneum

■ explain the function of smooth muscle in the walls of the alimentary canal

■ discuss the structures of the alimentary mucosa

■ outline the nerve supply of the alimentary canal.

The layers of the walls of the alimentary canal follow a consistent pattern from the oesophagus onwards. This basic structure does not apply so obviously to the mouth and the pharynx, which are considered later in the chapter.

In the organs from the oesophagus onwards, modifications of structure are found which are associated with specific functions. The basic structure is described here and any modifications in structure and function are described in the appropriate section.

The walls of the alimentary tract are formed by four layers of tissue:

- adventitia or serosa – outer covering
- muscle layer
- submucosa
- mucosa – lining.

Adventitia or serosa

This is the outermost layer. In the thorax it consists of *loose fibrous tissue* and in the abdomen the organs are covered by a serous membrane (serosa) called *peritoneum*.

Peritoneum

The peritoneum is the largest serous membrane of the body (Fig. 12.3A). It is a closed sac, containing a small amount of serous fluid, within the abdominal cavity. It is richly supplied with blood and lymph vessels, and contains many lymph nodes. It provides a physical barrier to local spread of infection, and can isolate an infective focus such as appendicitis, preventing involvement of other abdominal structures. It has two layers:

- the *parietal peritoneum*, which lines the abdominal wall
- the *visceral peritoneum*, which covers the organs (viscera) within the abdominal and pelvic cavities.

The parietal peritoneum lines the anterior abdominal wall.

The two layers of peritoneum are in close contact, and friction between them is prevented by the presence of serous fluid secreted by the peritoneal cells, thus the peritoneal cavity is only a potential cavity. A similar

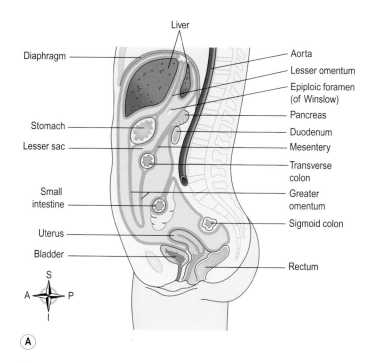

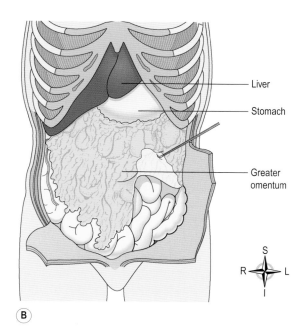

Figure 12.3 The peritoneum and associated structures. A. The peritoneal cavity (gold), the abdominal organs of the digestive system and the pelvic organs. **B.** The greater omentum.

arrangement is seen with the membranes covering the lungs, the pleura (p. 250). In the male, the peritoneal cavity is completely closed but in the female the uterine tubes open into it and the ovaries are the only structures inside (Ch. 18).

The arrangement of the peritoneum is such that the organs are invaginated (pushed into the membrane forming a pouch) into the closed sac from below, behind and above so that they are at least partly covered by the visceral layer, and attached securely within the abdominal cavity. This means that:

- pelvic organs are covered only on their superior surface
- the stomach and intestines, deeply invaginated from behind, are almost completely surrounded by peritoneum and have a double fold (the *mesentery*) that attaches them to the posterior abdominal wall. The fold of peritoneum enclosing the stomach extends beyond the greater curvature of the stomach, and hangs down in front of the abdominal organs like an apron (Fig. 12.3B). This is the *greater omentum*, which stores fat that provides both insulation and a long-term energy store
- the pancreas, spleen, kidneys and adrenal glands are invaginated from behind but only their anterior surfaces are covered and are therefore *retroperitoneal* (lie behind the peritoneum)
- the liver is invaginated from above and is almost completely covered by peritoneum, which attaches it to the inferior surface of the diaphragm
- the main blood vessels and nerves pass close to the posterior abdominal wall and send branches to the organs between folds of peritoneum.

Muscle layer

With some exceptions this consists of two layers of *smooth (involuntary) muscle*. The muscle fibres of the outer layer are arranged longitudinally, and those of the inner layer encircle the wall of the tube. Between these two muscle layers are blood vessels, lymph vessels and a plexus (network) of sympathetic and parasympathetic nerves, called the *myenteric plexus* (Fig. 12.2). These nerves supply the adjacent smooth muscle and blood vessels.

Contraction and relaxation of these muscle layers occurs in waves, which push the contents of the tract onwards. This type of contraction of smooth muscle is called *peristalsis* (Fig. 12.4) and is under the influence of sympathetic and parasympathetic nerves. Muscle contraction also mixes food with the digestive juices. Onward movement of the contents of the tract is controlled at various points by *sphincters*, which are thickened rings of circular muscle. Contraction of sphincters regulates forward movement. They also act as valves, preventing backflow in the tract. This control allows time for digestion and absorption to take place. ▓ 12.2

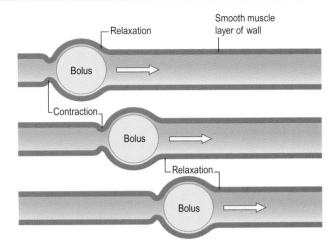

Figure 12.4 Movement of a bolus by peristalsis.

Submucosa

This layer consists of loose areolar connective tissue containing collagen and some elastic fibres, which binds the muscle layer to the mucosa. Within it are blood vessels and nerves, lymph vessels and varying amounts of lymphoid tissue. The blood vessels are arterioles, venules and capillaries. The nerve plexus is the *submucosal plexus* (Fig. 12.2), which contains sympathetic and parasympathetic nerves that supply the mucosal lining.

Mucosa

This consists of three layers of tissue:

- *mucous membrane* formed by columnar epithelium is the innermost layer, and has three main functions: *protection*, *secretion* and *absorption*
- *lamina propria* consisting of loose connective tissue, which supports the blood vessels that nourish the inner epithelial layer, and varying amounts of lymphoid tissue that protects against microbial invaders
- *muscularis mucosa*, a thin outer layer of smooth muscle that provides involutions of the mucosal layer, e.g. gastric glands (p. 299), villi (p. 302).

Mucous membrane

In parts of the tract that are subject to great wear and tear or mechanical injury, this layer consists of *stratified squamous epithelium* with mucus-secreting glands just below the surface. In areas where the food is already soft and moist and where secretion of digestive juices and absorption occur, the mucous membrane consists of *columnar epithelial cells* interspersed with mucus-secreting goblet cells (Fig. 12.5). Mucus lubricates the walls of the tract and provides a physical barrier that protects them from

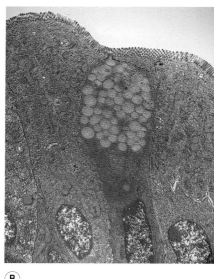

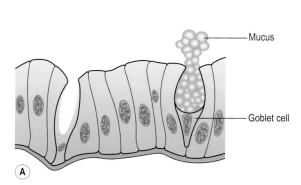

Mucus

Goblet cell

A

B

Figure 12.5 Columnar epithelium with a goblet cell. A. Diagram. **B.** Coloured transmission electron micrograph of a section through a goblet cell (pink and blue) of the small intestine.

the damaging effects of digestive enzymes. Below the surface in the regions lined with columnar epithelium are collections of specialised cells, or glands, which release their secretions into the lumen of the tract. The secretions include:

- *saliva* from the salivary glands
- *gastric juice* from the gastric glands
- *intestinal juice* from the intestinal glands
- *pancreatic juice* from the pancreas
- *bile* from the liver.

These are *digestive juices* and most contain enzymes that chemically break down food. Under the epithelial lining are varying amounts of lymphoid tissue that provide protection against ingested microbes.

Nerve supply

The alimentary canal and its related accessory organs are supplied by nerves from both divisions of the autonomic nervous system, i.e. both parasympathetic and sympathetic parts (Fig. 12.6). Their actions are generally antagonistic to each other and at any particular time one has a greater influence than the other, according to body needs, at that time. When digestion is required, this is normally through increased activity of the parasympathetic nervous system.

The parasympathetic supply. One pair of cranial nerves, the *vagus nerves*, supplies most of the alimentary canal and the accessory organs. Sacral nerves supply the most distal part of the tract. The effects of parasympathetic stimulation on the digestive system are:

- increased muscular activity, especially peristalsis, through increased activity of the myenteric plexus
- increased glandular secretion, through increased activity of the submucosal plexus (Fig. 12.2).

The sympathetic supply. This is provided by numerous nerves that emerge from the spinal cord in the thoracic and lumbar regions. These form plexuses (ganglia) in the thorax, abdomen and pelvis, from which nerves pass to the organs of the alimentary tract. The effects of sympathetic stimulation on the digestive system are to:

- decrease muscular activity, especially peristalsis, because there is reduced stimulation of the myenteric plexus
- decrease glandular secretion, as there is less stimulation of the submucosal plexus.

Mouth (Fig. 12.7)

Learning outcomes

After studying this section, you should be able to:

- list the principal structures associated with the mouth
- describe the structure of the mouth
- describe the structure and function of the tongue
- describe the structure and function of the teeth
- outline the arrangement of normal primary and secondary dentition.

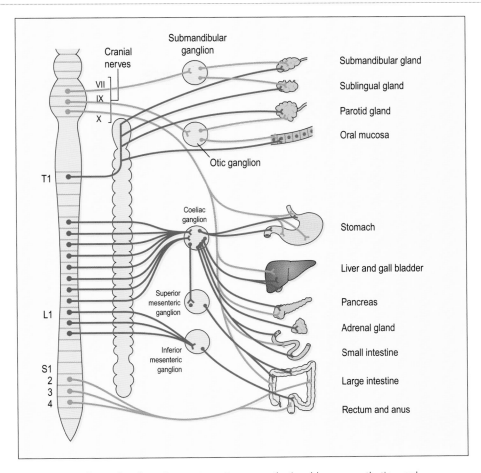

Figure 12.6 Autonomic nerve supply to the digestive system. Parasympathetic – blue; sympathetic – red.

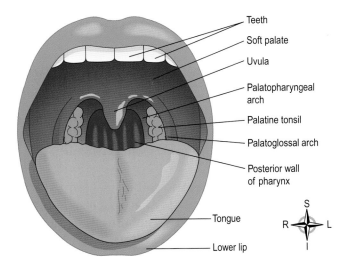

Figure 12.7 Structures seen in the widely open mouth.

The mouth or oral cavity is bounded by muscles and bones:

Anteriorly – by the lips
Posteriorly – it is continuous with the oropharynx
Laterally – by the muscles of the cheeks

Superiorly – by the bony hard palate and muscular soft palate
Inferiorly – by the muscular tongue and the soft tissues of the floor of the mouth.

The oral cavity is lined throughout with *mucous membrane*, consisting of stratified squamous epithelium containing small mucus-secreting glands.

The part of the mouth between the gums and the cheeks is the *vestibule* and the remainder of its interior is the *oral cavity*. The mucous membrane lining of the cheeks and the lips is reflected onto the gums or *alveolar ridges* and is continuous with the skin of the face.

The *palate* forms the roof of the mouth and is divided into the anterior *hard palate* and the posterior *soft palate* (Fig. 12.1). The hard palate is formed by the maxilla and the palatine bones. The soft palate, which is muscular, curves downwards from the posterior end of the hard palate and blends with the walls of the pharynx at the sides.

The *uvula* is a curved fold of muscle covered with mucous membrane, hanging down from the middle of the free border of the soft palate. Originating from the upper end of the uvula are four folds of mucous membrane, two passing downwards at each side to form membranous arches. The posterior folds, one on each side, are the *palatopharyngeal arches* and the two anterior folds are the *palatoglossal arches*. On each side, between the arches, is a collection of lymphoid tissue called the *palatine tonsil*.

Tongue

The tongue is composed of voluntary muscle. It is attached by its base to the *hyoid bone* (see Fig. 10.4, p. 244) and by a fold of its mucous membrane covering, called the *frenulum*, to the floor of the mouth (Fig. 12.8). The superior surface consists of stratified squamous epithelium, with numerous *papillae* (little projections). Many of these contain sensory receptors (specialised nerve endings) for the sense of taste in the *taste buds* (see Fig. 8.24, p. 206).

Blood supply

The main arterial blood supply to the tongue is by the *lingual branch* of the *external carotid artery*. Venous drainage is by the *lingual vein*, which joins the *internal jugular vein*.

Nerve supply

The nerves involved are:

- the *hypoglossal nerves* (12th cranial nerves), which supply the voluntary muscle
- the *lingual branch of the mandibular nerves*, which arise from the 5th cranial nerves, are the nerves of somatic (ordinary) sensation, i.e. pain, temperature and touch
- the *facial* and *glossopharyngeal nerves* (7th and 9th cranial nerves), the nerves of taste.

Functions of the tongue

The tongue plays an important part in:

- chewing (mastication)
- swallowing (deglutition)
- speech (p. 245)
- taste (p. 207).

Nerve endings of the sense of taste are present in the papillae and widely distributed in the epithelium of the tongue.

Teeth

The teeth are embedded in the alveoli or sockets of the alveolar ridges of the mandible and the maxilla (Fig. 12.9). Babies are born with two sets, or *dentitions*, the *temporary* or *deciduous teeth* and the *permanent teeth* (Fig. 12.10). At birth the teeth of both dentitions are present, in immature form, in the mandible and maxilla.

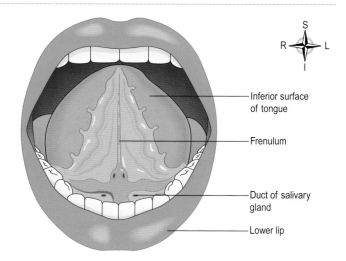

Figure 12.8 The inferior surface of the tongue.

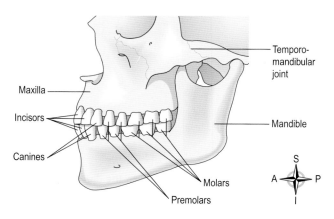

Figure 12.9 The permanent teeth and the jaw bones.

There are 20 temporary teeth, 10 in each jaw. They begin to erupt at about 6 months of age, and should all be present by 24 months (Table 12.1).

The permanent teeth begin to replace the deciduous teeth in the 6th year of age and this dentition, consisting of 32 teeth, is usually complete by the 21st year.

Functions of the teeth

Teeth have different shapes depending on their functions. *Incisors* and *canine* teeth are the cutting teeth and are used for biting off pieces of food, whereas the *premolar* and *molar* teeth, with broad, flat surfaces, are used for grinding or chewing food (Fig. 12.11).

Structure of a tooth (Fig. 12.12)

Although the shapes of the different teeth vary, the structure is the same and consists of:

- *the crown* – the part that protrudes from the gum
- *the root* – the part embedded in the bone

Table 12.1 Deciduous and permanent dentitions

Jaw	Molars	Premolars	Canine	Incisors	Incisors	Canine	Premolars	Molars
Deciduous teeth								
Upper	2	–	1	2	2	1	–	2
Lower	2	–	1	2	2	1	–	2
Permanent teeth								
Upper	3	2	1	2	2	1	2	3
Lower	3	2	1	2	2	1	2	3

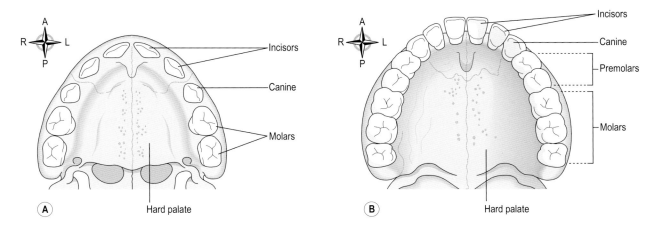

Figure 12.10 The roof of the mouth. A. The deciduous teeth – viewed from below. **B.** The permanent teeth – viewed from below.

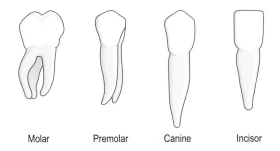

Figure 12.11 The shapes of the permanent teeth.

- *the neck* – the slightly narrowed region where the crown merges with the root.

In the centre of the tooth is the *pulp cavity* containing blood vessels, lymph vessels and nerves, and surrounding this is a hard ivory-like substance called *dentine*. The dentine of the crown is covered by a thin layer of very hard substance, *enamel*. The root of the tooth, on the other hand, is covered with a substance resembling bone, called *cementum*, which secures the tooth in its socket. Blood

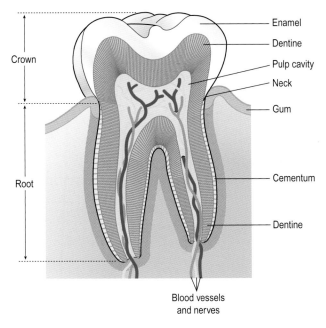

Figure 12.12 A section of a tooth.

vessels and nerves pass to the tooth through a small foramen (hole) at the apex of each root.

Blood supply

Most of the arterial blood supply to the teeth is by branches of the *maxillary arteries*. The venous drainage is by a number of veins which empty into the *internal jugular veins*.

Nerve supply

The nerve supply to the upper teeth is by branches of the *maxillary nerves* and to the lower teeth by branches of the *mandibular nerves*. These are both branches of the *trigeminal nerves* (5th cranial nerves) (Fig. 7.41, see p. 172).

Salivary glands (Fig. 12.13)

Learning outcomes

After studying this section, you should be able to:

■ describe the structure and the function of the principal salivary glands

■ explain the role of saliva in digestion.

Salivary glands release their secretions into ducts that lead to the mouth. There are three main pairs: the parotid glands, the submandibular glands and the sublingual glands. There are also numerous smaller salivary glands scattered around the mouth.

Parotid glands

These are situated one on each side of the face just below the external acoustic meatus (see Fig. 8.1, p. 192). Each gland has a *parotid duct* opening into the mouth at the level of the second upper molar tooth.

Submandibular glands

These lie one on each side of the face under the angle of the jaw. The two *submandibular ducts* open on the floor of the mouth, one on each side of the frenulum of the tongue.

Sublingual glands

These glands lie under the mucous membrane of the floor of the mouth in front of the submandibular glands. They have numerous small ducts that open into the floor of the mouth.

Structure of the salivary glands

The glands are all surrounded by a *fibrous capsule*. They consist of a number of *lobules* made up of small acini lined with secretory cells (Fig. 12.13B). The secretions are poured into ductules that join up to form larger ducts leading into the mouth.

Blood supply

Arterial supply is by various branches from the external carotid arteries and venous drainage is into the external jugular veins.

Composition of saliva

Saliva is the combined secretions from the salivary glands and the small mucus-secreting glands of the oral

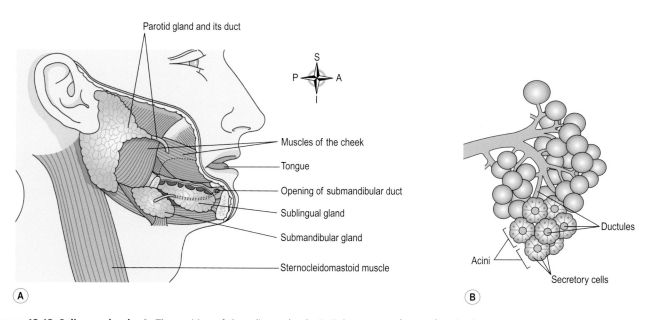

Figure 12.13 Salivary glands. A. The position of the salivary glands. **B.** Enlargement of part of a gland.

mucosa. About 1.5 litres of saliva is produced daily and it consists of:

- water
- mineral salts
- salivary amylase; a digestive enzyme
- mucus
- antimicrobial substances; immunoglobulins and the enzyme lysozyme.

Secretion of saliva

Secretion of saliva is controlled by the autonomic nervous system. Parasympathetic stimulation causes profuse secretion of watery saliva with a relatively low content of enzymes and other organic substances. Sympathetic stimulation results in secretion of small amounts of saliva rich in organic material, especially from the submandibular glands. Reflex secretion occurs when there is food in the mouth and the reflex can easily become *conditioned* so that the sight, smell and even the thought of food stimulates the flow of saliva.

Functions of saliva

Chemical digestion of polysaccharides
Saliva contains the enzyme *amylase* that begins the breakdown of complex sugars, including starches, reducing them to the disaccharide maltose. The optimum pH for the action of salivary amylase is 6.8 (slightly acid). Salivary pH ranges from 5.8 to 7.4 depending on the rate of flow; the higher the flow rate, the higher is the pH. Enzyme action continues during swallowing until terminated by the strongly acidic gastric juices (pH 1.5–1.8), which degrades the amylase.

Lubrication of food
The high water content means that dry food entering the mouth is moistened and lubricated by saliva before it can be made into a *bolus* ready for swallowing.

Cleaning and lubricating the mouth
An adequate flow of saliva is necessary to clean the mouth, and to keep it soft, moist and pliable. This helps to prevent damage to the mucous membrane by rough or abrasive food.

Non-specific defence
Lysozyme and immunoglobulins present in saliva combat invading microbes.

Taste
The taste buds are stimulated only by chemical substances in solution and therefore dry foods only stimulate the sense of taste after thorough mixing with saliva. The senses of taste and smell are closely linked and involved in the enjoyment, or otherwise, of food (see Ch. 8).

Pharynx

Learning outcome

After studying this section, you should be able to:

- describe the structure of the pharynx.

The pharynx is divided for descriptive purpose into three parts, the nasopharynx, oropharynx and laryngopharynx (see p. 245). The nasopharynx is important in respiration. The oropharynx and laryngopharynx are passages common to both the respiratory and the digestive systems. Food passes from the oral cavity into the pharynx then to the oesophagus below, with which it is continuous. The walls of the pharynx consist of three layers of tissue.

The *lining membrane* (mucosa) is stratified squamous epithelium, continuous with the lining of the mouth at one end and the oesophagus at the other. Stratified epithelial tissue provides a lining well suited to the wear and tear of swallowing ingested food.

The *middle layer* consists of connective tissue, which becomes thinner towards the lower end and contains blood and lymph vessels and nerves.

The *outer layer* consists of a number of involuntary muscles that are involved in swallowing. When food reaches the pharynx, swallowing is no longer under voluntary control.

Blood supply
The blood supply to the pharynx is by several branches of the facial arteries. Venous drainage is into the facial veins and the internal jugular veins.

Nerve supply
This is from the pharyngeal plexus and consists of parasympathetic and sympathetic nerves. Parasympathetic supply is mainly by the glossopharyngeal and vagus nerves and sympathetic from the cervical ganglia.

Oesophagus (Fig. 12.14)

Learning outcomes

After studying this section, you should be able to:

- describe the location of the oesophagus
- outline the structure of the oesophagus
- explain the mechanisms involved in swallowing, and the route taken by a bolus.

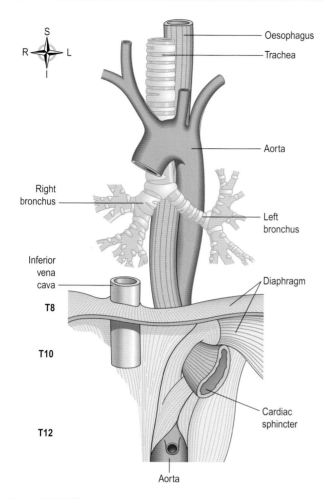

Figure 12.14 The oesophagus and some related structures.

The oesophagus is about 25 cm long and about 2 cm in diameter and lies in the median plane in the thorax in front of the vertebral column behind the trachea and the heart. It is continuous with the pharynx above and just below the diaphragm it joins the stomach. It passes between muscle fibres of the diaphragm behind the central tendon at the level of the 10th thoracic vertebra. Immediately the oesophagus has passed through the diaphragm it curves upwards before opening into the stomach. This sharp angle is believed to be one of the factors that prevents the regurgitation (backflow) of gastric contents into the oesophagus. The upper and lower ends of the oesophagus are closed by sphincters. The upper *cricopharyngeal* or *upper oesphageal sphincter* prevents air passing into the oesophagus during inspiration and the aspiration of oesophageal contents. The *cardiac* or *lower oesophageal sphincter* prevents the reflux of acid gastric contents into the oesophagus. There is no thickening of the circular muscle in this area and this sphincter is therefore 'physiological', i.e. this region can act as a sphincter without the presence of the anatomical features. When intra-abdominal pressure is raised, e.g. during

inspiration and defaecation, the tone of the lower oesophageal sphincter increases. There is an added pinching effect by the contracting muscle fibres of the diaphragm. ▨ **12.3**

Structure of the oesophagus

There are four layers of tissue as shown in Figure 12.2. As the oesophagus is almost entirely in the thorax the outer covering, the adventitia, consists of *elastic fibrous tissue* that attaches the oesophagus to the surrounding structures. The proximal third is lined by stratified squamous epithelium and the distal third by columnar epithelium. The middle third is lined by a mixture of the two.

Blood supply

Arterial. The thoracic region is supplied mainly by the paired oesophageal arteries, branches from the thoracic aorta. The abdominal region is supplied by branches from the inferior phrenic arteries and the left gastric branch of the coeliac artery.

Venous drainage. From the thoracic region venous drainage is into the azygos and hemiazygos veins. The abdominal part drains into the left gastric vein. There is a venous plexus at the distal end that links the upward and downward venous drainage, i.e. the general and portal circulations.

Functions of the mouth, pharynx and oesophagus

Formation of a bolus

When food is taken into the mouth it is chewed (masticated) by the teeth and moved around the mouth by the tongue and muscles of the cheeks (Fig. 12.15). It is mixed with saliva and formed into a soft mass or bolus ready

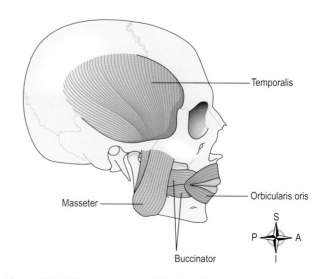

Figure 12.15 The muscles used in chewing.

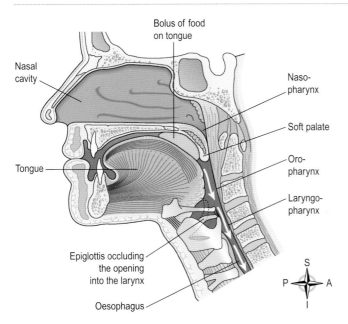

Nasal
cavity

Tongue

Bolus of food
on tongue

Naso-
pharynx

Soft palate

Oro-
pharynx

Laryngo-
pharynx

Epiglottis occluding
the opening
into the larynx

Oesophagus

Figure 12.16 Section of the face and neck showing the positions of structures during swallowing.

for swallowing. The length of time that food remains in the mouth largely depends on the consistency of the food. Some foods need to be chewed longer than others before the individual feels that the bolus is ready for swallowing. ▓ **12.4**

Swallowing (deglutition) (Fig. 12.16)
This occurs in three stages after chewing is complete and the bolus has been formed. It is initiated voluntarily but completed by a reflex (involuntary) action.

1. Oral stage. With the mouth closed, the voluntary muscles of the tongue and cheeks push the bolus backwards into the pharynx.

2. Pharyngeal stage. The muscles of the pharynx are stimulated by a reflex action initiated in the walls of the oropharynx and coordinated by the *swallowing centre* in the medulla. Involuntary contraction of these muscles propels the bolus down into the oesophagus. All other routes that the bolus could take are closed. The soft palate rises up and closes off the nasopharynx; the tongue and the pharyngeal folds block the way back into the mouth; and the larynx is lifted up and forward so that its opening is occluded by the overhanging epiglottis preventing entry into the airway (trachea). ▓ **12.5**

3. Oesophageal stage. The presence of the bolus in the pharynx stimulates a wave of peristalsis that propels the bolus through the oesophagus to the stomach. ▓ **12.2**

Peristaltic waves pass along the oesophagus only after swallowing begins (see Fig. 12.4). Otherwise the walls are relaxed. Ahead of a peristaltic wave, the cardiac sphincter guarding the entrance to the stomach relaxes to allow the

descending bolus to pass into the stomach. Usually, constriction of the cardiac sphincter prevents reflux of gastric acid into the oesophagus. Other factors preventing gastric reflux include:

- the attachment of the stomach to the diaphragm by the peritoneum
- the acute angle formed by the position of the oesophagus as it enters the fundus of the stomach, i.e. an acute cardio-oesophageal angle (see Fig. 12.18)
- increased tone of the cardiac sphincter when intra-abdominal pressure is increased and the pinching effect of diaphragm muscle fibres.

The walls of the oesophagus are lubricated by mucus which assists the passage of the bolus during the peristaltic contraction of the muscular wall.

Stomach

Learning outcomes

After studying this section, you should be able to:

- describe the location of the stomach with reference to surrounding structures
- explain the physiological significance of the layers of the stomach wall
- discuss the digestive functions of the stomach.

The stomach is a J-shaped dilated portion of the alimentary tract situated in the epigastric, umbilical and left hypochondriac regions of the abdominal cavity.

Organs associated with the stomach
(Fig. 12.17)

Anteriorly – left lobe of liver and anterior abdominal wall

Posteriorly – abdominal aorta, pancreas, spleen, left kidney and adrenal gland

Superiorly – diaphragm, oesophagus and left lobe of liver

Inferiorly – transverse colon and small intestine

To the left – diaphragm and spleen

To the right – liver and duodenum.

Structure of the stomach (Fig. 12.18)

The stomach is continuous with the oesophagus at the cardiac sphincter and with the duodenum at the pyloric sphincter. It has two curvatures. The *lesser curvature* is short, lies on the posterior surface of the stomach and is

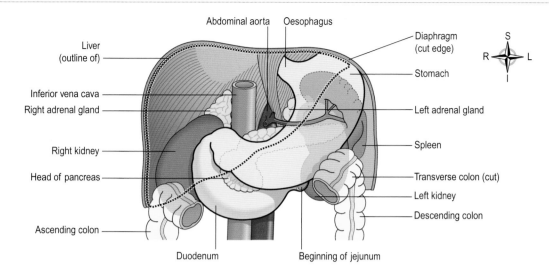

Figure 12.17 The stomach and its associated structures.

the downward continuation of the posterior wall of the oesophagus. Just before the pyloric sphincter it curves upwards to complete the J shape. Where the oesophagus joins the stomach the anterior region angles acutely upwards, curves downwards forming the *greater curvature* and then slightly upwards towards the pyloric sphincter.

The stomach is divided into three regions: the *fundus*, the *body* and the *pylorus*. At the distal end of the pylorus is the pyloric sphincter, guarding the opening between the stomach and the duodenum. When the stomach is inactive the pyloric sphincter is relaxed and open, and when the stomach contains food the sphincter is closed.

Walls of the stomach

The four layers of tissue that comprise the basic structure of the alimentary canal (Fig. 12.2) are found in the stomach but with some modifications.

Muscle layer. (Fig. 12.19). This consists of three layers of smooth muscle fibres:

- an outer layer of longitudinal fibres
- a middle layer of circular fibres
- an inner layer of oblique fibres.

In this respect, the stomach is different from other regions of the alimentary tract as it has three layers of muscle instead of two. This arrangement allows for the churning motion characteristic of gastric activity, as well as peristaltic movement. Circular muscle is strongest between the pylorus and the pyloric sphincter.

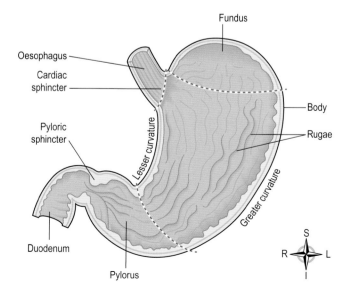

Figure 12.18 Longitudinal section of the stomach.

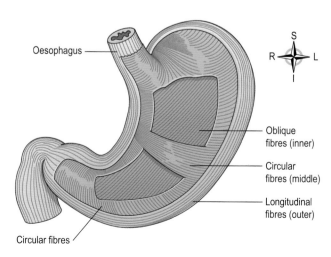

Figure 12.19 The muscle fibres of the stomach wall.
Sections have been removed to show the three layers.

Mucosa. When the stomach is empty the mucous membrane lining is thrown into longitudinal folds or *rugae*, and when full the rugae are 'ironed out' giving the surface a smooth, velvety appearance. Numerous *gastric glands* are situated below the surface in the mucous membrane and open on to it (Fig. 12.20). They consist of specialised cells that secrete *gastric juice* into the stomach.

Blood supply. Arterial supply to the stomach is by the left gastric artery, a branch of the coeliac artery, the right

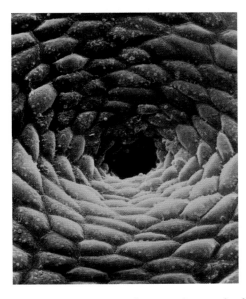

Figure 12.20 Coloured scanning electron micrograph of the mucous membrane lining the stomach showing the entrance to a gastric gland.

gastric artery and the gastroepiploic arteries. Venous drainage is through veins of corresponding names into the portal vein. Figures 5.38 and 5.40 (pp. 109 and 110) show these vessels.

Gastric juice and functions of the stomach

Stomach size varies with the volume of food it contains, which may be 1.5 litres or more in an adult. When a meal has been eaten the food accumulates in the stomach in layers, the last part of the meal remaining in the fundus for some time. Mixing with the gastric juice takes place gradually and it may be some time before the food is sufficiently acidified to stop the action of salivary amylase.

The gastric muscle generates a churning action that breaks down the bolus and mixes it with gastric juice, and peristaltic waves that propel the stomach contents towards the pylorus. When the stomach is active the pyloric sphincter closes. Strong peristaltic contraction of the pylorus forces *chyme*, gastric contents after they are sufficiently liquefied, through the pyloric sphincter into the duodenum in small spurts. Parasympathetic stimulation increases the motility of the stomach and secretion of gastric juice; sympathetic stimulation has the opposite effect. ▊ **12.6**

Gastric juice

About 2 litres of gastric juice are secreted daily by specialised secretory glands in the mucosa (Fig. 12.21). It consists of:

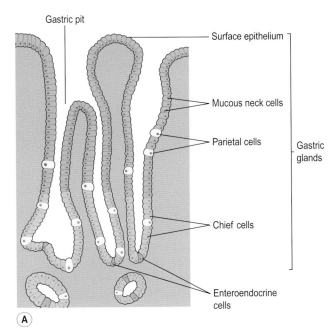

Gastric pit

Surface epithelium

Mucous neck cells

Parietal cells

Gastric glands

Chief cells

Enteroendocrine cells

(A)

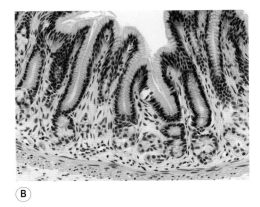

(B)

Figure 12.21 Structure of the gastric mucosa showing gastric glands. A. Diagram. **B.** Stained section of the pyloric region of the stomach (magnified x 150).

- water
- mineral salts
- mucus secreted by mucous neck cells in the glands and surface mucous cells on the stomach surface
- hydrochloric acid ⎫ secreted by *parietal cells*
- intrinsic factor ⎭ in the gastric glands
- inactive enzyme precursors: pepsinogens secreted by *chief cells* in the glands.

Functions of gastric juice

- *Water* further liquefies the food swallowed.
- *Hydrochloric acid*:
  - acidifies the food and stops the action of salivary amylase
  - kills ingested microbes
  - provides the acid environment needed for the action of pepsins.
- *Pepsinogens* are activated to *pepsins* by hydrochloric acid and by pepsins already present in the stomach. These enzymes begin the digestion of proteins, breaking them into smaller molecules. Pepsins have evolved to act most effectively at a very low pH, between 1.5 and 3.5. ▓ **12.7**
- *Intrinsic factor* (a protein) is necessary for the absorption of vitamin B_{12} from the ileum. (Deficiency leads to pernicious anemia p. 74.)
- *Mucus* prevents mechanical injury to the stomach wall by lubricating the contents. It also prevents chemical injury by acting as a barrier between the stomach wall and the corrosive gastric juice – hydrochloric acid is present in potentially damaging concentrations and pepsins would digest the gastric tissues.

Secretion of gastric juice

There is always a small quantity of gastric juice present in the stomach, even when it contains no food. This is known as fasting juice. Secretion reaches its maximum level about 1 hour after a meal then declines to the fasting level after about 4 hours.

There are three phases of secretion of gastric juice (Fig. 12.22).

1. Cephalic phase. This flow of juice occurs before food reaches the stomach and is due to reflex stimulation of the vagus (parasympathetic) nerves initiated by the sight, smell or taste of food. When the vagus nerves have been cut (vagotomy), this phase of gastric secretion stops. Sympathetic stimulation, e.g. during emotional states, also inhibits gastric activity.

2. Gastric phase. When stimulated by the presence of food the *enteroendocrine cells* in the pylorus (Fig. 12.21) and duodenum secrete the hormone *gastrin*, which passes directly into the circulating blood. Gastrin, circulating in the blood which supplies the stomach, stimulates the gastric glands to produce more gastric juice. In this way secretion of digestive juice is continued after completion of a meal and the end of the cephalic phase. Gastrin secretion is suppressed when the pH in the pylorus falls to about 1.5.

3. Intestinal phase. When the partially digested contents of the stomach reach the small intestine, two hormones, *secretin* and *cholecystokinin*, are produced by endocrine cells in the intestinal mucosa. They slow down the secretion of gastric juice and reduce gastric motility. By slowing the emptying rate of the stomach, the chyme in the duodenum becomes more thoroughly mixed with

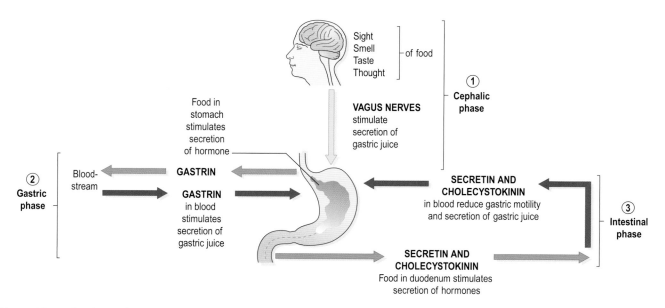

Figure 12.22 The three phases of secretion of gastric juice.

bile and pancreatic juice. This phase of gastric secretion is most marked following a meal with a high fat content.

The rate at which the stomach empties depends largely on the type of food eaten. A carbohydrate meal leaves the stomach in 2–3 hours, a protein meal remains longer and a fatty meal remains in the stomach longest.

Functions of the stomach

These include:

- temporary storage allowing time for the digestive enzymes, pepsins, to act
- chemical digestion – pepsins break proteins into polypeptides
- mechanical breakdown – the three smooth muscle layers enable the stomach to act as a churn, gastric juice is added and the contents are liquefied to chyme. Gastric motility and secretion are increased by parasympathetic nerve stimulation
- limited absorption – water, alcohol and some lipid-soluble drugs
- non-specific defence against microbes – provided by hydrochloric acid in gastric juice. Vomiting (Table 12.4) may occur in response to ingestion of gastric irritants, e.g. microbes or chemicals
- preparation of iron for absorption – the acid environment of the stomach solubilises iron salts, essential for iron absorption in the small intestine
- production and secretion of intrinsic factor needed for absorption of vitamin B_{12} in the terminal ileum
- regulation of the passage of gastric contents into the duodenum. When the chyme is sufficiently acidified and liquefied, the pylorus forces small jets of gastric contents through the pyloric sphincter into

the duodenum. The sphincter is normally closed, preventing backflow of chyme into the stomach

- secretion of the hormone gastrin (see above).

Small intestine (Figs 12.23 and 12.24)

Learning outcomes

After studying this section, you should be able to:

- describe the location of the small intestine, with reference to surrounding structures
- sketch a villus, labelling its component parts
- discuss the digestive functions of the small intestine and its secretions
- explain how nutrients are absorbed in the small intestine.

The small intestine is continuous with the stomach at the pyloric sphincter. The small intestine is about 2.5 cm in diameter, a little over 5 metres long and leads into the large intestine at the *ileocaecal valve*. It lies in the abdominal cavity surrounded by the large intestine. In the small intestine the chemical digestion of food is completed and absorption of most nutrients takes place. The small intestine comprises three continuous parts.

Duodenum. This is about 25 cm long and curves around the head of the pancreas. Secretions from the gall bladder and pancreas merge in a common structure – the *hepato-pancreatic ampulla* – and enter the duodenum at the *duodenal papilla*. The duodenal papilla is guarded by a ring of

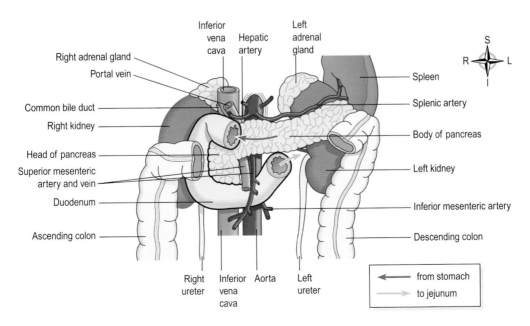

Figure 12.23 The duodenum and its associated structures.

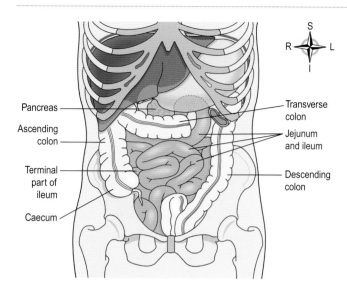

Figure 12.24 **The jejunum and ileum and their related structures.**

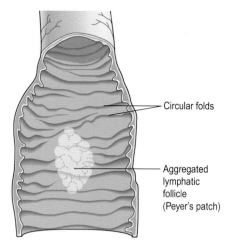

Figure 12.25 **Section of a small piece of small intestine (opened out), showing the permanent circular folds.**

smooth muscle, the *hepatopancreatic sphincter* (of Oddi) (see Fig. 12.38).

Jejunum. This is the middle section of the small intestine and is about 2 metres long.

Ileum. This terminal section is about 3 metres long and ends at the *ileocaecal valve*, which controls the flow of material from the ileum to the *caecum*, the first part of the large intestine, and prevents backflow.

Structure of the small intestine

The walls of the small intestine are composed of the four layers of tissue shown in Figure 12.2. Some modifications of the peritoneum and mucosa (mucous membrane lining) are described below.

Peritoneum
The *mesentery*, a double layer of peritoneum, attaches the jejunum and ileum to the posterior abdominal wall (see Fig. 12.3A). The attachment is quite short in comparison with the length of the small intestine, therefore it is fan shaped. The large blood vessels and nerves lie on the posterior abdominal wall and the branches to the small intestine pass between the two layers of the mesentery.

Mucosa
The surface area of the small intestine mucosa is greatly increased by permanent circular folds, villi and microvilli.

The *permanent circular folds*, unlike the rugae of the stomach, are not smoothed out when the small intestine is distended (Fig. 12.25). They promote mixing of chyme as it passes along.

The *villi* are tiny finger-like projections of the mucosal layer into the intestinal lumen, about 0.5–1 mm long

(Fig. 12.26). Their covering consists of columnar epithelial cells, or *enterocytes*, with tiny *microvilli* (1 μm long) on their free border. *Goblet cells* (see Fig. 12.5) that secrete mucus are interspersed between the enterocytes. These epithelial cells enclose a network of blood capilliaries and a central lymph capillary. Lymph capillaries are called *lacteals* because absorbed fat gives the lymph a milky appearance. Absorption and some final stages of digestion of nutrients take place in the enterocytes before entering the blood and lymph capillaries. ■ **12.8**

The *intestinal glands* are simple tubular glands situated below the surface between the villi. The epithelial cells of the glands migrate upwards to form the walls of the villi replacing those at the tips as they are rubbed off by the passage of intestinal contents. The entire epithelium is replaced every 3 to 5 days. During migration, epithelial cells produce digestive enzymes that lodge in the microvilli and, together with intestinal juice, complete the chemical digestion of carbohydrates, protein and fats.

Numerous *lymph nodes* are found in the mucosa at irregular intervals throughout the length of the small intestine. The smaller ones are known as *solitary lymphatic follicles*, and collections of about 20 or 30 larger nodes situated towards the distal end of the ileum are called *aggregated lymphatic follicles* (Peyer's patches, Fig. 12.25). These lymphatic tissues, packed with defensive cells, are strategically located to neutralise ingested antigens (Ch. 15).

Blood supply
The *superior mesenteric artery* supplies the whole of the small intestine. Venous drainage is by the *superior mesenteric vein* that joins other veins to form the portal vein (see Figs 5.40 and 5.41, pp. 110 and 111). The portal vein contains a high concentration of absorbed nutrients and this blood passes through the liver before entering the hepatic veins and, ultimately, into the inferior vena cava (see Fig. 12.36).

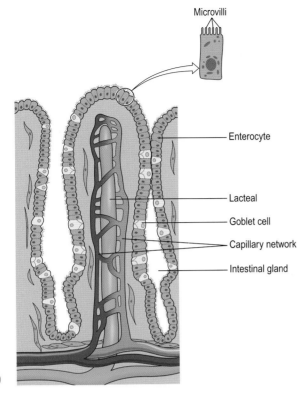

Microvilli

Enterocyte

Lacteal

Goblet cell

Capillary network

Intestinal gland

(A)

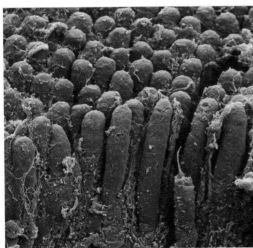

(B)

Figure 12.26 Villi. A. A highly magnified diagram of one complete villus in the small intestine. **B.** Coloured scanning electron micrograph showing many villi.

Intestinal juice

About 1500 mL of intestinal juice are secreted daily by the glands of the small intestine. It is slightly basic (alkaline) and consists of water, mucus and mineral salts.

Functions of the small intestine

The functions are:

- onward movement of its contents by peristalsis, which is increased by parasympathetic stimulation

- secretion of intestinal juice, also increased by parasympathetic stimulation
- completion of chemical digestion of carbohydrates, protein and fats in the enterocytes of the villi
- protection against infection by microbes that have survived the antimicrobial action of the hydrochloric acid in the stomach, by both solitary and aggregated lymph follicles
- secretion of the hormones cholecystokinin (CCK) and secretin
- absorption of nutrients.

Chemical digestion in the small intestine

When acid chyme passes into the small intestine it is mixed with *pancreatic juice*, *bile* and *intestinal juice*, and is in contact with the enterocytes of the villi. The digestion of all nutrients is completed:

- carbohydrates are broken down to monosaccharides
- proteins are broken down to amino acids
- fats are broken down to fatty acids and glycerol.

Pancreatic juice

Pancreatic juice is secreted by the exocrine pancreas (p. 308) and enters the duodenum at the duodenal papilla. It consists of:

- water
- mineral salts
- enzymes:
  - amylase
  - lipase
  - nucleases that digest DNA and RNA
- inactive enzyme precursors including:
  - trypsinogen
  - chymotrypsinogen.

Pancreatic juice is basic (alkaline, pH 8) because it contains significant quantities of bicarbonate ions, which are basic (alkaline) in solution. When acid stomach contents enter the duodenum they are mixed with pancreatic juice and bile and the pH is raised to between 6 and 8. This is the pH at which the pancreatic enzymes, amylase and lipase, act most effectively.

Functions

Digestion of proteins. Trypsinogen and chymotrypsinogen are inactive enzyme precursors activated by *enterokinase*, an enzyme in the microvilli, which converts them into the active proteolytic enzymes *trypsin* and *chymotrypsin*. These enzymes convert polypeptides to tripeptides, dipeptides and amino acids. It is important that they are produced as inactive precursors and are activated only upon their arrival in the duodenum, otherwise they would digest the pancreas.

303

Digestion of carbohydrates. *Pancreatic amylase* converts all digestible polysaccharides (starches) not acted upon by salivary amylase to disaccharides.

Digestion of fats. *Lipase* converts fats to fatty acids and glycerol. To aid the action of lipase, *bile salts* emulsify fats, i.e. reduce the size of the globules, increasing their surface area.

Control of secretion
The secretion of pancreatic juice is stimulated by secretin and CCK, produced by endocrine cells in the walls of the duodenum. The presence in the duodenum of acid chyme from the stomach stimulates the production of these hormones (see Fig. 12.22).

Bile

Bile, secreted by the liver, is unable to enter the duodenum when the hepatopancreatic sphincter is closed; therefore it passes from the *hepatic duct* along the *cystic duct* to the gall bladder where it is stored (see Fig. 12.38).

Bile has a pH of around 8 and between 500 and 1000 mL is secreted daily. It consists of:

- water
- mineral salts
- mucus
- bile salts
- bile pigments, mainly bilirubin
- cholesterol.

Functions
The functions of bile are explained further on page 311; in summary, these are:

- emulsification of fats in the small intestine – bile salts
- making cholesterol and fatty acids soluble, enabling their absorption along with the fat-soluble vitamins – bile salts
- excretion of *bilirubin* (a waste product from the breakdown of red blood cells), most of which is in the form of *stercobilin.*

Release from the gall bladder
After a meal, the duodenum secretes the hormones secretin and CCK during the intestinal phase of gastric secretion (p. 300). They stimulate contraction of the gall bladder and relaxation of the hepatopancreatic sphincter, expelling both bile and pancreatic juice through the duodenal papilla into the duodenum. Secretion is markedly increased when chyme entering the duodenum contains a high proportion of fat.

Intestinal secretions

The principal constituents of intestinal secretions are water, mucus and mineral salts.

Most of the digestive enzymes in the small intestine are contained in the enterocytes of the epithelium that covers the villi. Digestion of carbohydrate, protein and fat is completed by direct contact between these nutrients and the microvilli and within the enterocytes.

Chemical digestion associated with enterocytes
Alkaline intestinal juice (pH 7.8–8.0) assists in raising the pH of the intestinal contents to between 6.5 and 7.5. The enzymes that complete chemical digestion of food at the surface of the enterocytes are:

- peptidases
- lipase
- sucrase, maltase and lactase.

Peptidases such as trypsin break down polypeptides into smaller peptides and amino acids. Peptidases are secreted in an inactive form from the pancreas (to prevent them from digesting it) and must be activated by *enterokinase* in the duodenum.

The final stage of breakdown of all peptides to amino acids takes place at the surface of the enterocytes.

Lipase completes the digestion of emulsified fats to *fatty acids* and *glycerol* in the intestine.

Sucrase, maltase and *lactase* complete the digestion of carbohydrates by converting disaccharides such as sucrose, maltose and lactose to monosaccharides at the surface of the enterocytes.

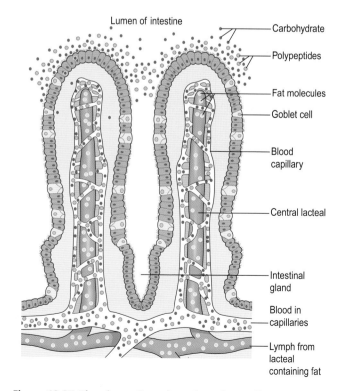

Figure 12.27 The absorption of nutrients into villi.

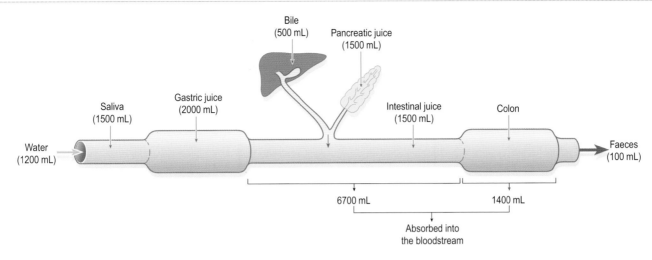

Figure 12.28 Average volumes of fluid ingested, secreted, absorbed and eliminated from the gastrointestinal tract daily.

Control of secretion

Mechanical stimulation of the intestinal glands by chyme is believed to be the main stimulus for the secretion of intestinal juice, although the hormone secretin may also be involved.

Absorption of nutrients (Fig. 12.27)

Absorption of nutrients from the small intestine through the enterocytes occurs by several processes, including diffusion, osmosis, facilitated diffusion and active transport. Water moves by osmosis; small fat-soluble substances, e.g. fatty acids and glycerol, are able to diffuse through cell membranes; while others are generally transported inside the villi by other mechanisms.

Monosaccharides and amino acids pass into the blood capillaries in the villi. Fatty acids and glycerol enter the lacteals and are transported along lymphatic vessels to the thoracic duct where they enter the circulation (Ch. 6).

A small number of proteins are absorbed unchanged, e.g. antibodies present in breast milk and oral vaccines, such as poliomyelitis vaccine.

Other nutrients such as vitamins, mineral salts and water are also absorbed from the small intestine into the blood capillaries. Fat-soluble vitamins are absorbed into the lacteals along with fatty acids and glycerol. Vitamin B_{12} combines with intrinsic factor in the stomach and is actively absorbed in the terminal ileum.

The surface area through which absorption takes place in the small intestine is greatly increased by the circular folds of mucous membrane and by the very large number of villi and microvilli present (Fig. 12.26). It has been calculated that the surface area of the small intestine is about five times that of the whole body surface.

Large amounts of fluid enter the alimentary tract each day (Fig. 12.28). Of this, only about 1500 mL is not absorbed by the small intestine, and passes into the large intestine. **12.9**

Large intestine, rectum and anal canal

Learning outcomes

After studying this section, you should be able to:

- identify the different sections of the large intestine

- describe the structure and functions of the large intestine, the rectum and the anal canal.

The large intestine is about 1.5 metres long, beginning at the *caecum* in the right iliac fossa and terminating at the *rectum* and *anal canal* deep within the pelvis. Its lumen is about 6.5 cm in diameter, larger than that of the small intestine. It forms an arch round the coiled-up small intestine (Fig. 12.29).

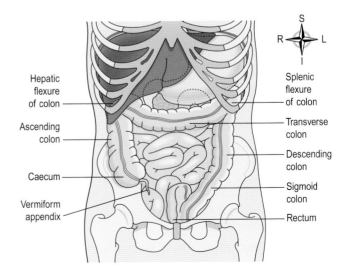

Figure 12.29 The parts of the large intestine and their positions.

305

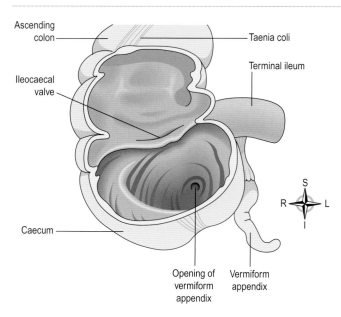

Figure 12.30 Interior of the caecum.

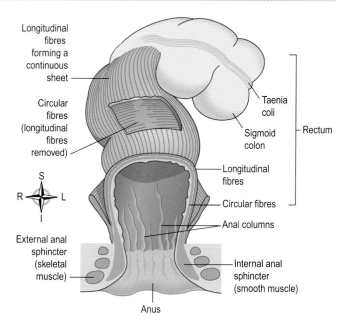

Figure 12.31 Arrangement of muscle fibres in the large intestine, rectum and anus. Sections have been removed to show the layers.

For descriptive purposes the large intestine is divided into the caecum, colon, sigmoid colon, rectum and anal canal.

The caecum
This is the first part of the large intestine (Fig. 12.30). It is a dilated region which has a blind end inferiorly and is continuous with the ascending colon superiorly. Just below the junction of the two the *ileocaecal valve* opens from the ileum. The *vermiform appendix* is a fine tube, closed at one end, which leads from the caecum. It is about 8–9 cm long and has the same structure as the walls of the large intestine but contains more lymphoid tissue. The appendix has no digestive function but can cause significant problems when it becomes inflamed (*appendicitis*, p. 325).

The colon
The colon has four parts which have the same structure and functions.

The ascending colon. This passes upwards from the caecum to the level of the liver where it curves acutely to the left at the *hepatic flexure* to become the transverse colon.

The transverse colon. This part extends across the abdominal cavity in front of the duodenum and the stomach to the area of the spleen where it forms the *splenic flexure* and curves acutely downwards to become the descending colon.

The descending colon. This passes down the left side of the abdominal cavity then curves towards the midline. At the level of the iliac crest it is known as the sigmoid colon.

The sigmoid colon. This part describes an S-shaped curve in the pelvic cavity that continues downwards to become the rectum.

The rectum
This is a slightly dilated section of the large intestine about 13 cm long. It leads from the sigmoid colon and terminates in the anal canal.

The anal canal
This is a short passage about 3.8 cm long in the adult and leads from the rectum to the exterior. Two sphincter muscles control the anus; the *internal sphincter*, consisting of smooth muscle, is under the control of the autonomic nervous system and the *external sphincter*, formed by skeletal muscle, is under voluntary control (Fig. 12.31). **12.10**

Structure
The four layers of tissue described in the basic structure of the gastrointestinal tract (Fig. 12.2) are present in the caecum, colon, the rectum and the anal canal. The arrangement of the longitudinal muscle fibres is modified in the caecum and colon. They do not form a continuous layer of tissue but are instead collected into three bands, called *taeniae coli*, which run lengthways along the caecum and colon. They stop at the junction of the sigmoid colon and the rectum. As these bands of muscle tissue are slightly shorter than the total length of the caecum and colon they give it a sacculated or puckered appearance (Fig. 12.31).

In the rectum the longitudinal muscle fibres spread out as in the basic structure and this layer therefore completely surrounds the rectum and anal canal. The anal sphincters are formed by thickening of the circular muscle layer.

In the submucosal layer there is more lymphoid tissue than in any other part of the alimentary tract, providing non-specific defence against invasion by resident and other potentially harmful microbes.

In the mucosal lining of the colon and the upper region of the rectum are large numbers of mucus-secreting goblet cells (see Fig. 12.5B) within simple tubular glands. They are not present beyond the junction between the rectum and the anal canal.

The lining membrane of the anal canal consists of stratified squamous epithelium continuous with the mucous membrane lining of the rectum above and which merges with the skin beyond the external anal sphincter. In the upper section of the anal canal the mucous membrane is arranged in 6–10 vertical folds, the *anal columns*. Each column contains a terminal branch of the superior rectal artery and vein.

Blood supply

Arterial supply is mainly by the superior and inferior mesenteric arteries (see Fig. 5.39, p. 109). The *superior mesenteric artery* supplies the caecum, ascending and most of the transverse colon. The *inferior mesenteric artery* supplies the remainder of the colon and the proximal part of the rectum. The *middle* and *inferior rectal arteries*, branches of the internal iliac arteries, supply the distal section of the rectum and the anus.

Venous drainage is mainly by the *superior* and *inferior mesenteric veins* which drain blood from the parts supplied by arteries of the same names. These veins join the splenic and gastric veins to form the portal vein (see Fig. 5.41, p. 111). Veins draining the distal part of the rectum and the anus join the *internal iliac veins*, meaning that blood from this region returns directly to the inferior cava, bypassing the portal circulation.

Functions of the large intestine, rectum and anal canal

Absorption

The contents of the ileum which pass through the ileocaecal valve into the caecum are fluid, even though a large amount of water has been absorbed in the small intestine. In the large intestine absorption of water, by osmosis, continues until the familiar semisolid consistency of faeces is achieved. Mineral salts, vitamins and some drugs are also absorbed into blood capillaries from the large intestine.

Microbial activity

The large intestine is heavily colonised by certain types of bacteria, which synthesise vitamin K and folic acid. They include *Escherichia coli*, *Enterobacter aerogenes*, *Streptococcus faecalis* and *Clostridium perfringens*. These microbes are commensals, i.e. normally harmless, in humans. However, they may become pathogenic if transferred to another part of the body, e.g. *E. coli* may cause cystitis if it gains access to the urinary bladder.

Gases in the bowel consist of some of the constituents of air, mainly nitrogen, swallowed with food and drink. Hydrogen, carbon dioxide and methane are produced by bacterial fermentation of unabsorbed nutrients, especially carbohydrate. Gases pass out of the bowel as *flatus* (wind).

Mass movement

The large intestine does not exhibit peristaltic movement as in other parts of the digestive tract. Only at fairly long intervals (about twice an hour) does a wave of strong peristalsis sweep along the transverse colon forcing its contents into the descending and sigmoid colons. This is known as *mass movement* and it is often precipitated by the entry of food into the stomach. This combination of stimulus and response is called the *gastrocolic reflex*.

Defaecation

Usually the rectum is empty, but when a mass movement forces the contents of the sigmoid colon into the rectum the nerve endings in its walls are stimulated by stretch. In infants, defaecation occurs by reflex (involuntary) action. However, during the second or third year of life children develop voluntary control of bowel function. In practical terms this acquired voluntary control means that the brain can inhibit the reflex until it is convenient to defaecate. The external anal sphincter is under conscious control through the *pudendal nerve*. Thus, defaecation involves involuntary contraction of the muscle of the rectum and relaxation of the internal anal sphincter. Contraction of the abdominal muscles and lowering of the diaphragm increase the intra-abdominal pressure (Valsalva's manoeuvre) and so assist defaecation. When the need to pass faeces is voluntarily postponed, it tends to fade until the next mass movement occurs and the reflex is initiated again. Repeated suppression of the reflex may lead to *constipation* (hard faeces, p. 282) as more water is absorbed.

Constituents of faeces. The faeces consist of a semisolid brown mass. The brown colour is due to the presence of stercobilin (p. 311 and Fig. 12.37).

Even though absorption of water takes place in the small and large intestines, water still makes up about 60–70% of the weight of the faeces. The remainder consists of:

- fibre (indigestible cellular plant and animal material)
- dead and live microbes
- epithelial cells shed from the walls of the tract
- fatty acids
- mucus secreted by the epithelial lining of the large intestine.

Mucus helps to lubricate the faeces and an adequate amount of dietary non-starch polysaccharide (NSP, fibre and previously known as roughage) ensures that the contents of the large intestine are sufficiently bulky to stimulate defaecation.

Pancreas (Fig. 12.32)

Learning outcome

After studying this section, you should be able to:

■ differentiate between the structures and functions of the exocrine and endocrine pancreas.

The pancreas is a pale grey gland weighing about 60 grams. It is about 12–15 cm long and is situated in the epigastric and left hypochondriac regions of the abdominal cavity (see Figs 3.37 and 3.38, p. 52). It consists of a broad head, a body and a narrow tail. The head lies in the curve of the duodenum, the body behind the stomach and the tail lies in front of the left kidney and just reaches the spleen. The abdominal aorta and the inferior vena cava lie behind the gland.

The pancreas is both an exocrine and endocrine gland.

The exocrine pancreas

This consists of a large number of *lobules* made up of small acini, the walls of which consist of secretory cells. Each lobule is drained by a tiny duct and these unite eventually to form the *pancreatic duct*, which extends along the whole length of the gland and opens into the duodenum. Just before entering the duodenum the pancreatic duct joins the *common bile duct* to form the hepatopancreatic ampulla. The duodenal opening of the ampulla is controlled by the hepatopancreatic sphincter (of Oddi) at the duodenal papilla.

The function of the exocrine pancreas is to produce *pancreatic juice* containing enzymes, some in the form of inactive precursors, that digest carbohydrates, proteins and fats (p. 303). As in the alimentary tract, parasympathetic stimulation increases the secretion of pancreatic juice and sympathetic stimulation depresses it.

The endocrine pancreas

Distributed throughout the gland are groups of specialised cells called the pancreatic islets (of Langerhans). The islets have no ducts so the hormones diffuse directly into the blood. The endocrine pancreas secretes the hormones *insulin* and *glucagon*, which are principally concerned with control of blood glucose levels (see Ch. 9).

Blood supply

The splenic and mesenteric arteries supply the pancreas, and venous drainage is by veins of the same names that join other veins to form the portal vein.

Liver

Learning outcomes

After studying this section, you should be able to:

■ describe the location of the liver in the abdominal cavity

■ describe the structure of a liver lobule

■ outline the functions of the liver.

The liver is the largest gland in the body, weighing between 1 and 2.3 kg. It is situated in the upper part of the abdominal cavity occupying the greater part of the right hypochondriac region, part of the epigastric region and extending into the left hypochondriac region. Its upper and anterior surfaces are smooth and curved to fit the under surface of the diaphragm (Fig. 12.33); its posterior surface is irregular in outline (Fig. 12.34).

Organs associated with the liver

Superiorly and anteriorly – diaphragm and anterior abdominal wall
Inferiorly – stomach, bile ducts, duodenum, hepatic flexure of the colon, right kidney and adrenal gland
Posteriorly – oesophagus, inferior vena cava, aorta, gall bladder, vertebral column and diaphragm
Laterally – lower ribs and diaphragm.

The liver is enclosed in a thin inelastic capsule and incompletely covered by a layer of peritoneum. Folds of peritoneum form supporting ligaments that attach the liver to

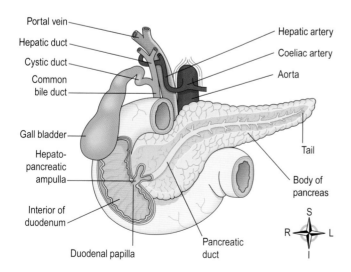

Portal vein
Hepatic duct
Cystic duct
Common bile duct
Gall bladder
Hepato-pancreatic ampulla
Interior of duodenum
Duodenal papilla
Hepatic artery
Coeliac artery
Aorta
Tail
Body of pancreas
Pancreatic duct

Figure 12.32 The pancreas in relation to the duodenum and biliary tract. Part of the anterior wall of the duodenum has been removed.

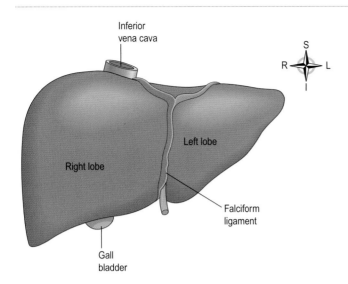

Figure 12.33 The liver. Anterior view.

the inferior surface of the diaphragm. It is held in position partly by these ligaments and partly by the pressure of the organs in the abdominal cavity.

The liver has four lobes. The two most obvious are the large *right lobe* and the smaller, wedge-shaped, *left lobe*. The other two, the *caudate* and *quadrate* lobes, are areas on the posterior surface (Fig. 12.34).

The portal fissure

This is the name given to the region on the posterior surface of the liver where various structures enter and leave the gland.

The *portal vein* enters, carrying blood from the stomach, spleen, pancreas and the small and large intestines. 12.11

The *hepatic artery* enters, carrying arterial blood. It is a branch from the coeliac artery, which branches from the abdominal aorta.

Nerve fibres, sympathetic and parasympathetic, enter here.

The *right* and *left hepatic ducts* leave, carrying bile from the liver to the gall bladder.

Lymph vessels leave the liver, draining lymph to abdominal and thoracic nodes.

Blood supply (see Figs 5.38 and 5.40)

The hepatic artery and the portal vein take blood to the liver (see Fig. 12.36). Venous return is by a variable number of hepatic veins that leave the posterior surface and immediately enter the inferior vena cava just below the diaphragm.

Structure

The lobes of the liver are made up of tiny functional units, called *lobules*, which are just visible to the naked eye (Fig. 12.35A). Liver lobules are hexagonal in outline and are formed by cuboidal cells, the *hepatocytes*, arranged in pairs of columns radiating from a central vein. Between two pairs of columns of cells are *sinusoids* (blood vessels with incomplete walls, Ch. 5) containing a mixture of blood from the tiny branches of the portal vein and hepatic artery (Fig. 12.35B). This arrangement allows the arterial blood and portal venous blood (with a high concentration of nutrients) to mix and come into close contact with the liver cells. Amongst the cells lining the sinusoids are hepatic macrophages (Kupffer cells) whose function is to ingest and destroy worn out blood cells and any foreign particles present in the blood flowing through the liver.

Blood drains from the sinusoids into *central* or *centrilobular veins*. These then merge with veins from other lobules, forming larger veins, until eventually they become the hepatic veins, which leave the liver and empty into the inferior vena cava. Figure 12.36 shows the system

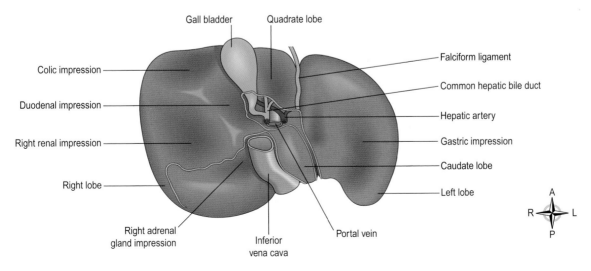

Figure 12.34 The liver. Inferior view (turned up to show the posterior surface).

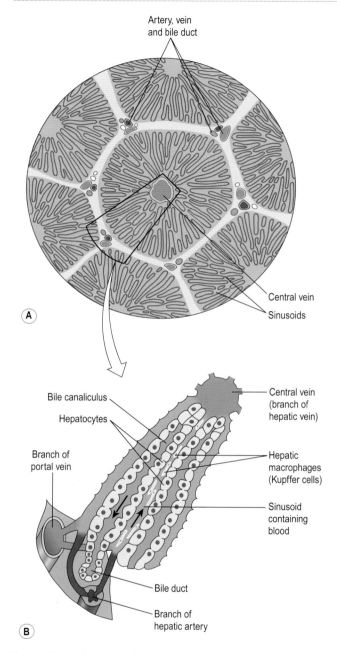

(A)

(B)

Figure 12.35 The liver lobule. A. A magnified transverse section of a liver lobule. **B.** Direction of the flow of blood and bile in a liver lobule.

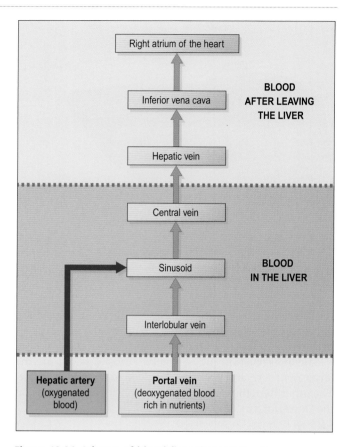

Figure 12.36 Scheme of blood flow through the liver.

Functions of the liver

The liver is an extremely active organ, which has many important functions that are described below.

Carbohydrate metabolism

The liver has an important role in maintaining plasma glucose levels. After a meal when levels rise, glucose is converted to glycogen for storage under the influence of the hormone insulin. Later, when glucose levels fall, the hormone glucagon stimulates conversion of glycogen into glucose again, keeping levels within the normal range (see Fig 12.39).

Fat metabolism

Stored fat can be converted to a form in which it can be used by the tissues to provide energy (see Fig. 12.44).

Protein metabolism

Deamination of amino acids. This process:

* removes the nitrogenous portion from amino acids that are not required for the formation of new protein; *urea* is formed from this nitrogenous portion and is excreted in urine
* breaks down nucleic acids (genetic material, e.g. DNA, see p. 438) to form *uric acid*, which is excreted in the urine.

of blood flow through the liver. One of the functions of the liver is to secrete bile. In Figure 12.35B it is seen that *bile canaliculi* run between the columns of liver cells. This means that each column of hepatocytes has a blood sinusoid on one side and a bile canaliculus on the other. The canaliculi join up to form larger bile canals until eventually they form the *right and left hepatic ducts*, which drain bile from the liver.

Lymphoid tissue and a network of lymph vessels are also present in each lobule.

Transamination. Removes the nitrogenous portion of amino acids and attaches it to other carbohydrate molecules forming new non-essential amino acids (see Fig. 12.42).

Synthesis of plasma proteins. These are formed from amino acids and include albumins, globulins and blood clotting factors (p. 62).

Breakdown of erythrocytes and defence against microbes

This is carried out by phagocytic hepatic macrophages (Kupffer cells) in the sinusoids although breakdown of red blood cells also takes place in the spleen and bone marrow.

Detoxification of drugs and toxic substances

These include ethanol (alcohol), waste products and microbial toxins. Some drugs are extensively inactivated by the liver and are not very effective when given by mouth (orally), e.g. glyceryl trinitrate. This is because after absorption from the alimentary tract, they travel in the blood to the liver where they are largely metabolised so that levels in the blood leaving the liver and which enters the systemic circulation are inadequate to achieve therapeutic effects. This is known as '*first pass metabolism*'.

Inactivation of hormones

These include insulin, glucagon, cortisol, aldosterone, thyroid and sex hormones.

Production of heat

The liver uses a considerable amount of energy, has a high metabolic rate and consequently produces a great deal of heat. It is the main heat-producing organ of the body.

Secretion of bile

The hepatocytes synthesise the constituents of bile from the mixed arterial and venous blood in the sinusoids. These include bile salts, bile pigments and cholesterol (see below).

Storage

Stored substances include:

- glycogen (see p. 315)
- fat-soluble vitamins: A, D, E, K
- iron, copper
- some water-soluble vitamins, e.g. vitamin B_{12}.

Composition of bile

Between 500 and 1000 mL of bile is secreted by the liver daily. Bile consists of:

- water
- mineral salts
- mucus

- bile pigments, mainly bilirubin
- bile salts
- cholesterol.

Functions of bile

Fat digestion. The bile acids, *cholic* and *chenodeoxycholic acid*, are synthesised by hepatocytes from cholesterol, then secreted into bile as sodium or potassium salts. In the small intestine they emulsify fats, aiding their digestion. Fatty acids are insoluble in water, which makes them very difficult to absorb through the intestinal wall. Bile salts make cholesterol and fatty acids more water-soluble, enabling both these and the fat-soluble vitamins (vitamins A, D, E and K) to be readily absorbed.

In the terminal ileum most of the bile salts are reabsorbed and return to the liver in the portal vein. This *enterohepatic circulation*, or recycling of bile salts, ensures that large amounts of bile salts enter the small intestine daily from a relatively small bile acid pool (Fig. 12.37).

Excretion of bilirubin. Bilirubin is one of the products of haemolysis of erythrocytes by hepatic macrophages (Kupffer cells) in the liver and by other macrophages in the spleen and bone marrow. Bilirubin is insoluble in water and is carried in the blood bound to the plasma protein albumin. In hepatocytes it is *conjugated* (combined) with glucuronic acid and becomes water-soluble enough to be excreted in bile. Microbes in the large

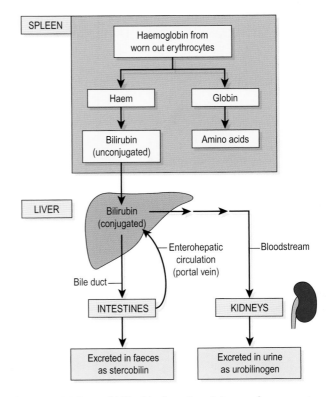

Figure 12.37 Fate of bilirubin from breakdown of worn-out erythrocytes.

intestine convert bilirubin into *stercobilin*, which is excreted in the faeces. Stercobilin colours and deodorises the faeces. A small amount is reabsorbed and excreted in urine as *urobilinogen* (Fig. 12.37). Jaundice is yellow pigmentation of the tissues, seen in the skin and conjunctiva, caused by excess blood bilirubin (p. 336).

Biliary tract

Learning outcomes

After studying this section, you should be able to:

■ describe the route taken by bile from the liver, to the gall bladder, and then to the duodenum

■ outline the structure and functions of the gall bladder.

Bile ducts (Fig. 12.38) ▓ **12.12**

The *right* and *left hepatic ducts* join to form the *common hepatic duct* just outside the portal fissure. The hepatic duct passes downwards for about 3 cm where it is joined by the *cystic duct* from the gall bladder. The cystic and hepatic ducts merge forming the *common bile duct*, which passes downwards behind the head of the pancreas. This is joined by the main pancreatic duct at the hepatopancreatic ampulla. It opens into the duodenum, at the duodenal papilla, which is controlled by the

hepatopancreatic sphincter (of Oddi). The common bile duct is about 7.5 cm long and has a diameter of about 6 mm.

Structure

The walls of the bile ducts have the same layers of tissue as those of the basic structure of the alimentary canal (Fig. 12.2). In the cystic duct the mucous membrane lining is arranged in irregular circular folds, which have the effect of a spiral valve. Bile passes through the cystic duct twice – once on its way into the gall bladder and again when it is expelled from the gall bladder into the common bile duct and then on to the duodenum.

Gall bladder

The gall bladder is a pear-shaped sac attached to the posterior surface of the liver by connective tissue. It has a *fundus* or expanded end, a *body* or main part and a *neck*, which is continuous with the cystic duct.

Structure

The wall of the gall bladder has the same layers of tissue as those of the basic structure of the alimentary canal, with some modifications.

Peritoneum. This covers only the inferior surface because the upper surface of the gall bladder is in direct contact with the liver and held in place by the visceral peritoneum that covers the liver.

Muscle layer. There is an additional layer of oblique muscle fibres.

Mucous membrane. This displays small rugae when the gall bladder is empty that disappear when it is distended with bile.

Blood supply

The *cystic artery*, a branch of the hepatic artery, supplies the gall bladder. Blood is drained away by the *cystic vein* that joins the portal vein.

Functions of the gall bladder

These include:

• reservoir for bile
• concentration of the bile by up to 10- or 15-fold, by absorption of water through the walls of the gall bladder
• release of stored bile.

When the muscle wall of the gall bladder contracts, bile passes through the bile ducts to the duodenum. Contraction is stimulated by the hormone cholecystokinin (CCK), secreted by the duodenum and the presence of fat and acid chyme in the duodenum.

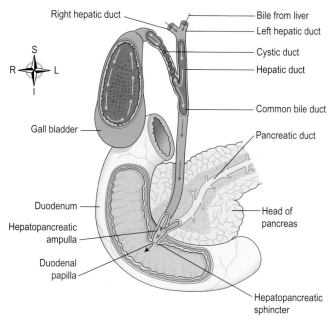

Figure 12.38 Direction of the flow of bile from the liver to the duodenum.

Relaxation of the hepatopancreatic sphincter (of Oddi) is caused by CCK and is a reflex response to contraction of the gall bladder.

Summary of digestion and absorption of nutrients

Learning outcomes

After studying this section, you should be able to:

■ list the principal digestive enzymes, their sites of action, their substrates and their products

■ describe the sites of absorption of the main nutrient groups.

Table 12.2 summarises the main digestive processes of the principal nutrient groups, the locations where these processes occur and the enzymes involved.

Metabolism

Learning outcomes

After studying this section, you should be able to:

■ discuss general principles of metabolism, including anabolism, catabolism, units of energy and metabolic rate

■ compare and contrast the metabolic rates of the body's main energy sources (carbohydrate, protein and fat)

■ describe in simple terms the central metabolic pathways; glycolysis, citric acid cycle and oxidative phosphorylation.

Metabolism constitutes all the chemical reactions that occur in the body, using nutrients to:

- provide energy by chemical oxidation of nutrients
- make new or replacement body substances.

Table 12.2 Summary showing the sites of digestion and absorption of nutrients

	Mouth	Stomach	Small intestine Digestion	Small intestine Absorption	Large intestine
Carbohydrate	*Salivary amylase:* digestible starches to disaccharides	*Hydrochloric acid:* denatures and stops action of salivary amylase	*Pancreatic amylase:* digestible starches to disaccharides *Sucrase, maltase, lactase* (in enterocytes): disaccharides to monosaccharides (mainly glucose)	Into blood capillaries of villi	–
Proteins		*Hydrochloric acid:* pepsinogen to pepsin *Pepsin:* proteins to polypeptides	*Enterokinase* (in enterocytes): chymotrypsinogen and trypsinogen (from pancreas) to chymotrypsin and trypsin *Chymotrypsin and trypsin:* polypeptides to di- and tripeptides *Peptidases* (in enterocytes): di- and tripeptides to amino acids	Into blood capillaries of villi	–
Fats	–	–	*Bile* (from liver): bile salts emulsify fats *Pancreatic lipase:* fats to fatty acids and glycerol *Lipases* (in enterocytes): fats to fatty acids and glycerol	Into the lacteals of the villi	–
Water	–	Small amount absorbed here		Most absorbed here	Remainder absorbed here
Vitamins	–	Intrinsic factor secreted for vitamin B_{12} absorption	–	Water-soluble vitamins absorbed into capillaries; fat-soluble ones into lacteals of villi	Bacteria synthesise vitamin K in colon; absorbed here

Two types of process are involved:

$$\text{large molecules} \underset{\text{anabolism}}{\overset{\text{catabolism}}{\rightleftharpoons}} \text{small molecules}$$

Catabolism. Catabolic processes break down large molecules into smaller ones releasing *chemical energy*, which is stored as adenosine triphosphate (ATP), and *heat*. Heat generated maintains core body temperature at the optimum level for chemical activity (36.8°C). Excess heat is lost, mainly through the skin (Ch. 14).

Anabolism. This is building up, or synthesis, of large molecules from smaller ones and requires a source of energy, usually ATP.

Metabolic pathways

Anabolism and catabolism usually involve a series of chemical reactions, known as metabolic pathways. These consist of 'small steps' that permit controlled, efficient and gradual transfer of energy from ATP rather than large intracellular 'explosions'. Metabolic pathways (see below) are switched on and off by hormones, providing control of metabolism and meeting individual requirements.

Both catabolic and anabolic processes occur continually in all cells. Very active tissues, such as muscle or liver, need a large energy supply to support their requirements.

Energy

The energy produced in the body may be measured and expressed in units of work (*joules*) or units of heat (*kilocalories*).

A kilocalorie (kcal) is the amount of heat required to raise the temperature of 1 litre of water by 1 degree Celsius (1°C). On a daily basis, the body's collective metabolic processes generate a total of about 3 million kilocalories.

$$1 \text{ kcal} = 4184 \text{ joules (J)} = 4.184 \text{ kilojoules (kJ)}$$

The nutritional value of carbohydrates, protein and fats eaten in the diet may be expressed in either *kilojoules per gram* or kcal per gram.

1 gram of carbohydrate provides 17 kilojoules (4 kcal)
1 gram of protein provides 17 kilojoules (4 kcal)
1 gram of fat provides 38 kilojoules (9 kcal)

Chapter 11 provides examples of foods providing these nutrients.

Energy balance

Energy balance is important as it determines changes in body weight. Body weight remains constant when energy intake is equal to energy use. When intake exceeds requirement, body weight increases, which may lead to obesity. Conversely, body weight decreases when nutrient intake does not meet energy requirements.

Table 12.3 Factors affecting metabolic rate

Factor	Effect on metabolic rate
Age	Gradually reduced with age
Gender	Higher in men than women
Height, weight	Relatively higher in larger people
Pregnancy, menstruation, lactation	Increased
Ingestion of food	Increased
Muscular activity, physical exertion	Increased
Elevated body temperature (fever)	Increased
Excess thyroid hormones	Increased
Starvation	Decreased
Emotional states	Increased

Metabolic rate 12.13

The metabolic rate is the rate at which energy is released from the fuel molecules inside cells. As most of the processes involved require oxygen and produce carbon dioxide as waste, the metabolic rate can be estimated by measuring oxygen uptake or carbon dioxide excretion.

The *basal metabolic rate* (BMR) is the rate of metabolism when the individual is at rest in a warm environment and is in the *postabsorptive state*, i.e. has not had a meal for at least 12 hours. In this state the release of energy is sufficient to meet only the essential needs of vital organs, such as the heart, lungs, nervous system and kidneys. Some of the many factors that affect metabolic rate are shown in Table 12.3. The postabsorptive state is important because the intake of food, especially protein, increases metabolic rate.

Central metabolic pathways

Much of the metabolic effort of cells is concerned with energy production to fuel cellular activities. Certain common pathways are central to this function. Fuel molecules enter these central energy-producing pathways and in a series of steps, during which a series of intermediate molecules are formed and energy is released, these fuel molecules are chemically broken down. The end results of these processes are production of energy and carbon dioxide and water (called *metabolic water*). Much of the energy is stored as ATP, although some is lost as heat. The carbon dioxide is excreted through the lungs and excess water excreted as urine.

The preferred fuel molecule is glucose, but alternatives should glucose be unavailable include amino acids, fatty acids, glycerol and occasionally nucleic acids. Each of these may enter the central energy-producing pathways and be converted to energy, carbon dioxide and water. There are three central metabolic pathways (see Fig. 12.44):

- glycolysis
- the citric acid (Krebs) cycle
- oxidative phosphorylation.

Products from glycolysis enter the citric acid cycle, and products from the citric acid cycle proceed to oxidative phosphorylation. The fates of the different fuel molecules entering the central metabolic pathways are discussed in the following sections.

Carbohydrate metabolism

Erythrocytes and neurones can use only glucose for fuel and therefore maintenance of blood glucose levels is needed to provide a constant energy source to these cells. Most other cells can also use other sources of fuel.

Digested carbohydrate, mainly glucose, is absorbed into the blood capillaries of the villi of the small intestine. It is transported by the portal circulation to the liver, where it is dealt with in several ways (Fig. 12.39):

- glucose may be oxidised to provide the chemical energy, in the form of ATP, necessary for the considerable metabolic activity which takes place in the liver itself (p. 310)
- some glucose may remain in the circulating blood to maintain the normal blood glucose of about 3.5–8 millimoles per litre (mmol/L) (63–144 mg/100 mL).

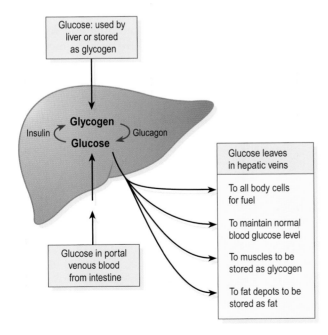

Figure 12.39 Summary of the source, distribution and use of glucose.

- some glucose, if in excess of the above requirements, may be converted by the hormone *insulin* to the insoluble polysaccharide, *glycogen*, in the liver and in skeletal muscles. The formation of glycogen inside cells is a means of storing carbohydrate without upsetting the osmotic equilibrium. Before it can be used to maintain blood levels or to provide ATP it must be broken down again into its constituent glucose units. Liver glycogen constitutes a store of glucose used for liver activity and to maintain the blood glucose level. Muscle glycogen stores provide the glucose requirement of muscle activity. *Glucagon*, *adrenaline* (*epinephrine*) and *thyroxine* are the main hormones associated with the breakdown of glycogen to glucose. These processes can be summarised:

$$\text{glucose} \xrightleftharpoons[\text{glucagon}]{\text{insulin}} \text{glycogen}$$

- carbohydrate in excess of that required to maintain the blood glucose level and glycogen stores in the tissues is converted to fat and stored in the fat depots.

All body cells require energy to carry out their metabolic processes including multiplication for replacement of worn out cells, muscle contraction and synthesis of glandular secretions. The oxidation of carbohydrate and fat provides most of the energy required by the body. When glycogen stores are low and more glucose is needed, the body can make glucose from non-carbohydrate sources, e.g. amino acids, glycerol. This is called *gluconeogenesis* (formation of new glucose).

Carbohydrate and energy release (Fig. 12.40)

Glucose is broken down in the body releasing energy, carbon dioxide and metabolic water. Catabolism of glucose occurs in a series of steps with a little energy being released at each stage. The total number of ATP molecules which may be generated from the complete breakdown of one molecule of glucose is 38, but for this to be achieved the process must occur in the presence of oxygen (aerobically). In the absence of oxygen (anaerobically) this number is greatly reduced; the process is therefore much less efficient. ▮ **12.14**

Aerobic respiration (catabolism). Aerobic catabolism of glucose can occur only when the oxygen supply is adequate, and is the process by which energy is released during prolonged, manageable exercise. When exercise levels become very intense, the energy requirements of muscles outstrip the oxygen supply, and anaerobic breakdown then occurs. Such high levels of activity can be sustained for only short periods, because there is accumulation of wastes (mainly lactic acid) and reduced efficiency of the energy production process.

The first stage of glucose catabolism is *glycolysis*. This is an anaerobic process that takes place in the cytoplasm

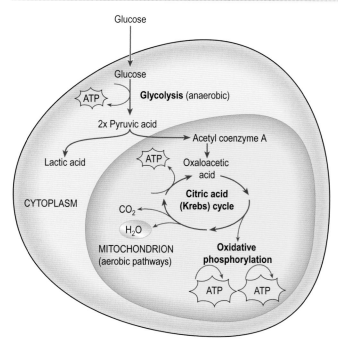

Figure 12.40 Oxidation of glucose.

of the cell. Through a number of intermediate steps one glucose molecule is converted to two molecules of pyruvic acid, with the net production of two molecules of ATP. The remainder of the considerable energy stores locked up in the original molecule of glucose is released only if there is enough oxygen to allow the pyruvic acid molecules to enter the biochemical roundabout called the *citric acid cycle* (Fig. 12.40). This takes place in the mitochondria of the cell and is oxygen dependent. For every two molecules of pyruvic acid entering the citric acid cycle, a further two molecules of ATP are formed but this is still far short of the maximum possible 38 ATP molecules. The remaining 34 molecules of ATP come from the third energy-generating process, *oxidative phosphorylation*, a process dependent on hydrogen atoms released during earlier stages of glucose breakdown. Oxidative phosphorylation, like the citric acid cycle, can occur only in the presence of oxygen and takes place in the mitochondria.

Anaerobic catabolism. When oxygen levels in the cell are low, the molecule of glucose still undergoes glycolysis and is split into two molecules of pyruvic acid, because glycolysis is an anaerobic process. However, the pyruvic acid does not enter the citric acid cycle or progress to oxidative phosphorylation; instead it is converted anaerobically to lactic acid. Build-up of lactic acid causes the pain and cramps of overexercised muscles. When oxygen levels are restored, lactic acid is reconverted to pyruvic acid, which may then enter the citric acid cycle.

Fate of the end products of carbohydrate metabolism

Lactic acid. Some of the lactic acid produced by anaerobic catabolism of glucose may be oxidised in the cells to carbon dioxide and water but first it must be changed back to pyruvic acid. If complete oxidation does not take place, lactic acid passes to the liver in the circulating blood where it is converted to glucose and may then take any of the pathways open to glucose (Fig. 12.39).

Carbon dioxide. This is excreted from the body as a gas by the lungs.

Metabolic water. This is added to the considerable amount of water already present in the body; excess is excreted as urine by the kidneys.

Protein metabolism

Dietary protein consists of a number of amino acids. About 20 amino acids have been named and nine of these are described as *essential* because they cannot be synthesised in the body. The others are *non-essential* amino acids because they can be synthesised by many tissues. The enzymes involved in this process are called *transaminases*. Digestion breaks down dietary protein into its constituent amino acids in preparation for absorption into the blood capillaries of the villi in the small intestine. Amino acids are transported in the portal circulation to the liver and then into the general circulation, thus making them available to all body cells and tissues. Different cells choose from those available the particular amino acids required for building or repairing their specific type of tissue and for synthesising their secretions, e.g. antibodies, enzymes or hormones.

Amino acids not required for building and repairing body tissues cannot be stored and are broken down in the liver (see deamination below).

Amino acid pool (Fig. 12.41)

A small pool of amino acids is maintained within the body. This is the source from which the body cells draw the amino acids they need to synthesise their own materials, e.g. new cells or cell components, secretions such as enzymes, hormones and plasma proteins.

Sources of amino acids
Exogenous. These are derived from dietary protein.

Endogenous. These are obtained from the breakdown of existing body proteins. In adults, about 80–100 g of protein are broken down and replaced each day. The entire intestinal mucosa is replaced about every 5 days.

Loss of amino acids
Deamination. Amino acids not needed by the body are broken down, or deaminated, mainly in the liver. The

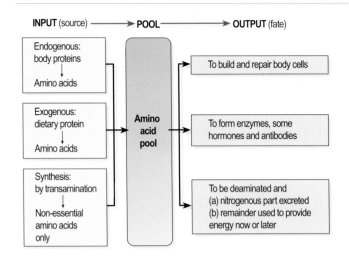

Figure 12.41 Sources and use of amino acids in the body.

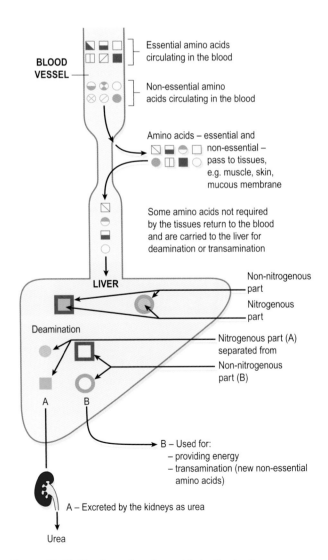

Figure 12.42 The fate of amino acids in the body.

nitrogenous part, the amino group (NH$_2$), is converted to ammonia (NH$_3$) and then combined with carbon dioxide forming *urea*, which is excreted in the urine. The remaining part is used to provide energy, as glucose by gluconeogenesis, or stored as fat, if in excess of immediate requirements.

Excretion. The faeces contain a considerable amount of protein within cells shed from the lining of the alimentary tract.

Endogenous and exogenous amino acids are mixed in the 'pool' and the body is said to be in *nitrogen balance* when the rate of removal from the pool is equal to the additions to it. Unlike carbohydrates, the body has no capacity for the storage of amino acids except for this relatively small pool. Figure 12.42 depicts what happens to amino acids in the body.

Amino acids and energy release (see Fig. 12.44)

Proteins, in the form of amino acids, are potential fuel molecules that are used by the body only when other energy sources are low, e.g. in starvation. To supply the amino acids for use as fuel, in extreme situations, the body breaks down muscle, its main protein source. Some amino acids can be converted directly to glucose, which enters glycolysis. Other amino acids are changed to intermediate compounds of the central metabolic pathways, e.g. acetyl coenzyme A or oxaloacetic acid, and therefore enter the system at a later stage.

Fat metabolism (Fig. 12.43)

Fat is synthesised from excess dietary carbohydrates and proteins, and stored in the fat depots, i.e. under the skin, in the omentum or around the kidneys.

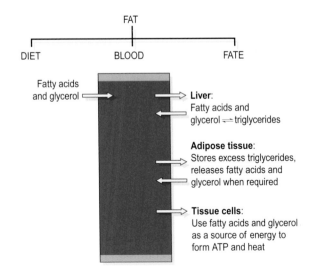

Figure 12.43 Sources, distribution and use of fats in the body.

Fats that have been digested and absorbed as fatty acids and glycerol into the lacteals are transported via the cisterna chyli and the thoracic duct of the lymphatic system (Ch. 6) to the bloodstream and so, by a circuitous route, to the liver. Fatty acids and glycerol circulating in the blood are used by the cells to provide energy and to synthesise some of their secretions. In the liver some fatty acids and glycerol are used to provide energy and heat, and some are recombined forming *triglycerides*, the form in which fat is stored. A triglyceride consists of three fatty acids chemically combined with a glycerol molecule (see Fig. 2.9, p. 27). When required, triglycerides are converted back to fatty acids and glycerol and used to provide energy. The end products of fat metabolism are chemical energy, heat, carbon dioxide and water.

Fatty acids and energy release

When body tissues are deprived of glucose, as occurs in prolonged fasting, starvation, energy-restricted diets or during strenuous exercise, the body uses alternative energy sources, mainly fat stores. Fatty acids may be converted to acetyl coenzyme A, and enter the energy production pathway in that form. One consequence of this is accumulation of *ketone bodies*, which are produced in the liver from acetyl coenzyme A when levels are too high for processing through the citric acid cycle (see Fig. 12.44). Ketone bodies then enter the blood and can be used by other body tissues, including the brain (which is usually glucose dependent) as a source of fuel. However, at high concentrations, ketone bodies are toxic, particularly to the brain. Ketone bodies include acetone and some weak organic acids. Normally levels are low because they are used as soon as they are produced. When production exceeds use, in the situations mentioned above, levels rise causing *ketosis*. Ketosis is associated with acidosis, which can lead to coma or even death if severe. Excretion of excess ketone bodies is via:

- the urine (ketonuria)
- the lungs, giving the breath a characteristic sweet smell of acetone or 'pear drops'.

In ketosis, compensation is required to maintain acid–base balance. This is achieved by buffer systems that excrete excess acid (hydrogen ions) by the lungs, through hyperventilation, or kidneys. In health, ketosis is self-limiting and ketone body production stops when fasting or exercise ceases. Ketoacidosis is associated with uncontrolled type 1 diabetes mellitus (p. 237).

Glycerol and energy release (Fig. 12.44)

The body converts glycerol from the degradation of fats into one of the intermediary compounds produced during glycolysis, and in this form it enters the central metabolic pathways.

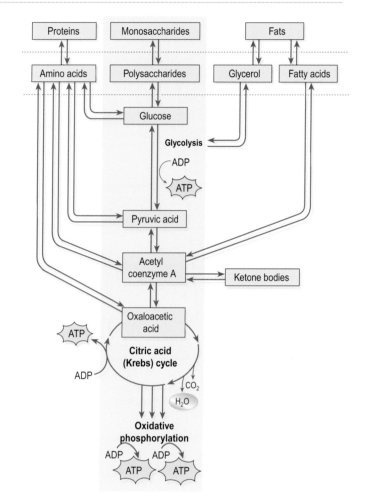

Figure 12.44 Summary of the fates of the three main energy sources in the central metabolic pathways.

Effects of ageing on the digestive system

Learning outcome

After studying this section you, should be able to:

■ describe the effects of ageing on the digestive system.

Loss of many teeth, e.g. through periodontal disease, may cause difficulty chewing which it turn restricts dietary choices. A reduction in the muscle mass of the tongue and lessened salivation can exacerbate this. The sensitivity of taste buds declines with age (p. 207).

Peristalsis within the alimentary canal reduces, which predisposes to constipation (p. 319). Other features of ageing such as lessened mobility or poor cognitive function also contribute to constipation unless dietary NSP (fibre) is increased and an adequate fluid intake is maintained.

Liver mass decreases with age and this is accompanied by a variable decline in its reserve capacity which can impair metabolism, including breakdown of drugs that may lead to toxicity.

In older adults there is a reduction in skeletal muscle mass and also responsiveness to hormones; including adrenaline, noradrenaline and thyroid hormones, contributing to a lower basal metabolic rate (BMR). Limited physical activity or inactivity also reduce BMR. A reduction in BMR that is not accompanied by a lower dietary intake predisposes to obesity and its consequences (p. 284).

Table 12.4 Common signs and symptoms of gastrointestinal disorders

Sign/symptom	Definition and description
Abdominal pain	This is caused by stretching of smooth muscle or organ capsules. The location is described with reference to the regions of the abdomen (see Fig. 3.38).
Anorexia	Loss of appetite which prevents or markedly reduces eating. When severe and ongoing, it is accompanied by weight loss.
Constipation	Passing faeces less frequently than normal and/or passing hard faeces. Normal frequency varies greatly between individuals between 3 times daily and 3 times per week.
Diarrhoea	Unusually frequent passing of loose or watery faeces. Normally most fluid in the GI tract is reabsorbed (see Fig. 12.28). Diarrhoea arises when water reabsorption from the intestines is reduced and/or intestinal motility is increased.
Dysphagia	Difficulty swallowing
Haematemesis	Vomiting of blood, either fresh blood or partly digested (described as 'coffee grounds').
Melaena	Passing blood in the faeces. Very small amounts are only found by testing for faecal occult (hidden) blood (FOB).
Nausea	Feeling of sickness, which usually precedes vomiting. It may be accompanied by profuse salivation and tachycardia.
Vomiting	An (involuntary) reflex in which there is forceful ejection of stomach contents through the mouth. Vomiting follows stimulation of, for example the pharynx, oesophagus, stomach or the vomiting centre in the medulla, e.g. by drugs. Co-ordinated by the medulla; the glottis closes, the diaphragm contacts, the upper oesophageal sphincter relaxes; strong waves of reverse peristalsis in the stomach then expel its contents upwards. If severe, consequences include disturbance of fluid, electrolyte and acid-base balance (metabolic alkalosis, as excessive H^+ is lost).

This section considers disorders of the digestive system. Table 12.4 lists some common signs and symptoms of gastrointestinal disorders.

Diseases of the mouth

Learning outcomes

After studying this section, you should be able to:

- discuss the main inflammatory and infectious conditions of the mouth
- outline the sites and effects of oral squamous cell carcinoma
- distinguish between cleft lip and cleft palate, including describing the anatomical abnormalities involved.

Inflammatory and infectious conditions

Injury may be caused to tissues in and around the mouth by food and other ingested substances, if they are corrosive, abrasive or excessively hot or cold. The mouth contains a large number and variety of normally harmless commensal micro-organisms. The antibacterial action of saliva helps to limit their growth, but the presence of dental plaque and residual foodstuffs, especially sugars, in the mouth can promote infection. Inflammation of the mouth is known as *stomatitis*, and inflammation of the gums as *gingivitis*.

Thrush (oral candidiasis)

This acute fungal infection is caused by the yeast *Candida albicans*, which occurs when the commensal microbe grows in white patches on the tongue and oral mucosa. In adults it causes opportunistic infection mainly in debilitated people and in those whose immunity is lowered by, e.g., steroids, antibiotics or cytotoxic drugs. In children it occurs most commonly in bottle-fed babies. *Chronic thrush* may develop, affecting the roof of the mouth in people who wear dentures. The fungus survives in fine grooves on the upper surface of the denture and repeatedly reinfects the oral mucosa. The same fungus is also responsible for sexually transmitted infections (p. 466).

Gingivitis

This is inflammation of the gums, which may be acute or, much more commonly, chronic. Chronic gingivitis is a common inflammatory condition that occurs in response to accumulation of bacterial plaque around the teeth. It causes bleeding gums and gradually destroys the tissues that support the teeth, which eventually loosen and may fall out.

Recurrent aphthous ulceration

This common condition features extremely painful ulcers that occur singly or in crops in any part of the mouth. The cause is unknown.

Viral infections

These are usually caused by one type of herpes simplex virus, HSV-1.

Acute herpetic gingivostomatitis. Inflammation of the mouth and gums is caused by herpes simplex-1 virus and is the most common oral virus infection. It is characterised by extensive and very painful ulceration.

Secondary or recurrent herpes lesions (cold sores). Lesions, caused by herpes simplex-1 virus, occur round the nose and on the lips. After an outbreak the viruses remain dormant within local nerves. Later outbreaks, usually at the same site, are precipitated by a variety of stimuli including exposure to UV rays (strong sunlight) and impaired immune response.

Tumours of the mouth

Squamous cell carcinoma

This is the most common type of malignant tumour in the mouth. It affects mainly older adults and carries a poor prognosis. The usual sites are the floor of the mouth and the edge of the tongue. Ulceration occurs frequently and there is early spread to surrounding tissues and cervical lymph nodes, in which case, the prognosis is poor.

Congenital disorders

Cleft palate and cleft lip (harelip)

During embryonic development, the roof of the mouth (hard palate) develops as two separate (right and left) halves; this occurs from the lips anteriorly to the uvula posteriorly. Before birth, these two halves normally fuse along the midline (Fig. 12.45A). If fusion is incomplete, a cleft (division) remains, which may be very minor, or it may be substantial. *Cleft lip* (Fig. 12.45B) ranges from a minor notch in the upper lip to a more extensive condition when the lip is completely split in one or two places and the nose is involved. In *cleft palate*, there is a gap between the two halves of the palate, which creates a channel of communication between the mouth and the nasal cavity (Fig. 12.45C). Contributing factors include genetic abnormalities, and certain drugs or poor nutrition between weeks 7 and 12 of pregnancy.

Drinking, eating and development of speech cannot take place normally until the defect has been surgically repaired.

Dental caries

Tooth decay starts with discolouration and then formation of cavities (caries). It arises when bacteria present in

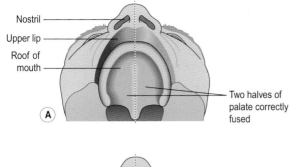

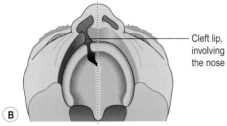

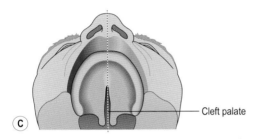

Figure 12.45 Cleft lip and cleft palate. A. Normal hard palate. **B.** Cleft lip. **C.** Cleft palate.

plaque on the teeth act on sugars forming acid, which may eventually destroy the hard parts of the teeth. Caries can be prevented by good oral hygiene.

Diseases of the pharynx

See tonsillitis and diphtheria (p. 262).

Diseases of salivary glands

Learning outcomes

After studying this section, you should be able to:

■ outline the pathophysiology of mumps

■ describe the most common tumours of the salivary glands.

Mumps

This is an acute inflammatory condition of the salivary glands, especially the parotids. It is caused by the mumps virus, one of the parainfluenza group. The virus is spread by inhalation of infected droplets. Viruses multiply elsewhere in the body before spreading to the salivary glands. The virus is most infectious for 1–2 days before and 5 days after symptoms appear. Complications may affect:

● the brain, causing meningitis (see Ch. 7) or meningoencephalitis

● the testes, causing orchitis (testicular inflammation) after puberty and sometimes atrophy of the glands and sterility.

In developed countries, children are usually vaccinated against mumps in their preschool years.

Tumours of the salivary glands

Salivary adenoma

This benign tumour occurs mainly in the parotid gland and is the most common tumour of the salivary glands. A second tumour may develop in the same gland several years after the first has been removed and it occasionally undergoes malignant change.

Carcinoma

Malignant tumours most commonly affect the parotid glands. Some forms have a tendency to infiltrate nerves in the surrounding tissues, causing severe pain. Lymph spread is to the cervical nodes.

Diseases of the oesophagus

Learning outcomes

After studying this section, you should be able to:

■ explain how oesophageal varices develop

■ discuss the main inflammatory conditions of the oesophagus

■ describe the main oesophageal tumours

■ define oesophageal atresia and tracheo-oesophageal fistula.

Oesophageal varices (Fig. 12.46)

In conditions such as cirrhosis (p. 334) or venous thrombosis, blood flow into the liver via the portal vein is impeded and blood pressure within the portal system rises (*portal hypertension*). This forces blood from the portal vein into anastomotic veins, which redirect (shunt) blood into the systemic venous circulation, bypassing the liver. Fifty percent or more of the portal blood may be shunted into anastomotic veins, leading to rising pressure in these veins too. One route taken by the shunted blood is into veins of the lower oesophagus, which become distended and weakened by the abnormally high volume of blood. *Varices* (localised dilations of veins) develop when

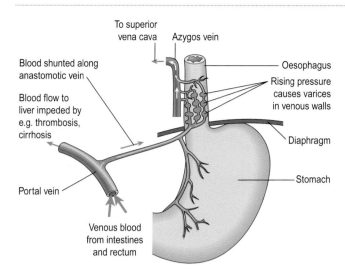

Figure 12.46 Oesophageal varices.

the weakest regions of the vessel wall bulge outwards into the lumen of the oesophagus, and, being thin walled and fragile, they are easily eroded or traumatised by swallowed food. Bleeding may be slight, but chronic, leading to iron deficiency anaemia (p. 74); however, sudden rupture can cause life-threatening haemorrhage.

Inflammatory and infectious conditions

Acute oesophagitis

This arises after caustic materials are swallowed and also if immunocompromised people acquire severe fungal infections, typically candidiasis (p. 320), or viral infections, e.g. herpes simplex. *Dysphagia* (difficulty in swallowing) is usually present. Following severe injury, healing often causes fibrosis, and there is a risk of oesophageal stricture developing later, as the fibrous tissue shrinks.

Gastro-oesophageal reflux disease (GORD)

This condition, the commonest cause of indigestion (or 'heartburn'), is caused by persistent regurgitation of acidic gastric juice into the oesophagus, causing irritation, inflammation and painful ulceration. Haemorrhage occurs when blood vessels are eroded. Persistent reflux leads to chronic inflammation and if damage is extensive, secondary healing with fibrosis occurs. Shrinkage of mature fibrous tissue may cause stricture of the oesophagus. This condition sometimes gives rise to Barrett's oesophagus (see below). Reflux of gastric contents is associated with:

- increase in the intra-abdominal pressure, e.g. in pregnancy, constipation and obesity
- low levels of secretion of the hormone gastrin, leading to reduced sphincter action at the lower end of the oesophagus
- the presence of hiatus hernia (p. 329).

Barrett's oesophagus

This condition develops after long-standing reflux oesophagitis. Columnar cells resembling those found in the stomach replace the squamous epithelium of the lower oesophagus. This is a premalignant state carrying an increased risk of subsequent malignancy.

Achalasia

This may occur at any age but is most common in middle life. Peristalsis of the lower oesophagus is impaired and the lower oesophageal sphincter fails to relax during swallowing, causing dysphagia, regurgitation of gastric contents and aspiration pneumonia. The oesophagus becomes dilated and the muscle layer hypertrophies. Autonomic nerve supply to the oesophageal muscle is abnormal, but the cause is not known.

Tumours of the oesophagus

Benign tumours are rare, accounting for only 5% of oesophageal tumours.

Malignant tumours

These occur more often in males than females. They are most common in the lower oesophagus but can arise at any level. Both types of tumour, described below, tend to begin as an ulcer that spreads round the circumference causing a stricture that results in dysphagia. By the time of diagnosis, local spread has usually occurred and the prognosis is very poor.

The geographical incidence of *squamous cell carcinoma* varies greatly worldwide. It is associated with long-term high alcohol intake and cigarette smoking. Other predisposing factors are believed to include obesity, low fruit and vegetable consumption, and chewing betel nuts or tobacco.

Adenocarcinoma usually develops from Barrett's oesophagus (see above).

Congenital abnormalities

The most common congenital abnormalities of the oesophagus are:

- *oesophageal atresia*, in which the lumen is narrow or blocked
- *tracheo-oesophageal fistula*, in which there is an opening (fistula) between the oesophagus and the trachea through which milk or regurgitated gastric contents are aspirated.

One or both abnormalities may be present. The causes are unknown.

Diseases of the stomach

Learning outcomes

After studying this section, you should be able to:

- compare the main features of chronic and acute gastritis

- discuss the pathophysiology of peptic ulcer disease

- describe the main tumours of the stomach and their consequences

- define the term congenital pyloric stenosis.

Gastritis

Inflammation of the stomach can be an acute or chronic condition.

Acute gastritis

This is usually a response to irritant drugs or alcohol. The drugs most commonly implicated are non-steroidal anti-inflammatory drugs (NSAIDs) including aspirin, even at low doses, although many others may also be involved. Other causes include the initial response to *Helicobacter pylori* infection (see below) and severe physiological stress, e.g. extensive burns and multiple organ failure.

There are varying degrees of severity. Mild cases can be asymptomatic or may present with nausea and vomiting associated with inflammatory changes of the gastric mucosa. Erosions, which are characterised by tissue loss affecting the superficial layers of the gastric mucosa may also occur. In more serious cases, multiple erosions may result in life-threatening haemorrhage causing *haematemesis* (vomiting of frank blood or black 'coffee grounds' when there has been time for digestion of blood to occur) and *melaena* (passing black tarry faeces), especially in older adults.

The outcome depends on the extent of the damage. In many cases recovery is uneventful after the cause is removed. Where there has been extensive tissue damage, healing is by fibrosis causing reduced elasticity and peristalsis.

Chronic gastritis

Chronic gastritis is a milder but longer-lasting condition. It is usually associated with *Helicobacter pylori* but is sometimes due to autoimmune disease or chemical injury. It is more common in later life.

Helicobacter-associated gastritis. *Helicobacter pylori* is a bacterium that can survive in the gastric mucosa and is commonly associated with gastric conditions, especially chronic gastritis and peptic ulcer disease.

Autoimmune chronic gastritis. This is a progressive disease. Destructive inflammatory changes that begin on the surface of the mucous membrane may extend to affect its whole thickness, including the gastric glands. When this stage is reached, secretion of hydrochloric acid and intrinsic factor are markedly reduced. The antigens are the gastric parietal cells and the intrinsic factor they secrete. When the parietal cells are destroyed as a result of this autoimmune condition, the inflammation subsides. The causes of the autoimmunity are not known but there is a familial predisposition and an association with thyroid disorders. Secondary consequences include:

- pernicious anaemia due to lack of intrinsic factor (p. 74)
- increased risk of cancer of the stomach.

Peptic ulcer disease

Ulceration involves the full thickness of the gastrointestinal mucosa and penetrates the muscle layer (Fig. 12.47). It is caused by disruption of the normal balance between the corrosive effect of gastric juice and the protective effect of mucus on the gastric epithelial cells. It may be viewed as an extension of the gastric erosions found in acute gastritis. The most common sites for ulcers are the stomach and the first few centimetres of the duodenum. More rarely they occur in the oesophagus and round the anastomosis of the stomach and small intestine, following gastrectomy. The incidence of peptic ulcers is greater in men than women and increases with age. The underlying causes are not known but there is a strong association with *H. pylori* infection. It is believed that *H. pylori,* some drugs, e.g. non-steroidal anti-inflammatory drugs (NSAIDs), and smoking may impair the gastric mucosal defences in some people. However, *H. pylori* is present in many people who show no signs of peptic ulcer disease.

If gastric mucosal protection is impaired, the epithelium can be exposed to gastric acid causing the initial cell

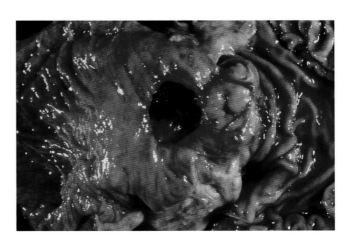

Figure 12.47 Peptic ulceration: a large duodenal ulcer.

damage that leads to ulceration. The main protective mechanisms are: a good blood supply, adequate mucus secretion and efficient epithelial cell replacement.

Blood supply. Reduced blood flow and ischaemia may be caused by cigarette smoking and severe stress, either physical or mental. In stressful situations the accompanying sympathetic activity causes constriction of the blood vessels supplying the alimentary tract.

Secretion of mucus. The composition and the amount of mucus may be altered, e.g.:

- by regular and prolonged use of aspirin and other anti-inflammatory drugs
- by the reflux of bile acids and salts
- in chronic gastritis.

Epithelial cell replacement. There is normally a rapid turnover of gastric and intestinal epithelial cells. This may be reduced:

- by raised levels of steroid hormones, e.g. in response to stress or when they are used as drugs
- in chronic gastritis
- by radiotherapy and cytotoxic drugs.

Acute peptic ulcers

These lesions may be single or multiple. They are found in many sites in the stomach and in the first few centimetres of the duodenum. Their development is often associated with acute gastritis, severe stress, e.g. severe illness, shock, burns, severe emotional disturbance and following major surgery. Healing without the formation of fibrous tissue usually occurs when the stressor is removed, although haemorrhage, which may be life-threatening, can be a complication.

Chronic peptic ulcers

These ulcers are 2–3 times more common in the duodenum than the stomach. They usually occur singly in the pylorus of the stomach or in the duodenum. *H. pylori* is found in 90% of people with duodenal ulcers and in 70% of those with gastric ulcers. The remaining gastric ulcers are almost entirely due to NSAIDs. Smoking predisposes to peptic ulceration and delays healing. Healing occurs with the formation of fibrous tissue and its subsequent shrinkage may cause:

- stricture of the lumen of the stomach
- gastric outflow obstruction or stenosis of the pyloric sphincter
- adhesions to adjacent structures, e.g. pancreas, liver, transverse colon.

Complications of peptic ulcers

Haemorrhage When a major artery is eroded a serious and possibly life-threatening haemorrhage may occur, causing shock (p. 118), haematemesis and/or melaena.

Perforation When an ulcer erodes through the full thickness of the wall of the stomach or duodenum their contents enter the peritoneal cavity, causing acute peritonitis (p. 325).

Infected inflammatory material may collect under the diaphragm, forming a *subphrenic abscess* (see Fig. 12.48) and the infection may spread through the diaphragm to the pleural cavity.

Anaemia Chronic persistent low level bleeding from an ulcer may lead to development of iron deficiency anaemia (p. 74).

Gastric outflow obstruction Also known as *pyloric stenosis*, fibrous tissue formed as an ulcer in the pyloric region heals, causes narrowing of the pylorus that obstructs outflow from the stomach and results in persistent vomiting.

Malignancy This is frequently associated with chronic gastritis caused by *H. pylori*.

Tumours of the stomach

Benign tumours of the stomach are rare.

Malignant tumours

This is a common malignancy that occurs more frequently in men than women and the incidence increases sharply after 50 years of age. The causes have not been established, but there appears to be a link with *Helicobacter pylori* infection in some 60–70% of cases. Smoking, alcohol and diets high in salted, smoked and pickled food have also been implicated. Local growth of the tumour gradually destroys the normal tissue so that achlorhydria (reduced hydrochloric acid secretion) and pernicious anaemia are frequently secondary features. As the tumour grows, the surface may ulcerate and become infected, especially when achlorhydria develops.

This condition carries a poor prognosis because spread has often already occurred prior to diagnosis. Local spread is to adjacent organs, e.g. the oesophagus, duodenum and pancreas and also to the peritoneal cavity when the outermost layer, the serosa, is affected. Spread via the blood is by the hepatic portal vein to the liver where tumour cells may lodge causing metastases. Lymphatic spread is also common, initially to nearby nodes and later to more distant ones.

Congenital pyloric stenosis

In this condition there is spasmodic constriction of the pyloric sphincter, characteristic projectile vomiting and failure to put on weight. In an attempt to overcome the spasms, hypertrophy of the muscle of the pylorus develops, causing pyloric obstruction 2–3 weeks after birth. The cause is not known but there is a familial tendency and this condition is more common in boys.

Diseases of the intestines

Diseases of the small and large intestines are described together because they have certain characteristics in common and some conditions affect both.

Appendicitis

The lumen of the appendix is very small and there is little room for swelling when it becomes inflamed. The initial cause of inflammation is not always clear. Microbial infection is commonly superimposed on obstruction by, for example, hard faecal matter (*faecoliths*), kinking or a foreign body. Inflammatory exudate, with fibrin and phagocytes, causes swelling and ulceration of the mucous membrane lining. In the initial stages, the pain of appendicitis is usually located in the central area of the abdomen. After a few hours, the pain typically shifts and becomes localised to the region above the appendix (the right iliac fossa). In mild cases the inflammation subsides and healing takes place. In more severe cases microbial growth progresses, leading to suppuration, abscess formation and further congestion. The rising pressure inside the appendix occludes first the veins, then the arteries and ischaemia develops, followed by gangrene and rupture.

Complications of appendicitis

Peritonitis. The peritoneum becomes acutely inflamed, the blood vessels dilate and excess serous fluid is secreted. It occurs as a complication of appendicitis when:

- microbes spread through the wall of the appendix and infect the peritoneum
- an appendix abscess (Fig. 12.48) ruptures and pus enters the peritoneal cavity

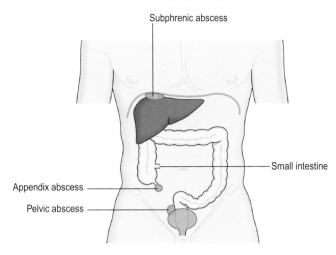

Figure 12.48 Abscess formation: complication of appendicitis.

- the appendix becomes gangrenous and ruptures, discharging its contents into the peritoneal cavity.

Abscess formation. The most common are:

- *subphrenic abscess*, between the liver and diaphragm, from which infection may spread upwards to the pleura, pericardium and mediastinal structures
- *pelvic abscess* from which infection may spread to adjacent structures (Fig. 12.48).

Adhesions. When healing takes place bands of fibrous scar tissue (adhesions) form and later shrinkage may cause:

- stricture or obstruction of the bowel
- limitation of the movement of a loop of bowel, which may twist around the adhesion causing a type of bowel obstruction called a volvulus (p. 330).

Gastrointestinal infections

The incidence of these diseases varies considerably but they represent a major cause of morbidity and mortality worldwide. Public health measures including clean, safe drinking water and effective sewage disposal, and safe food hygiene practices greatly reduce their spread: many are highly contagious. As many are spread by the faecal–oral route, meticulous handwashing after defaecation and contact between the hands and any potentially contaminated material is essential, especially in healthcare facilities. Contamination of drinking water results in diarrhoeal diseases that are a major cause of illness in all age groups and infant death in developing countries.

Typhoid and paratyphoid (enteric) fever

Typhoid and paratyphoid fevers are caused by *Salmonella typhi* and *S. paratyphi A* or *B*, respectively. Both are common in some tropical countries and both are spread by the faecal–oral route from food, water or fomites contaminated by individuals either suffering from the illness or who are carriers (see below).

The incubation period is about 10–14 days during which time bacteria invade the lymphoid tissue of the small intestine, especially the aggregated lymph follicles (Peyer's patches). Thereafter, the microbes spread via the blood to the liver, spleen and gallbladder. A bacteraemic period (febrile illness) follows accompanied by malaise, headache, drowsiness and aching limbs. The intestinal lymphoid tissue becomes acutely inflamed and ulcerated although healing usually follows. The spleen becomes enlarged (splenomegaly) and red spots are typically seen on the skin, especially of the chest and back.

Without treatment, severe, and often fatal, illness is common 2 weeks after the onset of illness. Complications due to spread of microbes during the bacteraemic phase include pneumonia, meningitis and typhoid cholecystitis in which microbes multiply in the gall bladder and are secreted in the bile, reinfecting the intestine (Fig. 12.49). Bacterial toxins can cause disorders of the heart (myocarditis, Ch. 5) and kidneys (nephritis, Ch.13). In the bowel, ulcers may perforate a blood vessel wall resulting in haemorrhage or erode the intestinal wall causing acute peritonitis.

A few individuals (up to 5%) may become carriers where there is asymptomatic but chronic infection of the gall bladder. Continued release of microbes into the bile for months or years after recovery leads to infection of the faeces; much less often the urinary system is also involved and microbes are released into the urine. Carriers may transmit the infection to others through contact with their infected faeces or urine.

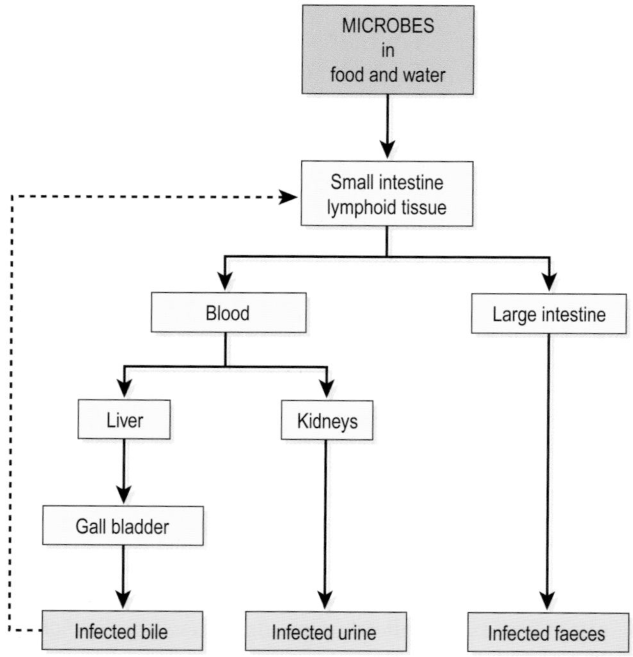

Paratyphoid fever follows a similar course but is usually milder and of shorter duration although the onset can be more sudden; complications are less frequent. Some people may become carriers, but fewer than in typhoid fever.

Other Salmonella infections

Salmonella typhimurium and *S. enteritidis* are the most common bacteria in this group. Generally the effects are confined to the gastrointestinal tract, unlike the *Salmonella* infections above. In addition to humans their hosts are domestic animals and birds. The microbes may be present in meat, poultry, eggs and milk, causing infection if cooking does not achieve sterilisation. Mice and rats also carry the organisms and may contaminate food before or after cooking.

The incubation period is 12–72 hours; enteritis is usually short lived and accompanied by acute abdominal pain and diarrhoea, which may cause dehydration and electrolyte imbalance. Sometimes vomiting is present. In children and debilitated older adults the infection may be severe or even fatal.

Escherichia coli (E. coli) food poisoning

Common sources of these bacteria include undercooked meat and unpasteurised milk; adequate cooking and pasteurization kill *E. coli*. The severity of the disease depends on the type of *E. coli* responsible; some types are more virulent than others. Outbreaks of *E. coli* food poisoning can cause fatalities, particularly in young children and older adults.

Staphylococcal food poisoning

After eating contaminated food, *Staphylococcus aureus* releases toxins that cause acute gastroenteritis (rather than the bacteria that cause the condition). Although cooking kills the bacteria, the toxins are heat resistant.

There is usually short-term acute inflammation with violent vomiting occurring 2–4 hours after ingestion, which may cause dehydration and electrolyte imbalance. Diarrhoea may not be significant. In most cases complete recovery occurs within 24 hours.

Clostridium perfringens food poisoning

These commensal bacteria are normally present in the intestines of humans and animals, but can cause food poisoning when ingested in large numbers. Meat may be contaminated at any stage between slaughter and the consumer. Outbreaks of food poisoning are associated with large-scale cooking, e.g. in institutions. Slow cooling after cooking and/or slow reheating allow microbial multiplication. When they reach the intestines, the bacteria release a toxin that causes watery diarrhoea and severe abdominal pain. The illness is usually self-limiting.

Figure 12.49 The routes of excretion of microbes in typhoid and paratyphoid (enteric) fever.

Antibiotic-associated diarrhoea

The bacterium *Clostridium difficile* is already present in the large intestine, but after antibiotic therapy many other commensal intestinal bacteria die. This allows *C. difficile* to take over and multiply, releasing toxins that damage the mucosa of the large intestine causing profound diarrhoea. Significant inflammation of the large intestine (colitis), which is often fatal in older adults and debilitated people, may occur as a complication.

Campylobacter food poisoning

These Gram-negative bacilli are a common cause of gastroenteritis accompanied by fever, acute pain and sometimes bleeding. They affect mainly young adults and children under 5 years. The bacteria are present in the intestines of birds and animals, and are spread in undercooked poultry and meat. They may also be spread in water and milk. Pets, such as cats and dogs, may be a source of infection. There is an association with Guillain–Barré syndrome (Ch. 7).

Cholera

Cholera is caused by *Vibrio cholerae*, which is spread by contaminated drinking water, faeces, vomit, food, hands and fomites. The only known hosts are humans. In some infected people, known as subclinical cases, no symptoms occur, although these people can transmit the condition to others while their infection remains. A very powerful toxin is released by the bacteria, which stimulates the intestinal glands to secrete large quantities of water, bicarbonate and chloride. This leads to persistent diarrhoea, severe dehydration and electrolyte imbalance, and may cause death due to hypovolaemic shock.

Dysentery

Bacillary dysentery. This infection of the large intestine is caused by bacteria of the *Shigella* group. The severity of the condition depends on the organisms involved. In the UK it is usually a relatively mild condition caused by *Shigella sonnei*. *Shigella dysenteriae* causes the most severe type of infection and it occurs mainly in developing countries. Children and older debilitated adults are particularly susceptible. The only host is humans and the organisms are spread by faecal contamination of food, drink, hands and fomites.

The intestinal mucosa becomes inflamed, ulcerated and oedematous with excess mucus secretion. In severe infections, the acute diarrhoea, that contains blood and excessive mucus, causes dehydration, electrolyte imbalance and anaemia. When healing occurs the mucous membrane is fully restored.

Amoebiasis (amoebic dysentery). This disease is caused by the protozoan *Entamoeba histolytica*. The only known hosts are humans and it is spread by faecal contamination of food, water, hands and fomites. Although many infected people do not develop symptoms they may become asymptomatic carriers.

The amoebae grow, divide and invade the mucosal cells, causing inflammation within the colon (colitis). Without treatment the condition frequently becomes chronic with mild, intermittent diarrhoea and abdominal pain. This may progress with ulceration of the colon accompanied by persistent and debilitating diarrhoea that contains mucus and blood. Complications are unusual but include severe haemorrhage from ulcers and liver abscesses.

Viral gastroenteritis

Several viruses, including rotavirus and norovirus, are known to cause vomiting and/or diarrhoea.

Rotavirus. This is a major cause of diarrhoea in young children. It is easily spread in healthcare facilities.

Norovirus. Also known as the '*winter vomiting virus*', this is responsible for outbreaks of acute but self-limiting enteritis with vomiting as the main symptom. Most common in the winter months, it spreads easily in families and in child and healthcare facilities. Spread is by the faecal–oral route but airborne transmission by inhalation may also occur.

Inflammatory bowel disease (IBD)

This term includes Crohn's disease and ulcerative colitis. A comparison of the main features is shown in Table 12.5; however, it is not always possible to distinguish these conditions in practice. Their aetiology is unknown but is thought to involve environmental and immune factors in genetically susceptible individuals. Both conditions typically have a pattern of relapse and remission.

Crohn's disease

This chronic inflammatory condition of the alimentary tract usually occurs in young adults. The terminal ileum and the rectum are most commonly affected but the disease may affect any part of the tract. There is chronic patchy inflammation with oedema of the full thickness of the intestinal wall, causing partial obstruction of the lumen, sometimes described as *skip lesions*. There are periods of remission of varying duration. The main symptoms are diarrhoea, abdominal pain and weight loss. Complications include:

- secondary infections, occurring when inflamed areas ulcerate
- fibrous adhesions and subsequent intestinal obstruction caused by the healing process
- fistulae between intestinal lesions and adjacent structures, e.g. loops of bowel, surface of the skin (p. 370)
- perianal fistulae, fissures and skin tags
- cancer of the small or large intestine.

Table 12.5 Comparison of the main features of Crohn's disease and ulcerative colitis

	Crohn's disease	Ulcerative colitis
Incidence	Usually between 20 and 40 years of age (mean 26 years); both sexes affected equally; smokers at higher risk	Usually between 20 and 40 years of age (mean 34 years); both sexes affected equally; smoking not a risk factor
Main sites of lesions	Anywhere in digestive tract from mouth to anus; common in terminal ileum	Rectum always involved, with variable spread along colon
Tissue involved	Entire thickness of the wall affected; ulcers and fistulae common	Only mucosa involved
Nature of lesions	'Skip' lesions, i.e. diseased areas interspersed with regions of normal tissue; ulcers and fistulae common	Continuous lesion; mucosa is red and inflamed
Prognosis	In severe cases, surgery may improve condition, but relapse rate very high, slightly increased risk of cancer	Surgical removal of entire colon cures the condition, significantly increased risk of cancer

Ulcerative colitis

This is a chronic inflammatory disease of the mucosa of the colon and rectum, which may ulcerate and become infected. It usually occurs in young adults and begins in the rectum. From there it may spread proximally to involve a variable proportion of the colon and, sometimes, the entire colon. The main symptom is bloody diarrhoea. There are periods of remission lasting weeks, months or years. Individuals may develop other systemic problems affecting, for example, the joints (ankylosing spondylitis, p. 433), skin and liver. In long-standing cases, cancer sometimes develops.

Toxic megacolon is an acute complication where the colon loses its muscle tone and dilates. There is a high risk of electrolyte imbalance, perforation and hypovolaemic shock, which may be fatal if untreated.

Diverticular disease

Diverticula are small pouches of mucosa that protrude (herniate) into the peritoneal cavity through the circular muscle fibres of the colon between the taeniae coli (Fig. 12.50). The walls consist of mucous membrane with a covering of visceral peritoneum. They occur at the weakest points of the intestinal wall, i.e. where the blood vessels enter, most commonly in the sigmoid colon.

The causes of *diverticulosis* (presence of diverticuli) are not known but it is associated with deficiency of dietary fibre. In Western countries, diverticulosis is fairly common after middle age but is usually asymptomatic.

Diverticulitis arises as a consequence of diverticulosis when faeces impact the diverticula. The walls become inflamed and oedematous as secondary infection develops. This reduces the blood supply causing ischaemic abdominal pain. Occasionally, rupture occurs resulting in peritonitis (p. 325).

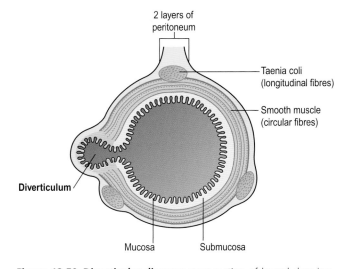

Figure 12.50 Diverticular disease: cross-section of bowel showing one diverticulum.

Tumours of the small and large intestines

Benign and malignant tumours of the small intestine are rare, especially compared with their occurrence in the stomach, large intestine and rectum.

Benign tumours

Benign neoplasms may form a broad-based mass or polyp, i.e. develop a pedicle. Occasionally polyps twist upon themselves, causing ischaemia, necrosis and, sometimes, gangrene. Malignant changes may occur in adenomas, which are mostly found in the large intestine. The incidence is high in developed countries.

Colorectal cancer

This is the most common malignancy of the alimentary tract in Western countries and, as a cause of cancer-related death, is second only to lung cancer in the UK.

The most important predisposing factor for colorectal cancer is thought to be diet. In cultures eating a high-fibre, low-fat diet, the disease is virtually unknown, whereas in Western countries, where large quantities of red meat and saturated animal fat and insufficient fibre are eaten, the disease is much more common. Slow movement of bowel contents may result in conversion of unknown substances present into carcinogenic agents. Genetic factors are also implicated. Predisposing diseases include ulcerative colitis and some benign tumours (usually adenomas).

The tumours are adenocarcinomas with about half arising in the rectum, one-third in the sigmoid colon and the remainder elsewhere in the colon. The tumour may be:

- a soft polypoid mass, projecting into the lumen of the colon or rectum with a tendency to ulceration, infection and bleeding
- a hard fibrous mass encircling the colon, causing narrowing of the lumen and, eventually, obstruction.

Local spread of intestinal tumours occurs early but may not be evident until there is severe ulceration and haemorrhage or obstruction. Spread can be outwards through the wall into the peritoneal cavity and adjacent structures.

Lymph-spread metastases occur in mesenteric lymph nodes, the peritoneum and other abdominal and pelvic organs. Pressure caused by enlarged lymph nodes may cause obstruction or damage other structures.

Blood-spread metastases are most common in the liver, brain and bones.

Hernias

A hernia is a protrusion of an organ or part of an organ through a weak point or aperture in the surrounding structures. In those affecting the digestive system, a piece of bowel protrudes through a weak point in either the musculature of the anterior abdominal wall or an existing opening (Fig. 12.51A). It occurs when there are intermittent increases in intra-abdominal pressure, most commonly in men who lift heavy loads at work. Outcomes include:

- spontaneous reduction, i.e. the loop of bowel slips back to its correct place when the intra-abdominal pressure returns to normal
- manual reduction, i.e. by applying gentle pressure over the abdominal swelling
- *strangulation* (Fig. 12.51B), when reduction is not possible and the venous drainage from the herniated loop of bowel is impaired, causing congestion, ischaemia and gangrene. In addition there is intestinal obstruction (p. 330).

Sites of hernias (Fig. 12.51A)

Inguinal hernia. The weak point is the inguinal canal, which contains the spermatic cord in the male and the

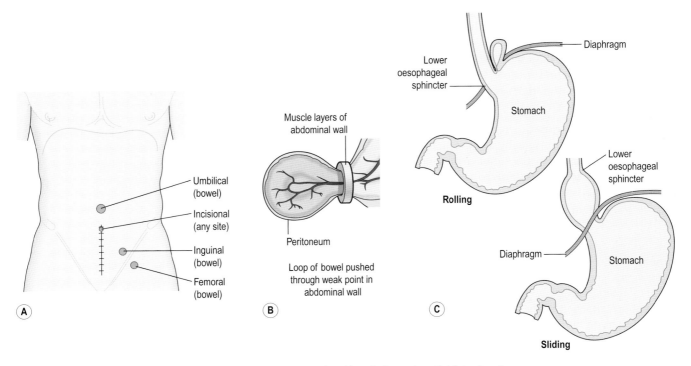

Figure 12.51 Hernias. A. Common sites of herniation. **B.** Strangulated hernia formation. **C.** Hiatus hernia.

round ligament in the female. It occurs more commonly in males than in females.

Femoral hernia. The weak point is the femoral canal through which the femoral artery, vein and lymph vessels pass from the pelvis to the thigh.

Umbilical hernia. The weak point is the umbilicus where the umbilical blood vessels from the placenta entered the fetus before birth.

Incisional hernia. This is caused by repeated stretching of fibrous (scar) tissue formed after previous abdominal surgery.

Hiatus hernia. This is the protrusion of a part of the fundus of the stomach through the oesophageal opening in the diaphragm (Fig. 12.51C). Although often asymptomatic, irritation of the oesophagus only occurs when there is reflux of acid gastric juice, especially when the individual lies flat or bends down. The long-term effects may be oesophagitis, fibrosis and narrowing of the oesophagus, causing dysphagia. Strangulation does not occur.

Rolling hiatus hernia An abnormally large opening in the diaphragm allows a pouch of stomach to 'roll' upwards into the thorax beside the oesophagus. This is associated with obesity and increased intra-abdominal pressure.

Sliding hiatus hernia Part of the stomach is pulled upwards into the thorax. The abnormality may be caused by shrinkage of fibrous tissue formed during healing of a previous oesophageal injury. The sliding movement of the stomach in the oesophageal opening is due to shortening of the oesophagus by muscular contraction during swallowing.

Peritoneal hernia. A loop of bowel may herniate through the epiploic foramen (of Winslow, Fig. 12.3A), the opening in the lesser omentum that separates the greater and lesser peritoneal sacs.

Congenital diaphragmatic hernia. Incomplete formation of the diaphragm, usually on the left side, allows abdominal organs such as the stomach and loops of intestine into the thoracic cavity, preventing normal development of the fetal lungs.

Volvulus

This occurs when a loop of bowel twists occluding its lumen resulting in obstruction. It is usually accompanied by *strangulation*, where there is interruption of the blood supply causing gangrene. It occurs in parts of the intestine that are attached to the posterior abdominal wall by the mesentery (a long double fold of visceral peritoneum. The most common site in adults is the sigmoid colon and in children the small intestine. Predisposing factors include:

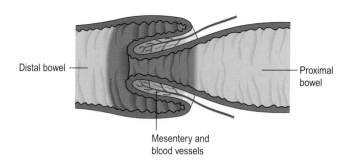

Distal bowel — — Proximal bowel

Mesentery and blood vessels

Figure 12.52 Intussusception.

- an unusually long mesentery
- heavy loading of the sigmoid colon with faeces
- a slight twist of a loop of bowel, causing gas and fluid to accumulate, which promotes further twisting
- adhesions formed following surgery or peritonitis.

Intussusception

In this condition a length of intestine is invaginated into itself causing intestinal obstruction (Fig. 12.52). It occurs most commonly in children when a piece of terminal ileum is pushed through the ileocaecal valve. The overlying mucosa bulges into the lumen, creating a partial obstruction and a rise in pressure inside the intestine proximal to the swelling. Strong peristaltic waves develop in an attempt to overcome the partial obstruction. These push the swollen piece of bowel into the lumen of the section immediately distal to it, creating the intussusception. The pressure on the veins in the invaginated portion is increased, causing congestion, further swelling, ischaemia and possibly gangrene. Complete intestinal obstruction may occur. In adults, tumours that bulge into the lumen, e.g. polyps, together with the strong peristalsis, may be the cause.

Intestinal obstruction

This is not a disease in itself but arises as a consequence of many other conditions. The summary below outlines effects and main causes of obstruction.

Mechanical causes
These include:

- constriction or blockage of the intestine by, for example, a strangulated hernia, intussusception, volvulus, peritoneal adhesions; partial obstruction (narrowing of the lumen) that suddenly becomes complete
- stenosis and thickening of the intestinal wall, e.g. in diverticulosis, Crohn's disease and malignant tumours; there is usually

a gradual progression from partial to complete obstruction

- physical causes where the obstruction is by, for example, a large gallstone or a tumour growing into the lumen
- pressure on the intestine from outside, e.g. from a large tumour in any pelvic or abdominal organ, such as a uterine fibroid; this is most likely to occur inside the confined space of the pelvic cavity.

Neurological causes of obstruction

Partial or complete loss of peristaltic activity produces the effects of obstruction. *Paralytic ileus* is the most common form. The mechanisms are not clear but there are well-recognised predisposing conditions including major surgery requiring considerable handling of the intestines and peritonitis.

Secretion of water and electrolytes continues although intestinal mobility is lost and absorption impaired. This causes distension and electrolyte imbalance, leading to hypovolaemic shock.

Vascular causes of obstruction

When the blood supply to a segment of bowel is cut off, ischaemia is followed by infarction and gangrene. The damaged bowel becomes unable to function. The causes may be:

- atheromatous changes in the blood vessel walls, with thrombosis (p. 119)
- embolism (p. 120)
- mechanical obstruction of the bowel, e.g. strangulated hernia (p. 329).

Effects of intestinal obstruction

Symptoms include abdominal pain, vomiting and constipation. When the upper gastrointestinal tract is affected vomiting may be profuse, although it may be absent in lower bowel obstruction. There are neither bowel sounds present nor passing of flatus (wind) as peristalsis ceases. Without treatment, irrespective of the cause, this condition is fatal.

Malabsorption

Impaired absorption of nutrients and water from the intestines is not a disease in itself, but the result of abnormal changes in one or more of the following:

- villi in the small intestine, e.g. coeliac disease, tropical sprue (see below)
- digestion of food
- absorption or transport of nutrients from the small intestine.

Intestinal conditions that impair normal digestion and/or absorption and transport of nutrients include:

- extensive resection of the small intestine

- 'blind loop syndrome' where there is microbial overgrowth in a blind end of intestine following surgery
- lymphatic obstruction by diseased or absent (following surgical excision) lymph nodes.

Coeliac disease

This disease is the main cause of malabsorption in Western countries. It is due to an abnormal, genetically determined autoimmune reaction to the protein gluten, present in wheat, barley and rye. When it is removed from the diet, there is complete remission of symptoms. There is marked villous atrophy, especially in the jejunum, and malabsorption characterised by the passage of loose, pale-coloured, fatty stools (*steatorrhoea*).

T-cell function may be disordered causing abnormal immune reactions to other antigens as well. Atrophy of the spleen is common and malignancy of the small intestine is a rarer consequence. Sometimes other autoimmune conditions are also present. It often presents in infants after weaning but can affect people of any age.

Tropical sprue

This disease is endemic in subtropical and tropical countries except Africa. After visiting an endemic area most travellers suffering from sprue recover, but others may not develop symptoms until months or even years later.

There is partial villous atrophy with malabsorption, chronic diarrhoea, a variable degree of weight loss and pernicious anaemia due to deficient absorption of vitamin B_{12} and folic acid. The cause is unknown but it may be that microbial infection is a factor.

Diseases of the pancreas

Learning outcomes

After studying this section, you should be able to:

- compare and contrast the causes and effects of acute and chronic pancreatitis
- outline the main pancreatic tumours and their consequences.

Pancreatitis

Proteolytic enzymes produced by the pancreas are secreted in inactive forms, which are not activated until they reach the intestine; this protects the pancreas from digestion by its own enzymes. If these precursor enzymes are activated while still in the pancreas, pancreatitis results.

Acute pancreatitis

The severity of the disease is directly related to the amount of pancreatic tissue involved. Mild forms are more common and damage only those cells near the ducts. Recovery is usually complete.

Severe forms cause widespread damage with necrosis and haemorrhage. Common complications include infection, suppuration, and local venous thrombosis. Pancreatic enzymes, especially amylase, enter and circulate in the blood, causing similar damage to other structures. In severe cases there is a high mortality rate.

The causes of acute pancreatitis are not clear but known predisposing factors are gallstones and excessive use of alcohol. Other associated conditions include:

- pancreatic cancer (see below)
- viral infections, notably mumps
- kidney and liver transplantation
- hypercalcaemia
- severe hypothermia
- drugs, e.g. corticosteroids, some cytotoxic agents.

Chronic pancreatitis

This is either due to repeated attacks of acute pancreatitis or may arise gradually without evidence of pancreatic disease. This form is associated with irreversible structural changes. It is more common in men and is frequently associated with fibrosis and distortion of the main pancreatic duct. There is intestinal malabsorption when pancreatic secretions are reduced and diabetes mellitus (p. 236) occurs when damage affects the β-islet cells.

Protein material secreted by the acinar cells blocks the tiny acinar ducts. This eventually leads to the formation of encapsulated cysts, which are a feature of acute and chronic pancreatitis.

The most common cause in the Western world is excessive alcohol consumption. In developing countries dietary factors and malnutrition have been implicated. It is also associated with cystic fibrosis.

Cystic fibrosis (see p. 266)

Tumours of the pancreas

Benign tumours are very rare.

Malignant tumours

These are relatively common and affect more men than women. There is an association with cigarette smoking, excessive alcohol intake, use of aspirin and co-existing conditions, e.g. diabetes mellitus and chronic pancreatitis.

They occur most frequently in the head of the pancreas, obstructing the flow of bile and pancreatic juice into the duodenum. Jaundice, sometimes accompanied by itching, develops. Weight loss is the result of impaired digestion and absorption of fat, although anorexia and metabolic effects of the tumour may also play a role.

Tumours in the body and tail of the gland rarely cause symptoms until the disease is advanced.

Irrespective of the site, metastases are often recognised before the primary tumour and therefore the prognosis is generally poor.

Diseases of the liver

Learning outcomes

After studying this section, you should be able to:

- compare and contrast the causes, forms and effects of chronic and acute hepatitis
- describe the main non-viral inflammatory conditions of the liver
- discuss the causes and consequences of liver failure
- describe the main liver tumours.

Liver tissue has a remarkable capacity for regeneration and therefore damage is usually extensive before it is evident. The effects of disease or toxic agents are seen when:

- regeneration of hepatocytes (liver cells) does not keep pace with damage, leading to hepatocellular failure
- there is a gradual replacement of damaged cells by fibrous tissue, leading to portal hypertension.

In most liver disease both conditions are present.

Acute hepatitis

Areas of necrosis develop as groups of hepatocytes die and the eventual outcome depends on the size and number of these areas. Causes of the damage may be a variety of conditions, including:

- viral infections
- toxic substances
- circulatory disturbances.

Viral hepatitis

Viral infections are the commonest cause of acute liver injury and different types are recognised. The types are distinguished serologically, i.e. by the antibodies produced to combat the infection. The severity of the ensuing disease caused by the different virus types varies considerably, but the pattern is similar. The viruses enter the liver cells, causing degenerative changes. An inflammatory reaction ensues, accompanied by production of an exudate containing lymphocytes, plasma cells and granulocytes. There is reactive hyperplasia of the hepatic macrophages (Kupffer cells) in the walls of the sinusoids.

As groups of cells die, necrotic areas of varying sizes develop, phagocytes remove the necrotic material and the lobules collapse. The basic lobule framework (Fig. 12.35) becomes distorted and blood vessels develop kinks. These changes interfere with the circulation of blood to the remaining hepatocytes and the resultant hypoxia causes further damage locally. Fibrous tissue develops in the damaged area and adjacent hepatocytes proliferate. The effect of these changes on the overall functioning of the liver depends on the size of the necrotic areas, the amount of fibrous tissue formed and the extent to which the blood and bile channels are distorted.

Hepatitis A

Previously known as 'infectious hepatitis', this type often occurs as epidemics in all parts of the world. It affects mainly children, causing a mild illness although it is often asymptomatic. Infection is spread by the faecal–oral route, e.g. via contaminated hands, food, water and fomites. Viruses are excreted in the faeces for 7–14 days before clinical symptoms appear and for about 7 days after. Symptoms may include general malaise followed by a period of jaundice (p. 336) that is accompanied by passing of dark urine and pale faeces. Antibodies develop and confer lifelong immunity after recovery. Subclinical disease may occur but not carriers.

Hepatitis B

Previously known as 'serum hepatitis', infection occurs at any age, but mostly in adults. The incubation period is from 50 to 180 days. The virus enters the blood and is spread by contaminated blood and blood products. People at greatest risk of infection are those who come in contact with blood and blood products in the course of their work, e.g. health-care workers. The virus is also spread by body fluids, i.e. saliva, semen, vaginal secretions, and from mother to fetus (vertical transmission). Others at risk include intravenous drug users and men who have sex with men. Antibodies are formed and immunity persists after recovery. Infection usually leads to severe illness lasting from 2 to 6 weeks, often followed by a protracted convalescence. Carriers may, or may not, have had clinical disease. Hepatitis B virus may cause massive liver necrosis and death. In less severe cases recovery may be complete. In others chronic hepatitis (see opposite) may develop; live viruses continue to circulate in the blood and other body fluids. The condition also predisposes to cirrhosis (see below) and liver cancer.

Hepatitis D. This virus contains no RNA and can only replicate in the presence of hepatitis B virus. It most often infects intravenous drug users who already have hepatitis B but also affects others with hepatitis B.

Box 12.1 Some hepatotoxic substances

Predictable group (dose related)	Unpredictable group (individual idiosyncrasy)
Alcohol	Phenothiazine compounds
Chloroform	Halothane
Cytotoxic drugs	Methyldopa
Tetracyclines	Indometacin
Anabolic steroids	Chlorpropamide
Paracetamol	Thiouracil
Some fungi	Sulphonamides

Hepatitis C

This virus is spread by blood and blood products, which accounts for the infection of many people with haemophilia. In countries, including the UK, where blood donors are now screened for the virus this route of transmission is now rare although it is prevalent in intravenous drug users. The infection is very frequently asymptomatic although a carrier state occurs. Infection is usually diagnosed later in life when cirrhosis (p. 334) or chronic liver failure becomes evident.

Toxic substances

Many drugs undergo chemical change in the liver before excretion in bile or by other organs. They may damage the liver cells in their original form or while in various intermediate stages. Some substances always cause liver damage (predictably toxic) while others only do so when hypersensitivity to normal doses develops (unpredictably toxic). In both types the extent of the damage depends on the size of the dose and/or the duration of exposure (Box 12.1).

Circulatory disturbances

The intensely active hepatocytes are particularly vulnerable to damage by hypoxia, which is usually due to impaired blood supply caused by:

- fibrosis in the liver following inflammation
- compression of the portal vein, hepatic artery or vein by a tumour
- acute general circulatory failure and shock
- venous congestion caused by acute or chronic right-sided heart failure (Ch. 5).

Chronic hepatitis

This is defined as any form of hepatitis which persists for more than 6 months. It may be caused by viruses, alcohol or drugs, but sometimes the cause is unknown.

Mild, persistent inflammation may follow acute viral hepatitis. There is usually little or no fibrosis.

There may be continuing progressive inflammation with cell necrosis and formation of fibrous tissue that may lead to cirrhosis of the liver. Distortion of the liver blood vessels causes localised hypoxia, leading to further hepatocyte damage. This condition is commonly associated with hepatitis B and C, some forms of autoimmunity and unpredictable (idiosyncratic) drug reactions.

Cirrhosis of the liver

This is the result of long-term injury caused by a variety of agents. The most common causes are:

- excessive alcohol consumption
- hepatitis B and C infections
- recurrent obstruction of the biliary tract.

Chronic liver damage results in inflammation, necrosis and, in time, affected tissue is replaced with fibrous tissue. Hyperplasia of hepatocytes occurs in areas adjacent to the damaged tissue in an attempt to compensate for destroyed cells, which leads to formation of nodules. The normal structure of the liver lobules becomes increasingly abnormal, usually over several years, which interferes with blood flow resulting in portal hypertension and its consequences (see p. 321), and impairment of liver cell function.

Liver failure may occur when cell regeneration is unable to keep pace with cell destruction, and there is increased risk of liver cancer developing.

Liver failure

This occurs when liver function is markedly impaired. It can be acute or chronic and may be the outcome of a wide variety of disorders, e.g.:

- acute viral hepatitis
- extensive necrosis due to poisoning, e.g. some drug overdoses, hepatotoxic chemicals, adverse drug reactions
- cirrhosis of the liver.

Liver failure has serious effects on other parts of the body.

Hepatic encephalopathy
This condition is characterised by apathy, disorientation, confusion and muscular rigidity, progressing to coma. The cells affected are the astrocytes in the brain and several factors may be involved, e.g.:

- nitrogenous bacterial metabolites absorbed from the colon, which are normally detoxified in the liver, reach the brain via the bloodstream
- other metabolites, normally present only in trace amounts, e.g. ammonia, may reach toxic concentrations and change the permeability of the cerebral blood vessels and the effectiveness of the blood–brain barrier
- hypoxia and electrolyte imbalance.

Blood coagulation defects
The liver fails to synthesise adequate supplies of blood clotting factors, i.e. prothrombin, fibrinogen and factors II, V, VII, IX and X; purpura, bruising and bleeding may occur.

Oliguria and renal failure
Portal hypertension may cause oesophageal varices (p. 321). If these rupture, severe haemorrhage may lead to a fall in blood pressure sufficient to reduce the renal blood flow, causing progressive oliguria and renal failure (p. 352).

Oedema and ascites
These may arise from one or both of the following factors:

- portal hypertension raises the capillary hydrostatic pressure in the organs drained by the tributaries of the portal vein (see Fig. 5.40, p. 110)
- diminished production of serum albumin and clotting factors reduces the plasma osmotic pressure.

Together these changes cause the movement of excess fluid into the interstitial spaces where it causes *oedema* (p. 125) as the fluid cannot leave the tissue. Eventually free fluid accumulates in the peritoneal cavity and the resultant *ascites* may be severe.

Jaundice
The following factors may cause jaundice as liver failure develops:

- inability of the hepatocytes to conjugate and excrete bilirubin
- obstruction to the movement of bile through the bile channels by fibrous tissue that has distorted the structural framework of liver lobules.

Tumours of the liver

Benign tumours are very rare.

Malignant tumours
Cancer of the liver is frequently associated with cirrhosis but the relationship between them is not clear. It may be that both cirrhosis and cancer are caused by the same agents or that the carcinogenic action of an agent is promoted by cirrhotic changes. Malignancy sometimes develops following hepatitis B and C. The most common sites of metastases are the abdominal lymph nodes, the peritoneum and the lungs.

Secondary malignant tumours (metastases) in the liver are more common than primary liver tumours. They usually spread there from primary tumours in the gastrointestinal tract, the lungs and the breast. These tumours tend to grow rapidly and are often the cause of death.

Diseases of the gall bladder and bile ducts

Learning outcomes

After studying this section, you should be able to:

- describe the causes and consequences of gallstones

- compare and contrast acute and chronic cholecystitis

- briefly outline the common sites and consequences of biliary tract tumours

- discuss the main causes and effects of jaundice.

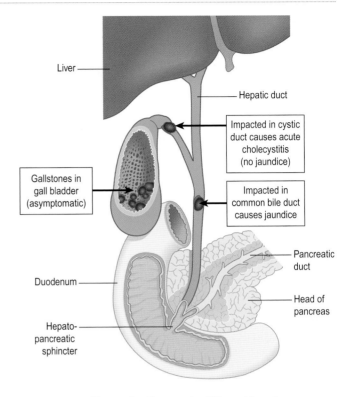

Figure 12.53 Effects of gallstones in different locations.

Gallstones (cholelithiasis)

Gallstones consist of deposits of the constituents of bile, most commonly cholesterol. Many small stones or one or more large stones may form but they do not necessarily produce symptoms. Predisposing factors include:

- changes in the composition of bile that affect the solubility of its constituents
- high blood cholesterol levels
- diabetes mellitus
- female gender
- obesity
- several pregnancies in young women, especially when accompanied by obesity.

Cholecystitis

This is usually associated with the presence of gallstones.

Acute cholecystitis

This is acute inflammation of the gall bladder that occurs when a gallstone becomes impacted (stuck) in the cystic duct (Fig. 12.53), often after a fatty meal. Strong peristaltic contractions of the smooth muscle in the wall of the cystic duct that occur in an attempt to move the stone onwards result in *biliary colic*, severe acute pain in the epigastrium or right hypochondrium. This does not cause jaundice because bile from the liver can still pass directly into the duodenum. However, bile is unable to leave the gall bladder and an inflammatory reaction follows.

This may be complicated by bacterial infection and distension of the gall bladder, which carries the risk of perforation and peritonitis.

Chronic cholecystitis

The onset is usually insidious, sometimes following repeated acute attacks. Gallstones are invariably present and there may be accompanying biliary colic. Secondary infection with suppuration may develop. Without treatment, ulceration of the tissues between the gall bladder and the duodenum or colon may occur with fistula formation and, later, fibrous adhesions. This condition is associated with cancer of the gall bladder.

Cholangitis

This is inflammation of bile ducts caused by bacterial infection which is typically accompanied by abdominal pain, fever and jaundice (because the flow of bile into the duodenum is blocked). Infection can spread upwards in the biliary tree to the liver (*ascending cholangitis*) causing liver abscesses.

Tumours of the biliary tract

Benign tumours are rare.

Malignant tumours

These are relatively rare and gallstones are nearly always present. Local spread to the liver, the pancreas and other adjacent organs is common. Lymph and blood spread lead to widespread metastases. The tumour has often spread by the time of diagnosis and, therefore, the prognosis is poor.

Jaundice

This is not a disease in itself, but yellowing of the skin and mucous membrane is a sign of abnormal bilirubin metabolism and excretion. Bilirubin, produced from the breakdown of haemoglobin, is normally conjugated in the liver and excreted in the bile (Fig. 12.37). Conjugation makes bilirubin water-soluble and greatly enhances its removal from the blood, an essential step in excretion.

Unconjugated bilirubin, which is fat-soluble, has a toxic effect on brain cells. However, it is unable to cross the blood–brain barrier until the plasma level rises above 340 μmol/L, but when it does it may cause neurological damage, seizures (fits) and cognitive impairment. Serum bilirubin may rise to 40–50 μmol/L before the yellow coloration of jaundice is evident in the skin and conjunctiva (normal 3–13 μmol/L). Jaundice is often accompanied by *pruritus* (itching) caused by the irritating effects of bile salts on the skin.

Jaundice develops when there is an abnormality of bilirubin processing and the different types are considered below.

Types of jaundice

Whatever stage in bilirubin processing is affected, the end result is rising blood bilirubin levels.

Pre-hepatic jaundice

This is due to increased haemolysis of red blood cells (see Fig. 12.37) that results in production of excess bilirubin. Because the excess bilirubin is unconjugated it cannot be excreted in the urine, which therefore remains normal in colour.

Neonatal haemolytic jaundice occurs in many babies, especially in those born prematurely where the normally high rate of haemolysis is coupled with a shortage of conjugating enzymes in the hepatocytes of the still immature liver.

Intra-hepatic jaundice

This is the result of damage to the liver itself by, e.g.:

- viral hepatitis (p. 332)
- toxic substances, such as drugs
- amoebiasis (amoebic dysentery) (p. 327)
- cirrhosis (p. 334).

Excess bilirubin accumulates in the liver. Because it is mainly in the conjugated form, it is water-soluble and excreted in the urine making it dark in colour.

Post-hepatic jaundice

Causes of obstruction to the flow of bile in the biliary tract include:

- gallstones in the common bile duct (Fig. 12.53)
- tumour of the head of the pancreas
- fibrosis of the bile ducts, following cholangitis or injury by the passage of gallstones.

In this situation excess bilirubin is also conjugated and is therefore excreted in the urine. The effects of raised serum bilirubin include:

- pruritus (itching)
- pale faeces due to absence of stercobilin (p. 311)
- dark urine due to the presence of increased amounts of bilirubin.

For a range of self-assessment exercises on the topics in this chapter, visit Evolve online resources: https://evolve.elsevier.com/Waugh/anatomy/

The urinary system

ANIMATIONS

The urinary system is the main excretory system and consists of the following structures:

- 2 *kidneys*, which secrete urine
- 2 *ureters* that convey the urine from the kidneys to the urinary bladder
- the *urinary bladder*, which collects and stores urine
- the *urethra* through which urine leaves the body. ▮ **13.1**

Figure 13.1 shows an overview of the urinary system. The urinary system plays a vital part in maintaining homeostasis of water and electrolytes within the body. The kidneys produce urine that contains metabolic waste products, including the nitrogenous compounds urea and uric acid, excess ions and some drugs. The main functions of the kidneys are:

- formation of urine, maintaining water, electrolyte and acid–base balance
- excretion of waste products
- production and secretion of *erythropoietin*, the hormone that stimulates formation of red blood cells (p. 66)
- production and secretion of *renin*, an important enzyme in the control of blood pressure (p. 225).

Urine is stored in the bladder and excreted by the process of *micturition*.

The first sections of this chapter explore the structures and functions of the organs of the urinary system and the impact of ageing on kidney function. In the final section the consequences of abnormal functioning of the various parts of the urinary system on body function are considered.

Kidneys

Learning outcomes

After studying this section, you should be able to:

- identify the organs associated with the kidneys
- outline the gross structure of the kidneys
- describe the structure of a nephron
- explain the processes involved in the formation of urine
- explain how body water and electrolyte balance is maintained.

The kidneys (Fig. 13.2) lie on the posterior abdominal wall, one on each side of the vertebral column, behind the peritoneum and below the diaphragm. They extend from the level of the 12th thoracic vertebra to the 3rd lumbar vertebra, receiving some protection from the lower rib cage. The right kidney is usually slightly lower than the left, probably because of the considerable space occupied by the liver.

Kidneys are bean-shaped organs, about 11 cm long, 6 cm wide, 3 cm thick and weigh 150 g. They are embedded in, and held in position by, a mass of fat. A sheath of fibrous connective tissue, the *renal fascia*, encloses the kidney and the renal fat.

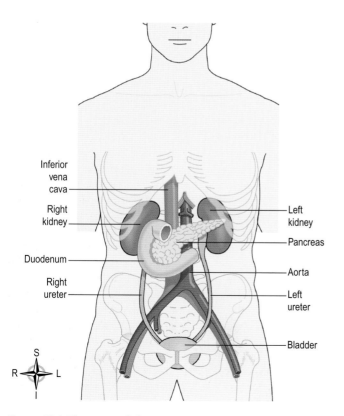

Figure 13.1 The parts of the urinary system (excluding the urethra) and some associated structures.

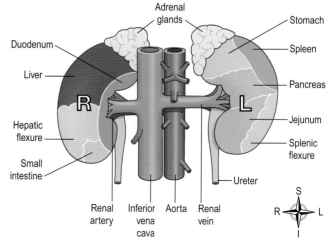

Figure 13.2 Anterior view of the kidneys showing the areas of contact with associated structures.

Organs associated with the kidneys

(Figs 13.1 and 13.2)

As the kidneys lie on either side of the vertebral column, each is associated with different structures.

Right kidney
Superiorly – the right adrenal gland
Anteriorly – the right lobe of the liver, the duodenum and the hepatic flexure of the colon
Posteriorly – the diaphragm, and muscles of the posterior abdominal wall.

Left kidney
Superiorly – the left adrenal gland
Anteriorly – the spleen, stomach, pancreas, jejunum and splenic flexure of the colon
Posteriorly – the diaphragm and muscles of the posterior abdominal wall.

Gross structure of the kidney ▦ 13.2

There are three areas of tissue that can be distinguished when a longitudinal section of the kidney is viewed with the naked eye (Fig. 13.3):

- an outer fibrous *capsule*, surrounding the kidney
- the *cortex*, a reddish-brown layer of tissue immediately below the capsule and outside the *renal pyramids*
- the *medulla*, the innermost layer, consisting of pale conical-shaped striations, the renal pyramids.

The *hilum* is the concave medial border of the kidney where the renal blood and lymph vessels, the ureter and nerves enter.

Urine formed within the kidney passes through a *renal papilla* at the apex of a pyramid into a *minor calyx*

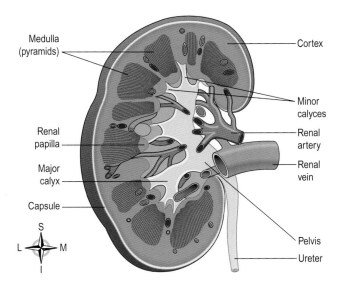

Figure 13.3 A longitudinal section of the right kidney.

Labels: Medulla (pyramids); Cortex; Renal papilla; Minor calyces; Renal artery; Renal vein; Major calyx; Capsule; Pelvis; Ureter

(Fig. 13.3). Several minor calyces merge into a *major calyx* and two or three major calyces combine forming the *renal pelvis*, a funnel shaped structure that narrows when it leaves the kidney as the ureter. The walls of the calyces and renal pelvis are lined with transitional epithelium and contain smooth muscle. Peristalsis, intrinsic contraction of smooth muscle, propels urine through the calyces, renal pelvis and ureters to the bladder.

Microscopic structure of the kidney
▦ 13.3

The kidney contains about 1–2 million functional units, the *nephrons*, and a much smaller number of *collecting ducts*. The collecting ducts transport urine through the pyramids to the calyces, giving the pyramids their striped appearance (Fig. 13.3). The collecting ducts are supported by connective tissue, containing blood vessels, nerves and lymph vessels.

The nephron (Fig. 13.4)
The nephron is essentially a tubule closed at one end that joins a collecting duct at the other end. The closed or blind end is indented to form the cup-shaped *glomerular capsule* (Bowman's capsule), which almost completely encloses a network of tiny arterial capillaries, the *glomerulus*. These resemble a coiled tuft and are shown in Figure 13.5. Continuing from the glomerular capsule, the remainder of the nephron is about 3 cm long and described in three parts:

- the proximal convoluted tubule
- the medullary loop (loop of Henle)
- the distal convoluted tubule, leading into a collecting duct.

The collecting ducts unite, forming larger ducts that empty into the minor calyces.

The kidneys receive about 20% of the cardiac output. After entering the kidney at the hilum, the renal artery divides into smaller arteries and arterioles. In the cortex an arteriole, the *afferent arteriole*, enters each glomerular capsule and then subdivides into a cluster of tiny arterial capillaries, forming the glomerulus. Between these capillary loops are connective tissue phagocytic *mesangial cells*, which are part of the monocyte–macrophage defence system (p. 70). The blood vessel leading away from the glomerulus is the *efferent arteriole*. The afferent arteriole has a larger diameter than the efferent arteriole, which increases pressure inside the glomerulus and drives filtration across the glomerular capillary walls (Fig. 13.6). The efferent arteriole divides into a second peritubular (meaning 'around tubules') capillary network, which wraps around the remainder of the tubule, allowing exchange between the fluid in the tubule and the bloodstream (Figs 13.4 and 13.7). This maintains the local supply of oxygen and nutrients and removes waste products. Venous blood drained from this capillary bed

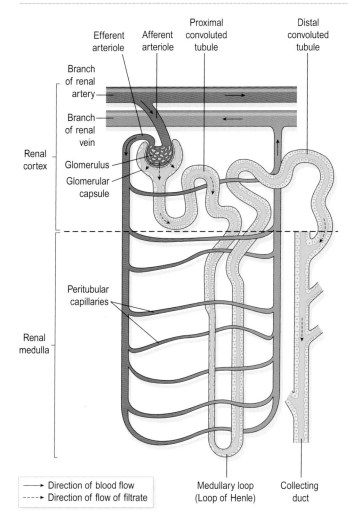

Figure 13.4 A nephron and associated blood vessels.

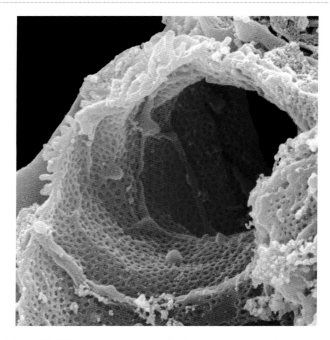

Figure 13.6 Coloured scanning electron micrograph of glomerular capillary.

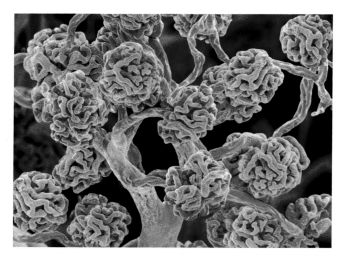

Figure 13.5 Coloured scanning electron micrograph of glomerular capillary tufts.

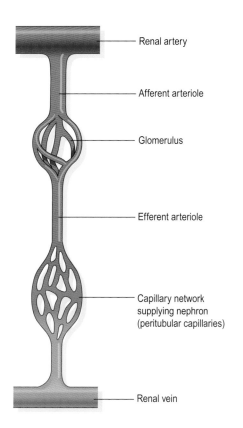

Figure 13.7 The series of blood vessels in the kidney.

340

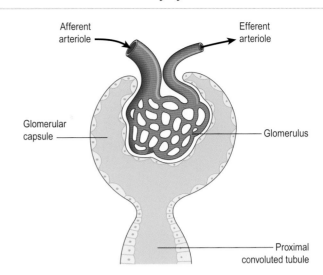

Figure 13.9 **The glomerulus and glomerular capsule.**

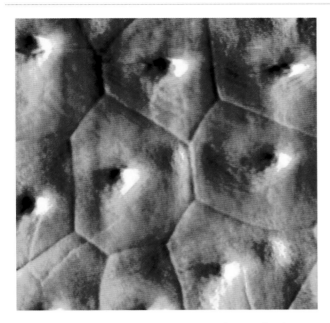

Figure 13.8 **Simple squamous epithelium of the collecting ducts. Coloured atomic force micrograph.**

eventually leaves the kidney in the renal vein, which empties into the inferior vena cava.

The walls of the glomerulus and the glomerular capsule consist of a single layer of flattened epithelial cells. The glomerular walls are more permeable than those of other capillaries. The remainder of the nephron and the collecting duct are formed by a single layer of simple squamous epithelium (Fig. 13.8).

Renal blood vessels are supplied by both sympathetic and parasympathetic nerves. The presence of both divisions of the autonomic nervous system controls renal blood vessel diameter and renal blood flow independently of autoregulation (p. 342).

Functions of the kidney

Formation of urine

The kidneys form urine, which passes to the bladder for storage prior to excretion. The composition of urine reflects exchange of substances between the nephron and the blood in the renal capillaries. Waste products of protein metabolism are excreted, water and electrolyte levels are controlled and pH (acid–base balance) is maintained by excretion of hydrogen ions. There are three processes involved in the formation of urine:

- filtration
- selective reabsorption
- secretion.

Filtration (Fig. 13.10) ■■ **13.4, 13.5**

This takes place through the semipermeable walls of the glomerulus (Fig. 13.9) and glomerular capsule. Water and

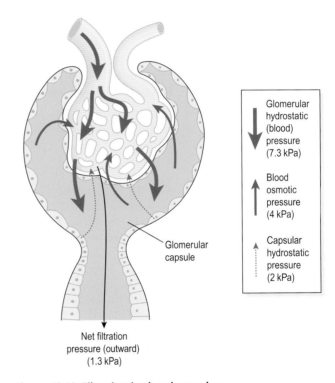

Figure 13.10 **Filtration in the glomerulus.**

other small molecules readily pass through, although some are reabsorbed later. Blood cells, plasma proteins and other large molecules are too large to filter through and therefore remain in the capillaries (Box 13.1). The filtrate in the glomerulus is very similar in composition to plasma with the important exceptions of plasma proteins and blood cells.

Filtration takes place because there is a difference between the blood pressure in the glomerulus and the pressure of the filtrate in the glomerular capsule. Because

---

Box 13.1 Constituents of glomerular filtrate and glomerular capillaries

Blood constituents in glomerular filtrate	Blood constituents remaining in glomerular capillaries
Water	Leukocytes
Mineral salts	Erythrocytes
Amino acids	Platelets
Ketoacids	Plasma proteins
Glucose	Some drugs (large molecules)
Some hormones	
Creatinine	
Urea	
Uric acid	
Some drugs (small molecules)	

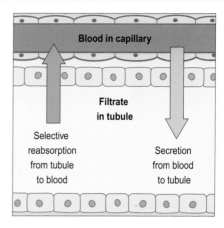

Figure 13.11 Directions of selective reabsorption and secretion in the nephron.

the efferent arteriole is narrower than the afferent arteriole, a *capillary hydrostatic pressure* of about 7.3 kPa (55 mmHg) builds up in the glomerulus. This pressure is opposed by the *osmotic pressure* of the blood, provided mainly by plasma proteins, about 4 kPa (30 mmHg), and by *filtrate hydrostatic pressure* of about 2 kPa (15 mmHg) in the glomerular capsule. The net *filtration pressure* is, therefore:

$$7.3 - (4 + 2) = 1.3 \text{ kPa, or}$$
$$55 - (30 + 15) = 10$$

The volume of filtrate formed by both kidneys each minute is called the *glomerular filtration rate* (GFR). In a healthy adult the GFR is about 125 mL/min, i.e. 180 litres of filtrate are formed each day by the two kidneys. Nearly all of the filtrate is later reabsorbed from the kidney tubules with less than 1%, i.e. 1–1.5 litres, excreted as urine. The differences in volume and concentration are due to selective reabsorption of some filtrate constituents and tubular secretion of others (see below).

Autoregulation. Renal blood flow, and therefore glomerular filtration, is protected by a mechanism called *autoregulation*, whereby renal blood flow is maintained at a constant pressure across a wide range of systolic blood pressures (from around 80–200 mmHg). Autoregulation operates independently of nervous control, i.e. if the nerve supply to the renal blood vessels is interrupted, autoregulation continues to operate. It is therefore a property inherent in renal blood vessels; it may be stimulated by changes in blood pressure in the renal arteries or by fluctuating levels of certain metabolites, e.g. prostaglandins.

In severe shock, when the systolic blood pressure falls below 80 mmHg, autoregulation fails and renal blood flow and the hydrostatic pressure decrease, impairing filtration within the glomeruli.

Selective reabsorption (Fig. 13.11) ▨ **13.6**

Most reabsorption from the filtrate back into the blood takes place in the proximal convoluted tubule, whose walls are lined with microvilli to increase surface area for absorption. Many substances are reabsorbed here, including some water, electrolytes and organic nutrients such as glucose. Some reabsorption is passive, but some substances, e.g. glucose, are actively transported. Only 60–70% of filtrate reaches the medullary loop. Much of this, especially water, sodium and chloride, is reabsorbed in the loop, so that only 15–20% of the original filtrate reaches the distal convoluted tubule, and the composition of the filtrate is now very different. More electrolytes are reabsorbed here, especially sodium, so the filtrate entering the collecting ducts is actually quite dilute. The main function of the collecting ducts is to reabsorb as much water as the body needs.

Active transport takes place at carrier sites in the epithelial membrane, using chemical energy to transport substances against their concentration gradients (p. 37).

Some ions, e.g. sodium and chloride, can be absorbed by both active and passive mechanisms depending on the site in the nephron.

Some constituents of glomerular filtrate (e.g. glucose, amino acids) do not normally appear in urine because they are completely reabsorbed unless blood levels are excessive.

Reabsorption of nitrogenous waste products, such as urea, uric acid and creatinine is very limited.

The kidneys' maximum capacity for reabsorption of a substance is the *transport maximum*, or renal threshold. For example, the normal blood glucose level is 3.5–8 mmol/L (63 to 144 mg/100 mL) and if this rises above the transport maximum of about 9 mmol/L (160 mg/100 mL), glucose appears in the urine. This occurs because all the carrier sites are occupied and the mechanism for active transport out of the tubules is overloaded. Other substances reabsorbed by active transport include sodium, calcium, potassium, phosphate and chloride.

The transport maximum, or renal threshold, of some substances varies according to body need at a particular time, and in some cases reabsorption is regulated by hormones.

Hormones that influence selective reabsorption 13.7

Parathyroid hormone. This is secreted by the parathyroid glands and together with *calcitonin* from the thyroid gland regulates the reabsorption of calcium and phosphate from the distal collecting tubules, so that normal blood levels are maintained. Parathyroid hormone increases the blood calcium level and calcitonin lowers it.

Antidiuretic hormone, ADH. This is secreted by the posterior pituitary. It increases the permeability of the distal convoluted tubules and collecting tubules, increasing water reabsorption. Secretion of ADH is controlled by a negative feedback system (Fig. 13.12).

Aldosterone. Secreted by the adrenal cortex, this hormone increases the reabsorption of sodium and water, and the excretion of potassium. Secretion is regulated through a negative feedback system (Fig. 13.13).

Atrial natriuretic peptide, ANP. This hormone is secreted by the atria of the heart in response to stretching of the atrial wall when blood volume is increased. It decreases reabsorption of sodium and water from the proximal convoluted tubules and collecting ducts. Secretion of ANP is also regulated by a negative feedback system (Fig. 13.14).

Tubular secretion (Fig. 13.11) 13.8

Filtration occurs as blood flows through the glomerulus. Substances not required and foreign materials, e.g. drugs including penicillin and aspirin, may not be entirely filtered out of the blood because of the short time it remains in the glomerulus. Such substances are cleared by secretion from the peritubular capillaries into the filtrate within the convoluted tubules. Tubular secretion of hydrogen ions (H^+) is important in maintaining normal blood pH.

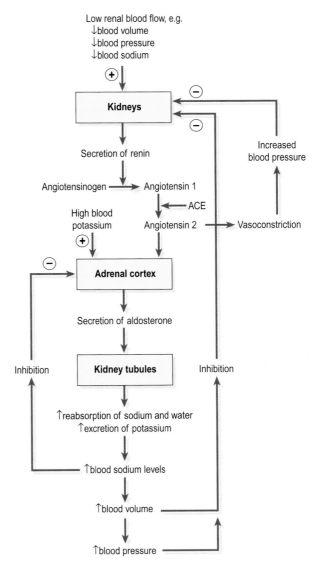

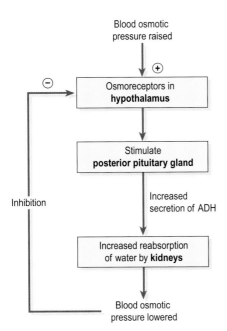

Figure 13.12 Negative feedback regulation of secretion of antidiuretic hormone (ADH).

Figure 13.13 Negative feedback regulation of aldosterone secretion. ACE = angiotensin converting enzyme.

Blood volume raised

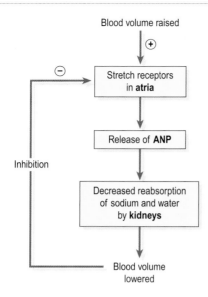

Figure 13.14 Negative feedback regulation of secretion of atrial natriuretic peptide (ANP).

Summary of urine formation

The three processes involved – filtration, selective reabsorption and tubular secretion – are described above and summarised in Figure 13.15.

Composition of urine

Urine is clear and amber in colour due to the presence of urobilin, a bile pigment altered in the intestine, reabsorbed then excreted by the kidneys (see Fig. 12.37, p. 311). The specific gravity is between 1020 and 1030, and the pH is around 6 (normal range 4.5–8). A healthy adult passes from 1000 to 1500 mL per day. The volume of urine produced and the specific gravity vary according to fluid intake and the amount of solute excreted. The constituents of urine are:

Water	96%			
Urea	2%			
Uric acid			Chlorides	
Creatinine			Phosphates	
Ammonia	} 2%		Sulphates	} 2%
Sodium			Oxalates	
Potassium				

Water balance and urine output

The source of most body water is dietary food and fluid although a small amount (called 'metabolic water') is formed by cellular metabolism. Water is excreted as the main constituent of urine, in expired air, faeces and through the skin as sweat. The amount lost in expired air and faeces is fairly constant; the amount of sweat produced is associated with environmental and body temperatures.

The balance between fluid intake and output is controlled by the kidneys. The minimum urinary output, i.e. the

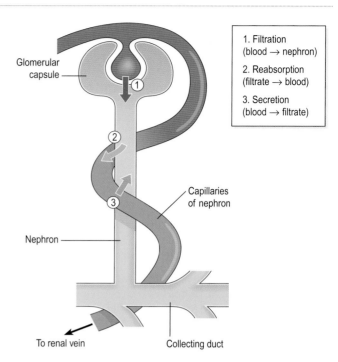

Figure 13.15 Summary of the three processes that form urine.

smallest volume required to excrete body waste products, is about 500 mL per day. Urinary volume in excess of this is controlled mainly by antidiuretic hormone (ADH) released into the blood by the posterior pituitary gland.

Sensory nerve cells in the hypothalamus (osmoreceptors) detect changes in the osmotic pressure of the blood. Nerve impulses from the osmoreceptors stimulate the posterior pituitary to release ADH. When the osmotic pressure is raised, i.e. the blood is becoming more concentrated, ADH output is increased and as a result, water reabsorption by the distal convoluted tubules and collecting ducts is increased, reducing the blood osmotic pressure and ADH output. This negative feedback mechanism maintains the blood osmotic pressure (and therefore sodium and water concentrations) within normal limits (see Fig. 13.12).

This negative feedback mechanism may be over-ridden even though there may be an excessive amount of a dissolved substance in the blood. For example, in diabetes mellitus when blood glucose levels exceed the transport capacity of the renal tubules the excess glucose remains in the filtrate, drawing water with it. Large volumes of urine are passed (*polyuria*), which may lead to dehydration despite increased ADH secretion. However acute thirst and increased water intake usually compensate for the polyuria, at least to some extent.

When blood volume is increased, stretch receptors in the atria of the heart are stimulated and cardiac muscle cells release atrial natriuretic hormone (ANP). This reduces reabsorption of sodium and water by the proximal convoluted tubules and collecting ducts, meaning that more sodium and water are excreted. In turn, this lowers blood volume and reduces atrial stretching, and through the negative feedback mechanism ANP secretion is switched off (see Fig. 13.14). Raised ANP levels also inhibit secretion of ADH and aldosterone, further promoting loss of sodium and water.

Electrolyte balance

Changes in the concentration of electrolytes in the body fluids may be due to changes in:

- the body water content, or
- electrolyte levels.

Several mechanisms maintain the balance between water and electrolyte concentration.

Sodium and potassium balance

Sodium is the most common cation (positively charged ion) in extracellular fluid and potassium is the most common intracellular cation.

Sodium is a constituent of almost all foods and, furthermore, salt is often added to food during cooking. This means that intake is usually in excess of the body's needs. It is excreted mainly in urine and sweat.

The amount of sodium excreted in sweat is usually insignificant unless sweating is excessive. This may occur when there is pyrexia (fever), a high environmental temperature or during sustained physical exercise. Normally the renin–angiotensin–aldosterone mechanism (described below) maintains the concentration of sodium and potassium within physiological limits. When excessive sweating is sustained, e.g. living in a hot climate or working in a hot environment, acclimatisation occurs in approximately 7 to 10 days and electrolyte secretion lost in sweat is reduced.

Sodium and potassium occur in high concentrations in digestive juices – sodium in gastric juice and potassium in pancreatic and intestinal juice. Normally these ions are reabsorbed by the colon, but following acute and prolonged diarrhoea they may be excreted in large quantities causing electrolyte imbalance.

Renin–angiotensin–aldosterone system. (Fig. 13.13) Sodium is a normal constituent of urine and its excretion is regulated by the hormone *aldosterone*, secreted by the adrenal cortex. Cells in the afferent arteriole of the nephron release the enzyme *renin* in response to sympathetic stimulation, low blood volume or by low arterial blood pressure. Renin converts the plasma protein *angiotensinogen*, produced by the liver, to angiotensin 1. *Angiotensin converting enzyme* (ACE), formed in small quantities in the lungs, proximal convoluted tubules and other tissues, converts angiotensin 1 into angiotensin 2, which is a very potent vasoconstrictor and increases blood pressure. Renin and raised blood potassium levels also stimulate the adrenal gland to secrete aldosterone. Water

is reabsorbed with sodium and together they increase the blood volume, which reduces renin secretion through the negative feedback mechanism. When sodium reabsorption is increased potassium excretion is increased, indirectly reducing intracellular potassium. Profound diuresis may lead to hypokalaemia (low blood potassium levels).

ANP. This hormone is also involved in the regulation of sodium levels (Fig. 13.14).

Calcium balance

Regulation of calcium levels is maintained by secretion of parathyroid hormone and calcitonin (see Ch. 9).

pH balance 13.9

In order to maintain normal blood pH (acid–base balance), the proximal convoluted tubules secrete hydrogen ions into the filtrate where they combine with buffers (p. 25):

- bicarbonate, forming carbonic acid
  ($H^+ + HCO_3^- \rightarrow H_2CO$)
- ammonia, forming ammonium ions
  ($H^+ + NH3 \rightarrow NH_4^+$)
- hydrogen phosphate, forming dihydrogen phosphate
  ($H^+ + HPO_3^{2-} \rightarrow H_2PO_3^-$

Carbonic acid is converted to carbon dioxide (CO_2) and water (H_2O), and the CO_2 is reabsorbed, maintaining the buffering capacity of the blood. Hydrogen ions are excreted in the urine as ammonium salts and hydrogen phosphate. The normal pH of urine varies from 4.5 to 8 depending on diet, time of day and other factors. Individuals whose diet contains a large amount of animal proteins tend to produce more acidic urine (lower pH) than vegetarians.

Ureters

Learning outcome

After studying this section, you should be able to:

■ outline the structure and function of the ureters.

The ureters carry urine from the kidneys to the urinary bladder (Fig. 13.16). They are about 25–30 cm long with a diameter of approximately 3 mm. The ureter is continuous with the funnel-shaped renal pelvis. It passes downwards through the abdominal cavity, behind the peritoneum in front of the psoas muscle into the pelvic cavity, and passes obliquely through the posterior wall of the bladder (Fig. 13.17). Because of this arrangement, as urine accumulates and the pressure in the bladder rises, the ureters are compressed and the openings into the

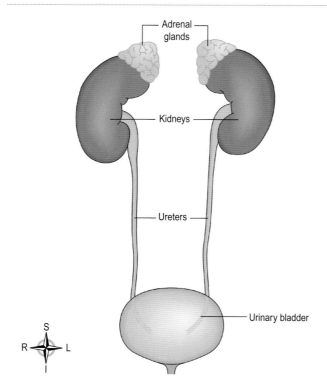

Figure 13.16 The ureters and their relationship to the kidneys and bladder.

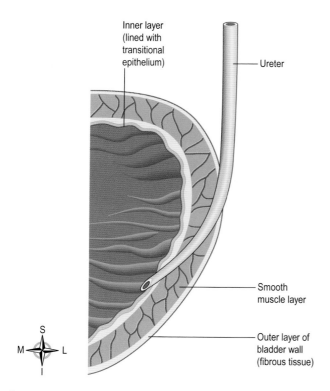

Figure 13.17 The position of the ureter where it passes through the bladder wall.

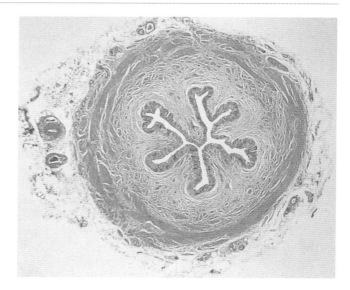

Figure 13.18 Cross-section of the ureter.

bladder are occluded. This prevents backflow (reflux) of urine into the ureters (towards the kidneys) as the bladder fills and also during micturition, when pressure increases as the muscular bladder wall contracts.

Structure 🎬 13.10

The walls of the ureters consist of three layers of tissue which are shown in cross-section in Figure 13.18:

* an outer covering of *fibrous tissue*, continuous with the fibrous capsule of the kidney
* a middle *muscular layer* consisting of interlacing smooth muscle fibres that form a functional unit round the ureter and an additional outer longitudinal layer in the lower third
* an inner layer, the *mucosa*, composed of transitional epithelium (see Fig. 3.15, p. 39).

Function

Peristalsis is an intrinsic property of the smooth muscle layer that propels urine along the ureter. Peristaltic waves occur several times per minute, increasing in frequency with the volume of urine produced, sending little spurts of urine along the ureter towards the bladder.

Urinary bladder

Learning outcome

After studying this section, you should be able to:

■ describe the structure of the bladder.

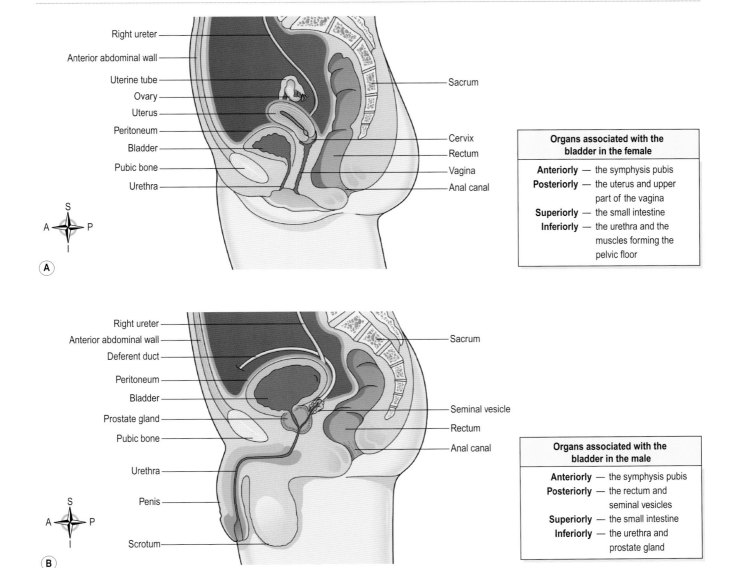

Organs associated with the bladder in the female	
Anteriorly — the symphysis pubis	
Posteriorly — the uterus and upper part of the vagina	
Superiorly — the small intestine	
Inferiorly — the urethra and the muscles forming the pelvic floor	

Organs associated with the bladder in the male	
Anteriorly — the symphysis pubis	
Posteriorly — the rectum and seminal vesicles	
Superiorly — the small intestine	
Inferiorly — the urethra and prostate gland	

Figure 13.19 The pelvic organs associated with the bladder and the urethra. A. The female. **B.** The male.

The urinary bladder is a reservoir for urine. It lies in the pelvic cavity and its size and position vary, depending on the volume of urine it contains. When distended, the bladder rises into the abdominal cavity.

Organs associated with the bladder

See Figure 13.19.

Structure (Fig. 13.20) ▐▐ **13.11**

The bladder is roughly pear shaped, but becomes more balloon shaped as it fills with urine. The posterior surface is the *base*. The bladder opens into the urethra at its lowest point, the *neck*.

The peritoneum covers only the superior surface before it turns upwards as the parietal peritoneum, lining the anterior abdominal wall. Posteriorly it surrounds the uterus in the female and the rectum in the male. The bladder wall is composed of three layers:

- the outer layer of loose connective tissue, containing blood and lymphatic vessels and nerves, covered on the upper surface by the peritoneum
- the middle layer, consisting of interlacing smooth muscle fibres and elastic tissue loosely arranged in three layers. This is called the *detrusor muscle* and when it contracts, it empties the bladder
- the inner mucosa, composed of transitional epithelium (Fig. 3.15, p. 39) that readily permits distension of the bladder as it fills.

When the bladder is empty the inner lining is arranged in folds, or rugae, which gradually disappear as it fills. The bladder is distensible but as it fills, awareness of the

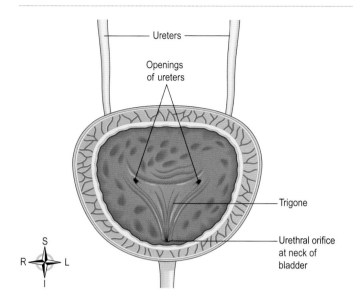

Figure 13.20 Section of the bladder showing the trigone.

need to pass urine is felt. The total capacity is rarely more than about 600 mL.

The three orifices in the bladder wall form a triangle or *trigone* (Fig. 13.20). The upper two orifices on the posterior wall are the openings of the ureters; the lower orifice is the opening into the urethra. The *internal urethral sphincter*, a thickening of the urethral smooth muscle layer in the upper part of the urethra, controls outflow of urine from the bladder. This sphincter is not under voluntary control.

Urethra

Learning outcome

After studying this section, you should be able to:

■ outline the structure and function of the urethra in males and females.

The urethra is a canal extending from the neck of the bladder to the exterior, at the external urethral orifice. It is longer in the male than in the female.

The male urethra is associated with both the urinary and reproductive systems, and is described in detail in Chapter 18.   **13.12**

The female urethra is approximately 4 cm long and 6 mm in diameter. It runs downwards and forwards behind the symphysis pubis and opens at the *external urethral orifice* just in front of the vagina. The external urethral orifice is guarded by the *external urethral sphincter*, which is under voluntary control.

The wall of the female urethra has two main layers: an outer muscle layer and an inner lining of mucosa, which

is continuous with that of the bladder. The muscle layer has two parts, an inner layer of smooth muscle that is under autonomic nerve control, and an outer layer of striated (voluntary) muscle surrounding it. The striated muscle forms the external urethral sphincter and is under voluntary control. The mucosa is supported by loose fibroelastic connective tissue containing blood vessels and nerves. Proximally it consists of transitional epithelium while distally it is composed of stratified epithelium.

Micturition

Learning outcome

After studying this section, you should be able to:

■ compare and contrast the process of micturition in infants and adults.

In infants, accumulation of urine in the bladder activates stretch receptors in the bladder wall generating sensory (afferent) impulses that are transmitted to the spinal cord, where a *spinal reflex* (p. 164) is initiated. This stimulates involuntary contraction of the detrusor muscle and relaxation of the internal urethral sphincter (Fig. 13.21), and expels urine from the bladder – this is *micturition* or voiding of urine.

When bladder control is established, the micturition reflex is still stimulated but sensory impulses also pass upwards to the brain and there is awareness of the need to pass urine as the bladder fills (around 300–400 mL in adults). By learned and conscious effort, contraction of the external urethral sphincter and muscles of the pelvic floor can inhibit micturition until it is convenient to pass urine (Fig. 13.22).

Urination can be assisted by increasing the pressure within the pelvic cavity, achieved by lowering the diaphragm and contracting the abdominal muscles. Over-distension of the bladder is extremely painful, and when this occurs there is a tendency for involuntary relaxation of the external sphincter to occur allowing a small amount of urine to escape, provided there is no mechanical obstruction. *Incontinence* is the involuntary loss of urine after bladder control has been established.

The effects of ageing of the urinary system

Learning outcome

After studying this section, you should be able to:

■ describe the effects of ageing on the urinary system.

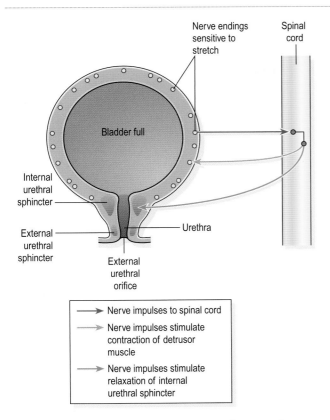

Figure 13.21 Reflex control of micturition when conscious effort cannot override the reflex action.

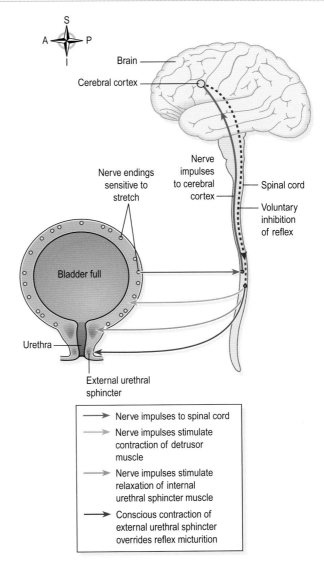

Figure 13.22 Control of micturition after bladder control is established.

The kidneys have a substantial functional reserve; the loss of one kidney does not cause problems in an otherwise healthy individual. The number of nephrons declines with age, glomerular filtration rate falls and the renal tubules function less efficiently; the kidneys become less able to concentrate urine.

These changes mean that older adults become more sensitive to alterations in fluid balance, and problems associated with fluid overload or dehydration are more prevalent. Elimination of drugs also becomes less efficient with declining kidney function which may lead to accumulation and toxicity.

The ability to inhibit contraction of the detrusor muscle declines and may result in the urgent need to pass urine and urinary frequency. Nocturia becomes increasingly

common in older adults. Incontinence (p. 356) is more prevalent in older adults affecting 15% of women and 10% of men over 65, figures which double by 85 years of age. Enlargement of the prostate gland is common in older men and may cause retention of urine and problems with micturition (see Ch. 18).

Diseases of the kidneys

Learning outcomes

After studying this section, you should be able to:

■ outline the principal effects of glomerulonephritis

■ describe the effects of diabetes mellitus and hypertension on kidney function

■ discuss the sources and consequences of kidney infections

■ explain the causes and implications of acute and chronic renal failure

■ describe the pathogenesis of kidney stones

■ list common congenital abnormalities of the kidneys

■ outline the development and spread of common kidney tumours.

As the kidneys have considerable functional reserve impairment of renal function does not become evident until the equivalent of more than one kidney is lost. This is why it is possible for a person with healthy kidneys to donate one for transplantation. Table 13.1 lists common signs and symptoms of renal disorders.

Glomerulonephritis (GN)

This term suggests inflammatory conditions of the glomerulus, but there are several types of GN and inflammatory changes are not always present. In many cases GN has an autoimmune component which leads to production of immune complexes that may lodge in the glomerular capillaries causing inflammation and impairment of glomerular filtration. Other immune mechanisms are also implicated in GN.

Classification of GN is based on a number of features: the cause, immunological characteristics and findings on microscopy. Microscopic distinction is based on:

• the extent of damage:
  – *diffuse*: affecting all glomeruli
  – *focal*: affecting some glomeruli
• appearance:
  – *proliferative*: increased number of cells in the glomeruli
  – *membranous*: thickening of the glomerular basement membrane.

Examples of different types of GN, their causes, features and prognoses are shown in Table 13.2.

Effects of glomerulonephritis

These depend on the type and are listed below.

Haematuria. This is usually painless and not accompanied by other symptoms. When microscopic, it may be

Table 13.1 Common signs and symptoms of disorders of the urinary system

Sign/symptom	Definition and description
Oliguria	Urine output less than 400 mL per day
Haematuria	Presence of blood in the urine. Leaky glomeruli allow red blood cells to escape from the glomerular capillaries and they cannot be reabsorbed from the filtrate as they are too large. Bleeding in the urinary tract also causes haematuria
Proteinuria	Presence of protein in the urine. This is abnormal and occurs when leaky glomeruli allow plasma proteins to escape into the filtrate but they are too large to be reabsorbed
Anuria	Absence of urine
Dysuria	Pain on passing urine, often described as a burning sensation
Glycosuria	Presence of sugar in the urine. This is abnormal and occurs in diabetes mellitus (see p. 236)
Ketonuria	Presence of ketones in the urine. This is abnormal and occurs in, e.g., starvation, diabetes mellitus
Nocturia	Passing urine during the night
Polyuria	Passing unusually large amounts of urine
Frequency of micturition	Requiring to pass, often small amounts of, urine frequently
Incontinence	Involuntary loss of urine (p. 356)

found on routine urinalysis when red blood cells have passed through damaged glomeruli into the filtrate.

Overt haematuria occurs when there is considerable escape of red blood cells into the renal tubules while smaller amounts give urine a smoky appearance.

Asymptomatic proteinuria. Damaged glomeruli may allow protein to escape from the blood into the filtrate, which may be asymptomatic and only found during routine urinalysis, however there are also other causes of asymptomatic proteinuria e.g. urinary tract infection. Significant proteinuria is associated with nephrotic syndrome (p. 351).

Acute nephritis. This is characterised by the presence of:

• oliguria (<400 mL urine/day in adults)
• hypertension
• haematuria
• uraemia (p. 353).

Loin pain, headache and malaise are also common.

Table 13.2 Glomerulonephritis: features and prognosis of different types

Type	Cause	Presenting features	Prognosis
Diffuse proliferative GN	Usually follows a transient infection, especially *β-haemolytic Streptococcus* but also other microbes	Acute nephritis Haematuria Proteinuria	Good in children; less good in adults, up to 40% develop hypertension or chronic renal failure
Focal proliferative GN	Associated with other systemic conditions, e.g. systemic lupus erythematosus (p. 434), infective endocarditis (p. 128)	Acute nephritis Haematuria Proteinuria	Variable
Membranous GN	Only sometimes has an identified cause such as infection, e.g. syphilis, malaria, hepatitis B; some drugs, e.g. penicillamine, gold, diamorphine; tumours	Nephrotic syndrome Haematuria Proteinuria	Variable, but most cases progress to chronic renal failure as sclerosis of glomeruli progresses
Minimal-change GN	Unknown	Nephrotic syndrome Haematuria Proteinuria	Good in children, but recurrences are common in adults

Nephrotic syndrome. (See below.)

Chronic renal failure. (p. 353) This occurs when nephrons are progressively and irreversibly damaged after the renal reserve is lost.

Nephrotic syndrome

This is not a disease in itself but is an important feature of several kidney diseases. The main characteristics are:

- marked proteinuria
- hypoalbuminaemia
- generalised oedema
- hyperlipidaemia.

When glomeruli are damaged, the permeability of the glomerular membrane increases and plasma proteins pass through into the filtrate. Albumin is the main protein lost because it is the most common and is the smallest of the plasma proteins. When the daily loss exceeds the rate of production by the liver there is a significant fall in the total plasma protein level. The consequent low plasma osmotic pressure leads to widespread oedema and reduced plasma volume (see Fig. 5.57, p. 125). This reduces the renal blood flow and stimulates the renin–angiotensin–aldosterone system (Fig. 13.13), causing increased reabsorption of water and sodium from the renal tubules. The reabsorbed water further reduces the blood osmotic pressure and increases the oedema. The key factor is the loss of albumin across the glomerular membrane and as long as this continues, the vicious circle is perpetuated (Fig. 13.23). Levels of nitrogenous waste products, i.e. uric acid, urea and creatinine, usually

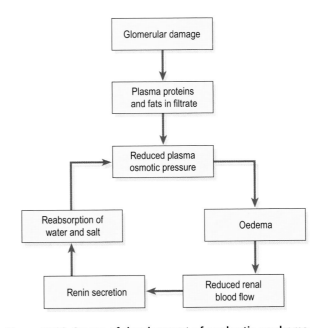

Figure 13.23 Stages of development of nephrotic syndrome.

remain normal. Hyperlipidaemia, especially hypercholesterolaemia, also occurs but the cause is unknown.

Nephrotic syndrome occurs in a number of diseases. In children the most common cause is minimal-change glomerulonephritis. In adults it may complicate:

- most forms of glomerulonephritis
- diabetic nephropathy (see below)
- systemic lupus erythematosus (p. 434)
- infections, e.g. malaria, syphilis, hepatitis B
- drugs, e.g. penicillamine, gold, captopril, phenytoin.

Diabetic nephropathy

Renal failure is the commonest cause of death in young people with diabetes mellitus (p. 236), especially if hypertension and severe, long-standing hyperglycaemia are also present. Diabetes causes damage to large and small blood vessels throughout the body, although the effects vary considerably between individuals. In the kidney, these are known collectively as *diabetic nephropathy* or *diabetic kidney* and include:

- progressive damage of glomeruli, proteinuria and nephrotic syndrome
- ascending infection leading to acute pyelonephritis
- atheroma (see Ch. 5) of the renal arteries and their branches leading to renal ischaemia and hypertension
- chronic renal failure (p. 353).

Hypertension and the kidneys

Hypertension can be the cause or the result of renal disease. Essential and secondary hypertension (p. 131) both affect the kidneys when renal blood vessel damage causes ischaemia. The reduced blood flow stimulates the renin–angiotensin–aldosterone system (see Fig. 13.13), raising the blood pressure still further.

Rising blood pressure is common in older adult (p. 117) and can cause gradual and progressive damage to the glomeruli, which may lead to renal failure after the renal reserve has been lost or to malignant hypertension.

Secondary hypertension

This can be caused by long-standing kidney diseases (described in this chapter) and may lead to chronic renal ischaemia, worsening hypertension and renal failure.

Malignant hypertension

Damage to arterioles spreads to the glomeruli with subsequent destruction of nephrons and leads to a further rise in blood pressure and a variable degree of renal impairment. Sometimes there are more serious effects; increased permeability of the glomeruli allows escape of plasma proteins and red blood cells into the filtrate causing proteinuria and haematuria, which may progress to renal failure.

Acute pyelonephritis

This is acute bacterial infection of the renal pelvis and calyces, which spreads to the kidney substance causing small abscesses. Bacteria usually reach the kidney by travelling up the urinary tract from the perineum but are sometimes blood-borne. This condition is accompanied by fever, malaise and loin pain.

Ascending infection. Upward spread of bacteria from the bladder (see cystitis, p. 356) is the most common cause of this condition. Reflux of infected urine into the ureters when the bladder contracts during micturition predisposes to upward spread of infection to the renal pelves and kidney substance. Normally the relative positions of the ureters and bladder (Fig. 13.16) prevents reflux that permits ascending access of bacteria to the kidneys.

Blood-borne infection. The kidneys are susceptible to blood-borne infection due to their large blood supply (20% of cardiac output). Bacteria may reach the kidney directly in septicaemia or travel there from distant sites e.g. a respiratory tract infection, infected wound or abscess.

Pathophysiology

Bacterial infection of the kidney tissues causes suppuration and destruction of nephrons. The prognosis depends on the amount of healthy kidney tissue remaining after the infection subsides. Necrotic tissue is eventually replaced by fibrous tissue but there may be some hypertrophy of healthy nephrons. The outcomes are healing; recurrence, especially if there is a structural abnormality of the urinary tract; and reflux nephropathy. Papillary necrosis is a rare complication, usually occurring if the condition is untreated.

Reflux nephropathy

Previously known as chronic pyelonephritis, this is almost always associated with reflux of urine from the bladder to the ureter allowing spread of infection upwards towards the kidneys. A congenital abnormality of the angle of insertion of the ureter into the bladder predisposes to this, but it is sometimes caused by an obstruction that develops later in life. Progressive damage to the renal papillae and collecting ducts may lead to chronic renal failure and concurrent hypertension is common.

Renal failure

Acute renal failure

The causes of acute renal failure are classified as:

- *prerenal*: the result of reduced renal blood flow, especially as a consequence of, e.g., severe and prolonged shock
- *renal*: due to damage to the kidney itself, e.g. acute tubular necrosis, glomerulonephritis
- *postrenal*: arises from obstruction to the outflow of urine, e.g. disease of the prostate gland, tumour of the bladder, uterus or cervix, large calculus (stone) in the renal pelvis.

There is a sudden and severe reduction in the glomerular filtration rate and kidney function that is often reversible over days or weeks if treated. Oliguria or anuria is accompanied by metabolic acidosis due to retention of H^+, electrolyte imbalance and accumulation of mainly nitrogenous

Box 13.2 Some causes of ATN

Ischaemia – severe shock, dehydration, haemorrhage, trauma; extensive burns; myocardial infarction; prolonged and complex surgery, especially in older people

Drugs – e.g. aminoglycoside antibiotics, non-steroidal anti-inflammatory drugs (NSAIDs), ACE inhibitors, lithium compounds, paracetamol overdose

Haemoglobinaemia – accumulation of haemoglobin, released by haemolysis of red blood cells, e.g. incompatible blood transfusion, malaria

Myoglobinaemia – accumulation of myoglobin released from damaged muscle raises blood levels, e.g. following crush injury.

Table 13.3 Polyuria in chronic renal failure

	Normal kidney	End-stage kidney
GFR	125 mL/min or 180 L/day	10 mL/min or 14 L/day
Reabsorption of water	>99%	Approx. 30%
Urine output	<1 mL/min or 1.5 L/day	Approx. 7 mL/min or 10 L/day

waste products. This occurs as a complication of conditions not necessarily associated with the kidneys.

Acute tubular necrosis (ATN)

This is the most common cause of acute renal failure. There is severe damage to the tubular epithelial cells caused by ischaemia or, less often, by nephrotoxic substances (Box 13.2).

Oliguria, severe oliguria (less than 100 mL of urine per day in adults) or *anuria* (see Table 13.1) may last for a few weeks, followed by profound diuresis. There is a reduction in glomerular filtration, selective reabsorption and secretion by the tubules, leading to:

- heart failure due to fluid overload
- generalised and pulmonary oedema
- accumulation of urea and other metabolic wastes
- electrolyte imbalance which may be exacerbated by the retention of potassium (hyperkalaemia) released from damaged cells anywhere in the body
- acidosis due to retention of hydrogen ions.

Profound diuresis (the diuretic phase) occurs during the healing process when the epithelial cells of the tubules have regenerated but are still incapable of selective reabsorption and secretion. Diuresis may lead to acute dehydration, complicating the existing high plasma urea, acidosis and electrolyte imbalance. If the patient survives the initial acute phase, a considerable degree of renal function is usually restored over several weeks (the recovery phase).

Chronic renal failure

Also known as chronic kidney disease (CKD), this is present when GFR has fallen to around 20% of normal. Onset is usually slow and asymptomatic, progressing over several years. The main causes are diabetes mellitus, glomerulonephritis and hypertension.

The effects on glomerular filtration rate (GFR), selective reabsorption and tubular secretion are significant.

GFR and filtrate volumes are greatly reduced, and reabsorption of water is seriously impaired. This results in production of up to 10 litres of urine per day (Table 13.3). Reduced glomerular filtration leads to accumulation of waste substances in the blood, notably urea and creatinine. When renal failure becomes evident, blood urea levels are raised and this is referred to as *uraemia*. Some of the signs and symptoms that may accompany this condition include nausea, vomiting, gastrointestinal bleeding, anaemia and pruritus (itching). Others are explained below.

Polyuria. Large volumes of dilute urine (with a low specific gravity) are passed, because water reabsorption is impaired. *Nocturia* is a common presenting symptom.

Acidosis. As the kidney buffer system that normally controls the pH of body fluids fails, hydrogen ions accumulate.

Electrolyte imbalance. This is also the result of impaired tubular reabsorption and secretion.

Anaemia. Deficiency of erythropoietin (p. 66) occurs after a few months, causing anaemia that is exacerbated by haemodialysis which damages red blood cells. If untreated, anaemia results in fatigue, and may also lead to dyspnoea and cardiac failure (p. 126). Tiredness and breathlessness are sometimes the initial symptoms of chronic renal failure.

Hypertension. This is often a consequence, if not a cause, of renal failure.

End-stage renal failure

When death is likely without renal replacement therapy, such as haemodialysis, peritoneal dialysis or a kidney transplant, the condition is referred to as *end-stage renal failure*. The excretory functions of the kidneys are lost, acid–base balance cannot be maintained and endocrine functions of the kidney are disrupted.

Towards the end of life anorexia, nausea and very deep (Kussmaul's) respirations occur as uraemia progresses. In the final stages there may be hiccoughs, itching, vomiting, muscle twitching, seizures, drowsiness and coma.

Renal calculi 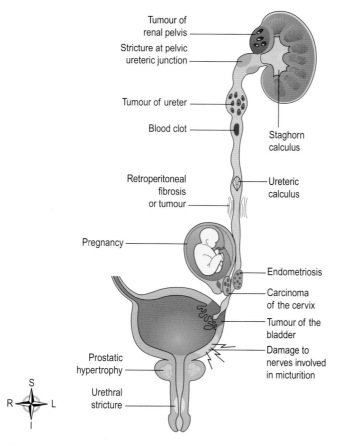 13.13

Calculi (stones) form in the kidneys and bladder when urinary constituents normally in solution, usually oxalate and phosphate salts, are precipitated. They are more common in males and after 30 years of age and often recur. Most originate in the collecting tubules or renal papillae. They then pass into the renal pelvis where they may increase in size. Some become too large to pass through the ureter and may obstruct the outflow of urine, causing kidney damage. Others pass to the bladder and are either excreted or increase in size and obstruct the urethra (Fig. 13.24). In developing countries and often in children, stones sometimes originate in the bladder. Predisposing factors include:

- *dehydration*: this leads to increased reabsorption of water from the tubules but does not change solute reabsorption, resulting in a low volume of highly concentrated filtrate in the collecting tubules
- *pH of urine*: when the normally acid filtrate becomes alkaline, some substances may be precipitated, e.g. phosphates. This occurs when the kidney buffering system is impaired and in some infections
- *infection*: necrotic material and pus provide foci upon which solutes in the filtrate may be deposited and the

products of infection may alter the pH of the urine. Infection sometimes leads to alkaline urine (see above)
- *metabolic conditions*: these include hyperparathyroidism (p. 233) and gout (p. 434).

Small calculi 13.14

These may pass through or become impacted in a ureter and damage the epithelium, leading to haematuria and after healing, fibrosis and stricture. In ureteric obstruction, which is usually unilateral, there is spasmodic contraction of the ureter, causing acute intermittent ischaemic pain (*renal colic*) as the smooth muscle of the ureter contracts over the stone in an attempt to move it. Stones reaching the bladder may be passed in urine or increase in size and eventually obstruct the urethra. Consequences include retention of urine and bilateral hydronephrosis (p. 355), infection proximal to the blockage, pyelonephritis and severe kidney damage.

Large calculi (staghorn calculus)

One large stone may form, usually over many years, filling the renal pelvis and the calyces (see Fig. 13.24). It causes stagnation of urine, predisposing to infection, hydronephrosis and occasionally kidney tumours. It may cause chronic renal failure.

Congenital abnormalities of the kidneys

Misplaced (ectopic) kidney

One or both kidneys may develop in abnormally low positions. Misplaced kidneys function normally if the blood vessels are long enough to provide an adequate blood supply but a kidney in the pelvic cavity may cause problems during pregnancy as the expanding uterus compresses renal blood vessels or the ureters. If the ureters become kinked there is increased risk of infection as there is a tendency for reflux and backflow to the kidney. There may also be difficulties during childbirth.

Polycystic disease

The *infantile form* is very rare and is usually fatal in early childhood.

Autosomal dominant polycystic kidney disease (ADPKD). This is inherited as an autosomal dominant condition (Ch. 17) that may become apparent any time between childhood and late adult life. Both kidneys are affected. Dilations (cysts) form at the junction of the distal convoluted tubules and collecting ducts. The cysts slowly enlarge and pressure causes ischaemia and destruction of nephrons. The disease is progressive and secondary hypertension is common; chronic renal failure affects

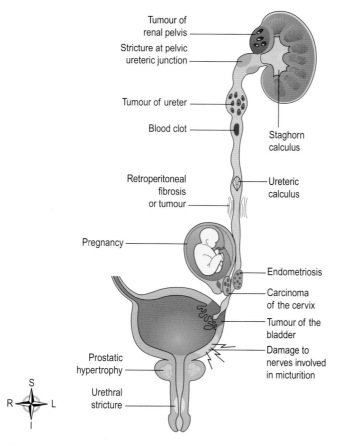

Figure 13.24 Summary of obstructions of the urinary tract.

about 50% of patients. Death may be due to chronic renal failure, cardiac failure or subarachnoid haemorrhage due to increased incidence of berry aneurysms of the circulus arteriosus (p. 105). Cysts may also develop in the liver, spleen and pancreas but are not associated with dysfunction of these organs.

Tumours of the kidney

Benign tumours are relatively uncommon.

Malignant tumours

These are most common in the bladder or kidney.

Renal adenocarcinoma

This tumour of tubular epithelium is more common after 50 years of age, and in males. Clinical features include haematuria, back or loin pain, anaemia, weight loss and fever. Local spread involves the renal vein and leads to early blood spread of tumour fragments, most commonly to the lungs and bones. The causes are unknown although there is an increased incidence in cigarette smokers.

Nephroblastoma (Wilms' tumour)

This is one of the most common malignant tumours in children under 10 years, usually occurring in the first 4 years. Clinical features include haematuria, hypertension, abdominal pain and, sometimes, intestinal obstruction. It is usually unilateral but rapidly becomes very large and invades the renal blood vessels, causing early blood spread to the lungs.

Diseases of the renal pelvis, ureters, bladder and urethra

Learning outcomes

After studying this section, you should be able to:

- describe the causes and implications of urinary obstruction

- explain the pathological features of urinary tract infections

- outline the characteristics of the main bladder tumours

- discuss the principal causes of urinary incontinence.

These structures are considered together because their combined functions are to collect and store urine prior to excretion. Obstruction and infection are the main problems (Fig. 13.24).

Obstruction to the outflow of urine

Hydronephrosis ▨ 13.15

This is dilation of the renal pelvis and calyces caused by accumulation of urine above an obstruction in the urinary tract (Fig. 13.24). It leads to destruction of the nephrons, fibrosis and atrophy of the kidney. One or both kidneys may be involved, depending on the cause and site. When there is an abnormality of the bladder or urethra, both kidneys are affected whereas an obstruction above the bladder is more common and affects only one kidney. The effects depend on the site and extent of the obstruction. Stasis of urine within the urinary tract predisposes to infection.

Complete sustained obstruction

In this condition hydronephrosis develops quickly, pressure in the nephrons rises and urine production stops. The most common causes are a large calculus or tumour. The outcome depends on whether one or both kidneys are involved (adequate renal function can be maintained by one kidney).

Partial or intermittent obstruction

This may progress undetected for many years. It leads to progressive hydronephrosis and is caused by, e.g.:

- a succession of renal calculi in a ureter, eventually moved onwards by peristalsis
- constriction of a ureter or the urethra by fibrous tissue, following epithelial inflammation caused by the passage of a stone or by infection
- a tumour in the urinary tract or in the abdominal or pelvic cavity
- enlarged prostate gland in the male.

Spinal lesions

When the nerve supply to the bladder is interrupted, e.g. transverse spinal cord lesions, micturition does not occur. When the bladder fills, the rise in pressure causes overflow incontinence (p. 356), back pressure into the ureters and hydronephrosis. Reflex micturition is usually re-established after a time, but loss of voluntary control may be irreversible. Pressure on the spinal cord and other abnormalities, e.g. spina bifida, can also impair micturition.

Urinary tract infections (UTIs)

Infection of any part of the urinary tract may spread upwards causing acute pyelonephritis (p. 352) and kidney damage.

Ureteritis

Inflammation of a ureter is usually due to the upward spread of infection in cystitis.

Cystitis

This is inflammation of the bladder and may be due to:

- upward spread of commensal bacteria of the bowel (*Escherichia coli* and *Streptococcus faecalis*) from the perineum via the urethra, especially in women
- trauma, with or without infection, following health-care interventions, e.g. radiotherapy, insertion of a urinary catheter or instrument into the bladder.

The effects of inflammation include oedema and small haemorrhages of the mucosa, which may be accompanied by *haematuria*. The sensory nerve endings in the bladder wall become hypersensitive and are stimulated when the bladder contains only small volumes of urine, leading to *frequency of micturition* and *dysuria*. The urine may appear cloudy and have an unpleasant smell. Lower abdominal pain often accompanies cystitis. If untreated, upward spread may cause acute pyelonephritis (see p. 352) or septicaemia.

Cystitis is *uncomplicated* when it occurs in otherwise healthy individuals with a normal urinary tract. When it affects people with structural or functional abnormalities of the urinary tract or those with pre-existing conditions, e.g. diabetes mellitus or urinary outflow obstruction, it is described as *complicated*. Complicated UTIs sometimes cause permanent renal damage, whereas this is very rare in uncomplicated infections. Recurrence is fairly common, especially in women, either when the original infection is not eradicated or reinfection occurs.

Predisposing factors. These include stasis of urine in the bladder and the shorter female urethra, which is close to the anus (Fig. 13.19A), and the moist perineal conditions there that may harbour commensal microbes. Sexual intercourse may cause trauma to the urethra and transfer of microbes from the perineum, especially in the female. Hormones associated with pregnancy relax perineal muscle, and cause relaxation and kinking of the ureters. Towards the end of pregnancy, pressure caused by the fetus may obstruct the outflow of urine. In the male, prostatitis provides a focus of local infection or an enlarged prostate gland may cause progressive urethral obstruction.

Urethritis

This is inflammation of the urethra and is described in Chapter 18.

Tumours of the bladder

It is not always clear whether bladder tumours are benign or malignant. Tumours are often multiple and recurrence is common. Predisposing factors include cigarette smoking, prolonged use of certain analgesics and occupational exposure to some chemicals, e.g. aniline dyes used in the textile and printing industries.

Transitional cell carcinomas

These tumours, also known as papillomas, arise from transitional epithelium and are often benign. They consist of a stalk with fine-branching fronds, which tend to break off causing painless bleeding and haemturia. Papillomas commonly recur, even when benign. Sometimes the tumour cells are well differentiated and non-invasive but in other cases they behave as carcinomas and invade surrounding blood and lymph vessels.

Solid tumours

These are all malignant to some degree. At an early stage the more malignant and solid tumours rapidly invade the bladder wall and spread in lymph and blood to other parts of the body. If the surface ulcerates there may be haemorrhage and necrosis.

Urinary incontinence

In this condition normal micturition (p. 348) is affected and there is involuntary loss of urine. Several types are recognised and described below. In addition to the mechanisms below, neurological abnormalities can also impair voluntary control of micturition, e.g. spinal cord injury, multiple sclerosis (p. 185).

Stress incontinence

This is leakage of urine when intra-abdominal pressure is raised, e.g. on coughing, laughing, sneezing or lifting. It usually affects women when there is weakness of the pelvic floor muscles or pelvic ligaments, e.g. after childbirth or as part of the ageing process. It occurs physiologically in young children before bladder control is achieved.

Urge incontinence

Leakage of urine follows a sudden and intense urge to void and there is inability to delay passing urine. This may be due to a urinary tract infection, calculus, tumour or hypersensitivity of the detrusor muscle.

Overflow incontinence

This occurs when there is chronic overfilling of the bladder and may be due to retention of urine due to incomplete voiding when there is obstruction of urinary outflow, e.g. enlarged prostate gland or urethral stricture and/or impaired contraction of the detrusor muscle during micturition. It may also arise as a complication of pelvic nerve damage caused by e.g. surgery, trauma, or when the cauda equina is compressed by a tumor or prolapsed intervertebral disc.

The bladder becomes distended and when the pressure inside overcomes the resistance of the external urethral sphincter, urine dribbles from the urethra. There may be difficulty initiating and/or maintaining micturition. Larger than normal residual volumes of urine in the bladder (>50–100 mL) predispose to infection.

For a range of self-assessment exercises on the topics in this chapter, visit Evolve online resources: https://evolve.elsevier .com/Waugh/anatomy/

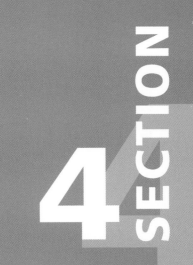

Protection and survival

The skin

ANIMATION

The skin

Learning outcomes

After studying this section, you should be able to:

■ describe the structure of the skin

■ explain the principal functions of the skin

■ compare and contrast the processes of primary and secondary wound healing.

The first part of this chapter explores the structure and functions of the skin, which is also known as the integumentary system. The effects of ageing on the skin are discussed in the following section. The chapter concludes with a review of common skin conditions.

The skin completely covers the body and is continuous with the membranes lining the body orifices. It:

● protects the underlying structures from injury and from invasion by microbes
● contains sensory nerve endings that enable discrimination of pain, temperature and touch
● is involved in the regulation of body temperature.

Structure of the skin

The skin is the largest organ in the body and has a surface area of about 1.5–2 m² in adults. In certain areas, it contains accessory structures: glands, hair and nails. There are two main layers; the *epidermis*, which covers the *dermis*. Between the skin and underlying structures is a subcutaneous layer composed of areolar tissue and adipose (fat) tissue.

Epidermis

This is the most superficial layer and is composed of *stratified keratinised squamous epithelium* (see Fig. 3.13, p. 39). It varies in thickness, being thickest on the palms of the hands and soles of the feet. There are no blood vessels or nerve endings in the epidermis, but its deeper layers are bathed in interstitial fluid from the dermis, which provides oxygen and nutrients, and drains away as lymph.

There are several layers (strata) of cells in the epidermis which extend from the deepest *germinative layer* to the most superficial *stratum corneum* (a thick horny layer) (Fig. 14.1). Epidermal cells originate in the germinative layer and undergo gradual change as they progress towards the skin surface. The cells on the surface are flat, thin, non-nucleated, dead cells, or *squames*, in which the cytoplasm has been replaced by the fibrous protein *keratin*. The surface cells are constantly rubbed off and replaced by those beneath. Complete replacement of the epidermis takes about a month.

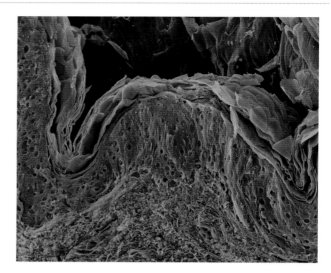

Figure 14.1 Coloured scanning electron micrograph of the skin showing the superficial stratum corneum (pale brown), above the lower layers of the epidermis (pink) and the dermis (grey brown).

Healthy epidermis depends upon three processes being synchronised:

● desquamation (shedding) of the keratinised cells from the surface
● effective keratinisation of cells approaching the surface
● continual cell division in the deeper layers with newly formed cells being pushed upwards to the surface.

Hairs, secretions from sebaceous glands and ducts of sweat glands pass through the epidermis to reach the surface.

Upward projections of the dermal layer, the *dermal papillae* (Fig. 14.2), anchor this securely to the more superficial epidermis and allow passage and exchange of nutrients and wastes to the lower part of the epidermis. This arrangement stabilises the two layers preventing damage due to shearing forces. *Blisters* develop when trauma causes separation of the dermis and epidermis, and serous fluid collects between the two layers.

In areas where the skin is subject to greater wear and tear, e.g. the palms and fingers of the hands and soles of the feet, the epidermis is thicker and hairs are absent. In these areas the dermal papillae are arranged in parallel lines giving the skin surface a ridged appearance. The pattern of ridges on the fingertips is unique to every individual and the impression made by them is the 'fingerprint'.

Skin colour is affected by various factors.

● Melanin, a dark pigment derived from the amino acid tyrosine and secreted by *melanocytes* in the deep germinative layer, is absorbed by surrounding epithelial cells. The amount is genetically determined and varies between different parts of the body,

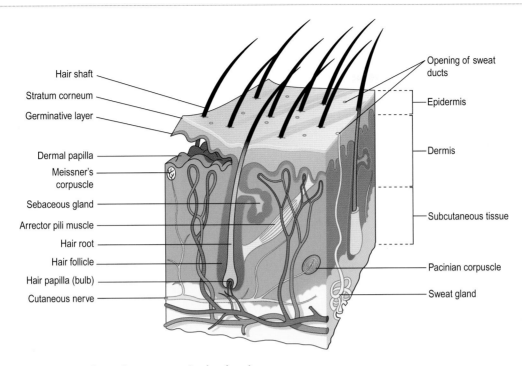

Figure 14.2 The skin showing the main structures in the dermis.

between people of the same ethnic origin and between ethnic groups. The number of melanocytes is fairly constant so the differences in colour depend on the amount of melanin secreted. It protects the skin from the harmful effects of ultraviolet rays in sunlight. Exposure to sunlight promotes synthesis of melanin.

- Normal saturation of haemoglobin (p. 66) and the amount of blood circulating in the dermis give white skin its pink colour. When oxygen saturation is very low, the skin may appear bluish (*cyanosis*).
- Excessive levels of bile pigments in blood and carotenes in subcutaneous fat give the skin a yellowish colour.

Dermis (Fig. 14.2)

The dermis is tough and elastic. It is formed from connective tissue and the matrix contains *collagen fibres* (see Fig. 3.16, p. 40) interlaced with *elastic fibres*. Rupture of elastic fibres occurs when the skin is overstretched, resulting in permanent *striae*, or stretch marks, that may be found in pregnancy and obesity. Collagen fibres bind water and give the skin its tensile strength, but as this ability declines with age, wrinkles develop. Fibroblasts (see Fig. 3.5, p. 34), macrophages (Fig. 3.17, p. 40) and mast cells are the main cells found in the dermis. Underlying its deepest layer is the subcutaneous layer containing areolar tissue and varying amounts of adipose (fat) tissue. The structures in the dermis are:

- blood and lymph vessels
- sensory nerve endings
- sweat glands and their ducts
- hairs, arrector pili muscles and sebaceous glands.

Blood and lymph vessels. Arterioles form a fine network with capillary branches supplying sweat glands, sebaceous glands, hair follicles and the dermis. Lymph vessels form a network throughout the dermis.

Sensory nerve endings. Sensory receptors (specialised nerve endings) sensitive to *touch, temperature, pressure* and *pain* are widely distributed in the dermis. Incoming stimuli activate different types of sensory receptors (Fig. 14.2, Box 14.1); for example, the Pacinian corpuscle is sensitive to deep pressure (Fig. 14.3). The skin is an important sensory organ through which individuals receive information about their environment. Nerve impulses, generated in the sensory receptors in the dermis, are transmitted to the spinal cord by sensory nerves (Fig. 14.4). From there impulses are conducted to the sensory area of the cerebrum where the sensations are perceived (see Fig. 7.22B, p. 158).

Box 14.1 Sensory receptors in the skin	
Sensory receptor	Stimulus
Meissner's corpuscle	Light pressure
Pacinian corpuscle	Deep pressure
Free nerve ending	Pain

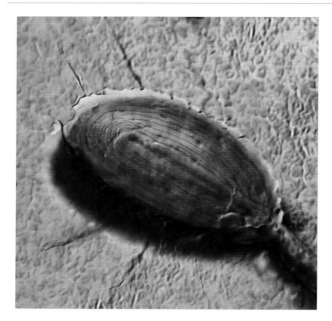

Figure 14.3 Pacinian corpuscle.

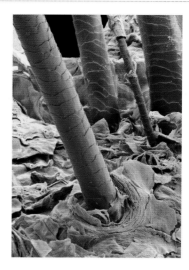

Figure 14.5 Coloured scanning electron micrograph of hair shafts growing through the skin.

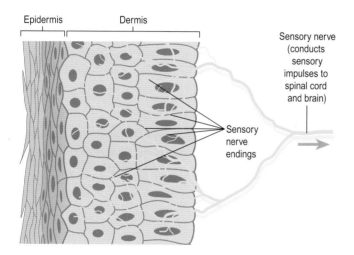

Figure 14.4 Sensory nerves in the dermis.

Sweat glands

These are widely distributed throughout the skin and are most numerous in the palms of the hands, soles of the feet, axillae and groins. They are formed from epithelial cells. The bodies of the glands lie coiled in the subcutaneous tissue. There are two types of sweat gland. Eccrine sweat glands are the more common type and open onto the skin surface through tiny pores, and the sweat produced here is a clear, watery fluid important in regulating body temperature. Apocrine glands open into hair follicles and become active at puberty. They may play a role in sexual arousal. These glands are found, for example, in the axilla. Bacterial decomposition of their secretions causes an unpleasant odour. A specialised example of this type of gland is the ceruminous gland of the outer ear, which secretes earwax (Ch. 8).

The most important function of sweat is in the regulation of body temperature (p. 367). Excessive sweating may lead to dehydration and serious depletion of sodium chloride unless intake of water and salt is appropriately increased. After 7–10 days' exposure to high environmental temperatures the amount of salt lost is substantially reduced but water loss remains high.

Hairs

These grow from *hair follicles*, downgrowths of epidermal cells into the dermis or subcutaneous tissue. At the base of the follicle is a cluster of cells called the *hair papilla* or *bulb*. The hair is formed by multiplication of cells of the bulb and as they are pushed upwards, away from their source of nutrition, the cells die and become keratinised. The part of the hair above the skin is the *shaft* and the remainder, the *root* (Fig. 14.2). Figure 14.5 shows hair growing through the skin and also desquamation, which roughens the skin surface; the roughened surface may harbour microbial growth although many are removed by the constant rubbing off of the topmost layers.

Hair colour is genetically determined and depends on the amount and type of melanin present. White hair is the result of the replacement of melanin by tiny air bubbles.

Arrector pili (Fig. 14.2). These are little bundles of smooth muscle fibres attached to the hair follicles. Contraction makes the hair stand erect and raises the skin around the hair, causing 'goose flesh'. The muscles are stimulated by sympathetic nerve fibres in response to fear and cold. Erect hairs trap air, which acts as an insulating layer. This is an efficient warming mechanism, especially when accompanied by shivering, i.e. involuntary contraction of skeletal muscles.

Sebaceous glands (Fig. 14.2). These consist of secretory epithelial cells derived from the same tissue as the hair follicles. They secrete an oily antimicrobial substance, *sebum*, into the hair follicles and are present in the skin of all parts of the body except the palms of the hands and the soles of the feet. They are most numerous in the scalp, face, axillae and groins. In regions of transition from one type of superficial epithelium to another, such as lips, eyelids, nipple, labia minora and glans penis, there are sebaceous glands that are independent of hair follicles, secreting sebum directly onto the surface.

Sebum keeps the hair soft and pliable and gives it a shiny appearance. On the skin it provides some water-proofing and acts as a bactericidal and fungicidal agent, preventing infection. It also prevents drying and cracking of skin, especially on exposure to heat and sunlight. The activity of these glands increases at puberty and is less at the extremes of age, rendering the skin of infants and older adults prone to the effects of excessive moisture (*maceration*).

Nails (Fig. 14.6)

Human nails are equivalent to the claws, horns and hooves of animals. Derived from the same cells as epidermis and hair these are hard, horny keratin plates that protect the tips of the fingers and toes.

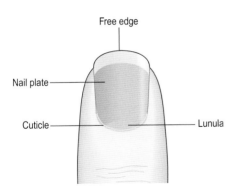

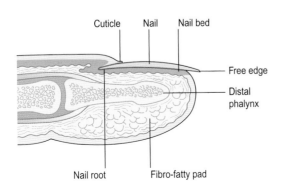

Figure 14.6 The nail and related skin.

The *root* of the nail is embedded in the skin and covered by the cuticle, which forms the hemispherical pale area called the *lunula*.

The *nail plate* is the exposed part that has grown out from the *nail bed*, the germinative zone of the epidermis.

Finger nails grow more quickly than toe nails and growth is faster when the environmental temperature is high.

Functions of the skin

Protection

The skin forms a relatively waterproof layer, provided mainly by its keratinised epithelium, which protects the deeper, more delicate structures. As an important non-specific defence mechanism it acts as a barrier against:

- invasion by micro-organisms
- chemicals
- physical agents, e.g. mild trauma, ultraviolet light
- dehydration.

The epidermis contains specialised immune cells called dendritic (Langerhans) cells, which are a type of macrophage. They phagocytose intruding antigens and travel to lymphoid tissue, where they present antigen to T-lymphocytes, thus stimulating an immune response (Ch. 15).

Abundant sensory nerve endings in the dermis enable perception, discrimination and location of internal and external stimuli. This allows responses to changes in the environment, e.g. by reflex action (withdrawal) to unpleasant or painful stimuli, protecting it from further injury (p. 164).

The pigment melanin protects against harmful ultraviolet rays in sunlight.

Regulation of body temperature

Body temperature remains fairly constant around 36.8°C across a wide range of environmental temperatures ensuring that the optimal range for enzyme activity required for metabolism is maintained. In health, variations are usually limited to between 0.5 and 0.75°C, although it rises slightly in the evening, during exercise and in women just after ovulation. To maintain this constant temperature, a negative feedback system regulates the balance between heat produced in the body and heat lost to the environment.

Heat production

When metabolic rate increases, body temperature rises, and when it decreases body temperature falls. Some of the energy released during metabolic activity is in the form of heat; the most active organs produce most heat. The principal organs involved are:

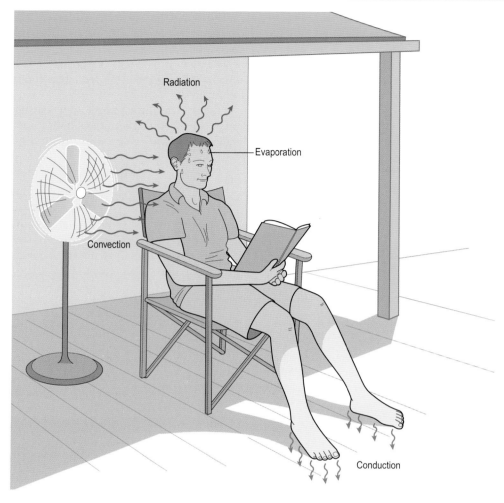

Figure 14.7 Mechanisms of heat loss.

- *skeletal muscles* – contraction of skeletal muscles produces a large amount of heat and the more strenuous the muscular exercise, the greater the heat produced. Shivering also involves skeletal muscle contraction, which increases heat production when there is the risk of body temperature falling below normal.
- *the liver* is very metabolically active, which produces heat as a by-product. Metabolic rate and heat production are increased after eating.
- *the digestive organs* that generate heat during peristalsis and the chemical reactions involved in digestion.

Heat loss

Most heat loss from the body occurs through the skin. Small amounts are lost in expired air, urine and faeces. Only heat loss through the skin can be regulated; heat lost by the other routes cannot be controlled.

Heat loss through the skin is affected by the difference between body and environmental temperatures, the amount of the body surface exposed and the type of clothes worn. Air insulates against heat loss when trapped in layers of clothing and between the skin and clothing. For this reason several layers of lightweight clothes provide more effective insulation against low environmental temperatures than one heavy garment.

Mechanisms of heat loss (Fig. 14.7). In *radiation*, the main mechanism, exposed parts of the body radiate heat away from the body. In *evaporation*, the body is cooled as body heat converts the water in sweat to water vapour. In *conduction*, clothes and other objects in direct contact with the skin take up heat. In *convection*, air passing over the exposed parts of the body is heated and rises, cool air replaces it and convection currents are set up. Convection also cools the body when clothes are worn, except when they are windproof.

Control of body temperature

The *temperature regulating centre* in the hypothalamus is sensitive to the temperature of circulating blood. This centre responds to decreasing temperature by sending nerve impulses to:

- arterioles in the dermis, which constrict decreasing blood flow to the skin
- skeletal muscles stimulating shivering.

As heat is conserved, body temperature rises and when it returns to the normal range again the negative feedback mechanism is switched off (see Fig. 1.5, p. 7).

Conversely when body temperature rises, heat loss is increased by dilation of arterioles in the dermis, increasing blood flow to the skin, and stimulation of the sweat glands causing sweating, until it falls into the normal range again when the negative feedback mechanism is switched off.

Activity of the sweat glands. When body temperature is increased by 0.25 to 0.5°C the sweat glands secrete sweat onto the skin surface. Evaporation of sweat cools the body, but is slower in humid conditions.

Loss of heat from the body by evaporation of water through the skin and expired air still occurs even when the environmental temperature is low. This is called *insensible water loss* (around 500 mL per day) and is accompanied by insensible heat loss.

Regulation of blood flow through the skin. The amount of heat lost from the skin depends largely on blood flow through dermal capillaries. As body temperature rises, the arterioles dilate and more blood enters the capillary network in the skin. The skin is warm and pink in colour. In addition to increasing the amount of sweat produced, the temperature of the skin rises and more heat is lost by radiation, conduction and convection.

If the environmental temperature is low or if heat production is decreased, the arterioles in the dermis are constricted. This reduces blood flow to the body surface, conserving heat. The skin appears paler and feels cool.

Fever

This is often the result of infection and is caused by release of chemicals (*pyrogens*) from inflammatory cells and invading bacteria. Pyrogens, e.g. *interleukin 1* (p. 379), act on the hypothalamus, which releases prostaglandins that reset the hypothalamic thermostat to a higher temperature. The body responds by activating heat-promoting mechanisms, e.g. shivering and vasoconstriction, until the new higher temperature is reached. When the thermostat is reset to the normal level, heat-loss mechanisms are activated. There is profuse sweating and vasodilation accompanied by warm, pink (flushed) skin until body temperature falls to the normal range again.

Hypothermia

This means a core (e.g. rectal) temperature below 35°C. At a core temperature below 32°C, compensatory mechanisms that restore body temperature normally fail, e.g. shivering is replaced by muscle rigidity and cramps, vasoconstriction fails and blood pressure, pulse and respiration rates fall. Confusion and disorientation occur. Death usually occurs when the temperature falls below 25°C.

Individuals at the extremes of age are prone to hypothermia as temperature regulation is less effective in the young and older adults.

Formation of vitamin D

7-Dehydrocholesterol is a lipid-based substance in the skin and is converted to vitamin D by sunlight. This vitamin is used with calcium and phosphate in the formation and maintenance of bone.

Cutaneous sensation

Sensory receptors are nerve endings in the dermis that are sensitive to touch, pressure, temperature or pain. Stimulation generates nerve impulses in sensory nerves that are transmitted to the cerebral cortex (see Fig. 7.22, p. 158). Some areas have more sensory receptors than others causing them to be especially sensitive, e.g. the lips and fingertips.

Absorption

This property is limited but substances that can be absorbed include:

- some drugs, in transdermal patches, e.g. hormone replacement therapy during the menopause, nicotine as an aid to smoking cessation
- some toxic chemicals, e.g. mercury.

Excretion

The skin is a minor excretory organ for some substances including:

- sodium chloride in sweat; excess sweating may lead to low blood sodium levels (hyponatraemia)
- urea, especially when kidney function is impaired
- aromatic substances, e.g. garlic and other spices.

Wound healing

Conditions required for wound healing

Systemic factors. These include good nutritional status and general health. Infection, impaired immunity, poor blood supply and systemic conditions, e.g. diabetes mellitus and cancer, reduce the rate of wound healing.

Local factors. Local factors that facilitate wound healing include a good blood supply to provide oxygen and nutrients and remove waste products, and freedom from contamination by, e.g., microbes, foreign bodies or toxic chemicals.

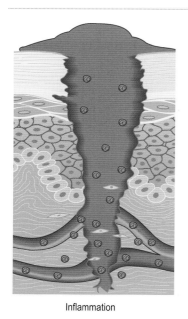
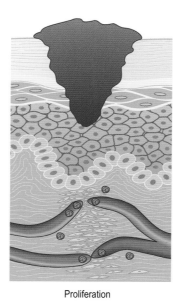
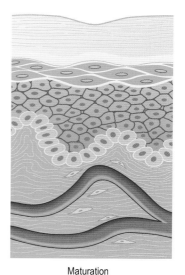
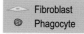

Inflammation   Proliferation   Maturation

Figure 14.8 Stages in primary wound healing.

Primary healing (healing by first intention)

This type of healing follows minimal destruction of tissue when the damaged edges of a wound are in close apposition, e.g. a surgical incision (Fig. 14.8). There are several overlapping stages in the repair process.

Inflammation. In the first few hours the cut surfaces become inflamed and blood clot (mainly fibrin, Fig. 4.15, p. 71) and cell debris fill the gap between them. Phagocytes, including macrophages, and fibroblasts migrate into the blood clot:

- phagocytes begin to remove the clot and cell debris, stimulating fibroblast activity
- fibroblasts secrete collagen fibres which begin to bind the wound margins together.

Proliferation. Epithelial cells proliferate across the wound, through the clot. The epidermis meets and grows upwards until full thickness is restored. The clot above the new tissue becomes the scab, which separates after 3–10 days. *Granulation tissue*, consisting of new capillary buds, phagocytes and fibroblasts, develops, invading the clot and restoring blood supply to the wound. Fibroblasts continue to secrete collagen fibres as the clot and any bacteria are removed by phagocytosis.

Maturation. The granulation tissue is replaced by fibrous scar tissue. Rearrangement of collagen fibres occurs and the strength of the wound increases. In time the scar becomes less vascular, appearing after a few months as a fine line.

The channels left when stitches are removed heal by the same process.

Secondary healing (healing by second intention)

This type of healing follows extensive tissue destruction or when the edges of a wound cannot be brought into apposition, e.g. varicose ulcers and pressure (decubitus) ulcers. The stages of secondary healing (Fig. 14.9) are the same as in primary healing (see above); healing time depends on effective removal of the cause and the size of the wound.

Inflammation. This develops on the surface of the healthy tissue and separation of necrotic tissue (*slough*) begins, due mainly to the action of phagocytes in the inflammatory exudate. The inflammatory process is described on page 377.

Proliferation. This begins as granulation tissue; consisting of capillary buds, phagocytes and fibroblasts; develops at the base of the cavity. Granulation tissue grows towards the surface, probably stimulated by macrophages and a range of locally released chemicals. Phagocytes in the plentiful blood supply reduce or prevent infection of the wound by ingesting bacteria after separation of the slough. Some fibroblasts in the wound develop a limited ability to contract, reducing the size of the wound and healing time. When granulation tissue reaches the level of the dermis, epithelial cells at the edges proliferate and grow towards the centre.

Maturation. This occurs by *fibrosis* (see below), in which scar tissue replaces granulation tissue, usually over several months until the full thickness of the skin is restored. Scar tissue is shiny and does not contain sweat glands, hair follicles or sebaceous glands.

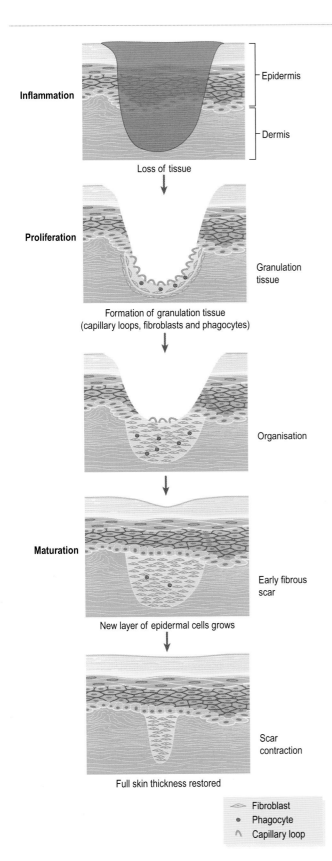

Inflammation

Epidermis

Dermis

Loss of tissue

Proliferation

Granulation tissue

Formation of granulation tissue
(capillary loops, fibroblasts and phagocytes)

Organisation

Maturation

Early fibrous scar

New layer of epidermal cells grows

Scar contraction

Full skin thickness restored

Fibroblast
Phagocyte
Capillary loop

Figure 14.9 Stages in secondary wound healing.

Fibrosis (scar formation)

Fibrous tissue is formed during healing by secondary intention, e.g. following chronic inflammation, persistent ischaemia, suppuration or extensive trauma. The process begins with formation of granulation tissue, then, over time, the inflammatory material is removed leaving only the collagen fibres secreted by the fibroblasts. Fibrous tissue may have long-lasting damaging effects.

Adhesions. These consist of fibrous tissue, which causes adjacent structures to stick together and may limit movement, e.g. between the layers of pleura, preventing inflation of the lungs or between loops of bowel, interfering with peristalsis.

Fibrosis of infarcts. Blockage of a vessel by a thrombus or an embolus causes an infarction. Fibrosis of one large infarct or of numerous small infarcts may follow, leading to varying degrees of organ dysfunction, e.g. in heart, brain, kidneys, liver.

Tissue shrinkage. This occurs as fibrous tissue ages. The effects depend on the site and extent of the fibrosis, e.g.:

- small tubes, such as blood vessels, air passages, ureters, the urethra and ducts of glands may become narrow or obstructed and lose their elasticity
- contractures (bands of shrunken fibrous tissue) may extend across joints, e.g. in a limb or digit there may be limitation of movement.

Complications of wound healing

In addition to the effects of adhesions, fibrosis of infarcts and tissue shrinkage described above, other complications are outlined below.

Infection. This arises from microbial contamination, usually by bacteria, and results in formation of pus (*suppuration*).

Pus consists of dead phagocytes, dead cells, cell debris, fibrin, inflammatory exudate and living and dead microbes. The most common pyogenic (pus-forming) pathogens are *Staphylococcus aureus* and *Streptococcus pyogenes*. Small amounts of pus form *boils* and larger amounts form *abscesses*. *S. aureus* produces the enzyme coagulase, which converts fibrinogen to fibrin, localising the pus. *S. pyogenes* produces toxins that break down tissue, spreading the infection. Healing, following pus formation, is by secondary intention (see above).

Superficial abscesses tend to rupture and discharge pus through the skin. Healing is usually complete unless tissue damage is extensive.

Deep abscesses have a variety of outcomes. There may be:

- early rupture with complete discharge of pus on to the surface, followed by healing

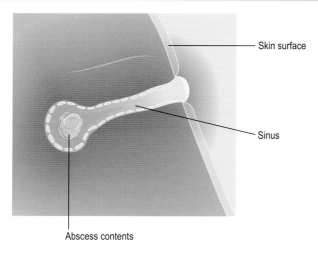

Figure 14.10 Sinus between an abscess and the body surface.

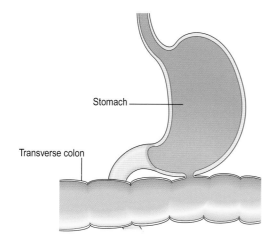

Figure 14.11 Fistula between the stomach and the colon.

- rupture and limited discharge of pus on to the surface, followed by the development of a chronic abscess with an infected open channel or *sinus* (Fig. 14.10)
- rupture and discharge of pus into an adjacent organ or cavity, forming an infected channel open at both ends, a *fistula* (Fig. 14.11)
- eventual removal of pus by phagocytes, followed by healing

- enclosure of pus by fibrous tissue that may become calcified, harbouring live organisms which may become a source of future infection, e.g. tuberculosis
- formation of adhesions (see above) between adjacent membranes, e.g. pleura, peritoneum
- shrinkage of fibrous tissue as it ages, which may reduce the lumen or obstruct a tube, e.g. oesophagus, bowel, blood vessel.

Effects of ageing on the skin

Learning outcome

After studying this section, you should be able to:

- describe the effects of ageing on the structure and function of the skin.

From the third decade, there are gradual changes in the structure and functioning of the skin which become much more prominent in old age. As the germinative layer becomes less active, the epidermis thins. The dermis also thins and there are fewer elastic and collagen fibres, which causes wrinkling and sagging. These changes may be accelerated by chronic exposure to strong sunlight, which is also associated with the development of malignant melanoma.

Sweat gland activity and temperature regulation become less efficient, putting older adults at greater risk in extreme temperatures making them increasingly prone to heatstroke and hypothermia. Less sebum is secreted making the skin dry and susceptible to continual exposure to moisture (maceration).

Production of vitamin D decreases predisposing older adults to deficiency and reduction in bone strength, especially when exposure to sunlight is limited.

Melanocytes become less active causing older adults to be more sensitive to sunlight and more prone to sunburn. In hair, when the pigment melanin is replaced by air bubbles, greying occurs. There are fewer active hair follicles and therefore hair thins although in some areas this is not the case; notably the eyebrows, nose and ears in males, and the face and upper lip in females.

Disorders of the skin

Infections

Viral infections

Human papilloma virus (HPV)

This causes *warts* or *veruccas* that are spread by direct contact, e.g. from another lesion or another infected individual. There is proliferation of the epidermis and development of a small firm growth, which is nearly always benign. Common sites are the hands, the face and soles of the feet.

Herpes viruses

Rashes seen in chickenpox and shingles (p. 184) are caused by the herpes zoster virus. Other herpes viruses cause *cold sores* (HSV1, p. 320) and *genital herpes* (HSV2, p. 466).

Bacterial infections

Impetigo

This is a highly infectious condition commonly caused by *Staphylococcus aureus*. Superficial pustules develop, usually round the nose and mouth. It is spread by direct contact and affects mainly children and immunosuppressed individuals. When caused by *Streptococcus pyogenes* (group A β-haemolytic streptococcus) the infection may be complicated by an immune reaction causing glomerulonephritis (p. 350) a few weeks later.

Cellulitis

This is a spreading infection caused by some anaerobic bacteria including *Streptococcus pyogenes* and *Clostridium perfringens* that enter through a break in the skin. Their spread is facilitated by the formation of enzymes that break down the connective tissue that normally isolates an area of inflammation. If untreated, the bacteria may enter the blood causing septicaemia.

In severe cases *necrotising fasciitis* may occur. There is rapid and progressive necrosis of subcutaneous tissue that usually includes the fascia in the affected area. Multiple organ failure is common and mortality is high.

Fungal infections (mycoses)

Ringworm and tinea pedis

These are superficial skin infections. In ringworm there is an outward spreading ring of inflammation. It most commonly affects the scalp, feet and groin and is easily spread to others. Tinea pedis (athlete's foot) affects the skin between the toes. Both infections are spread by direct contact.

Non-infective inflammatory conditions

Dermatitis (eczema)

Dermatitis is a common inflammatory skin condition that may be either acute or chronic. In acute dermatitis there is redness, swelling and exudation of serous fluid usually accompanied by *pruritus* (itching). This is often followed by crusting and scaling. If the condition becomes chronic, the skin thickens and may become leathery due to long-term scratching, which may cause infection.

Atopic dermatitis is associated with allergy and commonly affects atopic individuals, i.e. those prone to hypersensitivity disorders (p. 385). Children, who may also suffer from hay fever or asthma (pp. 262 and 264), are often affected.

Contact dermatitis may be caused by direct contact with irritants, e.g. cosmetics, soap, detergent, strong acids or alkalis, industrial chemicals or a hypersensitivity reaction (see Fig. 15.9, p. 386) to, e.g., latex, nickel, dyes and other chemicals.

Psoriasis

This common condition is genetically determined and characterised by exacerbations and periods of remission of varying duration. Proliferating cells of the basal layers of the epidermis progress more rapidly upwards through the epidermis resulting in incomplete maturation of the upper layer. Psoriasis is characterised by red, scaly plaques with a silvery surface (Fig. 14.12). Bleeding may occur when scales are scratched or rubbed off. The elbows, knees and scalp are common sites but other parts can also be affected. Trigger factors that lead to exacerbation of the condition include trauma, infection and sunburn. Sometimes psoriasis is associated with rheumatoid arthritis (p. 432).

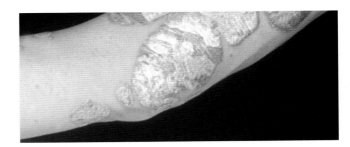

Figure 14.12 Psoriasis.

Acne vulgaris

This is commonest in adolescent males and thought to be caused by increased levels of testosterone after puberty. Sebaceous glands (in hair follicles) become blocked and then infected, leading to inflammation and pustule formation. In severe cases permanent scarring may result. The most common sites are the face, chest and upper back.

Pressure ulcers

Also known as *decubitus ulcers* or bedsores, these occur over 'pressure points', areas where the skin may be compressed for long periods between a bony prominence and a hard surface, e.g. a bed or chair. When this occurs, blood flow to the affected area is impaired and ischaemia develops. Initially the skin reddens, and later as ischaemia and necrosis occur, the skin sloughs and an ulcer forms that may then enlarge into a cavity. If infection occurs, this can result in septicaemia. Healing takes place by secondary intention (p. 368).

Predisposing factors

These may be:

- extrinsic, e.g. pressure, shearing forces, trauma, immobility, moisture, infection
- intrinsic, e.g. poor nutritional status, emaciation, incontinence, infection, concurrent illness, sensory impairment, poor circulation.

Burns

These may be caused by many types of trauma including: heat, cold, electricity, ionising radiation and corrosive chemicals, including strong acids or alkalis (bases). Local damage occurs disrupting the structure and functions of the skin.

Burns are classified according to their depth:

- *first degree* when only the epidermis is involved, the surface is moist and there are signs of inflammation including redness, swelling and pain. There are no blisters and tissue damage is minimal.
- *second degree* when the epidermis and upper dermis are affected. In addition to the signs and symptoms above, blistering is usually present.
- *third degree* (deep or full thickness) when the epidermis and dermis are destroyed. These burns are usually relatively painless as the sensory nerve endings in the dermis are destroyed. After a few days the destroyed tissue coagulates and forms an *eschar*, or thick scab, which sloughs off after 2 to 3 weeks. In *circumferential burns*, which encircle any area of the body, complications may arise from constriction of the part by eschar, e.g. respiratory impairment may follow circumferential burns of the chest, or

the circulation to the distal part of an affected limb may be seriously impaired. Skin grafting is required except for small injuries. Healing, which is prolonged, occurs by secondary intention (p. 368) and there is no regeneration of sweat glands, hair follicles or sebaceous glands. Resultant scar tissue often limits movement of affected joints. ▉ **14.1**

The extent of burns in adults is roughly estimated using the 'rule of nines' (Fig. 14.13). In adults, hypovolaemic shock usually develops when 15% of the surface area is affected. Fatality is likely in adults with third degree burns if the surface area affected is added to the patient's age and the total is greater than 80.

Complications of burns

Although burns affect the skin, when extensive, their systemic consequences can also be life-threatening or fatal.

Dehydration and hypovolaemia. These may occur in extensive burns when there is excessive leakage of water and plasma proteins from the damaged skin surface.

Shock. This may accompany severe hypovolaemia.

Hypothermia. This develops when excessive heat is lost in leakage from burns.

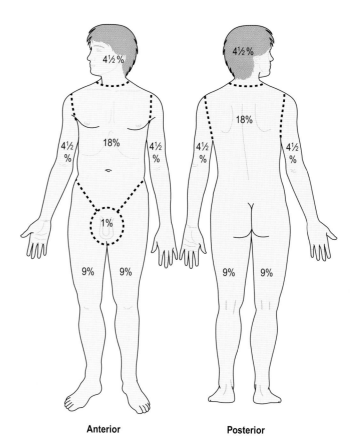

Figure 14.13 The 'rule of nines' for estimating the extent of burns in adults.

Infection. This occurs easily when subcutaneous tissue is exposed to the environment and may result in septicaemia.

Renal failure. This occurs when the kidney tubules cannot deal with the large amount of waste from haemolysed erythrocytes and damaged tissue.

Contractures. These may develop later as fibrous scar tissue contracts distorting joints, e.g. the hands, restricting their range of motion.

Malignant tumours

Basal cell carcinoma

This is the least malignant and most common type of skin cancer. It is associated with long-term exposure to sunlight and is therefore most likely to occur on sun-exposed sites, usually the head or neck. It appears as a shiny nodule and later this breaks down, becoming an ulcer with irregular edges, commonly called a *rodent ulcer*. Although this is locally invasive it seldom metastasises.

Malignant melanoma

This is malignant proliferation of melanocytes, usually originating in a mole that enlarges and may have an irregular outline (Fig. 14.14). It may ulcerate and bleed and most commonly affects young and middle-aged adults. Predisposing factors are a fair skin and recurrent episodes of intensive exposure to sunlight including repeated episodes of sunburn, especially in childhood. Sites for this tumour show a gender bias, with the lower leg being the commonest site in females and the upper back in males. Metastases usually develop early and are associated with a poor prognosis. Initial spread is usually to nearby

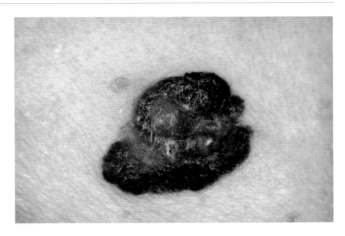

Figure 14.14 Malignant melanoma.

lymph nodes and is followed by blood-spread metastases in the liver, brain, lungs, bowel and bone marrow.

Kaposi's sarcoma

In this condition, which is usually AIDS-related, a malignant tumour arises in the walls of lymphatic vessels. A small red-blue patch or nodule develops, usually on the lower limbs but the mouth, oesophagus, stomach and intestines can also be affected. Without treatment skin lesions enlarge and become more numerous.

 For a range of self-assessment exercises on the topics in this chapter, visit Evolve online resources: https://evolve.elsevier.com/Waugh/anatomy/

Resistance and immunity

From the months spent in the womb to the end of life, every individual is under constant attack from an enormous range of potentially harmful invaders. These threats include such diverse entities as bacteria, viruses, cancer cells, parasites and foreign (non-self) cells, e.g. in tissue transplant. The body has therefore developed a wide selection of protective measures, which can be divided into two categories.

Non-specific defence mechanisms. These protect against any of an enormous range of possible dangers.

Specific defence mechanisms. These are grouped together under the term immunity. Resistance is directed against only one specific invader. In addition, *immunological memory* develops, which confers long-term immunity to specific infections. An *antigen* is anything that stimulates an immune response.

The later sections of the chapter describe the effects of ageing on the immune system, and consider some disorders of lymphatic system function.

Non-specific defence mechanisms

Learning outcomes

After studying this section, you should be able to:

■ identify the body's main non-specific defence cells

■ describe the functions and features of the inflammatory response

■ explain the process of phagocytosis

■ list the main antimicrobial substances of the body.

These are the first lines of general defence; they prevent entry and minimise further passage of microbes and other foreign material into the body.

There are five main non-specific defence mechanisms:

- defence at body surfaces
- phagocytosis
- natural antimicrobial substances
- the inflammatory response
- immunological surveillance.

Defence at body surfaces

Healthy, intact skin and mucous membranes provide an efficient physical barrier protecting the body's exposed surfaces. Few pathogens can establish themselves on healthy skin. Sebum and sweat secreted onto the skin surface contain antibacterial and antifungal substances.

Epithelial membranes lining body cavities and passageways exposed to the external environment (e.g. the respiratory, genitourinary and digestive tracts) are more delicate, but are also well defended. Epithelia produce antibacterial secretions, often acidic, containing antibodies and enzymes, as well as sticky mucus for trapping passing microbes.

Hairs in the nose act as a coarse filter, and the sweeping action of cilia in the respiratory tract (Fig. 10.12) moves mucus and inhaled foreign materials towards the throat. Then it is coughed up (*expectorated*) or swallowed.

The one-way flow of urine from the bladder minimises the risk of infection ascending through the urethra into the bladder. In the female, the acidity of vaginal secretions discourages microbial growth.

Phagocytosis 15.1

The process of phagocytosis (cell eating) is shown in Figure 4.11, page 69. Phagocytic defence cells such as macrophages and neutrophils are the body's first line of cellular defence. They actively migrate (chemotaxis, p. 68) to sites of inflammation and infection, because neutrophils themselves and invading microbes release chemicals that attract them (chemoattractants). Phagocytes attack and engulf their targets (Fig. 15.1). They indiscriminately digest and destroy foreign cells, antigenic material and damaged body cells and debris. They may also release chemicals toxic to invading microbes into the interstitial fluid. Macrophages have an important role as a link between the non-specific and specific defence mechanisms. After ingestion and digestion of an antigen, they act as *antigen-presenting cells*, displaying their antigen on their own cell surface to stimulate T-lymphocytes and activate the immune response (p. 379).

The body's population of fixed and roaming macrophages (the *monocyte-macrophage system*) is also discussed in Chapter 4.

Natural antimicrobial substances

Hydrochloric acid. This is present in high concentrations in gastric juice, and kills the majority of ingested microbes.

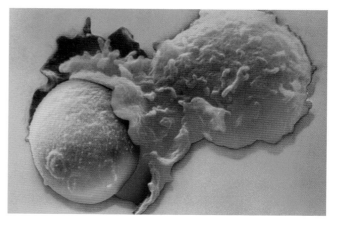

Figure 15.1 White blood cell (blue) phagocytosing a yeast cell (yellow).

Lysozyme. This antibacterial enzyme is present in granulocytes, tears, and other body secretions, but not in sweat, urine or cerebrospinal fluid. It destroys bacterial cell walls but does not affect viruses or other pathogens.

Antibodies. These protective proteins are found coating membranes and in body fluids, and inactivate bacteria (p. 381).

Saliva. This is secreted into the mouth and washes away food debris that may otherwise encourage bacterial growth. It contains antibodies, lysozyme and buffers to neutralise bacterial acids that promote dental decay.

Interferons. These chemicals are produced by T-lymphocytes, macrophages and body cells that have been invaded by viruses. They prevent viral replication within infected cells, and the spread of viruses to healthy cells.

Complement 15.2. Complement is a system of about 20 proteins found in the blood and tissues. It is activated by the presence of immune complexes (an antigen and antibody bound together) and by foreign sugars on bacterial cell walls. Complement:

- binds to, and damages, bacterial cell walls, destroying the microbe
- binds to bacterial cell walls, stimulating phagocytosis by neutrophils and macrophages
- attracts phagocytic cells such as neutrophils into an area of infection, i.e. stimulates chemotaxis.

The inflammatory response 15.3

This is the physiological response to tissue damage and is accompanied by a characteristic series of local changes (Fig. 15.2). Its purpose is protective: to isolate, inactivate and remove both the causative agent and damaged tissue, so that healing can take place. The cardinal signs of inflammation are *redness*, *heat*, *swelling* and *pain*.

Inflammatory conditions are recognised by their Latin suffix '-itis'; for example, appendicitis is inflammation of the appendix and laryngitis is inflammation of the larynx.

Causes of inflammation

Any form of tissue damage stimulates the inflammatory response, even in the absence of infection. The wide range of causative agents includes extremes of temperature, trauma, corrosive chemicals including extremes of pH, abrasion and infection by pathogens.

Acute inflammation

Acute inflammation is typically of short duration, e.g. days to a few weeks, and may range from mild to very severe, depending on the extent of the tissue damage. Most aspects of the inflammatory response are hugely

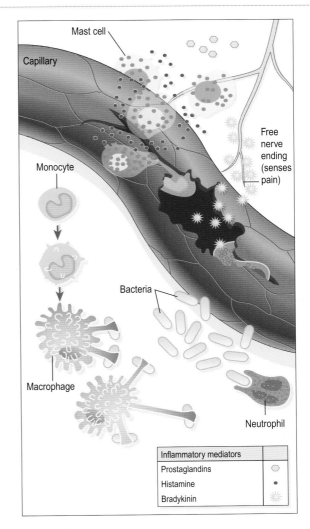

Inflammatory mediators	
Prostaglandins	⬡
Histamine	•
Bradykinin	✳

Figure 15.2 The inflammatory response.

beneficial, promoting removal of the harmful agent and setting the scene for healing to follow.

The acute inflammatory response is described here for convenience as a collection of separate events: increased blood flow, accumulation of tissue fluid, migration of leukocytes, increased core temperature, pain and suppuration. In reality, these events significantly overlap and develop together.

Some of the most important substances released in inflammation are summarised in Table 15.1.

Increased blood flow

Following injury, both the arterioles supplying the damaged area and the local capillaries dilate, increasing blood flow to the site.

This is caused mainly by the local release of a number of chemical mediators from damaged cells, e.g. histamine and serotonin. Increased blood flow to the area of tissue damage provides more oxygen and nutrients for the increased cellular activity that accompanies

Table 15.1 Summary of the principal substances released in inflammation

Substance	Made by	Trigger for release	Main pro-inflammatory actions
Histamine	Mast cells (in most tissues), basophils (blood); stored in cytoplasmic granules	Binding of antibody to mast cells and basophils	Vasodilation, itching, ↑ vascular permeability, degranulation, smooth muscle contraction (e.g. bronchoconstriction)
Serotonin (5-HT)	Platelets Mast cells and basophils (stored in granules) Also in CNS (acts as neurotransmitter)	When platelets are activated, and when mast cells/basophils degranulate	Vasoconstriction, ↑ vascular permeability
Prostaglandins (PGs)	Nearly all cells; not stored, but made from cell membranes as required	Many different stimuli, e.g. drugs, toxins, other inflammatory mediators, hormones, trauma	Diverse, sometimes opposing, e.g. fever, pain, vasodilation or vasoconstriction, ↑ vascular permeability
Heparin	Liver, mast cells, basophils (stored in cytoplasmic granules)	Released when cells degranulate	Anticoagulant (prevents blood clotting), which maintains blood supply (nutrients, O_2) to injured tissue and washes away microbes and wastes
Bradykinin	Tissues and blood	When blood clots, in trauma and inflammation	Pain Vasodilation

inflammation. Increased blood flow causes the increased temperature and reddening of an inflamed area, and contributes to the swelling (oedema) associated with inflammation.

Increased tissue fluid formation

One of the cardinal signs of inflammation is swelling of the tissues involved, which is caused by fluid leaving local blood vessels and entering the interstitial spaces.

This is partly due to increased capillary permeability caused by inflammatory mediators such as histamine, serotonin and prostaglandins, and partly due to elevated pressure inside the vessels because of increased blood flow. Most of the excess tissue fluid drains away in the lymphatic vessels, taking damaged tissue, dead and dying cells and toxins with it.

Plasma proteins, normally retained within the bloodstream, also escape into the tissues through the leaky capillary walls; this increases the osmotic pressure of the tissue fluid and draws more fluid out of the blood. These proteins include antibodies, which combat infection, and *fibrinogen*, a clotting protein. Fibrinogen in the tissues is converted by *thromboplastin* to fibrin, which forms an insoluble mesh within the interstitial space, walling off the inflamed area and helping to limit the spread of any infection. Some pathogens, e.g. *Streptococcus pyogenes*, which causes throat and skin infections, release toxins that break down this fibrin network and promote spread of infection into adjacent, healthy tissue.

Sometimes tissue oedema can be harmful. For instance, swelling around respiratory passages can obstruct breathing, and significant swelling often causes pain. On the other hand, the swelling around a painful, inflamed joint cushions it and limits movement, which encourages healing.

Migration of leukocytes

Loss of fluid from the blood thickens it, slowing flow and allowing the normally fast-flowing white blood cells to make contact with, and adhere to, the vessel wall. In the acute stages, the most important leukocyte is the neutrophil, which adheres to the blood vessel lining, squeezes between the endothelial cells and enters the tissues (diapedesis, see Fig. 4.10, p. 69), where its main function is in phagocytosis of antigens. Phagocyte activity is promoted by the raised temperatures (local and systemic) associated with inflammation.

After about 24 hours, macrophages become the predominant cell type at the inflamed site, and they persist in the tissues if the situation is not resolved, leading to chronic inflammation. Macrophages are larger and longer lived than neutrophils. They phagocytose dead/dying tissue, microbes and other antigenic material, and dead/dying neutrophils. Some microbes resist digestion and provide a possible source of future infection, e.g. *Mycobacterium tuberculosis* (p. 268).

Chemotaxis. This is the chemical attraction of leukocytes, including neutrophils and macrophages, to an area of inflammation.

It may be that chemoattractants act to retain passing leukocytes in the inflamed area, rather than actively attracting them from distant areas of the body. Chemoattractants include microbial toxins, chemicals released from leukocytes, prostaglandins from damaged cells and complement proteins.

Increased temperature

The increased temperature of inflamed tissues has the twin benefits of inhibiting the growth and division of microbes, whilst promoting the activity of phagocytes.

The inflammatory response may be accompanied by a rise in body temperature (fever, *pyrexia*), especially if there is bacterial infection. Body temperature rises when an endogenous pyrogen (interleukin 1) is released from macrophages and granulocytes in response to microbial toxins or immune complexes. Interleukin 1 is a chemical mediator that resets the temperature thermostat in the hypothalamus at a higher level, causing pyrexia and other symptoms that may also accompany systemic inflammation, e.g. fatigue and loss of appetite. Pyrexia increases the metabolic rate of cells in the inflamed area and, consequently, there is an increased need for oxygen and nutrients.

Pain

This occurs when local swelling compresses sensory nerve endings. It is exacerbated by chemical mediators of the inflammatory process, e.g. bradykinin and prostaglandins which potentiate the sensitivity of the sensory nerve endings to painful stimuli. Although pain is an unpleasant experience, it may indirectly promote healing, because it encourages protection of the damaged site.

Suppuration (pus formation)

Pus consists of dead phagocytes, dead cells, fibrin, inflammatory exudate and living and dead microbes. A localised collection of pus in the tissues is called an *abscess* (Fig. 14.10). The most common pyogenic (pus-forming) bacteria are *Staphylococcus aureus* and *Streptococcus pyogenes*.

Outcomes of acute inflammation

Resolution. This occurs when the cause has been successfully overcome. Damaged cells and residual fibrin are removed, being replaced with new healthy tissue, and repair is complete, with or without scar formation.

Development of chronic inflammation. Acute inflammation may become chronic if resolution is not complete, e.g. if live microbes remain at the site, as in some deepseated abscesses, wound infections and bone infections.

Chronic inflammation

The processes involved are very similar to those of acute inflammation but, because the process is of longer duration, considerably more tissue damage is likely. The inflammatory cells are mainly lymphocytes instead of neutrophils, and fibroblasts are activated, leading to the laying down of collagen, and *fibrosis*. If the body defences are unable to clear the infection, they may try to wall it off instead, forming nodules called *granulomas*, within which are collections of defensive cells. Tuberculosis is an example of an infection that frequently becomes chronic, leading to granuloma formation. The causative bacterium, *Mycobacterium tuberculosis*, is resistant to body defences and so pockets of organisms (Ghon foci, p. 269) are sealed up in granulomas within the lungs.

Chronic inflammation may either be a complication of acute inflammation (see above) or follow chronic exposure to an irritant. Fibrosis (scar formation) is discussed in Chapter 14.

Immunological surveillance

A population of lymphocytes, called natural killer (NK) cells, constantly patrol the body searching for abnormal cells. Cells that have been infected with a virus, or mutated cells that might become malignant, frequently display unusual markers on their cell membranes, which are recognised by NK cells. Having detected an abnormal cell, the NK cell immediately kills it. Although NK cells are lymphocytes, they are much less selective about their targets than the other two types discussed in this chapter (T- and B-cells).

Immunity

Learning outcomes

After studying this section, you should be able to:

- discuss the roles of the different types of T-lymphocyte in providing cell-mediated immunity

- describe the process of antibody-mediated immunity

- distinguish between artificially and naturally acquired immunity, giving examples of each

- distinguish between active and passive immunity, giving examples of each.

The body's first line of defence is its collection of non-specific defences, including phagocytes such as macrophages. If these are overwhelmed, activation of the powerful immune system follows. Immunity possesses three key attributes not seen with non-specific defences: specificity, memory and tolerance.

Specificity. Unlike mechanisms such as the inflammatory response and the phagocytic action of macrophages, which are triggered by a wide range of threats, an immune response is directed against one antigen and no others.

Memory. Again, unlike general defence mechanisms, an immune response against a particular antigen will usually generate immunological memory of that antigen. This means that the immune response on subsequent exposures to the same antigen is generally faster and more powerful.

Tolerance. The cells of the immune system are aggressive and potentially extremely destructive. Control of their activity is essential for protection of healthy body tissues. As immune cells travel around the body, they check the marker proteins that cells show on their cell membranes. Healthy body cells display the expected 'self' markers and are ignored by the patrolling immune cells. However, non-self cells, such as cancer cells, foreign (transplanted) cells or pathogens, possess different patterns of markers, which immediately activate the immune cell and usually lead to the destruction of the non-self cell.

Lymphocytes

Lymphocytes make up 20–30% of circulating white blood cells but at any one time most of them are found in lymphatic and other tissues rather than in the bloodstream. They include natural killer cells (p. 379) involved in immunological surveillance, T-cells (the majority) and B-cells. T- and B-cells are responsible for immunity (specific defence) and are produced in the bone marrow and some lymphatic tissues, although T-cells migrate to the thymus gland for final maturation.

For each of the millions of possible antigens that might be encountered in life, there is a corresponding T- and B-cell programmed to respond to it. There are, therefore, vast numbers of different T- and B-cells in the body, each capable of responding to only one antigen (antigen specificity).

T-cells

The hormone thymosin, produced by the thymus gland, is responsible for promoting T-cell maturation, which leads to the formation of fully specialised (differentiated), mature, functional T-cells. It is important to recognise that a mature T-cell has been programmed to recognise only one type of antigen, and during its subsequent travels through the body will react to no other antigen, however dangerous it might be. Thus, a T-cell manufactured to recognise the chickenpox virus will not react to a measles virus, a cancer cell, or a tuberculosis bacterium.

T-cells provide *cell-mediated immunity*, discussed below.

B-cells

These are both produced and matured in the bone marrow. They produce antibodies (immunoglobulins),

proteins designed to bind to, and destroy, an antigen. As with T-cells, each B-cell targets one specific antigen; the antibody released reacts with one type of antigen and no other. B-cells provide *antibody-mediated immunity*, discussed below.

Cell-mediated immunity 🎞 15.4

T-cells that have matured in the thymus gland are released into the circulation. When they encounter their antigen for the first time, they become sensitised to it. If the antigen has come from outside the body, it needs to be 'presented' to the T-cell on the surface of an antigen-presenting cell. There are different types of antigen-presenting cell, including macrophages. Macrophages are part of the non-specific defences, because they engulf and digest antigens indiscriminately, but they are a crucial 'link' cell between initial non-specific defences and the immune system. After digesting the antigen they transport the most antigenic fragment to their own cell membrane and display it on their surface (Fig. 15.3). They display (*present*) this antigen to the T-cell that has been processed to target that particular antigen, activating the T-cell.

If the antigen is an abnormal body cell, such as a cancer cell, it too will be displaying foreign (non-self) material on its cell membrane that will stimulate the T-cell. Whichever way the antigen is presented to the T-cell, it stimulates it to divide and proliferate (*clonal expansion*) (Fig. 15.3). Four main types of specialised T-cell are produced, each of which is still directed against the original antigen, but which will tackle it in different ways.

Cytotoxic T-cells

These directly inactivate any cells carrying antigens. They attach themselves to the target cell and release powerful toxins, which are very effective because the two cells are so close together. The main role of cytotoxic T-cells is in destruction of abnormal body cells, e.g. infected cells and cancer cells.

Helper T-cells

These are essential not only for cell-mediated immunity, but also antibody-mediated immunity. Their central role in immunity is emphasised in situations where they are destroyed, as by the human immunodeficiency virus (HIV). When helper T-cell numbers fall significantly, the whole immune system is compromised. T-helpers are the commonest of the T-cells; their main functions include:

- production of chemicals called *cytokines*, e.g. interleukins and interferons, which support and promote cytotoxic T-cells and macrophages
- cooperating with B-cells to produce antibodies; although B-cell are responsible for antibody

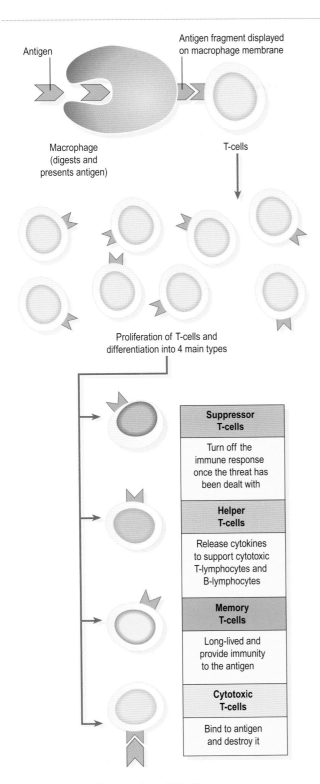

Figure 15.3 Clonal expansion of T-cells.

manufacture, they require to be stimulated by a helper T-cell first.

Suppressor T-cells

These cells act as 'brakes', turning off activated T- and B-cells. This limits the powerful and potentially damaging effects of the immune response. Suppressor T-cells are also thought to help prevent the development of auto-immunity (p. 385) and to protect the fetus in pregnancy.

Memory T-cells

These long-lived cells survive after the threat has been neutralised, and provide *cell-mediated immunity* by responding rapidly to another encounter with the same antigen.

Antibody-mediated (humoral) immunity ▨ 15.5

B-cells are much less mobile than T-cells, and spend much of their time in lymphoid tissue, e.g. the spleen and lymph nodes. B-cells, unlike T-cells, recognise and bind antigen particles without having to be presented with them by an antigen-presenting cell. Once its antigen has been detected and bound, and with the help of an activated helper T-cell, the B-cell enlarges and begins to divide (clonal expansion, Fig. 15.4). It produces two functionally distinct types of cell, plasma cells and memory B-cells.

Plasma cells

These secrete massive quantities of antibodies (immunoglobulins, Ig) into the blood. Antibodies are carried throughout the tissues. Plasma cells live no longer than a day and produce millions of molecules of only one type of antibody, which targets the specific antigen that originally bound to the B-cell. Antibodies:

- bind to antigens, labelling them as targets for other defence cells such as cytotoxic T-cells and macrophages
- bind to bacterial toxins, neutralising them
- activate complement (p. 377).

There are five main types of antibody, summarised in Table 15.2. ▨ 15.6

Memory B-cells

Like memory T-cells, these cells remain in the body long after the initial episode has been dealt with, and rapidly respond to another encounter with the same antigen by stimulating the production of antibody-secreting plasma cells. The interdependence of the two parts of the immune system is summarised in Figure 15.5.

The fact that the body does not normally develop immunity to its own cells is due to the fine balance that exists between the immune reaction and its suppression. *Autoimmune diseases* (p. 385) are due to the disturbance of this balance.

Acquired immunity

The immune response to an antigen following the first exposure (primary immunisation) is called the *primary*

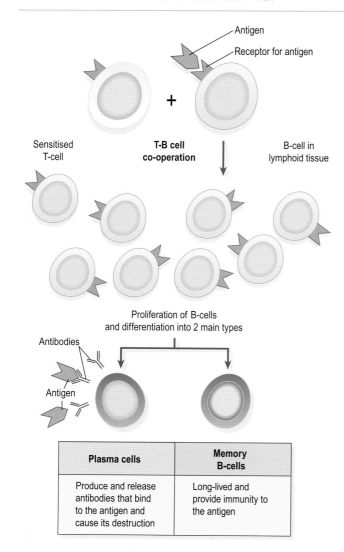

Figure 15.4 Clonal expansion of B-cells.

Plasma cells	Memory B-cells
Produce and release antibodies that bind to the antigen and cause its destruction	Long-lived and provide immunity to the antigen

Table 15.2 The five types of antibody

Type of antibody	Function
IgA	Found in body secretions like breast milk and saliva, and prevent antigens crossing epithelial membranes and invading deeper tissues
IgD	This is made by B-cells and displayed on their surfaces. Antigens bind here to activate B-cells
IgE	Found on cell membranes of, e.g., basophils and mast cells, and if it binds its antigen, activates the inflammatory response. This antibody is often found in excess in allergy
IgG	This is the largest and most common antibody type. It attacks many different pathogens, and crosses the placenta to protect the fetus
IgM	Produced in large quantities in the primary response and is a potent activator of complement

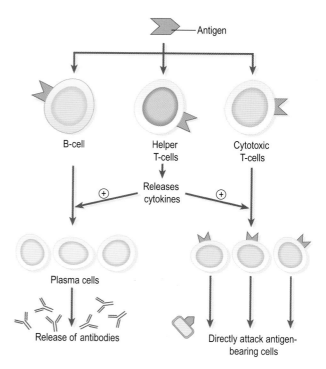

Figure 15.5 Interdependence of the T- and B-cell systems in the immune response.

response. Second and subsequent exposures give rise to a *secondary response* (Fig. 15.6).

The primary response. Exposure of the immune system to an antigen for the first time leads to a slow and delayed rise in antibody levels, peaking 1–2 weeks after infection. This delayed response reflects the time required to activate the T-cell system, which then stimulates B-cell division. Antibody levels start to fall once the infection is cleared, but if the immune system has responded well, it will have generated a population of long-lived memory B-cells, making the individual immune to future infection.

The secondary response. On subsequent exposures to the same antigen, the immune response is much faster and 10–15 times more powerful, because the memory B-cells generated after the first infection rapidly divide and antibody production begins almost immediately.

Immunity may be acquired *naturally* or *artificially* and both forms may be active or passive (Fig. 15.7). Active immunity means that the individual has responded to an antigen and produced his own antibodies, lymphocytes are activated and the memory cells formed provide long-lasting resistance. In passive immunity the individual is given antibodies produced by someone else. The

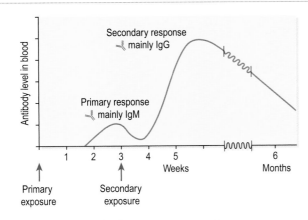

Figure 15.6 The antibody responses to antigen exposure.

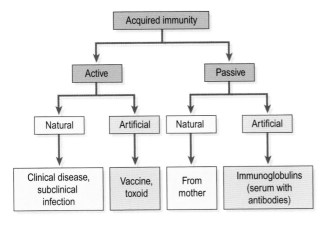

Figure 15.7 Summary of the types of acquired immunity.

antibodies break down with time, so passive immunity is relatively brief.

Active naturally acquired immunity

The body may be stimulated to produce its own antibodies by:

- *Having the disease*. During the course of the illness, B-cells develop into plasma cells that produce antibodies in sufficient quantities to overcome the infection. After recovery, the memory B-cells produced confer immunity to future infection by the same antigen.
- *Having a subclinical infection*. Sometimes the infection is not sufficiently severe to cause clinical disease but stimulates sufficient memory B-cells to establish immunity, e.g. hepatitis A, p. 333. In other cases, subclinical infection may be too mild to stimulate an adequate response for immunity to develop.

Active artificially acquired immunity

This type of immunity develops in response to the administration of dead or live artificially weakened pathogens (vaccines) or deactivated toxins (toxoids). The vaccines

Box 15.1 Diseases preventable by vaccination

- Anthrax
- Cholera
- Diphtheria
- Hepatitis B
- Measles
- Mumps
- Poliomyelitis
- Rubella
- Smallpox
- Tetanus
- Tuberculosis
- Typhoid
- Whooping cough

and toxoids retain the antigenic properties that stimulate the development of immunity but they cannot cause the disease. Many infectious diseases can be prevented by artificial immunisation. Examples are shown in Box 15.1.

Active immunisation against some infectious disorders gives lifelong immunity, e.g. diphtheria, whooping cough or mumps. In other infections the immunity may last for a number of years or for only a few weeks before revaccination is necessary. Apparent loss of immunity may be due to infection with a different strain of the same pathogen, which has different antigenic properties but causes the same clinical illness, e.g. viruses that cause the common cold and influenza. In older or poorly nourished individuals, lymphocyte production, especially B-cells, is reduced and the primary and secondary response may be inadequate.

Passive naturally acquired immunity

This type of immunity is acquired before birth by the passage of maternal antibodies across the placenta to the fetus, and to the baby in breast milk. The variety of different antibodies provided depends on the mother's active immunity. The baby's lymphocytes are not stimulated and this form of immunity is short lived.

Passive artificially acquired immunity

In this type, ready-made antibodies, in human or animal serum, are injected into the recipient. The source of the antibodies may be an individual who has recovered from the infection, or animals, commonly horses, that have been artificially actively immunised. Specific immunoglobulins (antiserum) may be administered *prophylactically* to prevent the development of disease in people who have been exposed to the infection, e.g. rabies, or *therapeutically* after the disease has developed.

Summary of the immune response to a bacterial infection

Figure 15.8 shows the main events that make up the body's integrated response to infection. Initially, nonspecific defence cells (neutrophils, natural killer cells and macrophages) accumulate at the site of infection, and attempt to limit bacterial expansion. If the threat is strong

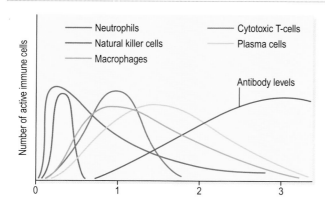

Figure 15.8 Summary of the defensive response to bacterial infection.

enough and many macrophages are involved, arriving T-cells are activated, producing populations of cytotoxic and helper T-cells, which in turn activate B-cells. As B-cells proliferate and differentiate into plasma cells, antibody levels progressively rise.

Ageing and immunity

Learning outcomes

After studying this section, you should be able to:

■ describe the effects of ageing on the immunity.

Immunity declines with advancing age, increasing the risk of infection in older adults and lengthening recovery times. The thymus gland progressively shrinks from its maximum size at puberty and may be only a quarter of that by age 50. This is linked to decreased T-cell responsiveness, and as the B-cell response is dependent upon T-cell function, antibody levels also fall with age. Levels of autoantibodies and incidence of autoimmunity increase in later life, and reduced function of natural killer cells is associated with increasing incidence of most types of cancer.

Abnormal immune function

Learning outcomes

After studying this section, you should be able to:

- describe, with examples, the four types of allergic response

- describe the basis of autoimmune disease

- discuss the specific examples of autoimmune disease

- discuss the cause and effects of acquired immune deficiency syndrome (AIDS).

Hypersensitivity (allergy) ▦ 15.7

Allergy is an inappropriate, powerful immune response to an antigen (allergen) that is usually harmless. Examples include house dust, animal dander and grass pollen. It is therefore usually the immune response that causes the damage to the body, not the allergen itself. Upon initial exposure to the allergen the individual becomes sensitised to it, and on second and subsequent exposures the immune system mounts a response entirely out of proportion to the perceived threat. It should be noted that these responses are exaggerated versions of normal immune function (secondary response, Fig. 15.6). Sometimes symptoms are mild, although annoying, e.g. the running nose and streaming eyes of hay fever. Occasionally the reaction can be extreme, overwhelming body systems and causing death, e.g. anaphylactic shock, see below.

There are four mechanisms of hypersensitivity, which are classified according to the parts of the immune system that are involved. They are summarised in Figure 15.9.

Type I, anaphylactic hypersensitivity

This occurs in individuals with very high levels of immunoglobulin E (IgE). When exposed to an allergen, e.g. house dust, these high levels of antibody activate mast cells and basophils (p. 69), which degranulate. The most important substance released is histamine, which constricts some smooth muscle, e.g. airway smooth muscle, causes vasodilation and increases vascular permeability (leading to exudation of fluid and proteins into the tissues). Examples of type I reactions include the serious situation of anaphylaxis. There is profound bronchoconstriction and shock (p. 118) due to extensive vasodilation. The condition can lead to death.

Type II, cytotoxic hypersensitivity

When an antibody reacts with an antigen on a cell surface, that cell is marked for destruction by the body's defence cells. This is the usual procedure in the elimination of, for example, bacteria, but if the antibodies are directed against self-antigens the result is destruction of the body's own tissues (autoimmune disease). Type II mechanisms cause other conditions, e.g. haemolytic disease of the newborn (p. 75) and transfusion reactions (p. 76).

Type III, immune-complex-mediated hypersensitivity

Antibody–antigen complexes (immune complexes) are usually cleared efficiently from the blood by phagocytosis. If they are not, for example when there is phagocyte failure or an excessive production of immune complexes (e.g. in chronic infections), they can be deposited in tissues, e.g. kidneys, skin, joints and the eye, where they set up an inflammatory reaction. The kidney is a common site of deposition because it receives a large proportion of the cardiac output and filters the blood. Immune complexes collecting here lodge in and block the glomeruli (p. 350), impairing kidney function (glomerulonephritis). Penicillin allergy is also a type III reaction; antibodies bind to penicillin (the antigen), and the symptoms are the result of deposition of immune complexes in tissues – rashes, joint pains and sometimes haematuria.

Type IV, delayed type hypersensitivity

Unlike types I–III, type IV hypersensitivity does not involve antibodies, but is an overreaction of T-cells to an antigen. When an antigen is detected by memory T-cells, it provokes clonal expansion of the T-cell (Fig. 15.3), and large numbers of cytotoxic T-cells are released to eliminate the antigen. Usually this system is controlled and the T-cell response is appropriate. If not, the actively aggressive cytotoxic T-cells damage normal tissues.

An example of this is contact dermatitis (p. 371). Graft and transplant rejection is also caused by T-cells; an incompatible skin graft, for instance, will become necrotic and slough off in the days following application of the graft.

Autoimmune disease

Normally, an immune response is mounted only against foreign (non-self) antigens, but occasionally the body fails to recognise its own tissues and attacks itself. The resulting autoimmune disorders, examples of type II hypersensitivity, include a number of relatively common conditions (Table 15.3).

Immunodeficiency

When the immune system is compromised, there is a tendency to recurrent infections, often by microbes not normally pathogenic in humans (*opportunistic infections*). Immunodeficiency is classified as *primary* (usually occurring in infancy and genetically mediated) or *secondary*, that is, acquired in later life as the result of another

Type	Characteristics

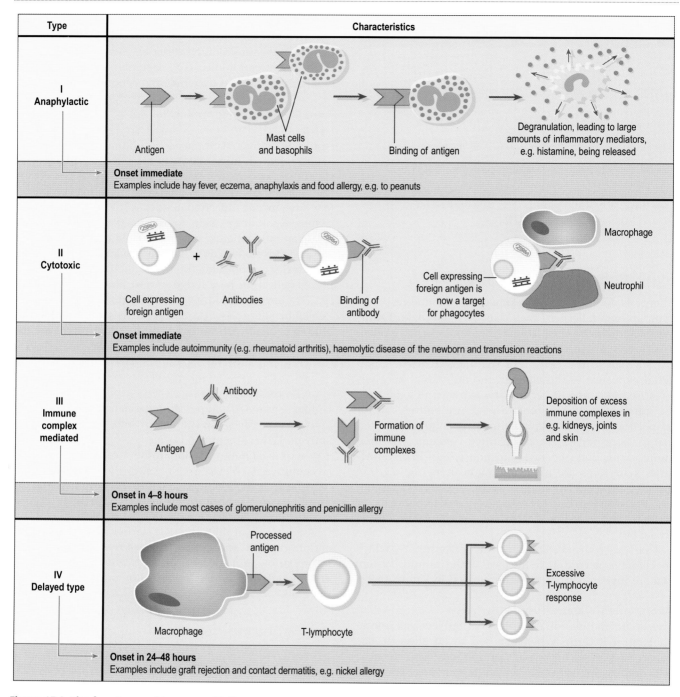

I Anaphylactic

Antigen — Mast cells and basophils — Binding of antigen — Degranulation, leading to large amounts of inflammatory mediators, e.g. histamine, being released

Onset immediate
Examples include hay fever, eczema, anaphylaxis and food allergy, e.g. to peanuts

II Cytotoxic

Cell expressing foreign antigen + Antibodies → Binding of antibody → Cell expressing foreign antigen is now a target for phagocytes — Macrophage — Neutrophil

Onset immediate
Examples include autoimmunity (e.g. rheumatoid arthritis), haemolytic disease of the newborn and transfusion reactions

III Immune complex mediated

Antibody — Antigen → Formation of immune complexes → Deposition of excess immune complexes in e.g. kidneys, joints and skin

Onset in 4–8 hours
Examples include most cases of glomerulonephritis and penicillin allergy

IV Delayed type

Macrophage — Processed antigen — T-lymphocyte → Excessive T-lymphocyte response

Onset in 24–48 hours
Examples include graft rejection and contact dermatitis, e.g. nickel allergy

Figure 15.9 The four types of hypersensitivity.

disease, e.g. protein deficiency, acute infection, chronic renal failure, bone marrow diseases, following splenectomy or acquired immune deficiency syndrome (AIDS).

Acquired immune deficiency syndrome (AIDS)

This condition is caused by the human immunodeficiency virus (HIV), an RNA retrovirus which produces the enzyme *reverse transcriptase* inside the cells of the infected person (host cells). This enzyme transforms viral RNA to DNA and this new DNA, called the provirus, is incorporated into the host cell DNA. The host cell then produces new copies of the virus that infect other host cells. When infected host cells divide, copies of the provirus are integrated into the DNA of daughter cells, spreading the disease within the body.

HIV has an affinity for cells that have a protein receptor called CD_4 in their membrane, including T-cells, monocytes, macrophages, some B-cells and, possibly,

Table 15.3 Common autoimmune disorders

Condition	Autoantibodies made against:
Rheumatoid arthritis (p. 432)	Synovial membrane of joints
Hashimoto's disease (p. 232)	Thyroglobulin
Graves' disease (p. 231)	TSH receptors on thyroid cells
Myasthenia gravis (p. 435)	Acetylcholine receptors of skeletal muscle
Glomerulonephritis (p. 350)	Glomerular membrane
Type 1 diabetes (p. 236)	Beta cells of the pancreas

cells in the gastrointestinal tract and neuroglial cells in the brain. CD_4 helper T-cells (Fig. 15.3) are the main cells involved. HIV establishes itself within the body's CD_4 cell populations and gradually destroys them, while at the same time it is protected from other body defence mechanisms. Because CD_4 cells are central to the body's immune system, both antibody-mediated and cell-mediated immunity are progressively eroded with the consequent development of widespread opportunistic infections, often by microbes of relatively low pathogenicity.

HIV has been isolated from semen, cervical secretions, lymphocytes, plasma, cerebrospinal fluid, tears, saliva, urine and breast milk. The secretions known to be especially infectious are semen, cervical secretions, blood and blood products.

Infection is spread by:

- sexual intercourse, vaginal and anal
- contaminated needles used:
  - during treatment of patients
  - when drug users share needles
- an infected mother to her child:
  - across the placenta before birth (vertical transmission)
  - during childbirth
  - in breast milk.

Stages of HIV infection. A few weeks after initial infection there may be an acute influenza-like illness with no specific features, followed by a period of 2 or more years without symptoms.

Chronic HIV infection may cause persistent generalised lymphadenopathy (PGL). Some patients may then develop AIDS-related complex (ARC) and experience chronic low-grade fever, diarrhoea, weight loss, anaemia and leukopenia.

AIDS is the most advanced stage of HIV infection, associated with a low CD_4 count and the presence of one or more characteristic infections, tumours or presentations:

- pneumonia, commonly caused by *Pneumocystis jirovecii* (formerly *Pneumocystis carinii*), but many other microbes may be involved
- persistent nausea, diarrhoea and weight loss due to recurrent infections of the alimentary tract by a wide variety of microbes
- meningitis, encephalitis and brain abscesses may be recurrent, either caused by opportunistic microbes or possibly by HIV
- neurological function may deteriorate, characterised by forgetfulness, loss of concentration, confusion, apathy, dementia, limb weakness, ataxia and incontinence (p. 356)
- skin conditions, often extensive, may occur, e.g. eczema, psoriasis, cellulitis, impetigo, warts, shingles and cold sores (see Ch. 14)
- generalised lymphadenopathy (p. 140)
- development of malignant tumours is not uncommon, because of the progressive failure of immunological surveillance as the virus destroys the T-cell population. Typical cancers include:
  - lymphoma (p. 141)
  - Kaposi's sarcoma, consisting of tumours under the skin and in internal organs (p. 373).

For a range of self-assessment exercises on the topics in this chapter, visit Evolve online resources: https://evolve.elsevier.com/Waugh/anatomy/

16 CHAPTER

The musculoskeletal system

The musculoskeletal system consists of the bones of the skeleton, their joints and the skeletal (voluntary) muscles that move the body. The characteristics and properties of joints, and of bone and muscle tissue, are discussed in this chapter. The effects of ageing on the musculoskeletal system are listed, and the illnesses section at the end of the chapter describes some disorders of bone, muscle and joints.

Bone

Learning outcomes

After studying this section, you should be able to:

■ state the functions of bones

■ list five types of bones and give an example of each

■ outline the general structure of a long bone

■ describe the structure of compact and spongy bone tissue

■ describe the development of bone

■ explain the process of bone healing and the factors that complicate it

■ outline the factors that determine bone growth.

Although bones are often thought to be static or permanent, they are highly vascular living structures that are continuously being remodelled.

Functions of bones

The functions of bones include:

• providing the body framework
• giving attachment to muscles and tendons
• allowing movement of the body as a whole and of parts of the body, by forming joints that are moved by muscles

• forming the boundaries of the cranial, thoracic and pelvic cavities, and protecting the organs they contain
• haemopoiesis, the production of blood cells in red bone marrow (p. 64)
• mineral storage, especially calcium phosphate – the mineral reservoir within bone is essential for maintenance of blood calcium levels, which must be tightly controlled.

Types of bones

Bones are classified as long, short, irregular, flat and sesamoid.

Long bones. These consist of a shaft and two extremities. As the name suggests, these bones are longer than they are wide. Most long bones are found in the limbs; examples include the femur, tibia and fibula.

Short, irregular, flat and sesamoid bones. These have no shafts or extremities and are diverse in shape and size. Examples include:

• short bones – carpals (wrist)
• irregular bones – vertebrae and some skull bones
• flat bones – sternum, ribs and most skull bones
• sesamoid bones – patella (knee cap).

Bone structure

Long bones

These have a *diaphysis* (shaft) and two *epiphyses* (extremities) (Fig. 16.1). The diaphysis is composed mainly of compact bone with a central medullary canal, containing fatty yellow bone marrow. The epiphyses consist of an outer covering of compact bone with *spongy (cancellous) bone* inside. The diaphysis and epiphyses are separated by *epiphyseal cartilages*, which ossify when growth is complete.

Long bones are almost completely covered by a vascular membrane, the *periosteum*, which has two layers. The outer layer is tough and fibrous, and protects the bone underneath. The inner layer contains osteoblasts and osteoclasts, the cells responsible for bone production and breakdown (see below), and is important in repair

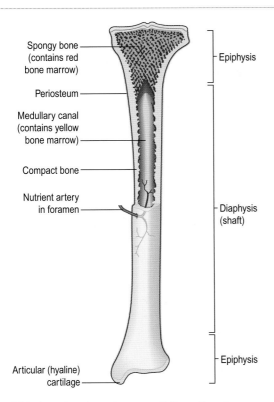

Figure 16.1 **A mature long bone:** partially sectioned.

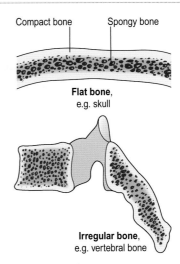

Figure 16.2 **Sections of flat and irregular bones.**

and remodelling of the bone. The periosteum covers the whole bone except within joint cavities, allows attachments of tendons and is continuous with the joint capsule. *Hyaline cartilage* replaces periosteum on bone surfaces that form joints. Thickening of a bone occurs by the deposition of new bone tissue under the periosteum.

Blood and nerve supply

One or more nutrient arteries supply the bone shaft; the epiphyses have their own blood supply, although in the mature bone the capillary networks arising from the two are heavily interconnected. The sensory nerve supply usually enters the bone at the same site as the nutrient artery, and branches extensively throughout the bone. Bone injury is, therefore, usually very painful.

Short, irregular, flat and sesamoid bones

These have a relatively thin outer layer of compact bone, with spongy bone inside containing red bone marrow (Fig. 16.2). They are enclosed by periosteum except the inner layer of the cranial bones where it is replaced by dura mater.

Microscopic structure of bone

Bone is a strong and durable type of connective tissue. Its major constituent (65%) is a mixture of calcium salts, mainly calcium phosphate. This inorganic matrix gives bone great hardness, but on its own would be brittle and prone to shattering. The remaining third is organic material, called *osteoid*, which is composed mainly of collagen. Collagen is very strong and gives bone slight flexibility. The cellular component of bone contributes less than 2% of bone mass.

Bone cells

There are three types of bone cell:

- osteoblast
- ostecyte
- osteoclast.

Osteoblasts

These bone-forming cells are responsible for the deposition of both inorganic salts and osteoid in bone tissue. They are therefore present at sites where bone is growing, repairing or remodelling, e.g.:

- in the deeper layers of periosteum
- in the centres of ossification of immature bone
- at the ends of the diaphysis adjacent to the epiphyseal cartilages of long bones
- at the site of a fracture.

As they deposit new bone tissue around themselves, they eventually become trapped in tiny pockets (*lacunae*, Fig. 16.3) in the growing bone, and differentiate into *osteocytes*.

Osteocytes

These are mature bone cells that monitor and maintain bone tissue, and are nourished by tissue fluid in the *canaliculi* that radiate from the *central canals*.

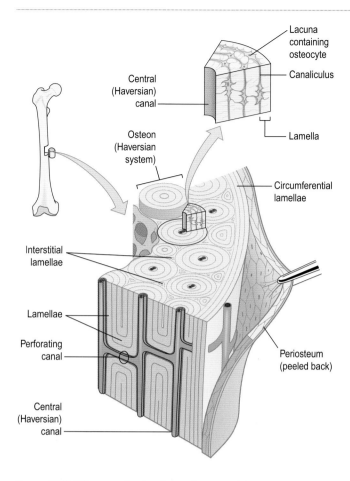

Figure 16.3 Microscopic structure of compact bone.

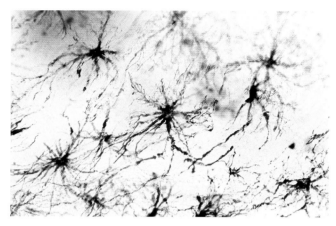

Figure 16.4 Light micrograph of osteocytes, showing the multiple fine processes that extend through bone canaliculi and allow each cell to communicate directly with its neighbours.

femur (thigh bone), they run from one epiphysis to the other. This gives the bone great strength.

The central canal contains nerves, lymphatics and blood vessels, and each central canal is linked with neighbouring canals by tunnels running at right angles between them, called *perforating canals*. The series of cylindrical plates of bone arranged around each central canal are called *lamellae*. Between the adjacent lamellae of the osteon are strings of little cavities called *lacunae*, in each of which sits an osteocyte. Lacunae communicate with each other through a series of tiny channels called *canaliculi*, which allows the circulation of interstitial fluid through the bone, and direct contact between the osteocytes, which extend fine processes into them (Fig. 16.4).

Between the osteons are *interstitial lamellae*, the remnants of older systems partially broken down during remodelling or growth of bone.

Spongy (cancellous, trabecular) bone

To the naked eye, spongy bone looks like a honeycomb. Microscopic examination reveals a framework formed from *trabeculae* (meaning 'little beams'), which consist of a few lamellae and osteocytes interconnected by canaliculi (Fig. 16.5). Osteocytes are nourished by interstitial fluid diffusing into the bone through the tiny canaliculi. The spaces between the trabeculae contain red bone marrow. In addition, spongy bone is lighter than compact bone, reducing the weight of the skeleton.

Development of bone tissue 🎞 16.1

Also called *osteogenesis* or *ossification*, this begins before birth and is not complete until about the 21st year of life. Long, short and irregular bones develop in the fetus from rods of cartilage, *cartilage models*. Flat bones develop from *membrane models* and sesamoid bones from *tendon models*.

Osteoclasts

These cells break down bone, releasing calcium and phosphate. They are very large cells with up to 50 nuclei, which have formed from the fusion of many monocytes (p. 69). The continuous remodelling of healthy bone tissue is the result of balanced activity of the bone's osteoblast and osteoclast populations. Osteoclasts are found in areas of the bone where there is active growth, repair or remodelling, e.g.:

- under the periosteum, maintaining bone shape during growth and to remove excess callus formed during healing of fractures (p. 394)
- round the walls of the medullary canal during growth and to canalise callus during healing.

Compact (cortical) bone

Compact bone makes up about 80% of the body bone mass. It is made up of a large number of parallel tube-shaped units called *osteons* (Haversian systems), each of which is made up of a central canal surrounded by a series of expanding rings, similar to the growth rings of a tree (Fig. 16.3). Osteons tend to be aligned the same way that force is applied to the bone, so for example in the

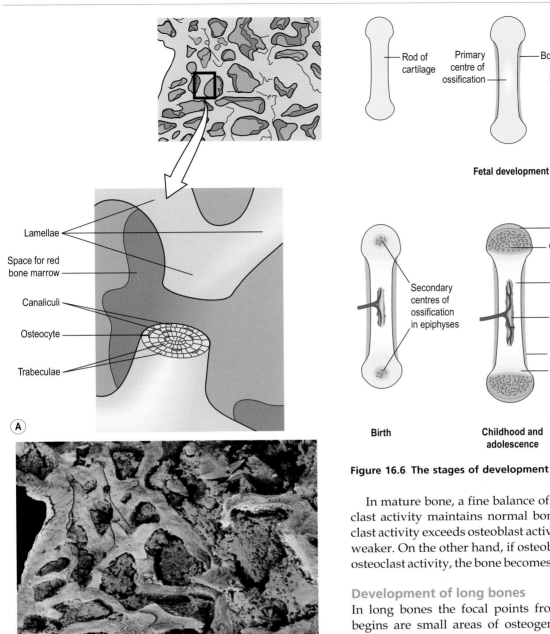

Lamellae

Space for red bone marrow

Canaliculi

Osteocyte

Trabeculae

(A)

(B)

Figure 16.5 Spongy bone. A. Microscopic structure of spongy bone. **B.** Electron micrograph of spongy bone showing bone marrow (orange) filling the spaces between trabeculae (grey/blue).

Rod of cartilage

Primary centre of ossification

Bony collar

Lengthening of diaphysis

Fetal development

Hyaline cartilage

Cancellous bone

Compact bone

Medullary canal

Periosteum

Epiphyseal cartilage

Secondary centres of ossification in epiphyses

Birth

Childhood and adolescence

Adult

Figure 16.6 The stages of development of a long bone.

In mature bone, a fine balance of osteoblast and osteoclast activity maintains normal bone structure. If osteoclast activity exceeds osteoblast activity, the bone becomes weaker. On the other hand, if osteoblast activity outstrips osteoclast activity, the bone becomes stronger and heavier.

Development of long bones

In long bones the focal points from which ossification begins are small areas of osteogenic cells, or *centres of ossification* in the cartilage model (Fig. 16.6). This is accompanied by development of a bone collar at about 8 weeks of gestation. Later the blood supply develops and bone tissue replaces cartilage as osteoblasts secrete osteoid in the shaft. The bone lengthens as ossification continues and spreads to the epiphyses. Around birth, secondary centres of ossification develop in the epiphyses, and the medullary canal forms when osteoclasts break down the central bone tissue in the middle of the shaft. During childhood, long bones continue to lengthen because the epiphyseal plate at each end of the bone, which is made of cartilage, continues to produce new cartilage on its diaphyseal surface (the surface facing the shaft of the bone, Fig. 16.7). This cartilage is then turned to bone. As long as cartilage production matches the rate of ossification, the bone continues to lengthen. At puberty, under

During ossification, osteoblasts secrete osteoid, which gradually replaces the initial model; then this osteoid is progressively calcified, also by osteoblast action. As the bone grows, the osteoblasts become trapped in the matrix of their own making and become osteocytes.

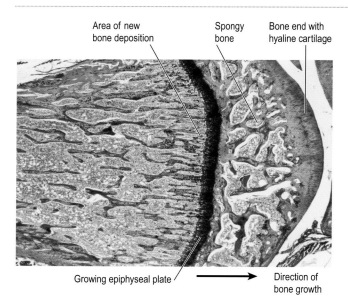

Area of new bone deposition   Spongy bone   Bone end with hyaline cartilage

Growing epiphyseal plate   →   Direction of bone growth

Figure 16.7 Light micrograph of the end of a growing bone, showing the epiphyseal plate.

the influence of sex hormones, the epiphyseal plate growth slows down, and is overtaken by bone deposition. Once the whole epiphyseal plate is turned to bone, no further lengthening of the bone is possible.

Hormonal regulation of bone growth

Hormones (see Ch. 9) that regulate the growth, size and shape of bones include the following.

- *Growth hormone* and the thyroid hormones, *thyroxine* and *tri-iodothyronine*, are especially important during infancy and childhood; deficient or excessive secretion of these results in abnormal development of the skeleton (p. 223).
- *Testosterone* and *oestrogens* influence the physical changes that occur at puberty and help maintain bone structure throughout life. Rising levels of these hormones are responsible for the growth spurt of puberty, but later stimulate closure of the epiphyseal plates (Fig. 16.7), so that bone growth lengthways stops (although bones can grow in thickness throughout life). Average adult male height is usually greater than female, because male puberty tends to occur at a later age than female puberty, giving a male child's bones longer to keep growing. Oestrogens are responsible for the wider female pelvis that develops during puberty, and for maintaining bone mass in the adult female. Falling oestrogen levels after menopause can put postmenopausal women at higher risk of bone fracture (osteoporosis, p. 431).
- *Calcitonin* and *parathyroid hormone* (p. 224) control blood levels of calcium by regulating its uptake into and release from bone. Calcitonin increases calcium uptake into bone (reducing blood calcium), and parathormone decreases it (increasing blood calcium).

Although the length and shape of bones does not normally change after ossification is complete, bone tissue is continually being remodelled and replaced when damaged. Osteoblasts continue to lay down osteoid and osteoclasts reabsorb it. The rate in different bones varies, e.g. the distal part of the femur is replaced over a period of 5 to 6 months.

Exercise and bone

Although bone growth lengthways permanently ceases once the epiphyseal plates have ossified, thickening of bone is possible throughout life. This involves the laying down of new osteons at the periphery of the bone through the action of osteoblasts in the inner layer of the periosteum. Weight-bearing exercise stimulates thickening of bone, strengthening it and making it less liable to fracture. Lack of exercise reverses these changes, leading to lighter, weaker bones.

Diet and bone

Healthy bone tissue requires adequate dietary calcium and vitamins A, C and D. Calcium, and smaller amounts of other minerals such as phosphate, iron and manganese, is essential for adequate mineralisation of bone. Vitamin A is needed for osteoblast activity. Vitamin C is used in collagen synthesis, and vitamin D is required for calcium and phosphate absorption from the intestinal tract.

Bone markings

Most bones have rough surfaces, raised protuberances and ridges that give attachment to muscle tendons and ligaments. These are not included in the following descriptions of individual bones unless they are of particular note, but many are marked on illustrations. Bone markings and related terminology are defined in Table 16.1.

Healing of bone ▮ 16.2

There are a number of terms used to classify bone fractures, including:

- *simple*: the bone ends do not protrude through the skin
- *compound*: the bone ends protrude through the skin
- *pathological*: fracture of a bone weakened by disease.

Following a fracture, the broken ends of bone are joined by the deposition of new bone. This occurs in several stages (Fig. 16.8).

1. A haematoma (collection of clotted blood) forms between the ends of bone and in surrounding soft tissues.
2. There follows development of acute inflammation and accumulation of inflammatory exudate, containing macrophages that phagocytose the haematoma and small dead fragments of bone

Table 16.1 Anatomical terminology related to bones

Term	Meaning
Articulating surface	The part of the bone that enters into the formation of a joint
Articulation	A joint between two or more bones
Bony sinus	A hollow cavity within a bone
Border	A ridge of bone separating two surfaces
Condyle	A smooth rounded projection of bone that forms part of a joint
Facet	A small, generally rather flat, articulating surface
Fissure or cleft	A narrow slit
Foramen (plural: foramina)	A hole in a structure
Fossa (plural: fossae)	A hollow or depression
Meatus	A tube-shaped cavity within a bone
Septum	A partition separating two cavities
Spine, spinous process or crest	A sharp ridge of bone
Styloid process	A sharp downward projection of bone that gives attachment to muscles and ligaments
Suture	An immovable joint, e.g. between the bones of the skull
Trochanter, tuberosity or tubercle	Roughened bony projections, usually for attachment of muscles or ligaments. The different names are used according to the size of the projection. Trochanters are the largest and tubercles the smallest

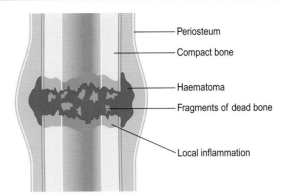

1. **Haematoma formation**

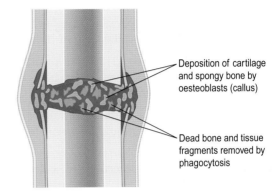

2. **Callus formation begins**

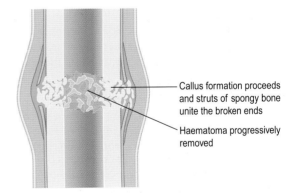

3. **Bone end reunited**

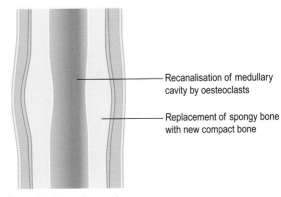

4. **Recanalisation and normal bone structure regained**

Figure 16.8 Stages in bone healing.

(this takes about 5 days). Fibroblasts migrate to the site; granulation tissue and new capillaries develop.
3. New bone forms as large numbers of osteoblasts secrete spongy bone, which unites the broken ends, and is protected by an outer layer of bone and cartilage; the new deposits of bone and cartilage is called a *callus*. Over the next few weeks, the callus matures, and the cartilage is gradually replaced with new bone.
4. Reshaping of the bone continues and gradually the medullary canal is reopened through the callus (in weeks or months). In time the bone heals completely with the callus tissue completely replaced with mature compact bone. Often the bone is thicker

395

and stronger at the repair site than originally, and a second fracture is more likely to occur at a different site.

Factors that delay healing of fractures

Tissue fragments between bone ends. Splinters of dead bone (*sequestrae*) and soft tissue fragments not removed by phagocytosis delay healing.

Deficient blood supply. This delays growth of granulation tissue and new blood vessels. Hypoxia also reduces the number of osteoblasts and increases the number of chondrocytes that develop from their common parent cells. This may lead to cartilaginous union of the fracture, which results in a weaker repair. The most vulnerable sites, because of their normally poor blood supply, are the neck of femur, the scaphoid and the shaft of tibia.

Poor alignment of bone ends. This may result in the formation of a large and irregular callus that heals slowly and often results in permanent disability.

Continued mobility of bone ends. Continuous movement results in fibrosis of the granulation tissue followed by fibrous union of the fracture.

Miscellaneous. These include infection (see below), systemic illness, malnutrition, drugs, e.g. corticosteroids and ageing.

Complications of fractures

Infection (osteomyelitis, p. 432). Pathogens enter through broken skin, although they may occasionally be blood-borne. Healing will not occur until the infection resolves.

Fat embolism. Emboli consisting of fat from the bone marrow in the medullary canal may enter the circulation through torn veins. They are most likely to lodge in the lungs and block blood flow through the pulmonary capillaries.

Axial skeleton

Learning outcomes

After studying this section, you should be able to:

- identify the bones of the skull (face and cranium)
- list the functions of the sinuses and fontanelles of the skull
- outline the characteristics of a typical vertebra
- describe the structure of the vertebral column
- explain the movements and functions of the vertebral column
- identify the bones forming the thoracic cage.

The bones of the skeleton are divided into two groups: the *axial skeleton* and the *appendicular skeleton* (Fig. 16.9).

The axial skeleton consists of the *skull, vertebral column, ribs* and *sternum*. Together the bones forming these structures constitute the central bony core of the body, the axis. The appendicular skeleton consists of the shoulder and pelvic girdles and the limb bones.

Skull (Figs 16.10 and 16.11)

The skull rests on the upper end of the vertebral column and its bony structure is divided into two parts: the cranium and the face.

Sinuses

Sinuses containing air are present in the sphenoid, ethmoid, maxillary and frontal bones. They all communicate with the nasal cavity and are lined with ciliated mucous membrane. They give resonance to the voice and reduce the weight of the skull, making it easier to carry.

Cranium

The cranium is formed by a number of flat and irregular bones that protect the brain. It has a *base* upon which the brain rests and a *vault* that surrounds and covers it. The periosteum lining the inner surface of the skull bones forms the outer layer of dura mater (p. 152). In the mature skull the joints (*sutures*) between the bones are immovable. The bones have numerous perforations (e.g. foramina, fissures) through which nerves, blood and lymph vessels pass. The bones of the cranium are:

- 1 frontal bone
- 2 parietal bones
- 2 temporal bones
- 1 occipital bone
- 1 sphenoid bone
- 1 ethmoid bone.

Frontal bone

This is the bone of the forehead. It forms part of the *orbital cavities* (eye sockets) and the prominent ridges above the eyes, the *supraorbital margins*. Just above the supraorbital margins, within the bone, are two air-filled cavities or *sinuses* lined with ciliated mucous membrane, which open into the nasal cavity.

The *coronal suture* joins the frontal and parietal bones and other sutures are formed with the sphenoid, zygomatic, lacrimal, nasal and ethmoid bones. The frontal bone originates in two parts joined in the midline by the *frontal suture* (see Fig. 16.18).

Parietal bones

These bones form the sides and roof of the skull. They articulate with each other at the *sagittal suture*, with the frontal bone at the coronal suture, with the occipital bone

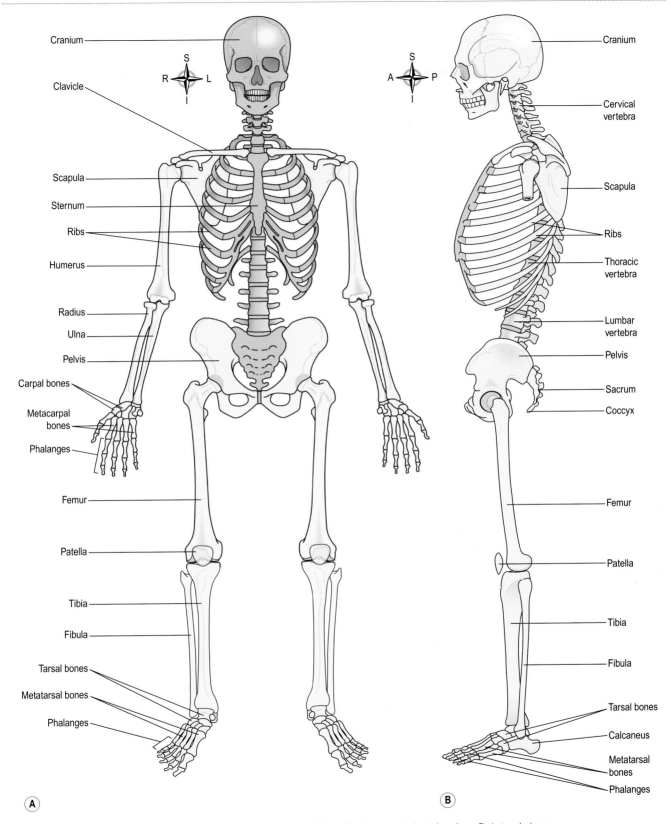

Figure 16.9 The skeleton. Axial skeleton in gold, appendicular skeleton in brown. **A.** Anterior view. **B.** Lateral view.

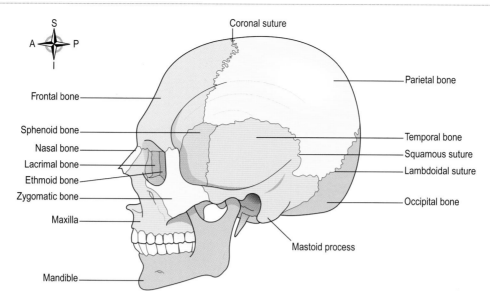

Figure 16.10 **The bones of the skull and their sutures (joints).**

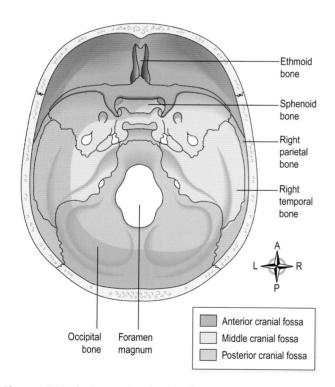

Figure 16.11 **The bones forming the base of the skull and the cranial fossae.** Viewed from above.

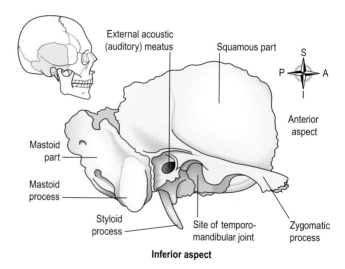

Figure 16.12 **The right temporal bone.** Lateral view.

zygomatic bones. The *squamous part* is the thin fan-shaped area that articulates with the parietal bone. The *zygomatic process* articulates with the zygomatic bone to form the zygomatic arch (cheekbone).

The *mastoid part* contains the mastoid process, a thickened region easily felt behind the ear. It contains a large number of very small air sinuses that communicate with the middle ear and are lined with squamous epithelium.

The *petrous portion* forms part of the base of the skull and contains the organs of hearing (the spiral organ) and balance.

The temporal bone articulates with the mandible at the *temporomandibular joint*, the only movable joint of the skull. Immediately behind this articulating surface is

at the *lambdoidal suture* and with the temporal bones at the *squamous sutures*. The inner surface is concave and is grooved to accommodate the brain and blood vessels.

Temporal bones (Fig. 16.12)

These bones lie one on each side of the head and form sutures with the parietal, occipital, sphenoid and

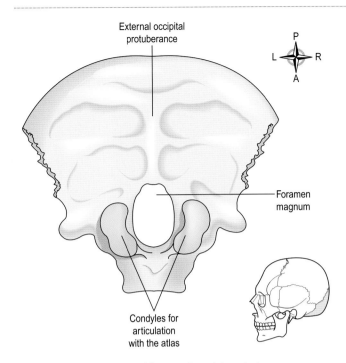

Figure 16.13 The occipital bone. Viewed from below.

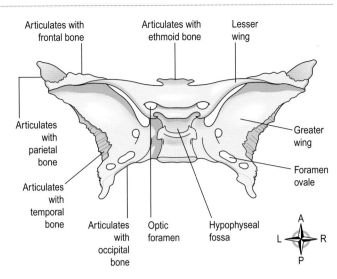

Figure 16.14 The sphenoid bone. Viewed from above.

the *external acoustic meatus* (auditory canal), which passes inwards towards the petrous portion of the bone.

The styloid process projects from the lower process of the temporal bone, and supports the hyoid bone and muscles associated with the tongue and pharynx.

Occipital bone (Fig. 16.13)

This bone forms the back of the head and part of the base of the skull. It forms sutures with the parietal, temporal and sphenoid bones. Its inner surface is deeply concave and the concavity is occupied by the occipital lobes of the cerebrum and by the cerebellum. The occiput has two articular condyles that form condyloid joints (p. 414) with the first bone of the vertebral column, the *atlas*. This joint permits nodding movements of the head. Between the condyles is the *foramen magnum* (meaning 'large hole') through which the spinal cord passes into the cranial cavity.

Sphenoid bone (Fig. 16.14)

This bone occupies the middle portion of the base of the skull and it articulates with the occipital, temporal, parietal and frontal bones (Fig. 16.11). It links the cranial and facial bones, and cross-braces the skull. On the superior surface in the middle of the bone is a little saddle-shaped depression, the *hypophyseal fossa* (*sella turcica*) in which the *pituitary gland* rests. The body of the bone contains some fairly large air sinuses lined with ciliated mucous membrane with openings into the nasal cavity. The optic nerves pass through the *optic foramina* on their way to the brain.

Ethmoid bone (Fig. 16.15)

The ethmoid bone occupies the anterior part of the base of the skull and helps to form the orbital cavity, the nasal septum and the lateral walls of the nasal cavity. On each side are two projections into the nasal cavity, the *superior* and *middle conchae* or *turbinated processes*. It is a very delicate bone containing many air sinuses lined with ciliated epithelium and with openings into the nasal cavity. The horizontal flattened part, the *cribriform plate*, forms the roof of the nasal cavity and has numerous small foramina through which nerve fibres of the *olfactory nerve* (sense of smell) pass upwards from the nasal cavity to the brain.

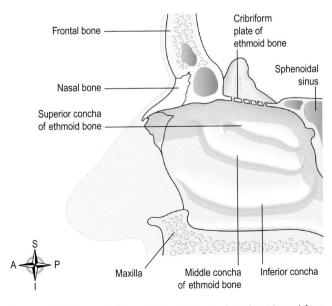

Figure 16.15 Lateral view of the right nasal cavity. Viewed from the left.

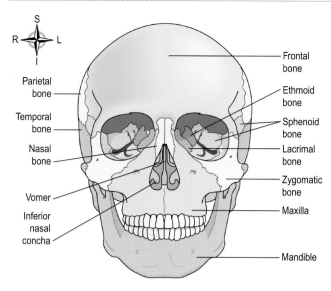

Figure 16.16 The bones of the face. Anterior view.

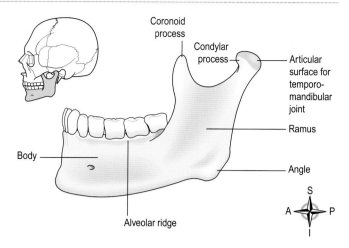

Figure 16.17 The left mandible. Lateral view.

There is also a very fine *perpendicular plate* of bone that forms the upper part of the *nasal septum*.

Face

The skeleton of the face is formed by 13 bones in addition to the frontal bone already described. Figure 16.16 shows the relationships between the bones:

- 2 zygomatic (cheek) bones
- 1 maxilla
- 2 nasal bones
- 2 lacrimal bones
- 1 vomer
- 2 palatine bones
- 2 inferior conchae
- 1 mandible.

Zygomatic (cheek) bones
The zygomatic bone originates as two bones that fuse before birth. They form the prominences of the cheeks and part of the floor and lateral walls of the orbital cavities.

Maxilla (upper jaw bone)
This originates as two bones that fuse before birth. The maxilla forms the upper jaw, the anterior part of the roof of the mouth, the lateral walls of the nasal cavity and part of the floor of the orbital cavities. The *alveolar ridge*, or *process*, projects downwards and carries the upper teeth. On each side is a large air sinus, the *maxillary sinus*, lined with ciliated mucous membrane and with openings into the nasal cavity.

Nasal bones
These are two small flat bones that form the greater part of the lateral and superior surfaces of the bridge of the nose.

Lacrimal bones
These two small bones are posterior and lateral to the nasal bones and form part of the medial walls of the orbital cavities. Each is pierced by a foramen for the passage of the *nasolacrimal duct* that carries the tears from the medial canthus of the eye to the nasal cavity.

Vomer
The vomer is a thin flat bone that extends upwards from the middle of the hard palate to form most of the inferior part of the nasal septum. Superiorly it articulates with the perpendicular plate of the ethmoid bone.

Palatine bones
These are two small L-shaped bones. The horizontal parts unite to form the posterior part of the hard palate and the perpendicular parts project upwards to form part of the lateral walls of the nasal cavity. At their upper extremities they form part of the orbital cavities.

Inferior conchae
Each concha is a scroll-shaped bone, which forms part of the lateral wall of the nasal cavity and projects into it below the middle concha. The superior and middle conchae are parts of the ethmoid bone. The conchae collectively increase the surface area in the nasal cavity, allowing inspired air to be warmed and humidified more effectively.

Mandible (lower jaw bone, Fig. 16.17)
This is the lower jaw, the only movable bone of the skull. It originates as two parts that unite at the midline. Each half consists of two main parts: a *curved body* with the *alveolar ridge* containing the lower teeth and a *ramus*, which projects upwards almost at right angles to the posterior end of the body.

At the upper end the ramus divides into the *condylar process* which articulates with the temporal bone to form

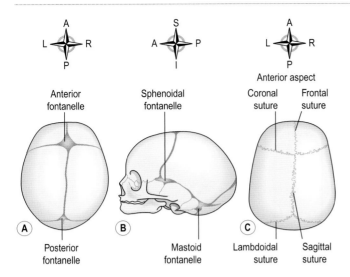

Figure 16.18 The skull showing the fontanelles and sutures.
A. Fontanelles viewed from above. **B.** Fontanelles viewed from the side. **C.** Main sutures viewed from above when ossification is complete.

the *temporomandibular* joint (see Fig. 16.12) and the *coronoid process*, which gives attachment to muscles and ligaments that close the jaw. The point where the ramus joins the body is the *angle* of the jaw.

Hyoid bone

This is an isolated horseshoe-shaped bone lying in the soft tissues of the neck just above the *larynx* and below the *mandible* (see Fig. 10.4). It does not articulate with any other bone, but is attached to the styloid process of the temporal bone by ligaments. It supports the larynx and gives attachment to the base of the tongue.

Fontanelles of the skull (Fig. 16.18)

At birth, ossification of the cranial sutures is incomplete. The skull bones do not fuse earlier to allow for moulding of the baby's head during childbirth. Where three or more bones meet there are distinct membranous areas, or *fontanelles*. The two largest are the *anterior fontanelle*, not fully ossified until the child is between 12 and 18 months old, and the *posterior fontanelle*, usually ossified 2–3 months after birth.

Functions of the skull

The various parts of the skull have specific and different functions:

- the *cranium* protects the brain
- the *bony eye sockets* protect the eyes and give attachment to the muscles that move them
- the *temporal bone* protects the delicate structures of the inner ear
- the sinuses in some face and skull bones give resonance to the voice

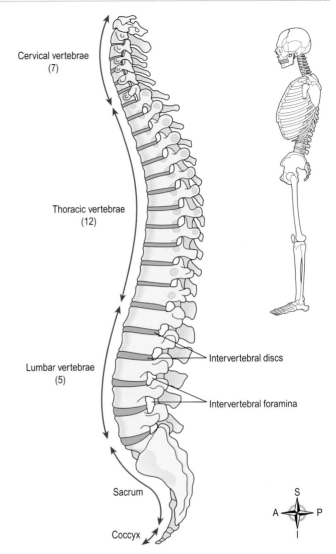

Figure 16.19 The vertebral column. Lateral view.

- the bones of the face form the walls of the posterior part of the nasal cavities and form the upper part of the air passages
- the *maxilla* and the *mandible* provide alveolar ridges in which the teeth are embedded
- the mandible, controlled by muscles of the lower face, allows chewing.

Vertebral column (Fig. 16.19) 16.3

There are 26 bones in the vertebral column. Twenty-four separate vertebrae extend downwards from the occipital bone of the skull; then there is the *sacrum*, formed from five fused vertebrae, and lastly the *coccyx*, or tail, which is formed from between three and five small fused vertebrae. The vertebral column is divided into different regions. The first seven vertebrae, in the neck, form the cervical spine; the next 12 vertebrae are the thoracic spine,

401

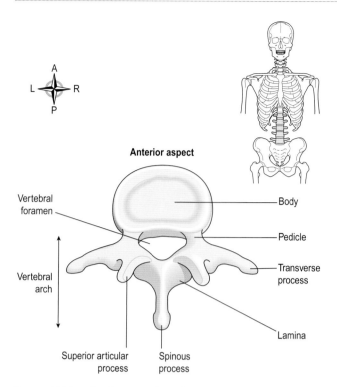

Figure 16.20 A lumbar vertebra showing the features of a typical vertebra. Viewed from above.

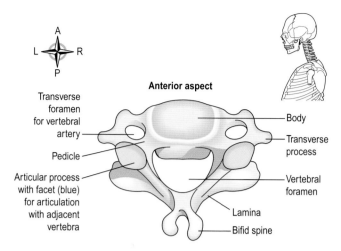

Figure 16.21 A cervical vertebra, showing typical features. Viewed from above.

and the next five the lumbar spine, the lowest vertebra of which articulates with the sacrum. Each vertebra is identified by the first letter of its region in the spine, followed by a number indicating its position. For example, the topmost vertebra is C1, and the third lumbar vertebra is L3.

The movable vertebrae have many characteristics in common, but some groups have distinguishing features.

Characteristics of a typical vertebra (Fig. 16.20)

The body. This is the broad, flattened, largest part of the vertebra. When the vertebrae are stacked together in the vertebral column, it is the flattened surfaces of the body of each vertebra that articulate with the corresponding surfaces of adjacent vertebrae. However, there is no direct bone-to-bone contact since between each pair of bones is a tough pad of fibrocartilage called the *intervertebral disc*. The bodies of the vertebrae lie to the front of the vertebral column, increasing greatly in size towards the base of the spine, as the lower spine has to support much more weight than the upper regions.

The vertebral (neural) arch. This encloses a large *vertebral foramen*. It lies behind the body, and forms the posterior and lateral walls of the vertebral foramen. The lateral walls are formed from plates of bone called *pedicles*, and the posterior walls are formed from *laminae*. Projecting

from the regions where the pedicle meets the lamina is a lateral prominence, the *transverse process*, and where the two laminae meet at the back is a process called the *spinous process*. These bony prominences can be felt through the skin along the length of the spine. The vertebral arch has four articular surfaces: two articulate with the vertebra above and two with the one below. The vertebral foramina form the vertebral (neural) canal that contains the spinal cord.

Region-specific vertebral characteristics

Cervical vertebrae (Fig. 16.21)

These are the smallest vertebrae. The transverse processes have a foramen through which a vertebral artery passes upwards to the brain. The first two cervical vertebrae, the *atlas* and the *axis*, are atypical.

The first cervical vertebra (C1), the *atlas*, is the bone on which the skull rests. Below the atlas is the *axis*, the second cervical vertebra (C2).

The atlas (Fig. 16.22A) is essentially a ring of bone, with no distinct body or spinous process, although it has two short transverse processes. It possesses two flattened facets that articulate with the occipital bone; these are condyloid joints (p. 414) and they permit nodding of the head.

The axis (Fig. 16.22B) sits below the atlas, and has a small body with a small superior projection called the *odontoid process* (also called the dens, meaning tooth). This occupies part of the posterior foramen of the atlas above, and is held securely within it by the transverse ligament (Fig. 16.22C). The head pivots (i.e. turns from side to side) on this joint.

The 7th cervical vertebra, C7, is also known as the *vertebra prominens*. It possesses a long spinous prominence terminating in a swollen tubercle, which is easily felt at the base of the neck.

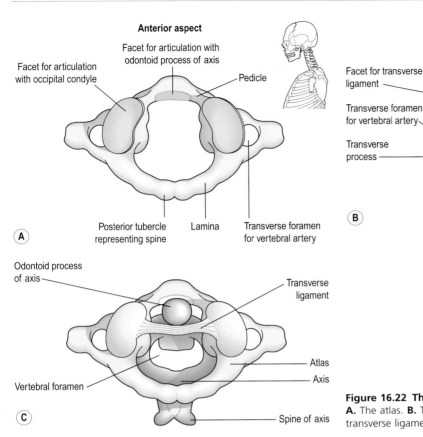

Anterior aspect

Facet for articulation with odontoid process of axis

Facet for articulation with occipital condyle

Pedicle

Posterior tubercle representing spine

Lamina

Transverse foramen for vertebral artery

(A)

Anterior aspect

Facet for transverse ligament

Transverse foramen for vertebral artery

Transverse process

Odontoid process

Facet for atlas

Pedicle

Body

Lamina

Spinous process

(B)

Odontoid process of axis

Transverse ligament

Vertebral foramen

Atlas

Axis

Spine of axis

(C)

Figure 16.22 The upper cervical vertebrae. Viewed from above. **A.** The atlas. **B.** The axis. **C.** The atlas and axis in position showing the transverse ligament.

Thoracic vertebrae (Fig. 16.23)

The 12 thoracic vertebrae are larger than the cervical vertebrae because this section of the vertebral column has to support more body weight. The bodies and transverse processes have facets for articulation with the ribs.

Lumbar vertebrae (Fig. 16.20)

These are the largest of the vertebrae because they have to support the weight of the upper body. They have substantial spinous processes for attachment of the muscles of the lower back.

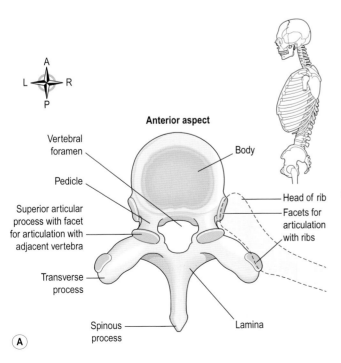

Anterior aspect

Vertebral foramen

Pedicle

Superior articular process with facet for articulation with adjacent vertebra

Transverse process

Spinous process

Body

Head of rib

Facets for articulation with ribs

Lamina

(A)

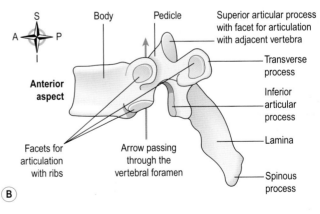

Body

Pedicle

Superior articular process with facet for articulation with adjacent vertebra

Transverse process

Inferior articular process

Lamina

Spinous process

Anterior aspect

Facets for articulation with ribs

Arrow passing through the vertebral foramen

(B)

Figure 16.23 A thoracic vertebra. A. Viewed from above. **B.** Viewed from the side.

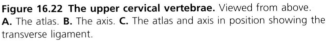

403

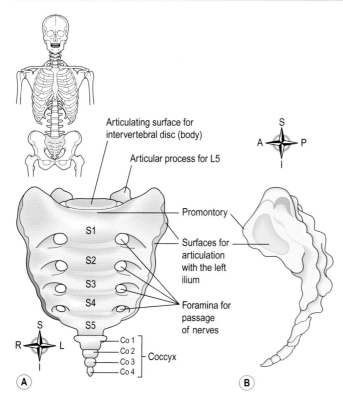

Figure 16.24 The sacrum and coccyx. **A.** Anterior view. **B.** Lateral view.

Sacrum (Fig. 16.24)

This consists of five rudimentary vertebrae fused to form a triangular or wedge-shaped bone with a concave anterior surface. The upper part, or base, articulates with the 5th lumbar vertebra. On each side it articulates with the ilium to form a *sacroiliac joint,* and at its inferior tip it articulates with the coccyx. The anterior edge of the base, the *promontory,* protrudes into the pelvic cavity. The vertebral foramina are present, and on each side of the bone there is a series of foramina for the passage of nerves.

Coccyx (Fig. 16.24)

This consists of the four terminal vertebrae fused to form a very small triangular bone, the broad base of which articulates with the tip of the sacrum.

Features of the vertebral column

Intervertebral discs

The bodies of adjacent vertebrae are separated by *intervertebral discs,* consisting of an outer rim of fibrocartilage (*annulus fibrosus*) and a central core of soft gelatinous material (*nucleus pulposus*) (Fig. 16.25). They are thinnest in the cervical region and become progressively thicker towards the lumbar region, as spinal loading increases. The posterior longitudinal ligament in the vertebral canal helps to keep them in place. They have a shock-absorbing function and the cartilaginous joints they form contribute to the flexibility of the vertebral column as a whole.

Intervertebral foramina

When two adjacent vertebrae are viewed from the side, a foramen formed by a gap between adjacent vertebral pedicles can be seen.

Throughout the length of the column there is an intervertebral foramen on each side between every pair of vertebrae, through which the spinal nerves, blood vessels and lymph vessels pass (Fig. 16.26).

Ligaments of the vertebral column (Fig. 16.25)

These ligaments hold the vertebrae together and keep the intervertebral discs in position.

The *transverse ligament* holds the odontoid process of the axis in the correct position in relation to the atlas (Fig. 16.22C).

The *anterior longitudinal ligament* extends the whole length of the column and lies in front of the vertebral bodies.

The *posterior longitudinal ligament* lies inside the vertebral canal and extends the whole length of the vertebral

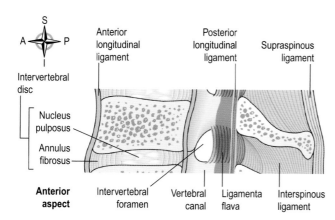

Figure 16.25 Section of the vertebral column showing the ligaments, intervertebral discs and intervertebral foramina.

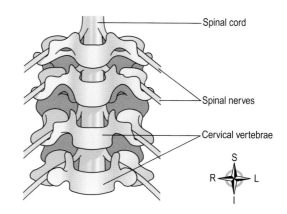

Figure 16.26 Lower cervical vertebrae separated to show the spinal cord and spinal nerves emerging through the intervertebral foramina. Anterior view.

column in close contact with the posterior surface of the bodies of the bones.

The *ligamenta flava* connect the laminae of adjacent vertebrae.

The *ligamentum nuchae* and the *supraspinous ligament* connect the spinous processes, extending from the occiput to the sacrum.

Curves of the vertebral column (Fig. 16.27)

When viewed from the side, the vertebral column presents four curves: two *primary* and two *secondary*.

The fetus in the uterus lies curled up so that the head and the knees are more or less touching. This position shows the *primary curvature*. The secondary *cervical curve* develops when the child can hold up their head (after about 3 months) and the secondary *lumbar curve* develops when able to stand (after 12–15 months). The thoracic and sacral primary curves are retained.

Movement of the vertebral column

Movement between the individual bones of the vertebral column is very limited. However, the movements of the column as a whole are quite extensive and include *flexion* (bending forward), *extension* (bending backward), *lateral flexion* (bending to the side) and *rotation*. There is more movement in the cervical and lumbar regions than elsewhere.

Functions of the vertebral column

These include:

- collectively the vertebral foramina form the vertebral canal, which provides a strong bony protection for the delicate spinal cord lying within it
- the pedicles of adjacent vertebrae form intervertebral foramina, one on each side, providing access to the spinal cord for spinal nerves, blood vessels and lymph vessels
- the numerous individual bones with their intervertebral discs allow movement of the whole column
- support of the skull
- the intervertebral discs act as shock absorbers, protecting the brain
- formation of the axis of the trunk, giving attachment to the ribs, shoulder girdle and upper limbs, and the pelvic girdle and lower limbs.

Thoracic cage (Fig. 16.28)

The thorax (thoracic cage) is formed by the sternum anteriorly, twelve pairs of ribs forming the lateral bony cages, and the twelve thoracic vertebrae.

Sternum (breast bone, Fig. 16.29)

This flat bone can be felt just under the skin in the middle of the front of the chest.

The *manubrium* is the uppermost section and articulates with the clavicles at the *sternoclavicular joints* and with the first two pairs of ribs.

The *body* or *middle portion* gives attachment to the ribs.

The *xiphoid process* is the inferior tip of the bone. It gives attachment to the diaphragm, muscles of the anterior

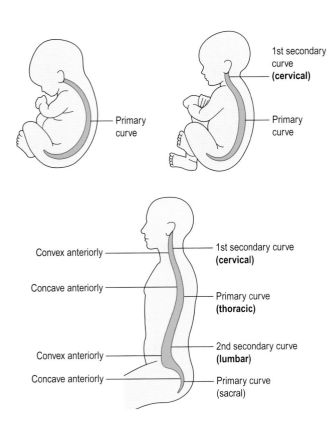

Figure 16.27 Development of the spinal curves.

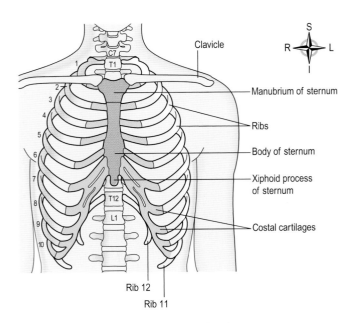

Figure 16.28 The thoracic cage. Anterior view.

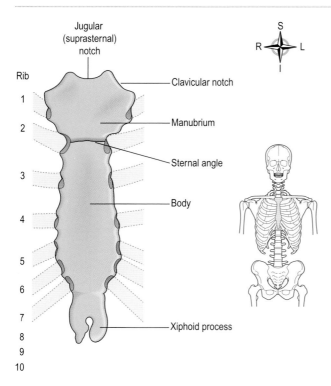

Figure 16.29 The sternum and its attachments. Anterior view.

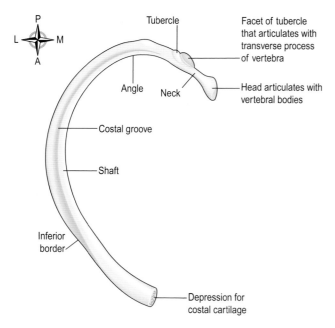

Figure 16.30 A typical rib. Viewed from below.

abdominal wall and the *linea alba* (literally 'white line'; Fig. 16.62).

Ribs

The 12 pairs of ribs form the lateral walls of the thoracic cage (Fig. 16.28). They are elongated curved bones (Fig. 16.30) that articulate posteriorly with the vertebral column. Anteriorly, the first seven pairs of ribs articulate directly with the sternum and are known as the *true ribs*. The next three pairs articulate only indirectly. In both cases, *costal cartilages* attach the ribs to the sternum. The lowest two pairs of ribs, referred to as *floating ribs*, do not join the sternum at all, their anterior tips being free.

Each rib forms up to three joints with the vertebral column. Two of these joints are formed between facets on the head of the rib and facets on the bodies of two vertebrae, the one above the rib and the one below. Ten of the ribs also form joints between the tubercle of the rib and the transverse process of (usually) the lower vertebra.

The inferior surface of the rib is deeply grooved, providing a channel along which intercostal nerves and blood vessels run. Between each rib and the one below are the intercostal muscles, which move the rib cage during breathing.

Because of the arrangement of the ribs, and the quantity of cartilage present in the ribcage, it is a flexible structure that can change its shape and size during breathing. The first rib is firmly fixed to the sternum and to the 1st thoracic vertebra, and does not move during inspiration. Because it is a fixed point, when the intercostal muscles contract, they pull the entire ribcage upwards towards the first rib. The mechanism of breathing is described on page 225.

Appendicular skeleton

Learning outcomes

After studying this section, you should be able to:

- identify the bones forming the appendicular skeleton

- state the characteristics of the bones forming the appendicular skeleton

- outline the differences in structure between the male and female pelves.

The appendicular skeleton consists of the:

- shoulder girdle with the upper limbs
- pelvic girdle with the lower limbs (Fig. 16.9).

Shoulder girdle and upper limb

The upper limb forms a joint with the trunk via the shoulder (pectoral) girdle.

Shoulder girdle

The shoulder girdle consists of two clavicles and two scapulae.

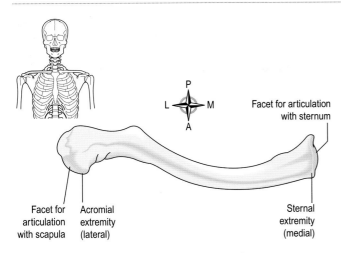

Figure 16.31 The right clavicle. Viewed from above.

Clavicle (collar bone, Fig. 16.31)

The clavicle is an S-shaped long bone. It articulates with the manubrium of the sternum at the *sternoclavicular joint* and forms the *acromioclavicular joint* with the *acromion process* of the scapula. The clavicle provides the only bony link between the upper limb and the axial skeleton.

Scapula (shoulder blade, Fig. 16.32)

The scapula is a flat triangular-shaped bone, lying on the posterior chest wall superficial to the ribs and separated from them by muscles.

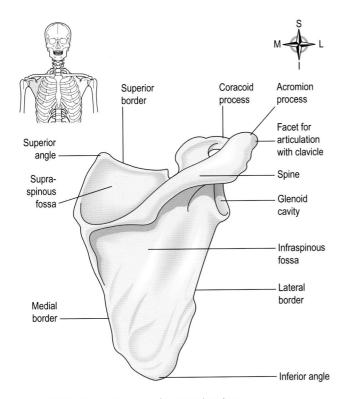

Figure 16.32 The right scapula. Posterior view.

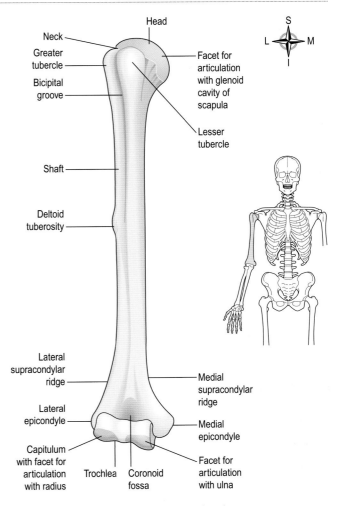

Figure 16.33 The right humerus. Anterior view.

At the lateral angle is a shallow articular surface, the *glenoid cavity*, which, with the *head of the humerus*, forms the *shoulder joint*.

On the posterior surface runs a rough ridge called the *spine*, which extends beyond the lateral border of the scapula and overhangs the glenoid cavity. The prominent overhang, which can be felt through the skin as the highest point of the shoulder, is called the *acromion process* and forms a joint with the clavicle, the *acromioclavicular joint*, a slightly movable synovial joint that contributes to the mobility of the shoulder girdle. The *coracoid process*, a projection from the upper border of the bone, gives attachment to muscles that move the shoulder joint.

The upper limb

Humerus (Fig. 16.33)

This is the bone of the upper arm. The head sits within the glenoid cavity of the scapula, forming the shoulder joint. Distal to the head are two roughened projections of bone, the *greater* and *lesser tubercles*, and between them there is a deep groove, the *bicipital groove* or *intertubercular*

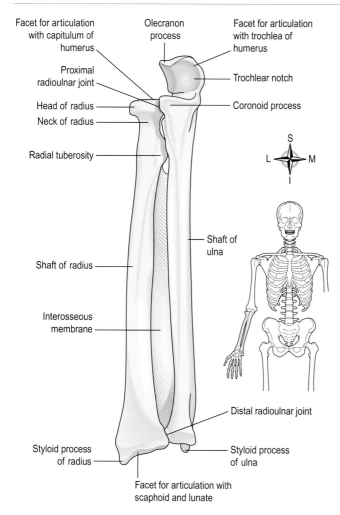

Figure 16.34 The right radius and ulna with the interosseous membrane. Anterior view.

sulcus, occupied by one of the tendons of the biceps muscle.

The distal end of the bone presents two surfaces that articulate with the radius and ulna to form the elbow joint.

Ulna and radius (Fig. 16.34)

These are the two bones of the forearm. The ulna is longer than and medial to the radius and when the arm is in the anatomical position, i.e. with the palm of the hand facing forward, the two bones are parallel. They articulate with the humerus at the *elbow joint*, the carpal bones at the *wrist joint* and with each other at the *proximal* and *distal radioulnar* joints. In addition, an interosseous membrane, a fibrous joint, connects the bones along their shafts, stabilising their association and maintaining their relative positions despite forces applied from the elbow or wrist.

Carpal (wrist) bones (Fig. 16.35)

There are eight carpal bones arranged in two rows of four. From outside inwards they are:

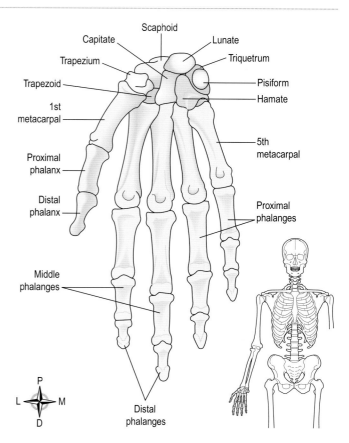

Figure 16.35 The bones of the right hand, wrist and fingers. Anterior view.

- *proximal row*: scaphoid, lunate, triquetrum, pisiform
- *distal row*: trapezium, trapezoid, capitate, hamate.

These bones are closely fitted together and held in position by ligaments that allow a limited amount of movement between them. The bones of the proximal row are associated with the wrist joint and those of the distal row form joints with the metacarpal bones. Tendons of muscles lying in the forearm cross the wrist and are held close to the bones by strong fibrous bands, called retinacula (see Fig. 16.50).

Metacarpal bones (bones of the hand)

These five bones form the palm of the hand. They are numbered from the thumb side inwards. The proximal ends articulate with the carpal bones and the distal ends with the phalanges.

Phalanges (finger bones)

There are 14 phalanges, three in each finger and two in the thumb. They articulate with the metacarpal bones and with each other, by hinge joints.

Pelvic girdle and lower limb

The lower limb forms a joint with the trunk at the pelvic girdle.

The pelvic girdle

The pelvic girdle is formed from two innominate (hip) bones. The *pelvis* is the term given to the basin-shaped structure formed by the pelvic girdle and its associated sacrum.

Innominate (hip) bones (Fig. 16.36)

Each hip bone consists of three fused bones: the *ilium*, *ischium* and *pubis*. On its lateral surface is a deep depression, the *acetabulum*, which forms the hip joint with the almost-spherical head of femur.

The *ilium* is the upper flattened part of the bone and it presents the *iliac crest*, the anterior curve of which is called the *anterior superior iliac spine*. The ilium forms a synovial joint with the sacrum, the *sacroiliac joint*, a strong joint capable of absorbing the stresses of weight bearing and which tends to become fibrosed in later life.

The *pubis* is the anterior part of the bone and it articulates with the pubis of the other hip bone at a cartilaginous joint, the *symphysis pubis*.

The *ischium* is the inferior and posterior part. The rough inferior projections of the ischia, the *ischial tuberosities*, bear the weight of the body when seated.

The union of the three parts takes place in the *acetabulum*.

The pelvis (Fig. 16.37)

The pelvis is formed by the hip bones, the sacrum and the coccyx. It is divided into upper and lower parts by the *brim of the pelvis*, consisting of the promontory of the sacrum and the iliopectineal lines of the innominate bones. The *greater* or *false pelvis* is above the brim and the lesser or *true pelvis* is below.

Differences between male and female pelves (Fig. 16.38). The shape of the female pelvis allows for the passage of the baby during childbirth. In comparison with the male pelvis, the female pelvis has lighter bones, is more shallow and rounded and is generally roomier.

The lower limb

Femur (thigh bone, Fig. 16.39)

The femur is the longest and heaviest bone of the body. The head is almost spherical and fits into the *acetabulum*

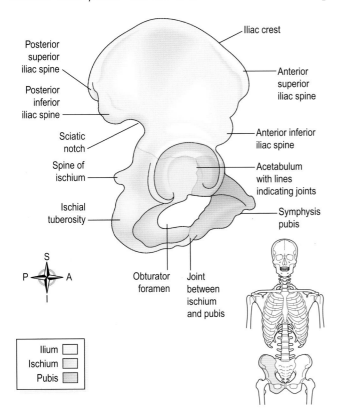

Figure 16.36 The right hip bone. Lateral view.

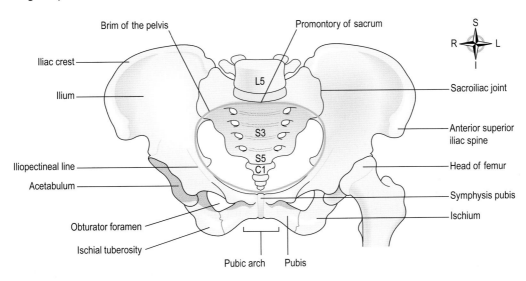

Figure 16.37 The bones of the pelvis and the upper part of the left femur.

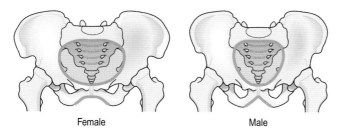

Female   Male

Figure 16.38 The difference in shape of the male and female pelves.

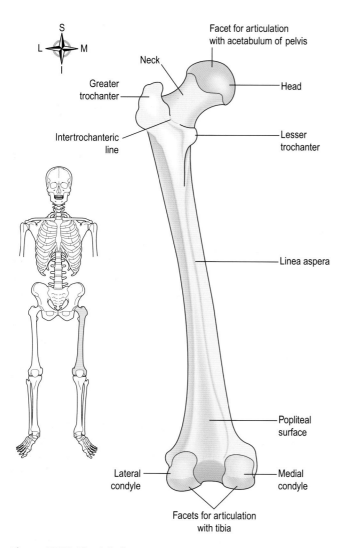

Figure 16.39 The left femur. Posterior view.

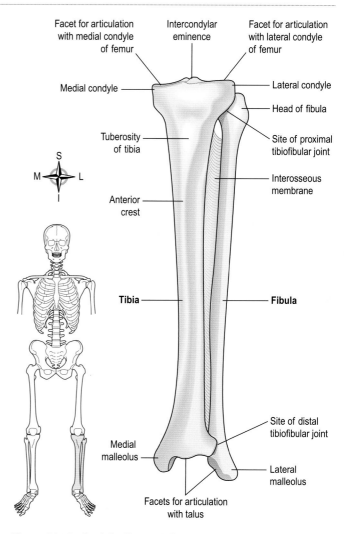

Figure 16.40 The left tibia and fibula with the interosseous membrane. Anterior view.

and patella, form the knee joint. The femur transmits the weight of the body through the bones below the knee to the foot.

Tibia (shin bone, Fig. 16.40)

The tibia is the medial of the two bones of the lower leg. The proximal extremity is broad and flat and presents two *condyles* for articulation with the femur at the knee joint. The head of the fibula articulates with the inferior aspect of the lateral condyle, forming the proximal tibiofibular joint.

The distal extremity of the tibia forms the *ankle joint* with the talus and the fibula. The *medial malleolus* is a downward projection of bone medial to the ankle joint.

Fibula (Fig. 16.40)

The fibula is the long slender lateral bone in the leg. The head or upper extremity articulates with the lateral

of the hip bone to form the *hip joint*. The neck extends outwards and slightly downwards from the head to the shaft and most of it is within the capsule of the hip joint.

The posterior surface of the lower third forms a flat triangular area called the *popliteal surface*. The distal extremity has two articular *condyles*, which, with the tibia

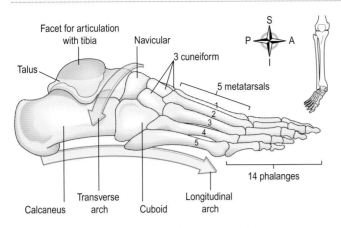

Figure 16.41 The bones of the left foot. Lateral view.

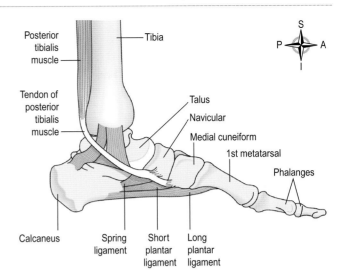

Figure 16.42 The tendons and ligaments supporting the arches of the left foot. Medial view.

condyle of the tibia, forming the proximal tibiofibular joint, and the lower extremity articulates with the tibia, and projects beyond it to form the *lateral malleolus*. This helps to stabilise the ankle joint.

Patella (knee cap)

This is a roughly triangular-shaped sesamoid bone associated with the knee joint. Its posterior surface articulates with the patellar surface of the femur in the knee joint and its anterior surface is in the *patellar tendon*, i.e. the tendon of the quadriceps femoris muscle.

Tarsal (ankle) bones (Fig. 16.41)

The seven tarsal bones forming the posterior part of the foot (ankle) are the talus, calcaneus, navicular, cuboid and three cuneiform bones. The talus articulates with the tibia and fibula at the ankle joint. The calcaneus forms the heel of the foot. The other bones articulate with each other and with the metatarsal bones.

Metatarsals (bones of the foot, Fig. 16.41)

These are five bones, numbered from inside out, which form the greater part of the dorsum (sole) of the foot. At their proximal ends they articulate with the tarsal bones and at their distal ends, with the phalanges. The enlarged distal head of the 1st metatarsal bone forms the 'ball' of the foot.

Phalanges (toe bones, Fig. 16.41)

There are 14 phalanges arranged in a similar manner to those in the fingers, i.e. two in the great toe (the *hallux*) and three in each of the other toes.

Arches of the foot. The arrangement of bones in the foot, supported by associated ligaments and action of associated muscles, gives the sole of the foot an arched or curved shape (Figs 16.41 and 16.42). The curve running from heel to toe is called the *longitudinal* arch, and the curve running across the foot is called the *transverse* arch.

In the normal longitudinal arch, only the calcaneus and the distal ends of the metatarsals should touch the ground, the bones in between being lifted clear. This gives the conventional footprint shape. If, however, the concavity of the sole is lost because of sagging ligaments or tendons, the arch sinks and much more of the sole of the foot is in contact with the ground: this is called *flat foot*. Because the arches of the foot are important in distributing the weight of the body evenly whilst upright, whether stationary or moving, the flat foot loses the springiness of normal foot structure and leads to sore feet when standing, walking or running for long periods. As there are movable joints between all the bones of the foot, very strong muscles and ligaments are necessary to maintain the strength, resilience and stability of the foot during walking, running and jumping.

Posterior tibialis muscle This is the most important muscular support of the longitudinal arch. It lies on the posterior aspect of the lower leg, originates from the middle third of the tibia and fibula and its tendon passes behind the medial malleolus to be inserted into the navicular, cuneiform, cuboid and metatarsal bones. It acts as a sling or 'suspension apparatus' for the arch.

Short muscles of the foot This group of muscles is mainly concerned with the maintenance of the longitudinal and transverse arches. They make up the fleshy part of the sole of the foot.

Plantar calcaneonavicular ligament ('spring' ligament) This is a very strong thick ligament stretching from the calcaneus to the navicular bone. It plays an important part in supporting the medial longitudinal arch.

Plantar ligaments and interosseous membranes These structures support the lateral and transverse arches.

Joints

Learning outcomes

After studying this section, you should be able to:

- state the characteristics of fibrous and cartilaginous joints

- list the different types of synovial joint

- outline the movements possible at five types of synovial joint

- describe the structure and functions of a typical synovial joint.

- describe the structure and movements of the following synovial joints: shoulder, elbow, wrist, hip, knee and ankle.

A joint is the site at which any two or more bones articulate or come together. Joints allow flexibility and movement of the skeleton and allow attachment between bones.

Fibrous joints

The bones forming these joints are linked with tough, fibrous material. Such an arrangement often permits no movement. For example, the joints between the skull bones, the *sutures*, are completely immovable (Fig. 16.43), and the healthy tooth is cemented into the mandible by the periodontal ligament. The tibia and fibula in the leg are held together along their shafts by a sheet of fibrous tissue called the interosseous membrane (Fig. 16.40). This fibrous joint allows a limited amount of movement and stabilises the alignment of the bones.

Cartilaginous joints

These joints are formed by a pad of tough fibrocartilage that acts as a shock absorber. The joint may be immovable, as in the cartilaginous epiphyseal plates, which in the growing child links the diaphysis of a long bone to the epiphysis. Some cartilaginous joints permit limited movement, as between the vertebrae, which are separated by

the intervertebral discs (Fig. 16.44), or at the symphysis pubis (Fig. 16.37), which is softened by circulating hormones during pregnancy to allow for expansion during childbirth.

Synovial joints

Synovial joints are characterised by the presence of a space or capsule between the articulating bones (Fig. 16.45). The ends of the bones are held close together by a sleeve of fibrous tissue, and lubricated with a small amount of fluid. Synovial joints are the most moveable of the body.

Characteristics of a synovial joint

All synovial joints have certain characteristics in common (Fig. 16.45).

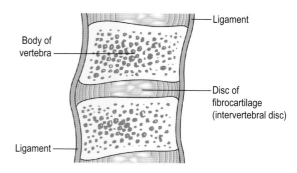

Figure 16.44 The cartilaginous joint between adjacent vertebral bodies.

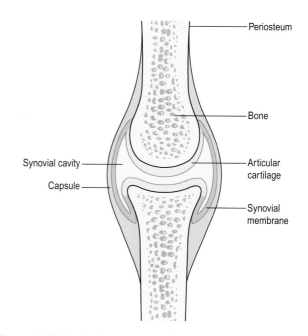

Figure 16.45 The basic structure of a synovial joint.

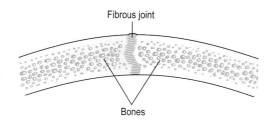

Figure 16.43 Suture (fibrous joint) of the skull.

Articular or hyaline cartilage

The parts of the bones in contact with each other are coated with hyaline cartilage (see Fig. 3.22A). This provides a smooth articular surface, reduces friction and is strong enough to absorb compression forces and bear the weight of the body. The cartilage lining, which is up to 7 mm thick in young people, becomes thinner and less compressible with age. This leads to increasing stress on other structures in the joint. Cartilage has no blood supply and receives its nourishment from synovial fluid.

Capsule or capsular ligament

The joint is surrounded and enclosed by a sleeve of fibrous tissue which holds the bones together. It is sufficiently loose to allow freedom of movement but strong enough to protect it from injury.

Synovial membrane

This epithelial layer lines the capsule and covers all non-weight-bearing surfaces inside the joint. It secretes synovial fluid.

Synovial fluid. This is a thick sticky fluid, of egg-white consistency, which fills the synovial cavity. It:

- nourishes the structures within the joint cavity
- contains phagocytes, which remove microbes and cellular debris
- acts as a lubricant
- maintains joint stability
- prevents the ends of the bones from being separated, as does a little water between two glass surfaces.

Little sacs of synovial fluid or *bursae* are present in some joints, e.g. the knee. They act as cushions to prevent friction between a bone and a ligament or tendon, or skin where a bone in a joint is near the surface.

Other intracapsular structures

Some joints have structures within the capsule to pad and stabilise the joint, e.g. fat pads and menisci in the knee joint. If these structures do not bear weight they are covered by synovial membrane.

Extracapsular structures

- *Ligaments* that blend with the capsule stabilise the joint.
- *Muscles* or their *tendons* also provide stability and stretch across the joints they move. When the muscle contracts it shortens, pulling one bone towards the other.

Nerve and blood supply

Nerves and blood vessels crossing a joint usually supply the capsule and the muscles that move it.

Table 16.2 Movements possible at synovial joints

Movement	Definition
Flexion	Bending, usually forward but occasionally backward, e.g. knee joint
Extension	Straightening or bending backward
Abduction	Movement away from the midline of the body
Adduction	Movement towards the midline of the body
Circumduction	Movement of a limb or digit so that it describes the shape of a cone
Rotation	Movement round the long axis of a bone
Pronation	Turning the palm of the hand down
Supination	Turning the palm of the hand up
Inversion	Turning the sole of the foot inwards
Eversion	Turning the sole of the foot outwards

Movements at synovial joints

Movement at any given joint depends on various factors, such as the tightness of the ligaments holding the joint together, how well the bones fit and the presence or absence of intracapsular structures. Generally, the more stable the joint, the less mobile it is. The main movements possible are summarised in Table 16.2 and Figure 16.46.

Types of synovial joint

Synovial joints are classified according to the range of movement possible (Table 16.2) or to the shape of the articulating parts of the bones involved.

Ball and socket joints

The head of one bone is ball-shaped and articulates with a cup-shaped socket of another. The joint allows for a wide range of movement, including flexion, extension, adduction, abduction, rotation and circumduction. Examples include the shoulder and hip.

Hinge joints

The articulating ends of the bones fit together like a hinge on a door, and movement is therefore restricted to flexion and extension. The elbow joint is one example, permitting only flexion and extension of the forearm. Other hinge joints include the knee, ankle and the joints between the phalanges of the fingers and toes (interphalangeal joints).

Gliding joints

The articular surfaces are flat or very slightly curved and glide over one another, but the amount of movement

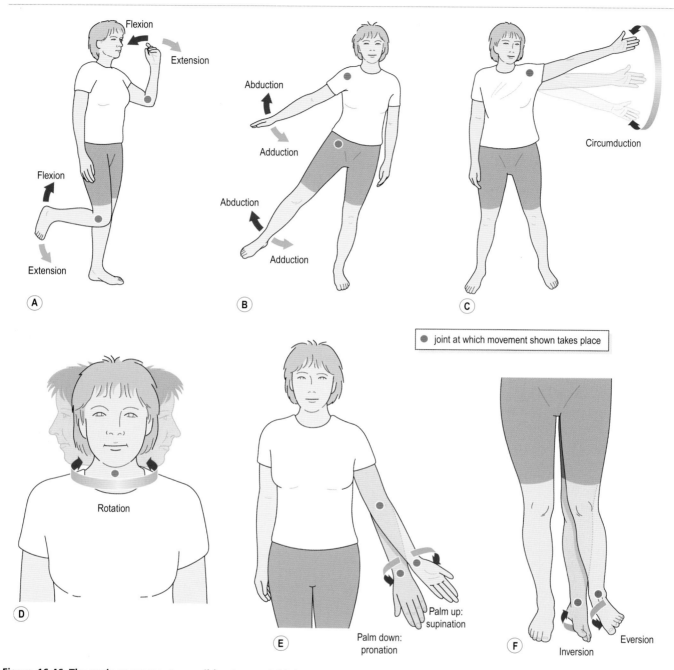

Figure 16.46 The main movements possible at synovial joints.

possible is very restricted; this group of joints is the least movable of all the synovial joints. Examples include the joints between the carpal bones in the wrist, the tarsal bones in the foot, and between the processes of the spinal vertebrae (note that the joints between the vertebral bodies are the cartilaginous discs; Fig. 16.44).

Pivot joints

These joints allow a bone or a limb to rotate. One bone fits into a hoop-shaped ligament that holds it close to another bone and allows it to rotate in the ring thus

formed. For example, the head rotates on the pivot joint formed by the dens of the axis held within the ring formed by the transverse ligament and the odontoid process of the atlas (Fig. 16.22).

Condyloid joints

A condyle is a smooth, rounded projection on a bone and in a condyloid joint it sits within a cup-shaped depression on the other bone. Examples include the joint between the condylar process of the mandible and the temporal bone, and the joints between the metacarpal and phalangeal bones of the hand, and between the metatarsal and phalangeal bones of the foot. These joints permit flexion, extension, abduction, adduction and circumduction.

Saddle joints

The articulating bones fit together like a man sitting on a saddle. The most important saddle joint is at the base of the thumb, between the trapezium of the wrist and the first metacarpal bone (Fig. 16.35). The range of movement is similar to that at a condyloid joint but with additional flexibility; *opposition* of the thumb, the ability to touch each of the fingertips on the same hand, is due to the nature of the thumb joint.

Main synovial joints of the limbs 16.4

All synovial joints have the characteristics described above, so only their distinctive features are included in this section.

Shoulder joint (Fig. 16.47)

This ball and socket joint is the most mobile in the body, and consequently is the least stable and prone to dislocation, especially in children. It is formed by the glenoid cavity of the scapula and the head of the humerus, and is well padded with protective bursae. The capsular ligament is very loose inferiorly to allow for the free movement normally possible at this joint. The glenoid cavity is deepened by a rim of fibrocartilage, the *glenoidal labrum*, which provides additional stability without limiting movement. The tendon of the long head of the *biceps muscle* is held in the intertubercular (bicipital) groove of the humerus by the transverse humeral ligament. It extends through the joint cavity and attaches to the upper rim of the glenoid cavity.

Synovial membrane forms a sleeve round the part of the tendon of the long head of the biceps muscles within the capsular ligament and covers the glenoidal labrum.

The joint is stabilised partly by a number of ligaments (the glenohumoral, coracohumeral and transverse humeral) but mainly by the muscles (and their tendons) present in the shoulder. Some of these muscles collectively are called the *rotator cuff*, and rotator cuff injury is a common cause of shoulder pain (p. 435). The stability of the joint may be reduced if these structures, together with the tendon of the biceps muscle, are stretched by repeated dislocations of the joint.

Muscles and movements (see Fig. 16.65)

The muscles that move the arm are described in more detail on page 427, and Table 16.3 summarises the muscles and movements possible at the shoulder joint.

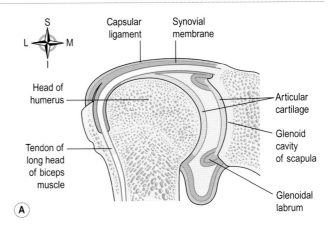

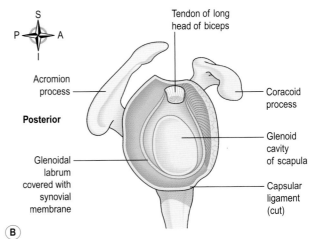

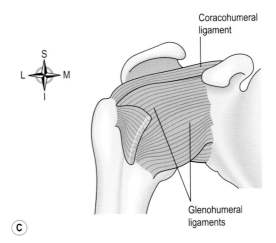

Figure 16.47 The right shoulder joint. A. Section viewed from the front. **B.** The position of glenoidal labrum with the humerus removed, viewed from the side. **C.** The supporting ligaments viewed from the front.

Elbow joint (Fig. 16.48)

This hinge joint is formed by the trochlea and the capitulum of the humerus, and the trochlear notch of the ulna and the head of the radius. It is an extremely stable joint

Table 16.3 Muscles and movements at the shoulder joint

Extension	Latissimus dorsi, teres major
Flexion	Coracobrachialis, pectoralis major
Abduction	Deltoid
Adduction	Latissimus dorsi, pectoralis major
Lateral rotation	Teres minor, posterior part of deltoid
Medial rotation	Latissimus dorsi, pectoralis major, teres major and anterior part of deltoid
Circumduction	Combination of actions of above muscles

because the humeral and ulnar surfaces interlock, and the capsule is very strong.

Extracapsular structures consist of anterior, posterior, medial and lateral strengthening ligaments, which contribute to joint stability.

Muscles and movements (see Fig. 16.65)

Because of the structure of the elbow joint, the only two movements it allows are flexion and extension. The biceps is the main flexor of the forearm, aided by the brachialis; the triceps extends it.

Proximal and distal radioulnar joints

The *proximal radioulnar joint* is a pivot joint formed by the rim of the head of the radius rotating in the radial notch of the ulna, and is in the same capsule as the elbow joint. The *annular ligament* is a strong extracapsular ligament that encircles the head of the radius and keeps it in contact with the radial notch of the ulna (Fig. 16.48B).

The distal *radioulnar joint* is a pivot joint between the distal end of the radius and the head of the ulna (Fig. 16.49).

Note, in addition, the presence of a fibrous membrane linking the bones along their shafts; this interosseous membrane (Fig. 16.34) is a type of fibrous joint and prevents separation of the bones when force is applied at either end, i.e. at the wrist or elbow.

Muscles and movements (see Fig. 16.65)

The forearm may be pronated (turned palm down) or supinated (turned palm up). Pronation is caused by the action of the pronator teres (p. 428) and supination by the supinator and biceps muscles (p. 427-8).

Wrist joint (Fig. 16.49)

This is a condyloid joint between the distal end of the radius and the proximal ends of the scaphoid, lunate and triquetrum. A disc of white fibrocartilage separates the

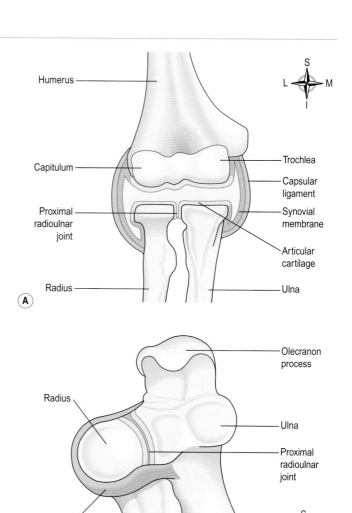

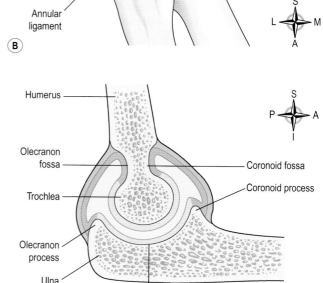

Figure 16.48 The right elbow and proximal radioulnar joints.
A. Section viewed from the front. **B.** The proximal radioulnar joint, viewed from above. **C.** Section of the elbow joint, partly flexed, viewed from the right side.

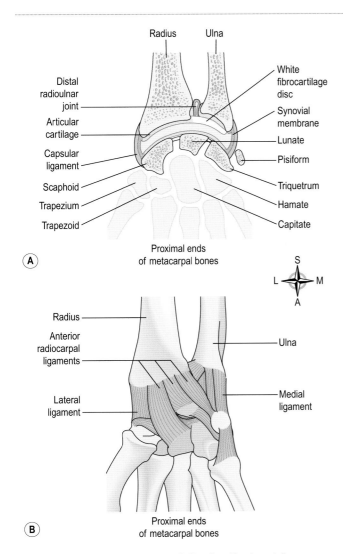

Figure 16.49 The right wrist and distal radioulnar joints.
Anterior view. **A.** Section. **B.** Supporting ligaments.

Table 16.4 Muscles and movements at the wrist joint

Flexion	Flexor carpi radialis, flexor carpi ulnaris
Extension	Extensors carpi radialis (longus and brevis), extensor carpi ulnaris
Adduction	Flexor carpi radialis, extensor carpi radialis
Abduction	Flexor carpi ulnaris, extensor carpi ulnaris

the phalanges. Movement at the hand and finger joints is controlled by muscles in the forearm and smaller muscles within the hand. There are no muscles in the fingers; finger movements are produced by tendons extending from muscles in the forearm and the hand.

The joint at the base of the thumb is a saddle joint, unlike the corresponding joints of the other fingers, which are condyloid. This means that the thumb is more mobile than the fingers and the thumb can be flexed, extended, circumducted, abducted and adducted. In addition, the thumb can be moved across the palm to touch the tips of each of the fingers on the same hand (opposition), giving great manual dexterity and allowing, for example, the holding of a pen and the fine manipulation of objects held in the hand.

The joints between the metacarpals and finger bones allow movement of the fingers. The fingers may be flexed, extended, adducted, abducted and circumducted, with the first finger more flexible than the others. The finger joints are hinge joints, and allow only flexion and extension.

The *flexor retinaculum* is a strong fibrous band that stretches across the front of the carpal bones, forming the *carpal tunnel*. The tendons of flexor muscles of the wrist joint and the fingers and the median nerve pass through the carpal tunnel, the retinaculum holding them close to the bones. Synovial membrane forms sleeves around these tendons in the carpal tunnel and extends some way into the palm of the hand. Synovial sheaths also enclose the tendons on the flexor surfaces of the fingers. Their synovial fluid prevents friction that might damage the tendons as they move over the bones (Fig. 16.50).

The *extensor retinaculum* is a strong fibrous band that extends across the back of the wrist. Tendons of muscles that extend the wrist and finger joints are encased in synovial membrane under the retinaculum. The synovial fluid secreted prevents friction.

ulna from the joint cavity and articulates with the carpal bones. It also separates the inferior radioulnar joint from the wrist joint.

Extracapsular structures consist of medial and lateral ligaments and anterior and posterior radiocarpal ligaments.

Muscles and movements (see Fig. 16.65)
The wrist can be flexed, extended, abducted and adducted. The muscles that perform these movements are described in more detail on page 428. Table 16.4 summarises the main muscles that move the wrist.

Joints of the hands and fingers

There are synovial joints between the carpal bones, between the carpal and metacarpal bones, between the metacarpal bones and proximal phalanges and between

Hip joint (Fig. 16.51)

This ball and socket joint is formed by the cup-shaped acetabulum of the innominate (hip) bone and the almost spherical head of the femur. The capsular ligament encloses the head and most of the neck of the femur. The

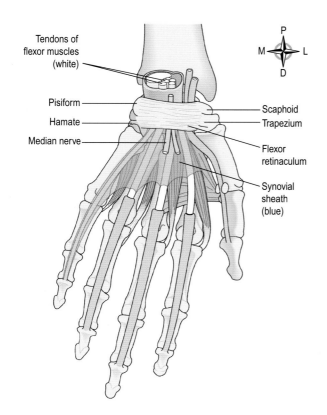

Figure 16.50 The carpal tunnel and synovial sheaths in the wrist and hand in blue; tendons in white. Palmar view, left hand.

cavity is deepened by the *acetabular labrum*, a ring of fibrocartilage attached to the rim of the acetabulum, which stabilises the joint without limiting its range of movement. The hip joint is necessarily a sturdy and powerful joint, since it bears all body weight when standing. It is stabilised by its surrounding musculature, but its ligaments are also important. The three main external ligaments are the *iliofemoral*, *pubofemoral* and *ischiofemoral* ligaments (Fig. 16.51B). Within the joint, the ligament of the head of the femur (*ligamentum teres*) attaches the femoral head to the acetabulum (Fig. 16.51A and C).

Muscles and movements (see Fig. 16.66)

The lower limb can be extended, flexed, abducted, adducted, rotated and circumducted at the hip joint (Table 16.5).

Knee joint (Fig. 16.52)

This is the body's largest and most complex joint. It is a hinge joint formed by the condyles of the femur, the condyles of the tibia and the posterior surface of the patella. The anterior part of the capsule is formed by the tendon of the quadriceps femoris muscle, which also supports the patella. Intracapsular structures include two *cruciate ligaments* that cross each other, extending from the

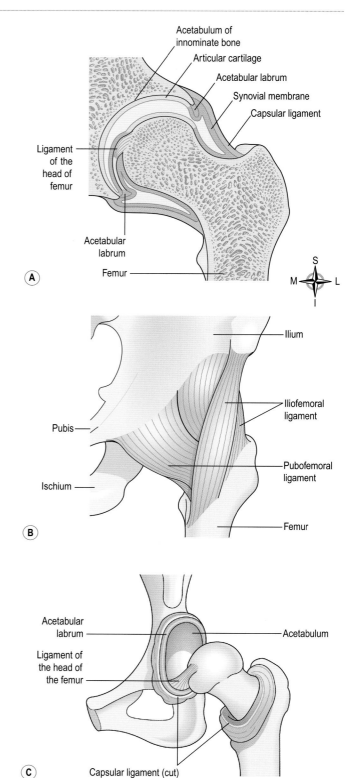

Figure 16.51 The left hip joint. Anterior view. **A.** Section. **B.** Supporting ligaments. **C.** Head of femur and acetabulum separated to show acetabular labrum and ligament of head of femur.

Table 16.5 Muscles and movements at the hip joint

Flexion	Psoas, iliacus, sartorius
Extension	Gluteus maximus, hamstrings
Abduction	Gluteus medius and minimus, sartorius
Adduction	Adductor group (longus, brevis and magnus)
Medial rotation	Gluteus medius and minimus, adductor group
Lateral rotation	Gluteus maximus, quadratus femoris, obturators

intercondylar notch of the femur to the *intercondylar eminence* of the tibia. They help to stabilise the joint.

Semilunar cartilages or *menisci* are incomplete discs of white fibrocartilage lying on top of the articular condyles of the tibia. They are wedge shaped, being thicker at their outer edges, and provide stability. They prevent lateral displacement of the bones, and cushion the moving joint by shifting within the joint space according to the relative positions of the articulating bones.

Bursae and pads of fat are numerous. They prevent friction between a bone and a ligament or tendon and between the skin and the patella. Synovial membrane covers the cruciate ligaments and the pads of fat. The menisci are not covered with synovial membrane because they are weight bearing. External ligaments provide further support, making it a hard joint to dislocate. The main ligaments are the patellar ligament, an extension of the quadriceps tendon, the popliteal ligaments at the back of the knee and the collateral ligaments to each side.

Muscles and movements (see Fig. 16.66)

Possible movements at this joint are flexion, extension and a rotatory movement that 'locks' the joint when it is fully extended. When the joint is locked, it is possible to stand upright for long periods of time without tiring the knee extensors. The main muscles extending the knee are the quadriceps femoris, and the principal flexors are the gastrocnemius and hamstrings.

Ankle joint (Fig. 16.53)

This hinge joint is formed by the distal end of the tibia and its malleolus (medial malleolus), the distal end of the fibula (lateral malleolus) and the talus. Four important ligaments strengthen this joint: the deltoid and the anterior, posterior, medial and lateral ligaments.

Muscles and movements (see Fig. 16.66)

The movements of *inversion* and *eversion* occur between the tarsal bones and not at the ankle joint. Ankle joint

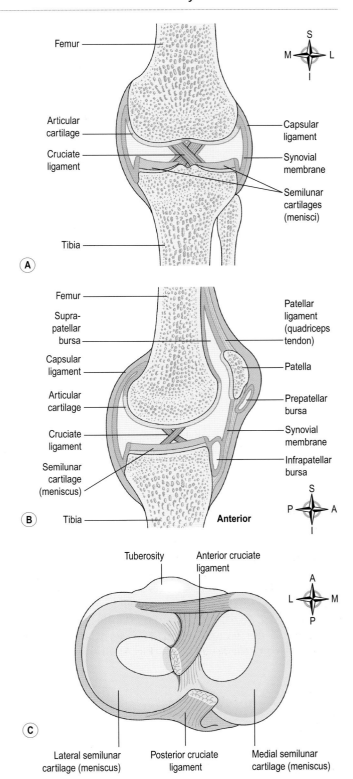

Figure 16.52 The left knee joint. A. Section viewed from the front. **B.** Section viewed from the side. **C.** The superior surface of the tibia, showing the semilunar cartilages and the cruciate ligaments.

419

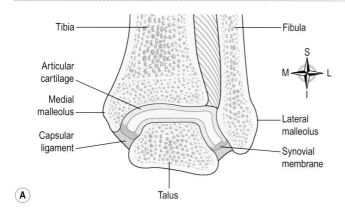

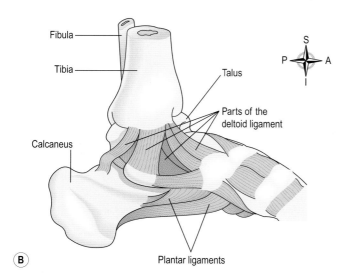

Figure 16.53 The left ankle joint. A. Section viewed from the front. **B.** Supporting ligaments, medial view.

Table 16.6 Muscles and movements at the ankle joint	
Dorsiflexion (lifting toes towards calf)	Anterior tibialis and toe extensors
Plantar flexion (rising on tiptoe)	Gastrocnemius, soleus and toe flexors

movements and the related muscles are shown in Table 16.6.

Joints of the feet and toes

There are a number of synovial joints between the tarsal bones, between the tarsal and metatarsal bones, between the metatarsals and proximal phalanges and between the phalanges. Movements are produced by muscles in the leg with long tendons that cross the ankle joint, and by muscles of the foot. The tendons crossing the ankle joint

are wrapped in synovial sheaths and held close to the bones by strong transverse ligaments. They move smoothly within their sheaths as the joints move. In addition to moving the joints of the foot, these muscles support the arches of the foot and help to maintain balance.

Skeletal muscle

Learning outcomes

After studying this section, you should be able to:

- identify the main characteristics of skeletal muscle

- relate the structure of skeletal muscle fibres to their contractile activity

- describe the nature of muscle tone and fatigue

- discuss the factors that affect the performance of skeletal muscle

- name the main muscles of the body regions described in this section

- outline the functions of the main muscles described in this section.

Muscle cells are specialised contractile cells, also called *fibres*. The three types of muscle tissue, *smooth, cardiac* and *skeletal*, each differ in structure, location and physiological function. Smooth muscle and cardiac muscle are not under voluntary control and are discussed elsewhere (smooth muscle and cardiac muscle p. 43-4). Skeletal muscles, which are under voluntary control, are attached to bones via their tendons (Fig. 16.54A) and move the skeleton. Like cardiac (but not smooth) muscle, skeletal muscle is *striated* (striped), and the stripes are seen in a characteristic banded pattern when the cells are viewed under the microscope (Fig. 16.54B, Fig. 16.55).

Organisation of skeletal muscle (Fig. 16.54)

A skeletal muscle may sometimes contain hundreds of thousands of muscle fibres as well as blood vessels and nerves. Throughout the muscle, providing internal structure and scaffolding, is an extensive network of connective tissue. The entire muscle is covered in a connective tissue sheath called the *epimysium*. Within the muscle, the cells are collected into separate bundles called fascicles, and each *fascicle* is covered in its own connective tissue sheath called the *perimysium*. Within the fascicles, the individual muscle cells are each wrapped in a fine connective tissue layer called the *endomysium*. Each of these connective tissue layers runs the length of the muscle. They bind the fibres into a highly organised structure,

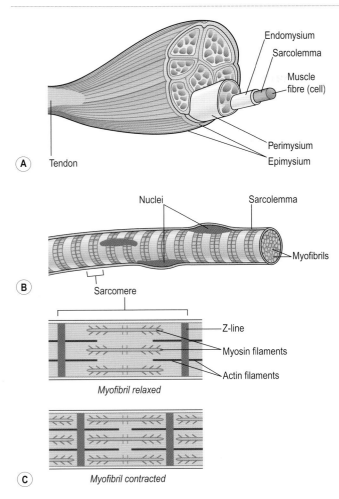

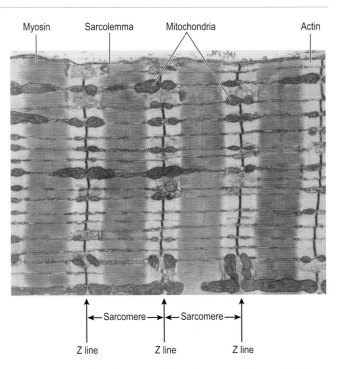

Figure 16.55 Coloured transmission electron micrograph of part of a skeletal muscle cell, showing the characteristic banding pattern and multiple mitochondria.

Figure 16.54 Organisation within a skeletal muscle.
A. A skeletal muscle and its connective tissue. **B.** A muscle fibre (cell). **C.** A myofibril, relaxed and contracted.

and blend together at each end of the muscle to form the *tendon*, which secures the muscle to bone. Often the tendon is rope-like, but sometimes it forms a broad sheet called an *aponeurosis*, e.g. the occipitofrontalis muscle (see Fig. 16.58). The multiple connective tissue layers throughout the muscle are important for transmitting the force of contraction from each individual muscle cell to its points of attachment to the skeleton.

The fleshy part of the muscle is called the *belly*.

Skeletal muscle cells (fibres)

Contraction of a whole skeletal muscle occurs because of coordinated contraction of its individual fibres.

Structure

Under the microscope, skeletal muscle cells are seen to be roughly cylindrical in shape, lying parallel to one another, with a distinctive banded appearance consisting of alternate dark and light stripes (Figs 16.54B and 16.55).

Individual fibres may be very long, up to 35 cm in the longest muscles. Each cell has several nuclei (because the cells are so large), found just under the cell membrane (the *sarcolemma*). The cytoplasm of muscle cells, also called *sarcoplasm*, is packed with tiny filaments running longitudinally along the length of the muscle; these are the contractile filaments. There are also many mitochondria (Fig. 16.55), essential for producing adenosine triphosphate (ATP) from glucose and oxygen to power the contractile mechanism. Also present is a specialised oxygen-binding substance called *myoglobin*, which is similar to the haemoglobin of red blood cells and stores oxygen within the muscle. In addition, there are extensive intracellular stores of calcium, which is released into the sarcoplasm by nervous stimulation of muscle and is essential for the contractile activity of the myofilaments.

Actin, myosin and sarcomeres. There are two types of contractile myofilament within the muscle fibre, called thick and thin, arranged in repeating units called sarcomeres (Figs 16.54C and 16.55). The thick filaments, which are made of the protein *myosin*, correspond to the dark bands seen under the microscope. The thin filaments are made of the protein *actin*. Where only these are present, the bands are lighter in appearance.

Each sarcomere is bounded at each end by a dense stripe, the *Z line*, to which the actin fibres are attached, and lying in the middle of the sarcomere are the myosin filaments, overlapping with the actin.

421

Contraction

The skeletal muscle cell contracts in response to stimulation from a nerve fibre, which supplies the muscle cell usually about halfway along its length. The name given to a synapse between a motor nerve and a skeletal muscle fibre is the *neuromuscular junction*. When the action potential spreads from the nerve along the sarcolemma, it is conducted deep into the muscle cell through a special network of channels that run through the sarcoplasm, and releases calcium from the intracellular stores. Calcium triggers the binding of myosin to the actin filament next to it, forming so-called cross-bridges. ATP then provides the energy for the two filaments to slide over each other, pulling the Z lines at each end of the sarcomere closer to one another, shortening the sarcomere (Fig. 16.54C). This is called the *sliding filament theory*. If enough fibres are stimulated to do this at the same time, the whole muscle will shorten (contract). ▓ **16.5**

The muscle relaxes when nerve stimulation stops. Calcium is pumped back into its intracellular storage areas, which breaks the cross-bridges between the actin and myosin filaments. They then slide back into their starting positions, lengthening the sarcomeres and returning the muscle to its original length.

The neuromuscular junction ▓ **16.6**

The axons of motor neurones, carrying impulses to skeletal muscle to produce contraction, divide into a number of fine filaments terminating in minute pads called synaptic knobs. The space between the synaptic knob and the muscle cell is called the synaptic cleft. Stimulation of the motor neurone releases the neurotransmitter acetylcholine (ACh), which diffuses across the synaptic cleft and binds to acetylcholine receptors on the postsynaptic membrane on the *motor end plate* (the area of the muscle membrane directly across the synaptic cleft, Fig. 16.56). Acetylcholine causes contraction of the muscle cell.

Motor units

Each muscle fibre is stimulated by only one synaptic knob, but since each motor nerve has many synaptic knobs, it stimulates a number of muscle fibres. Figure 16.57 shows an electron micrograph of a motor nerve and two of its motor end plates.

One nerve fibre and the muscle fibres it supplies constitute a *motor unit*. Nerve impulses cause serial contraction of motor units in a muscle, and each unit contracts to its full capacity. The *strength* of the contraction depends on the *number* of motor units in action at a particular time.

Some motor units contain large numbers of muscle fibres, i.e. one nerve serves many muscle cells. This arrangement is associated with large-scale, powerful movements, such as in the legs or upper arms. Fine, delicate control of muscle movement is achieved when one motor unit contains very few muscle fibres, as in the muscles controlling eye movement.

Action of skeletal muscle

When individual muscle cells in a muscle shorten, they pull on the connective tissue framework running through the whole muscle, and the muscle develops a degree of tension (tone).

Muscle tone

When a muscle fibre contracts, it obeys the *all-or-none law*, i.e. the whole fibre either contracts completely or not at all. The degree of contraction achieved by a whole muscle depends therefore on the number of fibres within it that are contracting at any one time, as well as how often they

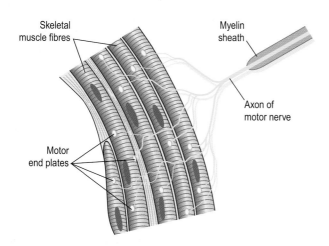

Figure 16.56 The neuromuscular junction.

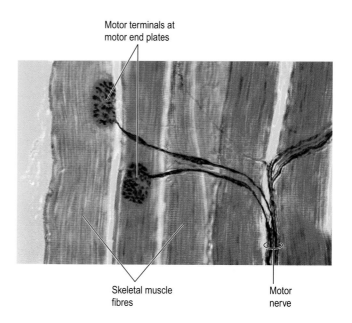

Figure 16.57 The neuromuscular junction. Colour transmission electron micrograph of a motor neurone and two of its motor end plates.

are stimulated. Powerful contractions involve a larger proportion of available fibres than weaker ones; to lift a heavy weight, more active muscle fibres are required than to lift a lighter one. *Muscle tone* is a sustained, partial muscle contraction that allows posture to be maintained without fatiguing the muscles involved. For instance, keeping the head upright requires constant activity of the muscles of the neck and shoulders. Groups of muscle fibres within these muscles take it in turns to contract, so that at any one time, some fibres are contracted and others are resting. This allows the effort required to hold the head upright to be distributed throughout the muscles involved. Good muscle tone protects joints and gives a muscle firmness and shape, even when relaxed.

Muscle fatigue

To work at sustained levels, muscles need an adequate supply of oxygen and fuel such as glucose. Fatigue occurs when a muscle works at a level that exceeds these supplies. The muscle response decreases with fatigue.

The chemical energy (ATP) that muscles require is usually derived from the breakdown of carbohydrate and fat; protein may be used if supplies of fat and carbohydrate are exhausted. An adequate oxygen supply is needed to fully release all the energy stored within these fuel molecules; without it, the body uses anaerobic metabolic pathways (p. 316) that are less efficient and lead to lactic acid production. Fatigue (and muscle pain) resulting from inadequate oxygen supply, as in strenuous exercise, occurs when lactic acid accumulates in working muscles. Fatigue may also occur because energy stores are exhausted, or due to physical injury to muscle, which may occur after prolonged episodes of strenuous activity, e.g. marathon running.

Muscle recovery

After exercise, muscle needs a period of time to recover, to replenish its ATP and glycogen stores and to repair any damaged fibres. For some time following exercise, depending on the degree of exertion, the *oxygen debt* remains (an extended period of increased oxygen demand), as the body converts lactic acid to pyruvic acid and replaces its energy stores.

Factors affecting skeletal muscle performance

Skeletal muscle performs better when it is regularly exercised. Training improves endurance and power. Anaerobic training, such as weightlifting, increases muscle bulk because it increases the size of individual fibres within the muscle (hypertrophy).

The action of skeletal muscles

In order to move a body part, the muscle or its tendon must stretch across at least one joint. When it contracts, the muscle then pulls one bone towards another. For example, when the elbow is bent during flexion of the forearm, the main mover is the biceps brachii, which is anchored on the scapula at one end and on the radius at the other. When it contracts, its shortening pulls on the radius, moving the forearm up toward the upper arm and bending the elbow.

This example also illustrates another feature of muscle arrangement: that of *antagonistic pairs*. Many muscles/muscle groups of the body are arranged so that their actions oppose one another. Using the example of bending the elbow, when the main flexors on the front of the upper arm contract, the muscles at the back of the upper arm must simultaneously relax to prevent injury.

Isometric and isotonic contraction 16.7

Contraction of a muscle usually results in its shortening, as happens for instance to the biceps muscle if the forearm is used to pick up a cup. The power generated by the muscle is used to lift the manageable weight, and tension in the muscle remains constant. In this situation, the contraction is said to be isotonic (iso = same; tonic = tension). However, imagine trying to lift an 80 kg man with one hand. Most people would be unable to perform this task, but the muscles of the arm and shoulder would still be working hard as they attempted it. In this situation, because the resistance from the man's weight is too great for him to be moved by the efforts of the lifter, the muscles would be unable to shorten, and the power generated increases the muscle tension instead. This is *isometric* contraction (iso = same; metric = length).

Muscle terminology

Muscles are named according to various characteristics (Table 16.7), and becoming familiar with the principal ones makes it much easier to identify unfamiliar muscles.

The *origin* of a muscle is (usually) its proximal attachment; this is generally the bone that remains still when the muscle contracts, giving it an anchor to pull against. The *insertion* is (usually) the distal attachment site, generally on the bone that is moved when the muscle contracts.

Principal skeletal muscles

This section considers the main muscles that move the limbs, as well as the major muscles of the face and neck, back, chest, pelvic floor and abdominal wall.

Muscles of the face and neck (Fig. 16.58)

Muscles of the face

Many muscles are involved in changing facial expression and with movement of the lower jaw during chewing and speaking. Only the main muscles are described here. Except where indicated the muscles are present in pairs, one on each side.

Occipitofrontalis (unpaired). This consists of a posterior muscular part over the occipital bone (*occipitalis*), an anterior part over the frontal bone (*frontalis*) and an extensive flat tendon or aponeurosis that stretches over the dome of the skull and joins the two muscular parts. It raises the eyebrows.

Levator palpebrae superioris. This muscle extends from the posterior part of the orbital cavity to the upper eyelid. It raises the eyelid.

Orbicularis oculi. This muscle surrounds the eye, eyelid and orbital cavity. It closes the eye and when strongly contracted 'screws up' the eyes.

Buccinator. This flat muscle of the cheek draws the cheeks in towards the teeth in chewing and in forcible expulsion of air from the mouth ('the trumpeter's muscle').

Orbicularis oris (unpaired). This muscle surrounds the mouth and blends with the muscles of the cheeks. It closes the lips and, when strongly contracted, shapes the mouth for whistling.

Masseter. This broad muscle extends from the zygomatic arch to the angle of the jaw. In chewing it draws the mandible up to the maxilla, closing the jaw, exerting considerable pressure on the food.

Temporalis. This muscle covers the squamous part of the temporal bone. It passes behind the zygomatic arch to be inserted into the coronoid process of the mandible. It closes the mouth and assists with chewing.

Pterygoid. This muscle extends from the sphenoid bone to the mandible. It closes the mouth and pulls the lower jaw forward.

Table 16.7 Muscle terminology		
Characteristic	**Example**	**Comment**
Shape	Trapezius	Trapezium shaped
Fibre direction	Oblique muscles of abdomen	Fibres run obliquely
Muscle position	Tibialis	Found close to tibia in the leg
Movement produced	Extensor carpi ulnaris	Attached to the carpal bones of the wrist and the ulna, and extends the wrist
Number of points of attachment	Biceps brachii	Bi = 2; this muscle has two points of attachment at the shoulder
Bones to which muscle is attached	Carpi radialis muscles	Attached to the carpal bones of the wrist and the radius of the forearm

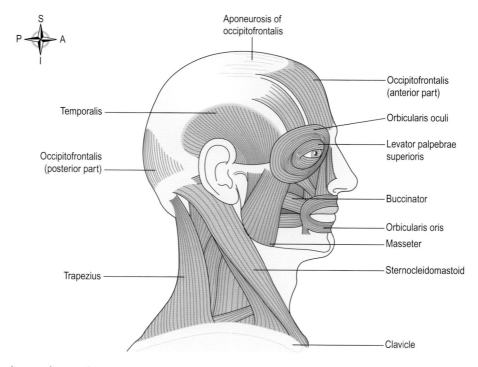

Figure 16.58 The main muscles on the right side of the face, head and neck.

Muscles of the neck

There are many muscles in the neck, but only the two largest are considered here.

Sternocleidomastoid. This muscle arises from the manubrium of the sternum and the clavicle and extends upwards to the mastoid process of the temporal bone. It assists in turning the head from side to side and is also an accessory muscle in respiration. When the muscle on one side contracts it draws the head towards the shoulder. When both contract at the same time they flex the cervical vertebrae or draw the sternum and clavicles upwards when the head is maintained in a fixed position, e.g. in forced respiration.

Trapezius. This muscle covers the shoulder and the back of the neck. The upper attachment is to the occipital protuberance, the medial attachment is to the transverse processes of the cervical and thoracic vertebrae and the lateral attachment is to the clavicle and to the spinous and acromion processes of the scapula. It pulls the head backwards, squares the shoulders and controls the movements of the scapula when the shoulder joint is in use.

Muscles of the trunk

These muscles stabilise the association between the appendicular and axial skeletons at the pectoral girdle, and stabilise and allow movement of the shoulders and upper arms.

Muscles of the back

There are six pairs of large muscles in the back, in addition to those forming the posterior abdominal wall (Figs 16.59–16.61). The arrangement of these muscles is the same on each side of the vertebral column. They are:

- trapezius (see above)
- latissimus dorsi
- teres major
- psoas (p. 429)
- quadratus lumborum
- sacrospinalis.

Latissimus dorsi. This arises from the posterior part of the iliac crest and the spinous processes of the lumbar and lower thoracic vertebrae. It passes upwards across the back then under the arm to be inserted into the bicipital groove of the humerus. It adducts, medially rotates and extends the arm.

Teres major. This originates from the inferior angle of the scapula and is inserted into the humerus just below the shoulder joint. It extends, adducts and medially rotates the arm.

Quadratus lumborum. This muscle originates from the iliac crest, then it passes upwards, parallel and close to the vertebral column and it is inserted into the 12th rib

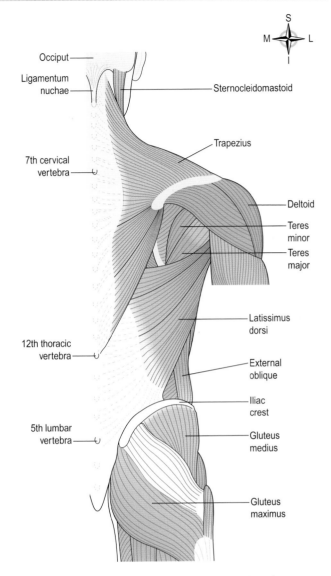

Figure 16.59 The main muscles of the back. Right side.

(Fig. 16.60). Together the two muscles fix the lower rib during respiration and cause extension of the vertebral column (bending backwards). If one muscle contracts it causes lateral flexion of the lumbar region of the vertebral column.

Sacrospinalis (erector spinae). This is a group of muscles lying between the spinous and transverse processes of the vertebrae (Fig. 16.61). They originate from the sacrum and are finally inserted into the occipital bone. Their contraction causes extension of the vertebral column.

Muscles of the abdominal wall

Five pairs of muscles form the abdominal wall (Figs 16.62 and 16.63). From the surface inwards they are:

- rectus abdominis
- external oblique

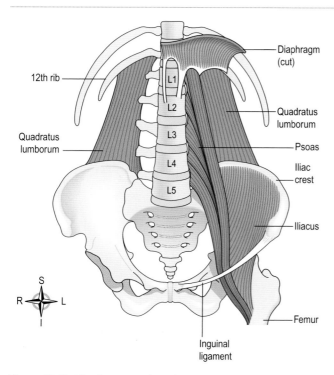

Figure 16.60 The deep muscles of the posterior abdominal wall. Anterior view.

- internal oblique
- transversus abdominis
- quadratus lumborum (see above).

The main function of these paired muscles is to form the strong muscular anterior wall of the abdominal cavity. When the muscles contract together they:

- compress the abdominal organs
- flex the vertebral column in the lumbar region (Fig. 16.61).

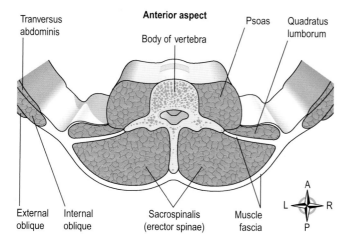

Figure 16.61 Transverse section of the posterior abdominal wall: a lumbar vertebra and its associated muscles.

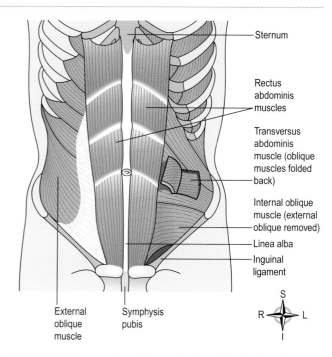

Figure 16.62 The muscles of the anterior abdominal wall.

Contraction of the muscles on one side only bends the trunk towards that side. Contraction of the oblique muscles on one side rotates the trunk.

The anterior abdominal wall is divided longitudinally by a very strong midline tendinous cord, the *linea alba* (meaning 'white cord') which extends from the xiphoid process of the sternum to the symphysis pubis.

Rectus abdominis. This is the most superficial muscle. It is broad and flat, originating from the transverse part of the pubic bone then passing upwards to be inserted into the lower ribs and the xiphoid process of the sternum. Medially the two muscles are attached to the linea alba.

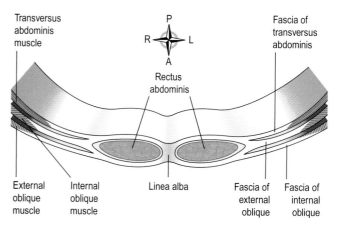

Figure 16.63 Transverse section of the muscles and fasciae of the anterior abdominal wall.

External oblique. This muscle extends from the lower ribs downwards and forward to be inserted into the iliac crest and, by an aponeurosis, to the linea alba.

Internal oblique. This muscle lies deep to the external oblique. Its fibres arise from the iliac crest and by a broad band of fascia from the spinous processes of the lumbar vertebrae. The fibres pass upwards towards the midline to be inserted into the lower ribs and, by an aponeurosis, into the linea alba. The fibres are at right angles to those of the external oblique.

Transversus abdominis. This is the deepest muscle of the abdominal wall. The fibres arise from the iliac crest and the lumbar vertebrae and pass across the abdominal wall to be inserted into the linea alba by an aponeurosis. The fibres are at right angles to those of the rectus abdominis.

Inguinal canal

This canal is 2.5–4 cm long and passes obliquely through the abdominal wall. It runs parallel to and immediately in front of the transversalis fascia and part of the inguinal ligament (Fig. 16.60). In the male it contains the *spermatic cord* and in the female, the *round ligament*. It constitutes a weak point in the otherwise strong abdominal wall through which herniation may occur.

Muscles of the thorax

These muscles are concerned with respiration, and are discussed in Chapter 10.

Muscles of the pelvic floor (Fig. 16.64)

The pelvic floor is divided into two identical halves that unite along the midline. Each half consists of fascia and muscle. The muscles are the levator ani and the coccygeus.

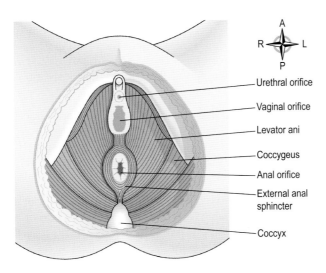

Figure 16.64 The muscles of the female pelvic floor.

The pelvic floor supports the organs of the pelvis and maintains continence, i.e. it resists raised intrapelvic pressure during micturition and defaecation.

Levator ani. This is a pair of broad flat muscles, forming the anterior part of the pelvic floor. They originate from the inner surface of the true pelvis and unite in the midline. Together they form a sling that supports the pelvic organs.

Coccygeus. This is a paired triangular sheet of muscle and tendinous fibres situated behind the levator ani. They originate from the medial surface of the ischium and are inserted into the sacrum and coccyx. They complete the formation of the pelvic floor, which is perforated in the male by the urethra and anus, and in the female by the urethra, vagina and anus.

Muscles of the shoulder and upper limb (Fig. 16.65)

These muscles stabilise the association between the appendicular and axial skeletons at the pectoral girdle, and stabilise and allow movement of the shoulders and upper arms.

Deltoid. These muscle fibres originate from the clavicle, acromion process and spine of scapula and radiate over the shoulder joint to be inserted into the deltoid tuberosity of the humerus. It forms the fleshy and rounded contour of the shoulder and its main function is movement of the arm. The anterior part causes flexion, the middle or main part abduction and the posterior part extends and laterally rotates the shoulder joint.

Pectoralis major. This lies on the anterior thoracic wall. The fibres originate from the middle third of the clavicle and from the sternum and are inserted into the lip of the intertubercular groove of the humerus. It draws the arm forward and towards the body, i.e. flexes and adducts.

Coracobrachialis. This lies on the upper medial aspect of the arm. It arises from the coracoid process of the scapula, stretches across in front of the shoulder joint and is inserted into the middle third of the humerus. It flexes the shoulder joint.

Biceps. This lies on the anterior aspect of the upper arm. At its proximal end it is divided into two parts (heads), each of which has its own tendon. The short head rises from the coracoid process of the scapula and passes in front of the shoulder joint to the arm. The long head originates from the rim of the glenoid cavity and its tendon passes through the joint cavity and the bicipital groove of the humerus to the arm. It is retained in the bicipital groove by a transverse humeral ligament that stretches across the groove. The distal tendon crosses the elbow joint and is inserted into the radial tuberosity. It helps to stabilise and flex the shoulder joint and at the elbow joint it assists with flexion and supination.

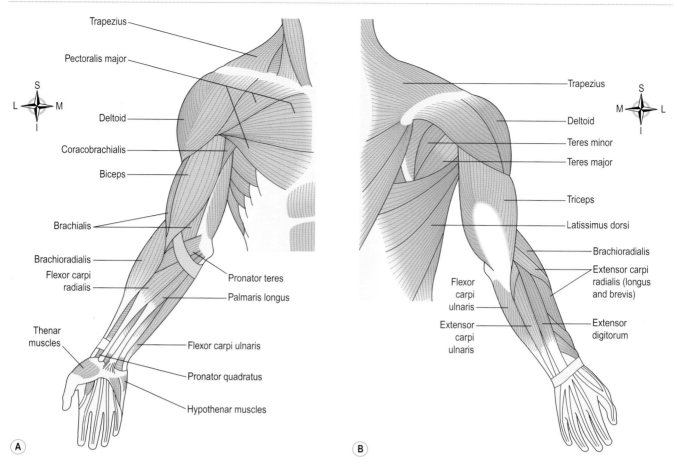

Figure 16.65 The main muscles of the right shoulder and upper limb. A. Anterior view. **B.** Posterior view.

Brachialis. This lies on the anterior aspect of the upper arm deep to the biceps. It originates from the shaft of the humerus, extends across the elbow joint and is inserted into the ulna just distal to the joint capsule. It is the main flexor of the elbow joint.

Triceps. This lies on the posterior aspect of the humerus. It arises from three heads, one from the scapula and two from the posterior surface of the humerus. The insertion is by a common tendon to the olecranon process of the ulna. It helps to stabilise the shoulder joint, assists in adduction of the arm and extends the elbow joint.

Brachioradialis. The brachioradialis spans the elbow joint, originating on the distal end of the humerus and inserts on the lateral epicondyle of the radius. Contraction flexes the elbow joint.

Pronator quadratus. This square-shaped muscle is the main muscle causing pronation of the hand and has attachments on the lower sections of both the radius and the ulna.

Pronator teres. This lies obliquely across the upper third of the front of the forearm. It arises from the medial epicondyle of the humerus and the coronoid process of the

ulna and passes obliquely across the forearm to be inserted into the lateral surface of the shaft of the radius. It rotates the radioulnar joints, changing the hand from the anatomical to the writing position, i.e. pronation.

Supinator. This lies obliquely across the posterior and lateral aspects of the forearm. Its fibres arise from the lateral epicondyle of the humerus and the upper part of the ulna and are inserted into the lateral surface of the upper third of the radius. It rotates the radioulnar joints, often with help from the biceps, changing the hand from the writing to the anatomical position, i.e. supination. It lies deep to the muscles shown in Figure 16.65.

Flexor carpi radialis. This lies on the anterior surface of the forearm. It originates from the medial epicondyle of the humerus and is inserted into the second and third metacarpal bones. It flexes the wrist joint, and when acting with the extensor carpi radialis, abducts the joint.

Flexor carpi ulnaris. This lies on the medial aspect of the forearm. It originates from the medial epicondyle of the humerus and the upper parts of the ulna and is inserted into the pisiform, the hamate and the fifth metacarpal bones. It flexes the wrist, and when acting with the extensor carpi ulnaris, adducts the joint.

Extensor carpi radialis longus and brevis. These lie on the posterior aspect of the forearm. The fibres originate from the lateral epicondyle of the humerus and are inserted by a long tendon into the second and third metacarpal bones. They extend and abduct the wrist.

Extensor carpi ulnaris. This lies on the posterior surface of the forearm. It originates from the lateral epicondyle of the humerus and is inserted into the fifth metacarpal bone. It extends and adducts the wrist.

Palmaris longus. This muscle resists shearing forces that might pull the skin and fascia of the palm away from the underlying structures, and flexes the wrist. Its origin is on the medial epicondyle of the humerus, and it inserts on tendons on the palm of the hand.

Extensor digitorum. This muscle originates on the lateral epicondyle of the humerus and spans both the elbow and wrist joints; in the wrist, it divides into four tendons, one for each finger. Action of this muscle can extend any of the joints across which it passes, i.e. the elbow, wrist or finger joints.

Muscles that control finger movements. Large muscles in the forearm that extend to the hand give power to the hand and fingers, but not the delicacy of movement needed for fine and dexterous finger control. Smaller muscles, which originate on the carpal and metacarpal bones, control tiny and precise finger movements via tendinous attachments on the phalanges; muscle fibres do not extend into the fingers.

Muscles of the hip and lower limb (Fig. 16.66)

The biggest muscles of the body are found here, since their function is largely in weight bearing. The lower parts of the body are designed to transmit the force of body weight in walking, running, etc., evenly throughout weight-bearing structures, and act as shock absorbers.

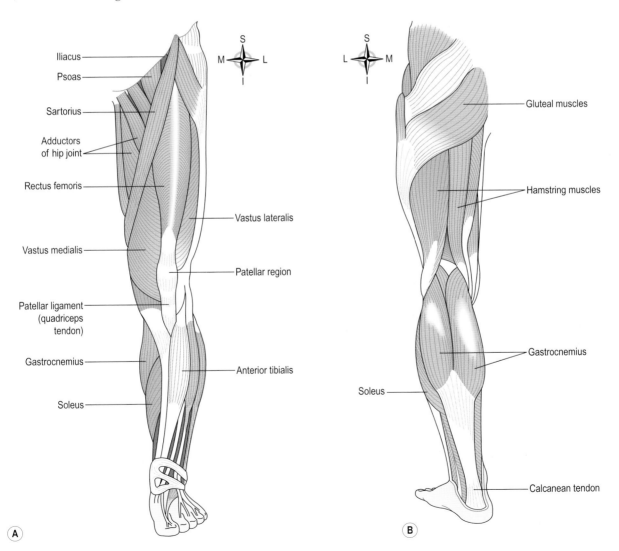

Figure 16.66 The main muscles of the left lower limb. A. Anterior view. **B.** Posterior view.

Psoas. This arises from the transverse processes and bodies of the lumbar vertebrae. It passes across the flat part of the ilium and behind the inguinal ligament to be inserted into the femur. Together with the iliacus it flexes the hip joint (see Fig. 16.60).

Iliacus. This lies in the iliac fossa of the innominate bone. It originates from the iliac crest, passes over the iliac fossa and joins the tendon of the psoas muscle to be inserted into the lesser trochanter of the femur. The combined action of the iliacus and psoas flexes the hip joint.

Quadriceps femoris. This is a group of four muscles lying on the front and sides of the thigh. They are the *rectus femoris* and three *vasti*: lateralis, medialis and intermedius (this last muscle is not shown in Figure 16.66 because it lies deep to the other two). The rectus femoris originates from the ilium and the three vasti from the upper end of the femur. Together they pass over the front of the knee joint to be inserted into the tibia by the patellar tendon. Only the rectus femoris flexes the hip joint. Together, the group acts as a very strong extensor of the knee joint.

Obturators. The obturators, deep muscles of the buttock, have their origins in the rim of the obturator foramen of the pelvis and insert into the proximal femur. Their main function lies in lateral rotation at the hip joint.

Gluteals. These consist of the *gluteus maximus*, *medius* and *minimus*, which together form the fleshy part of the buttock. They originate from the ilium and sacrum and are inserted into the femur. They cause extension, abduction and medial rotation at the hip joint.

Sartorius. This is the longest muscle in the body and crosses both the hip and knee joints. It originates from the anterior superior iliac spine and passes obliquely across the hip joint, thigh and knee joint to be inserted into the medial surface of the upper part of the tibia. It is associated with flexion and abduction at the hip joint and flexion at the knee.

Adductor group. This lies on the medial aspect of the thigh. They originate from the pubic bone and are inserted into the linea aspera of the femur. They adduct and medially rotate the thigh.

Hamstrings. These lie on the posterior aspect of the thigh. They originate from the ischium and are inserted into the upper end of the tibia. They are the *biceps femoris*, *semimembranosus* and *semitendinosus muscles*. They flex the knee joint.

Gastrocnemius. This forms the bulk of the calf of the leg. It arises by two heads, one from each condyle of the femur, and passes down behind the tibia to be inserted into the calcaneus by the *calcanean tendon* (*Achilles tendon*). It crosses both knee and ankle joints, causing flexion at the knee and plantarflexion (rising onto the ball of the foot) at the ankle.

Anterior tibialis. This originates from the upper end of the tibia, lies on the anterior surface of the leg and is inserted into the middle cuneiform bone by a long tendon. It is associated with dorsiflexion of the foot.

Soleus. This is one of the main muscles of the calf of the leg, lying immediately deep to the gastrocnemius. It originates from the heads and upper parts of the fibula and the tibia. Its tendon joins that of the gastrocnemius so that they have a common insertion into the calcaneus by the calcanean (Achilles) tendon. It causes plantarflexion at the ankle and helps to stabilise the joint when standing.

Ageing and the musculoskeletal system

Learning outcome

After reading this section, you should be able to:

- describe the effects of ageing on the structure and function of the musculoskeletal system.

Bone tissue in old age becomes lighter and less dense, so fractures are more likely. This natural process is called *osteopenia* and begins between the ages of 30 and 40. Oestrogen protects against the loss of bone mass, and there is a significant acceleration in the process in post-menopausal women, predisposing to osteoporosis (p. 431). Compaction of the intervertebral discs reduces the length of the spinal column and leads to a shortening in stature.

Cartilage and other connective tissues stiffen and may degenerate with age, leading to reduced flexibility and mobility of joints and predisposing to osteoarthritis (p. 434). Skeletal muscle fibres become smaller, less elastic and take longer to repair following injury. Damaged muscle may be replaced with fibrous tissue, which is inelastic and reduces the strength of contraction. Exercise tolerance reduces because each cell stores less glucose and myoglobin, and as cardiovascular function declines, regulation of blood supply to muscle becomes less efficient. In addition, older adults cannot lose the heat generated by working muscle as effectively as younger people.

Regular exercise throughout life can significantly slow these age-related changes.

Diseases of bone

Osteoporosis

In this condition, bone density (the amount of bone tissue) is reduced because its deposition does not keep pace with resorption (Fig. 16.67). Although the bone is adequately mineralised, it is fragile and microscopically abnormal, with loss of internal structure. Peak bone mass occurs around 35 years and then gradually declines in both sexes. Lowered oestrogen levels after the menopause are associated with a period of accelerated bone loss in women. Thereafter bone density in women is less than in men for any given age. A range of environmental factors and diseases are also associated with decreased bone mass and are implicated in development of osteoporosis (Box 16.1). Some can be influenced by changes in lifestyle. Exercise and calcium intake during childhood and adolescence are thought to be important in determining eventual bone mass of an individual, and therefore the risk of osteoporosis in later life. As bone mass decreases, susceptibility to fractures increases. Immobility causes reversible osteoporosis, the extent of which

corresponds to the length and degree of immobility. For instance, during prolonged periods of unconsciousness, osteoporotic changes are uniform throughout the skeleton, but immobilisation of a particular joint following fracture leads to local osteoporotic changes in involved bones only.

Common features of osteoporosis are:

- skeletal deformity – gradual loss of height with age, caused by compression of vertebrae
- bone pain
- fractures – especially of the hip (neck of femur), wrist (Colles' fracture) and vertebrae.

Paget's disease

Paget's disease is a disorder of bone remodelling, where the normal balance between bone building and bone breakdown becomes disorganised and both osteoblasts and osteoclasts become abnormally active. The bone deposited is soft and structurally abnormal. This predisposes to deformities (Fig. 16.68) and fractures, commonly of the pelvis, femur, tibia and skull. Most cases occur after 40 years of age and the incidence increases with age. The cause is unknown and it often goes undetected until complications arise. The disease increases the risk of osteoarthritis (p. 434) and osteosarcoma.

Rickets and osteomalacia

In both conditions, bone is inadequately mineralised, usually because of vitamin D deficiency, or sometimes because of defective vitamin D metabolism. Rickets occurs in children, whose bones are still growing, leading to characteristic bowing and deformity of the lower limbs. Adults still require vitamin D for normal turnover of bone, and deficiency leads to osteomalacia, which is associated with increased risk of fracture and bone pain.

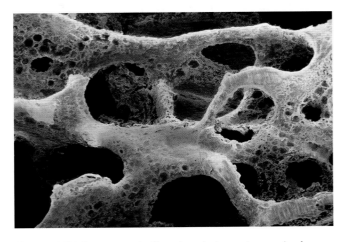

Figure 16.67 Osteoporosis. Scanning electron micrograph of spongy bone.

Box 16.1 Causes of decreased bone mass

Risk factors	**Drugs**
Female gender	Corticosteroids
Increasing age	
White ethnic origin	**Diseases**
Family history	Cushing's syndrome
Lack of exercise/	Hyperparathyroidism
immobility	Type 1 diabetes mellitus
Diet (low calcium)	Rheumatoid arthritis
Smoking	Chronic renal failure
Excess alcohol intake	Chronic liver disease
Early menopause/	Anorexia nervosa
oophorectomy	Certain cancers
Thin build (small bones)	

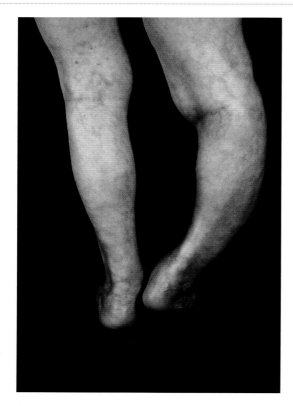

Figure 16.68 Severe leg deformity in Paget's disease.

Deficiency may be caused by poor diet, malabsorption, or by limited exposure to sunlight (needed for normal vitamin D metabolism).

Osteomyelitis

This is bacterial infection of bone and may follow an open fracture or surgical procedures, which allow microbial entry through broken skin. It may also be a consequence of blood-borne infection from a focus elsewhere, such as the ear, throat or skin; this is most commonly seen in children. If promptly and adequately treated, the infection can resolve without permanent damage, but if not, it may become chronic, with sinus formation draining pus to the skin, fever and pain.

Developmental abnormalities of bone

Achondroplasia
This is caused by a genetic abnormality that prevents the proper ossification of bones that develop from cartilage models, such as the long bones of the limbs, leading to short limbs and characteristic dwarfism.

Osteogenesis imperfecta ('brittle bone syndrome')
This is a group of conditions in which there is a congenital defect of collagen synthesis, resulting in failure of ossification. The bones are brittle and fracture easily, either spontaneously or following very slight trauma.

Tumours of bone

Benign tumours

Single or multiple tumours may develop for unknown reasons in bone and cartilage. They may cause pathological fractures or pressure damage to soft tissues, e.g. a benign vertebral tumour may damage the spinal cord or a spinal nerve. Benign tumours of cartilage have a tendency to undergo malignant change.

Malignant tumours

Metastatic tumours
The most common malignancies of bone are metastases of primary carcinomas of the breast, lungs, thyroid, kidneys and prostate gland. The usual sites are those with the best blood supply, i.e. spongy bone, especially the bodies of the lumbar vertebrae and the epiphyses of the humerus and femur. Tumour fragments are spread in blood, and possibly along the walls of the veins from pelvic tumours to vertebrae. Tumour growth erodes and weakens normal bone tissue, leading to pain, pathological fractures and destruction of normal bone architecture.

Primary tumours
Primary malignant tumours of bone are relatively rare. *Osteosarcoma* is rapidly growing and often highly malignant. It is commonest in adolescence and usually develops in the medullary canal of long bones, especially the femur. It occasionally occurs in elderly people, generally in association with Paget's disease, and involving the vertebrae, skull and pelvis.

Disorders of joints

Learning outcomes

After studying this section, you should be able to:

■ relate the features of the diseases in this section to abnormal anatomy and physiology

■ compare and contrast the features of rheumatoid arthritis and osteoarthritis.

The tissues involved in diseases of the synovial joints are synovial membrane, hyaline cartilage and bone.

Inflammatory joint disease (arthritis)

Rheumatoid arthritis (RA, rheumatoid disease)

This is a chronic progressive inflammatory autoimmune disease mainly affecting peripheral synovial joints. It is a systemic disorder in which inflammatory changes affect not only joints but also many other sites including the heart, blood vessels and skin.

It is more common in females than males and can affect all ages, including children (Still's disease), although it usually develops between the ages of 35 and 55 years. The cause is not clearly understood but autoimmunity may be initiated by microbial infection, possibly by viruses, in genetically susceptible people. Risk factors include:

- age – risk increases with age
- gender – premenopausal women are affected three times as commonly as men
- genetic risk – there is a strong familial link in some cases, and some markers on the surface membranes of white blood cells have also been associated with higher risk of the disease.

Up to 90% of affected individuals have rheumatoid factor (RF-autoantibodies) in their body fluids. High levels of RF, especially early in the disease, are strongly associated with accelerated and more severe disease. Symptoms include joint pain and stiffness, particularly in the morning and after rest. Joints can be visibly swollen, hot and tender.

Acute exacerbations of rheumatoid arthritis are usually accompanied by fever, and are interspersed with periods of remission. The joints most commonly affected are those of the hands (Fig. 16.69) and feet, but in severe cases most synovial joints may be involved. With each exacerbation there is additional and cumulative damage to the joints, leading to increasing deformity, pain and loss of function. The early changes, which may be reversible, include hypertrophy and hyperplasia of synovial cells and fibrinous inflammatory effusion into the joint. Progression of the disease usually leads to permanent tissue damage. Growth of inflammatory granulation tissue, called *pannus*, distorts the joint and destroys articular cartilage, exposing the bone below and causing further damage. Fibrosis of the pannus reduces joint mobility. Pain, stiffness and deformity severely restrict the use of affected joints, and as a result the associated muscles start to waste. About a third of patients, usually those with the most aggressive form of the disease, develop nodules of connective tissue (rheumatoid nodules), usually in the forearm or elbow. Extra-articular symptoms can include anaemia, peripheral neuropathy, cardiac abnormalities, pleurisy and vasculitis.

In the later stages of the disease, the inflammation and fever are less marked. The extent of disability varies from slight to severe. Table 16.8 highlights differences between osteoarthritis and rheumatoid arthritis.

Other types of polyarthritis

Polyarthritis means inflammation of more than one joint. This group of autoimmune inflammatory arthritic diseases has many characteristics similar to RA but the rheumatoid factor is absent. The causes are not known but genetic features may be involved.

Ankylosing spondylitis. This tends to occur in young adults, and affects the joints of the vertebral column. Calcification of the intervertebral joints and laying down of new bone leads to reduced spinal flexibility and permanent deformity.

Psoriatic arthritis. This occurs in a proportion of people who suffer from psoriasis (p. 371), especially if the nails are involved. The joints most commonly affected are those of the fingers and toes.

Reiter's syndrome (polyarthritis with urethritis and conjunctivitis). This syndrome may be precipitated by *Chlamydia trachomatis* infection; the affected joints are usually those of the lower limb.

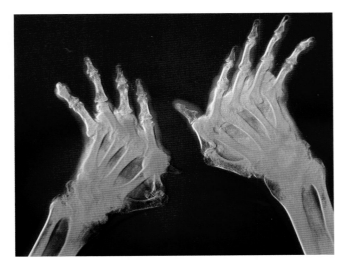

Figure 16.69 Severe deformity of the hands in rheumatoid arthritis.

Table 16.8 Features of the two main types of arthritis

	Osteoarthritis	Rheumatoid arthritis
Type of disease	Degenerative	Inflammatory and autoimmune
Tissue affected	Articular cartilage	Synovial membrane
Age of onset	Late middle age	Any age, mainly 30–55 years, occasionally children
Joints affected	Weight bearing, e.g. hip, knee; often only a single joint	Small, e.g. hands, feet; often many joints

Rheumatic fever. Rheumatic fever (p. 128) is a diffuse inflammatory condition that affects many connective tissues. Polyarthritis is a common presenting feature, often involving the wrists, elbows, knees and ankles. Unlike cardiac effects (p. 128), arthritis usually resolves spontaneously without complications.

Infective arthritis

Joint infection (septic arthritis) usually results from a blood-borne systemic infection (septicaemia, mainly staphylococcal), although it may also be caused by a penetrating joint injury. Often the joint has been damaged by pre-existing disease, making it more susceptible to infection. Normally, only one joint is involved, which becomes acutely inflamed, and the patient is likely to be ill from the associated septicaemia. Complete resolution is possible if treatment is prompt, but permanent joint damage occurs early in the disease.

Osteoarthritis (osteoarthrosis, OA)

This is a degenerative non-inflammatory disease that results in pain and restricted movement of affected joints. Osteoarthrosis is the more appropriate name but is less commonly used. In its early stages, OA is often asymptomatic. It is very common, with the majority of over-65s showing some degree of osteoarthritic changes. Articular cartilage gradually becomes thinner because its renewal does not keep pace with its breakdown. Eventually the bony articular surfaces come in contact and the bones begin to degenerate. Bone repair is abnormal and the articular surfaces become misshapen, reducing mobility of the joint. Chronic inflammation develops with effusion (collection of fluid) into the joint, possibly due to irritation caused by tissue debris not removed by phagocytes. Sometimes there is abnormal outgrowth of cartilage at the edges of bones that becomes ossified, forming *osteophytes*.

In most cases, the cause of OA is unknown (primary OA), but risk factors include excessive repetitive use of the affected joints, female gender, increasing age, obesity and heredity. Secondary OA occurs when the joint is already affected by disease or abnormality, e.g. trauma or gout. Osteoarthritis usually develops in late middle age and affects large weight-bearing joints, i.e. the hips, knees and joints of the cervical and lower lumbar spine. In many cases only one joint is involved.

Traumatic injury to joints

Sprains, strains and dislocations

These damage the soft tissues, tendons and ligaments round the joint without penetrating the joint capsule. In dislocations there may be additional damage to intracapsular structures by stretching, e.g. to the long head of biceps muscle in the shoulder joint, the cruciate ligaments in the knee joint, or the ligament of head of femur in the hip joint. If repair is incomplete there may be some loss of stability, which increases the risk of repeated injury.

Penetrating injuries

These may be caused by a compound fracture of one of the articulating bones, or trauma. Healing may be uneventful or delayed by the presence of fragments of damaged or torn joint tissue (bone, cartilage or ligaments), which cannot be removed or repaired by normal body mechanisms and prevent full joint recovery. Infection is another risk. Chronic inflammation can lead to permanent degenerative changes in the joint.

Gout

This condition is caused by the deposition of sodium urate crystals in joints and tendons, provoking an acute inflammatory response. Risk factors include male gender, obesity, heredity, hyperuricaemia and high alcohol intake. *Primary* gout, the commonest form, occurs almost always in men and is associated with reduced ability to excrete urate or increased urate production. *Secondary* gout occurs usually as a consequence of diuretic treatment or kidney failure, both of which reduce urate excretion.

In many cases only one joint is involved (monoarthritis) and it is typically red, hot and extremely painful. The sites most commonly affected are the metatarsophalangeal joint of the big toe and the ankle, knee, wrist and elbow joints. Episodes of arthritis lasting days or weeks are interspersed with periods of remission. After repeated acute attacks, permanent damage may occur with chronic deformity and loss of function of the affected joints. Gout is sometimes complicated by the development of renal calculi.

Connective tissue diseases

This group of chronic autoimmune disorders has common features. They:

- affect many systems of the body, especially the joints, skin and subcutaneous tissues
- tend to occur in early adult life
- usually affect more females than males.

They include the following:

- *Systemic lupus erythematosus* (SLE) – the affected joints are usually the hands, knees and ankles. A characteristic red 'butterfly' rash may occur on the face. Kidney involvement is common and can result in glomerulonephritis that may be complicated by chronic renal failure.
- *Systemic sclerosis* (*scleroderma*) – in this group of disorders there is progressive thickening of connective tissue. There is increased production of collagen that affects many organs. In the skin there is dermal

fibrosis and tightness that impairs the functioning of joints, especially of the hands. It also affects the walls of blood vessels, intestinal tract and other organs.

- Rheumatoid arthritis (p. 432).
- Ankylosing spondylitis (p. 433).
- Reiter's syndrome (p. 433).

Carpal tunnel syndrome

This occurs when the median nerve is compressed in the wrist as it passes through the carpal tunnel (see Fig. 16.50). It is common, especially in women, between the ages of 30 and 50 years. There is pain and numbness in the hand and wrist affecting the thumb, index and middle fingers, and half of the ring finger. Many cases are idiopathic or secondary to other conditions, e.g. rheumatoid arthritis, diabetes mellitus, acromegaly and hypothyroidism. Repetitive flexion and extension of the wrist joint also cause the condition, e.g. following prolonged keyboard use.

Diseases of muscle

Learning outcomes

After studying this section, you should be able to:

- list the causes of the diseases in this section
- compare and contrast the characteristics of different types of muscular dystrophy.

Myasthenia gravis

This autoimmune condition of unknown origin affects more women than men, usually aged between 20 and 40 years. Antibodies are produced that bind to and block the acetylcholine receptors of the neuromuscular junction. The transmission of nerve impulses to muscle fibres is therefore blocked. This causes progressive and extensive muscle weakness, although the muscles themselves are normal. Extrinsic and eyelid muscles are affected first, causing *ptosis* (drooping of the eyelid) or *diplopia* (double vision), followed by those of the neck (possibly affecting chewing, swallowing and speech) and limbs. There are periods of remission, relapses being precipitated by, for example, strenuous exercise, infections or pregnancy.

Muscular dystrophies

In this group of inherited diseases there is progressive degeneration of groups of muscles. The main differences in the types are age of onset, rate of progression and groups of muscles involved.

Duchenne muscular dystrophy

Inheritance of this condition is sex linked (p. 444).

Signs and symptoms may not appear until about 5 years of age. Wasting and weakness begin in muscles of the lower limbs then spread to the upper limbs, progressing rapidly without remission. Death usually occurs in adolescence, often from respiratory failure, cardiac arrhythmias or cardiomyopathy.

Facioscapulohumeral dystrophy

This disease affects both sexes. It usually begins in adolescence and the younger the age of onset the more rapidly it progresses. Muscles of the face and shoulders are affected first. This is a chronic condition that usually progresses slowly and may not cause complete disability. Life expectancy is normal.

Myotonic dystrophy

This disease usually begins in adult life and affects both genders. Muscles contract and relax slowly, often seen as difficulty in releasing an object held in the hand. Muscles of the tongue and the face are first affected, then muscles of the limbs. Systemic conditions associated with myotonic dystrophy include:

- cataracts (p. 211)
- atrophy of the gonads
- cardiomyopathy
- glucose intolerance.

The disease progresses without remission and with increasing disability. Death usually occurs in middle age from respiratory or cardiac failure.

Rotator cuff injury

The rotator cuff muscles (p. 415) stabilise and strengthen the shoulder joint. Injury here is common, leading to pain and restricted mobility of the shoulder. Healing can take months or even years.

For a range of self-assessment exercises on the topics in this chapter, visit Evolve online resources: https://evolve.elsevier.com/Waugh/anatomy/

Introduction to genetics

All living organisms, including human beings, need to reproduce, so that at the end of their life span they have produced at least one, often several, other individuals to replace themselves. This ensures the continuation of their species. Offspring inherit from their parents a copy of all information needed to develop into a functioning organism; this information is carried as deoxyribonucleic acid (DNA), mainly within the cell nucleus. DNA is organised into functional units called genes, which themselves are part of much bigger structures, the chromosomes. Collectively, all the genetic material in a cell is called its *genome*. Genetics is the study of genes, and advancing knowledge in this area has a profound effect on many aspects of daily life, e.g. for genetic counselling in families carrying inherited diseases and the production of human insulin from genetically engineered micro-organisms.

The Human Genome project, an international collaboration, was initiated in 1990. Its aim was to identify and sequence every gene on every chromosome, and to be able to draw a map of each chromosome, showing the position of all its genes. It has yielded a great deal of important information regarding human genetic disorders.

At the end of the chapter, the effects of ageing on chromosomes, cell division and heredity are considered, and this is followed by a section on some common genetic abnormalities.

Chromosomes, genes and DNA

Learning outcomes

After studying this section, you should be able to:

- explain the structural relationship between chromosomes, genes and DNA

- describe the molecular structure of DNA

- explain the terms autosomes and sex chromosomes

- define the terms genome, haploid, diploid and karyotype.

Chromosomes

Nearly every body cell contains, within its nucleus, an identical copy of the entire complement of the individual's genetic material. Two important exceptions are red blood cells (which have no nucleus) and the gametes or sex cells. In a resting cell, the *chromatin* (genetic material, see Fig. 3.8) is diffuse and hard to see under the microscope, but when the cell prepares to divide, it is collected into highly visible, compact, sausage-shaped structures called *chromosomes*. Each chromosome is one of a pair, one inherited from the mother and one from the father, so the

human cell has 46 chromosomes that can be arranged as 23 pairs. A cell with 23 pairs of chromosomes is termed *diploid*. Gametes (spermatozoa and ova) with only half of the normal complement, i.e. 23 chromosomes instead of 46, are described as *haploid*. Chromosomes belonging to the same pair are called *homologous* chromosomes. The complete set of chromosomes from a cell is its *karyotype* (Fig. 17.1). ▓ **17.1**

Each pair of chromosomes is numbered, the largest pair being no. 1. The first 22 pairs are collectively known as *autosomes*, and the chromosomes of each pair contain the same amount of genetic material. The chromosomes of pair 23 are called the *sex chromosomes* (Fig. 17.2) because they determine the individual's gender. Unlike autosomes, these two chromosomes are not necessarily the same size; the Y chromosome is much shorter than the X and is carried only by males. A child inheriting two X chromosomes (XX), one from each parent, is female, and a child inheriting an X from his mother and a Y from his father (XY) is male. ▓ **17.2**

Each end of the chromosome is capped with a length of DNA called a *telomere*, which seals the chromosome and is structurally essential. During replication, the telomere is shortened, which would damage the chromosome, and so it is repaired with an enzyme called *telomerase*. Reduced telomerase activity with age is related to cell *senescence* (p. 445).

Genes

Along the length of the chromosomes are the genes. Each gene contains information in code that allows the cell to make (almost always) a specific protein, the so-called *gene product*. Each gene codes for one specific protein, and research puts the number of genes in the human genome at between 25 000 and 30 000.

Genes normally exist in pairs, because the gene on one chromosome is matched at the equivalent site (locus) on the other chromosome of the pair.

DNA

Genes are composed mainly of very long strands of DNA; the total length of DNA in each cell is about a metre. Because this is packaged into chromosomes, which are micrometres (10^{-6} m) long, this means that the DNA must be tightly wrapped up to condense it into such a small space.

DNA is a double-stranded molecule, made up of two chains of *nucleotides*. Nucleotides consist of three subunits:

- a sugar
- a phosphate group
- a base.

The DNA molecule is sometimes likened to a twisted ladder, with the uprights formed by alternating chains of

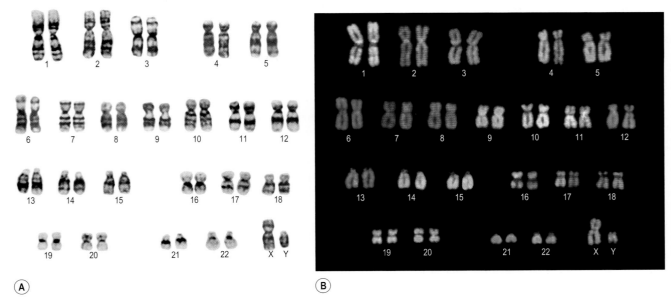

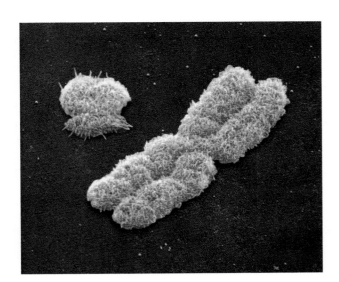

(A)   (B)

Figure 17.1 Chromosomal complement (karyotype) of a normal human male, showing 22 pairs of autosomes and sex chromosomes (XY, pair 23).

Figure 17.2 Coloured scanning electron micrograph of replicated human sex chromosomes: Y upper left, X centre.

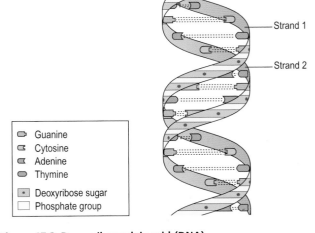

Figure 17.3 Deoxyribonucleic acid (DNA).

sugar and phosphate units (Fig. 17.3). In DNA, the sugar is deoxyribose, thus DNA. The bases are linked to the sugars, and each base binds to another base on the other sugar/phosphate chain, forming the rungs of the ladder. The two chains are twisted around one another, giving a double helix (twisted ladder) arrangement. The double helix itself is further twisted and wrapped in a highly organised way around structural proteins called *histones*, which are important in maintaining the heavily coiled three-dimensional shape of the DNA. The term given to the DNA–histone material is *chromatin*. The chromatin is supercoiled and packaged into the chromosomes shortly before the cell divides (Fig. 17.4).

The genetic code

DNA carries a huge amount of information that determines all biological activities of an organism, and which is transmitted from one generation to the next. The key to how this information is kept is found in the bases within DNA. There are four bases:

- adenine (A)
- guanine (G)
- thymine (T)
- cytosine (C).

439

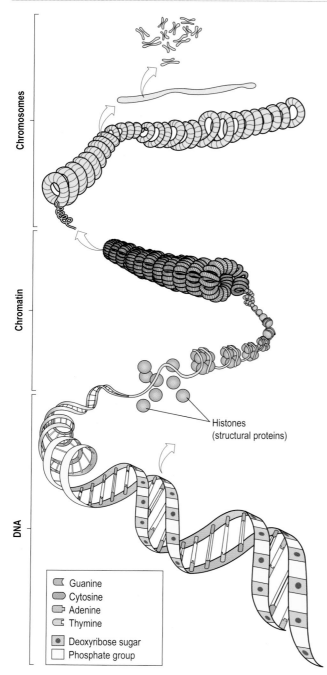

Guanine
Cytosine
Adenine
Thymine
Deoxyribose sugar
Phosphate group

Histones
(structural proteins)

Chromosomes

Chromatin

DNA

Figure 17.4 The structural relationship between DNA, chromatin and chromosomes.

They are arranged in a precise order along the DNA molecule, making a base code that can be read when protein synthesis is required. Each base along one strand of DNA pairs with a base on the other strand in a precise and predictable way. This is known as *complementary base pairing*. Adenine always pairs with thymine (and vice versa), and cytosine and guanine always go together. The bases on opposite strands run down the middle of the helix and bind to one another with hydrogen bonds (Fig. 17.3).   **17.3**

Mitochondrial DNA

Each body cell has, on average, 5000 mitochondria (p. 33) that hold a quantity of DNA (mitochondrial DNA), which codes, for example, for enzymes important in energy production. This DNA is passed from one generation to another via the ovum (p. 463), so the offspring's complement of mitochondrial DNA is inherited from the mother. Certain rare inherited disorders that arise from faulty mitochondrial DNA are therefore passed through generations via the maternal line.

Mutation

Mutation means an inheritable alteration in the normal genetic make-up of a cell. Most mutations occur spontaneously, because of the countless millions of DNA replications and cell divisions that occur normally throughout life. Others may be caused by external factors, such as X-rays, ultraviolet rays or exposure to certain chemicals. Any factor capable of mutating DNA is called a *mutagen* (p. 55). Most mutations are immediately repaired by an army of enzymes present in the cell nucleus, and therefore cause no permanent problems.

Sometimes the mutation is lethal, because it disrupts some essential cellular function, causing cell death and the mutation is destroyed along with the cell. Often, the mutated cell is detected by immune cells and destroyed because it is abnormal (p. 379). Other mutations do not kill the cell but alter its function in some way that may cause disease, e.g. in cancer (p. 55). A persistent mutation in the genome that has not led to cell death can be passed from parent to child and may cause inherited disease, e.g. phenylketonuria (p. 446) or cystic fibrosis (p. 266).

Protein synthesis

Learning outcomes

After studying this section, you should be able to:

■ describe the origin and structure of mRNA

■ explain the mechanism of transcription

■ outline the mechanism of translation.

DNA holds the cell's essential biological information, written within the base code in the centre of the double helix. The products of this information are almost always proteins. Proteins are essential to all aspects of body function, forming the major structural elements of the body as well as the enzymes (p. 28) essential for all biochemical

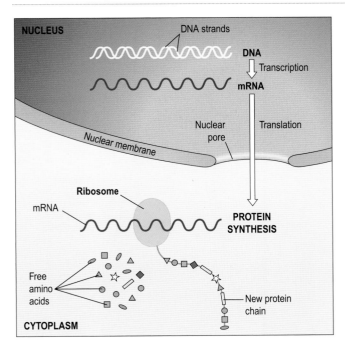

Figure 17.5 The relationship between DNA, RNA and protein synthesis.

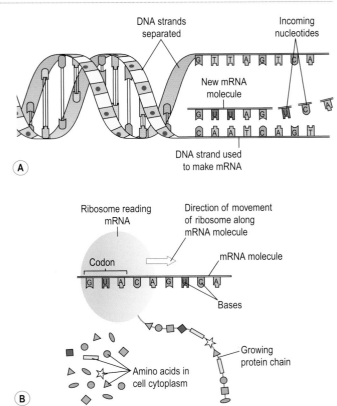

Figure 17.6 Transcription (A) and translation (B).

processes within it. The building blocks of human proteins are about 20 different amino acids. As the cell's DNA is too big to leave the nucleus, an intermediary molecule is needed to carry the genetic instructions from the nucleus to the cytoplasm, where proteins are made. This is called *messenger (m)*RNA. Protein synthesis is summarised in Figure 17.5.

Messenger ribonucleic acid (mRNA)

mRNA is a single-stranded chain of nucleotides synthesised in the nucleus from the appropriate gene, whenever the cell requires to make the protein for which that gene codes. There are three main differences between the structures of RNA and DNA:

- it is single instead of double stranded
- it contains the sugar ribose instead of deoxyribose
- it uses the base uracil instead of thymine.

Using the DNA as a template, a piece of mRNA is made from the gene to be used. This process is called *transcription*. The mRNA then leaves the nucleus through the nuclear pores and carries its information to the ribosomes in the cytoplasm.

Transcription 17.4

Because the code is buried within the DNA molecule, the first step is to open up the helix to expose the bases. Only the gene to be transcribed is opened; the remainder of the chromosome remains coiled. Opening up the helix exposes both base strands, but the enzyme that makes the

mRNA uses only one of them, so the mRNA molecule is single, not double stranded. As the enzyme moves along the opened DNA strand, reading its code, it adds the complementary base to the mRNA. Therefore, if the DNA base is cytosine, guanine is added to the mRNA molecule (and vice versa); if it is thymine, adenine is added; if it is adenine, uracil is added (remember there is no thymine in RNA, but uracil instead) (Fig. 17.6A). When the enzyme gets to a 'stop' signal, it terminates synthesis of the mRNA molecule, and the mRNA is released. The DNA is zipped up again by other enzymes, and the mRNA then leaves the nucleus.

Translation 17.5

Translation is synthesis of the final protein using the information carried on mRNA. It takes place on free ribosomes (p. 34) in the cytoplasm and those attached to rough endoplasmic reticulum. First, the mRNA attaches to the ribosome. The ribosome then 'reads' the base sequence of the mRNA (Fig. 17.6B).

Because proteins are built from up to 20 different amino acids, it is not possible to use the four bases individually in a simple one-to-one code. To give enough options, the base code in RNA is read in triplets, giving a possible 64 base combinations, which allows a coded instruction for each amino acid as well as other codes, e.g. stop and start instructions. Each of these specific triplet sequences is called a *codon*; for example, the base sequence ACA (adenine, cytosine, adenine) codes for the amino acid cysteine.

The first codon is a start codon, which initiates protein synthesis. The ribosome slides along the mRNA, reading the codons and adding the appropriate amino acids to the growing protein molecule as it goes. The ribosome continues assembling the new protein molecule until it arrives at a stop codon, at which point it terminates synthesis and releases the new protein. Some new proteins are used within the cell itself, and others are exported, e.g. insulin synthesised by pancreatic β-islet cells is released into the bloodstream.

Gene expression

Although all nucleated cells (except gametes) have an identical set of genes, each cell type uses only those genes related directly to its own particular function. For example, the only cell type *containing* haemoglobin is the red blood cell, although all body cells carry the haemoglobin gene. This selective gene expression is controlled by various regulatory substances, and the genes not needed by the cell are kept switched off.

Cell division

Learning outcomes

After studying this section, you should be able to:

- explain the mechanism of DNA replication

- compare and contrast the processes of mitosis and meiosis

- describe the basis of genetic diversity from generation to generation.

Most body cells are capable of division, even in adulthood. Cell division usually leads to production of two identical diploid daughter cells, *mitosis* (p. 35) and is important in body growth and repair. Production of gametes is different in that the daughter cells have only half the normal chromosome number – 23 instead of 46, i.e. they are haploid. Gametes are produced by a form of cell division called *meiosis*. DNA replication takes place before mitosis and meiosis.

DNA replication

DNA is the only biological molecule capable of self-replication. Mistakes in copying may lead to production of non-functioning or poorly functional cells, or cells that do not respond to normal cell controls (this could lead to the development of a tumour). Accurate copying of DNA is therefore essential.

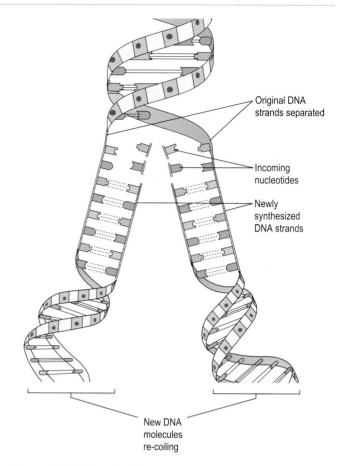

Original DNA strands separated

Incoming nucleotides

Newly synthesized DNA strands

New DNA molecules re-coiling

Figure 17.7 DNA replication.

The initial step in DNA replication is the unfolding of the double helix and the unzipping of the two strands to expose the bases, as happens in transcription. Both strands of the parent DNA molecule are copied. The enzyme responsible for DNA replication moves along the base sequence on each strand, reading the genetic code and adding the complementary base to the newly forming chain. This means that each strand of opened bases becomes a double strand and the end result is two identical DNA molecules (Fig. 17.7). As each new double strand is formed, other enzymes cause it to twist and coil back into its normal highly folded form.

Mitosis

This is described on page 35.

Meiosis

Meiosis is the final step in gamete production. On fertilisation, when the male gamete (sperm cell) and the female gamete (ovum) unite, the resulting zygote is diploid, because each gamete was haploid.

Unlike mitosis, meiosis involves two distinct cell divisions rather than one (Fig. 17.8). Additionally, meiosis

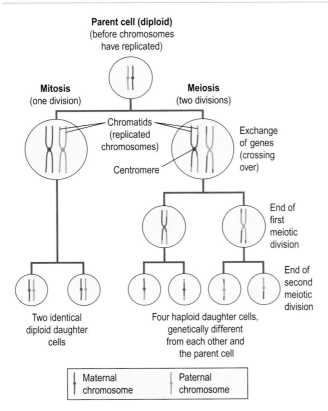

Figure 17.8 Mitosis and meiosis, showing only one pair of chromosomes for clarity.

In the figure: Parent cell (diploid) (before chromosomes have replicated); Mitosis (one division); Meiosis (two divisions); Chromatids (replicated chromosomes); Centromere; Exchange of genes (crossing over); End of first meiotic division; End of second meiotic division; Two identical diploid daughter cells; Four haploid daughter cells, genetically different from each other and the parent cell; Maternal chromosome; Paternal chromosome.

mitosis, producing two genetically unique diploid daughter cells.

Second meiotic division

For a gamete to be produced, the amount of genetic material present in the two daughter cells following the first meiotic division must be halved. This is accomplished by a second division (Fig. 17.8). The centromeres separate and the two sister chromatids travel to opposite ends of the cell, which then divides. Each of the four haploid daughter cells now has only one chromosome from each original pair. Fusion with another gamete creates a zygote (fertilised ovum), a diploid cell which can then go on to grow and develop into a human being by mitosis.

The genetic basis of inheritance

Learning outcomes

After studying this section, you should be able to:

- describe the basis of autosomal inheritance, including the relevance of recessive and dominant genes

- explain how sex-linked characteristics are passed from one generation to the next.

produces four daughter cells, not two, all different from the parent cells and from each other. This is the basis of genetic diversity and the uniqueness of each human individual.

First meiotic division

This stage (Fig. 17.8) produces two genetically different daughter cells.

DNA replication occurred beforehand, so each pair of chromosomes is now four chromatids, and they gather together into a tight bundle. Because the chromosomes are so tightly associated, it is possible for them to exchange genes. This process is called *crossing over* **17.6**, and results in the four chromatids acquiring different combinations of genes. Following crossing over, the pairs of chromosomes then separate in preparation for the first meiotic division, and transfer of maternal and paternal chromosomes to either daughter cell is random. This means that the two daughter cells have an unpredictable assortment of maternal and paternal DNA, giving rise to a huge number of possible combinations of chromosomes in them. This explains why a child inherits a combination of its mother's and father's characteristics and why children from the same parents can be very different from one another.

Each pair of chromosomes separates and one travels to each end of the cell, guided by a spindle as in

Mixing up of parental genes during meiosis leads to the huge genetic variety of the human race. It is important to understand how genes interact to produce inherited characteristics.

Autosomal inheritance

Each of a pair of homologous chromosomes contains genes for the same traits. For example, the ability to roll one's tongue is coded for on a single gene. Because one chromosome of each pair is inherited from the father and one from the mother, an individual has two genes controlling the ability to roll the tongue. Such paired genes are called *alleles*. Corresponding alleles contain genes concerned with the same trait, but they need not be identical. An individual may have:

- two identical forms of the gene (*homozygous*)
- two different forms of the gene (*heterozygous*).

One copy of the tongue-rolling gene may code for the ability to roll the tongue, but the corresponding gene on the other chromosome of the pair may be a different form and code for inability to tongue roll. This simple example involves only two forms of the same gene, but other characteristics are more complex. Eye colour is a diverse trait with a wide range of pigment colours and patterns possible, and is controlled by more than one gene.

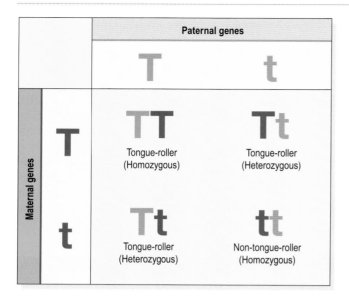

Figure 17.9 Autosomal inheritance. Example shows all possible combinations of tongue-rolling genes in children of parents heterozygous for the trait. T: dominant gene (tongue rolling); t: recessive gene (non-tongue rolling).

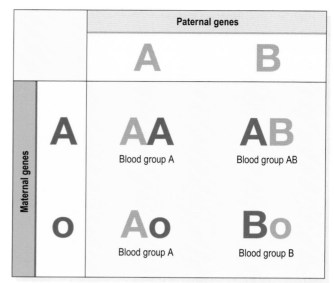

Figure 17.10 Co-dominant inheritance of ABO blood groups.

Should an individual inherit a tongue-rolling gene from one parent, and the non-rolling gene from the other, he will still be able to roll his tongue. This is because the tongue-rolling form of the gene is *dominant*, and takes priority over the non-rolling gene, which is *recessive*. Dominant genes are always *expressed* (active) in preference over recessive genes, and only one copy of a dominant gene is required for that characteristic to be expressed. A recessive gene can only be expressed if it is present on both chromosomes, i.e. individuals unable to tongue-roll have two copies of the recessive, non-rolling gene.

Individuals homozygous for a gene have two identical copies, of either the dominant or the recessive form. Heterozygous individuals have one dominant and one recessive gene. **17.7**

Punnett squares **17.8**

The probability of inheriting either form of a gene depends upon parental make-up. Simple autosomal inheritance can be illustrated using a Punnett square. Figure 17.9 shows all the possible combinations of the tongue-rolling gene in children whose parents are heterozygous for the trait. Using this example, there is a 3 in 4 (75%) chance that the child of these parents will be a tongue roller (TT or Tt), and only a 1 in 4 chance that they would inherit two recessive genes (tt), making them a non-roller.

Prediction of the probability that a baby will be born with an inherited disease, e.g. cystic fibrosis, page 266, forms the basis of genetic counselling.

Co-dominance

For some traits, there can be more than two alleles that code for it, and more than one allele can be dominant.

An example of this is the inheritance of A and B type antigens on the surface of red blood cells, determined clinically as the ABO system of blood grouping (p. 67). There are three possible alleles here: one allele codes for production of A type antigens (A), one allele codes for production of B type antigens (B) and a third allele codes for no antigen at all (o). An individual may have any combination of two of these three alleles: AA, AB, BB, Ao, Bo, or oo. Both A and B are dominant, and both express themselves wherever they are present. This is called co-dominance. O is recessive, and so only expresses itself in a homozygous recessive genotype. This means that individuals with an oo genotype have neither A nor B antigens on their red cell surface and are blood group O. An individual with genotype AB has both A and B and is blood group AB. An individual with genotype Ao or AA has only A type antigens and is blood group A; someone with genotype Bo or BB has only B type antigens and is blood group B.

Figure 17.10 shows a Punnett square illustrating the possible blood types of children produced by a mother with genotype AO (phenotype blood group A) and a father with genotype AB (phenotype blood group AB).

Sex-linked inheritance **17.9**

Figure 17.2 shows clearly that the Y chromosome is much smaller than the X chromosome. It is not surprising then to find that the Y chromosome carries only 86 genes compared with the X chromosome's 2000, and the vast majority of genes on the X-chromosome are not matched on the Y. This means that a male has only one copy of most of the genes on his sex chromosomes. Traits coded for on the section of the X chromosome that has no corresponding material on the Y are said to be sex linked. The gene that codes for normal colour vision is one example, and is therefore carried on X chromosomes only. It is the dominant form of the gene. There is a rare, recessive form of this gene, which is faulty and codes for red–green colour blindness. If a female inherits a faulty copy of the gene, she is statistically likely to have a normal gene on her other X chromosome, giving normal colour vision. A female carrying the colour blindness gene, even though she is not colour blind, may pass the faulty gene on to her children and is said to be a *carrier*. If the gene is abnormal in a male, he will be colour blind because, having only one X-chromosome, he has only one copy of the gene. Inheritance of colour blindness is shown in Figure 17.11. This illustrates the possible genetic combinations of the children of a carrier mother (one normal gene and one faulty gene) and a normal father (one normal gene).

There is a 50% chance of a son being colour blind, a 50% chance of a son having normal vision, a 50% chance of a daughter being a carrier (with normal vision herself) and a 50% chance of a daughter being normal.

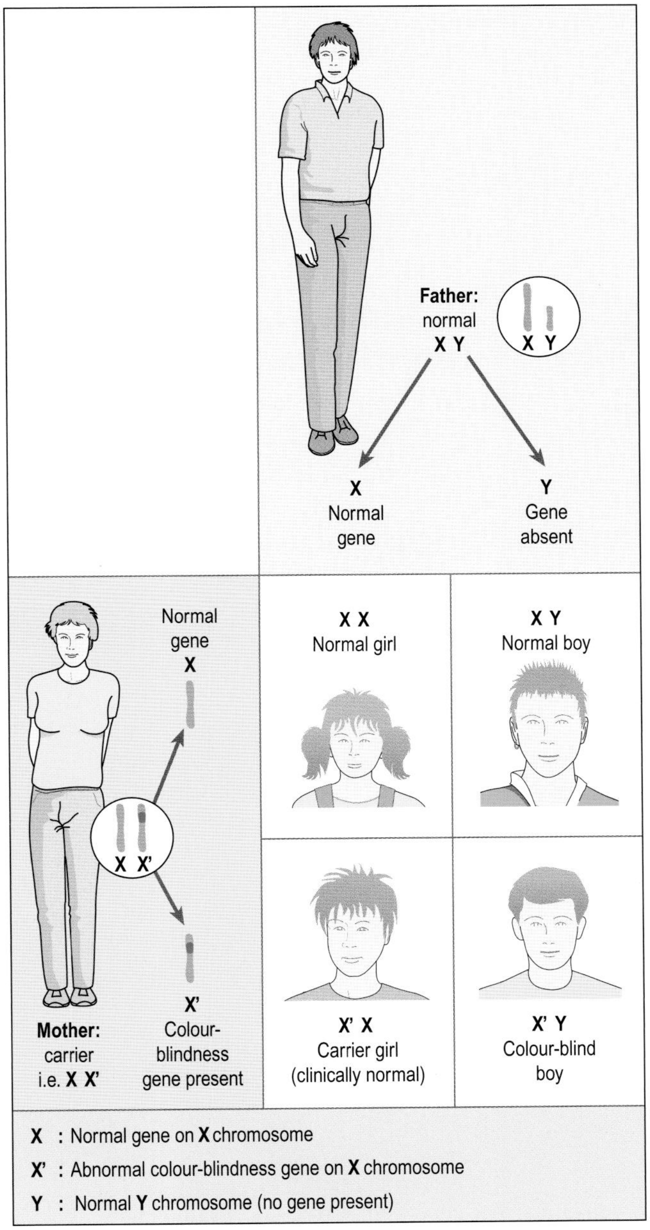

Figure 17.11 Inheritance of sex-linked red–green colour blindness gene between generations.

Ageing and genetics

Learning outcomes

At the end of this section, you should be able to:

- describe the main effects of ageing on the genetic material of cells
- outline the genetic mechanisms of senescence.

Ageing and DNA

Cumulative exposure over a lifetime to potential mutagens as well as a diminishing ability to repair DNA means the cell's genome gradually accumulates mutations, which can lead to diminished function and increased risk of disease, e.g. cancer. Mitochondrial DNA is more prone to mutations than nuclear DNA and as it ages and develops 'wear and tear' damage, it causes progressive impairment of cell function.

Cell senescence (ageing). The number of times a cell can divide is somewhere between 50 and 60 divisions. One important factor in this is thought to relate to the effects of ageing on telomerase function. Telomerase is the enzyme that repairs the telomeres (chromosome tips) following DNA replication. It declines in function with age. This restricts the number of cell replications possible, since without effective telomerase activity, the chromosomes become progressively shorter with each division and eventually become too short to be replicated and the cell can no longer divide.

Genetic basis of disease

Learning outcomes

After studying this section, you should be able to:

■ outline the link between cancer and cell mutation

■ distinguish between genetic disorders caused by gene mutation and chromosomal abnormalities, giving examples of each.

Cancer

Cancer (malignant growth of new tissue, p. 55) is caused by mutation (p. 440) of cellular DNA, causing its growth pattern to become disorganised and uncontrolled.

Inherited disease

Box 17.1 lists a number of diseases with an inherited component.

Gene mutations

Many diseases, such as cystic fibrosis (p. 266) and haemophilia (p. 79), are passed directly from parent to child via a faulty gene. Many of these genes have been located by mapping of the human genome, e.g. the gene for cystic fibrosis is carried on chromosome 7. Other diseases, e.g. asthma, some cancers and cardiovascular disease, have a genetic component (run in the family). In these cases, a single faulty gene has not been identified, and inheritance is not as predictable as when a single gene is responsible. The likelihood of an individual developing the disease depends not only on their genetic make-up, but also on the influence of other factors, such as lifestyle and environment.

Phenylketonuria

In this disorder, an example of an *inborn error of metabolism*, the gene responsible for producing the enzyme phenylalanine hydroxylase is faulty, and the enzyme is absent. This enzyme normally converts phenylalanine to tyrosine in the liver, but in its absence phenylalanine accumulates in the liver and overflows into the blood (Fig. 17.12). In high quantities, phenylalanine is toxic to the central nervous system and, if untreated, results in brain damage and mental retardation within a few

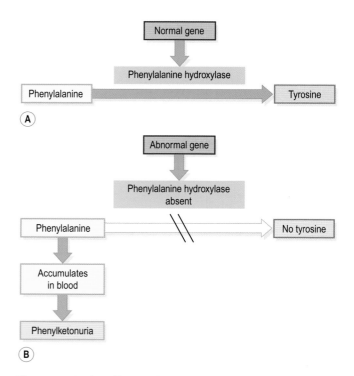

Figure 17.12 Phenylketonuria. A. Gene function normal. **B.** Abnormal gene.

Box 17.1 Some disorders with an inherited component

Single gene disorders
Phenylketonuria
Duchenne muscular dystrophy (p. 435)
Huntington disease
Haemophilia (p. 79)
Achondroplasia (p. 432)
Some cancers, including a proportion of breast, ovarian and bowel cancers
Myotonic dystrophy
Cystic fibrosis (p. 266)
Polycystic kidney disease (p. 354)

More complex inheritance: more than one gene likely to be involved, leading to increased susceptibility and 'running in families'. Lifestyle and other factors involved in determining risk.
Asthma (p. 264)
Cleft lip (p. 320)
Hypertension (p. 131)
Atheroma (p. 120)
Some cancers, e.g. breast and gastric cancer
Types I and II diabetes mellitus (p. 236)
Epilepsy
Schizophrenia
Neural tube defects, e.g. spina bifida (p. 188)

months. Because there are low levels of tyrosine, which is needed to make melanin, depigmentation occurs and affected children are fair skinned and blonde. The incidence of this disease is now low in developed countries because screening of newborn babies detects the condition and treatment is provided.

Mitochondrial abnormalities

Mitochondrial DNA contains only 37 genes but defects in these genes can cause inherited disorders with a very wide range of potentially fatal signs and symptoms, most commonly involving the CNS and skeletal or cardiac muscle. Spontaneous mutations in this DNA can also occur in maturity, leading to onset of disease in adults. There is evidence that mitochondrial mutations may be associated with some forms of important diseases, e.g. diabetes mellitus, Parkinson disease and Alzheimer disease.

Chromosomal abnormalities

Sometimes a fault during meiosis produces a gamete carrying abnormal chromosomes – too many, too few, abnormally shaped, or with segments missing. Often, these aberrations are lethal and a pregnancy involving such a gamete miscarries in the early stages. Non-lethal conditions include Down syndrome and cri-du-chat syndrome.

Down syndrome

In this disorder, there are three copies of chromosome 21 (trisomy 21), meaning that an extra chromosome is present, caused by failure of chromosomes to separate normally during meiosis. People with Down syndrome are usually short of stature, with pronounced eyelid folds and flat, round faces. The tongue may be too large for the mouth and habitually protrudes. Learning disability is present, ranging from mild to severe. Life expectancy is shorter than normal, with a higher than average incidence of cardiovascular and respiratory disease, and a high incidence of early dementia. Down syndrome is associated with increasing maternal age, especially over 35 years.

Cri-du-chat syndrome

Cri-du-chat (cat's cry) refers to the characteristic meowing cry of an affected child. This syndrome is caused when part of chromosome 5 is missing, and is associated with learning disabilities and anatomical abnormalities, including gastrointestinal and cardiovascular problems.

Abnormalities of the sex chromosomes

If the sex chromosomes fail to separate normally during meiosis, the daughter cells will have an incorrect number, either too many or too few. A child born with such an abnormality will not follow normal sexual development without treatment, and may have additional problems such as learning disability.

Turner syndrome. This is usually associated with having only one sex chromosome, an X, as well as 22 normal pairs of autosomes. The karyotype is therefore usually XO, and affected individuals are female. They have female external genitalia and ovaries, but are infertile because the ovaries fail to develop during fetal life, and secondary sexual characteristics do not develop at puberty unless oestrogen treatment is given. Other features include short stature and coarctation of the aorta (in 15%, p. 130). Intelligence is usually normal.

Klinefelter syndrome. The karyotype in this condition is XXY, so affected individuals are male, with 47 chromosomes instead of 46. This condition is commoner than Turner syndrome and is associated with a greater than average height and mild learning disability. The genitalia are male but the testes are underdeveloped and affected individuals are infertile. At puberty, development of feminine characteristics such as enlarged breasts (gynaecomastia) and rounded hips is common, and there is no development of male secondary sexual characteristics unless testosterone treatment is given.

For a range of self-assessment exercises on the topics in this chapter, visit Evolve online resources: https://evolve.elsevier.com/Waugh/anatomy/

The reproductive systems

ANIMATIONS

The ability to reproduce is one of the properties distinguishing living from non-living matter. The more primitive the animal, the simpler the process of reproduction. In mammals, including humans, the process is one of sexual reproduction, in which the male and female organs differ anatomically and physiologically, and the new individual develops from the fusion of two different sex cells (gametes).The male gametes are called *spermatozoa* and the female gametes are called *ova*.

The first sections of this chapter explain the structure and functions of the female and male reproductive systems, including the production of gametes. The next sections give a brief overview of fetal development, beginning with the fusion of two gametes (fertilisation), and the effects of ageing on reproductive function. Finally, some significant reproductive disorders are described.

Female reproductive system

Learning outcomes

After studying this section, you should be able to:

- describe the main structures of the external genitalia

- explain the structure and function of the vagina

- describe the location, structure and function of the uterus and the uterine tubes

- discuss the process of ovulation and the hormones that control it

- outline the changes that occur in the female at puberty, including the physiology of menstruation

- describe the structure and function of the female breast.

The functions of the female reproductive system are:
- formation of ova
- reception of spermatozoa
- provision of suitable environments for fertilisation and fetal development
- parturition (childbirth)
- lactation, the production of breast milk, which provides complete nourishment for the baby in its early life.

The female reproductive organs, or genitalia, include both external and internal organs (Fig. 18.1).

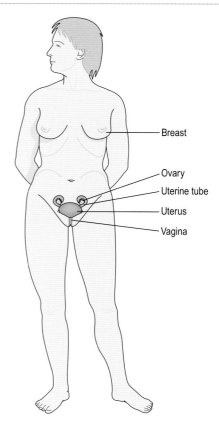

Figure 18.1 The female reproductive organs. Faint lines indicate the positions of the lower ribs and the pelvis.

External genitalia (vulva) 18.1

The external genitalia (Fig. 18.2) are known collectively as the vulva, and consist of the labia majora and labia minora, the clitoris, the vaginal orifice, the vestibule, the hymen and the vestibular glands (Bartholin's glands).

Labia majora
These are the two large folds forming the boundary of the vulva. They are composed of skin, fibrous tissue and fat and contain large numbers of sebaceous and eccrine sweat glands. Anteriorly the folds join in front of the symphysis pubis, and posteriorly they merge with the skin of the perineum. At puberty, hair grows on the mons pubis and on the lateral surfaces of the labia majora.

Labia minora
These are two smaller folds of skin between the labia majora, containing numerous sebaceous and eccrine sweat glands.

The cleft between the labia minora is the *vestibule*. The vagina, urethra and ducts of the greater vestibular glands open into the vestibule.

Clitoris

The clitoris corresponds to the penis in the male and contains sensory nerve endings and erectile tissue.

Vestibular glands 18.2

The vestibular glands (Bartholin's glands) are situated one on each side near the vaginal opening. They are about the size of a small pea and their ducts open into the vestibule immediately lateral to the attachment of the hymen. They secrete mucus that keeps the vulva moist.

Blood supply, lymph drainage and nerve supply

Arterial supply. This is by branches from the internal pudendal arteries that branch from the internal iliac arteries and by external pudendal arteries that branch from the femoral arteries.

Venous drainage. This forms a large plexus which eventually drains into the internal iliac veins.

Lymph drainage. This is through the superficial inguinal nodes.

Nerve supply. This is by branches from pudendal nerves.

Perineum

The perineum is a roughly triangular area extending from the base of the labia minora to the anal canal. It consists of connective tissue, muscle and fat. It gives attachment to the muscles of the pelvic floor (p. 427).

Internal genitalia

The internal organs of the female reproductive system (Figs 18.3 and 18.4) lie in the pelvic cavity and consist of the vagina, uterus, two uterine tubes and two ovaries.

Vagina 18.3

The vagina is a fibromuscular tube lined with stratified squamous epithelium (Fig. 3.39) opening into the vestibule at its distal end, and with the uterine cervix protruding into its proximal end. It runs obliquely upwards and backwards at an angle of about 45° between the bladder in front and rectum and anus behind. In the adult, the anterior wall is about 7.5 cm long and the posterior wall about 9 cm long. The difference is due to the angle of insertion of the cervix through the anterior wall.

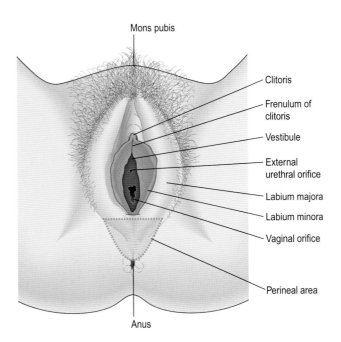

Figure 18.2 The external genitalia of the female.

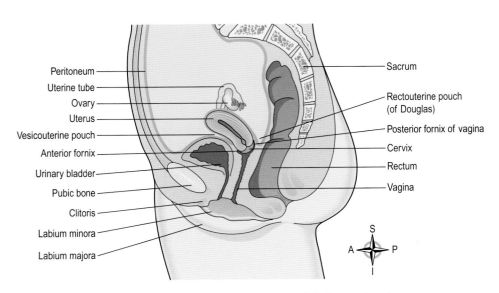

Figure 18.3 Lateral view of the female reproductive organs in the pelvis and their associated structures.

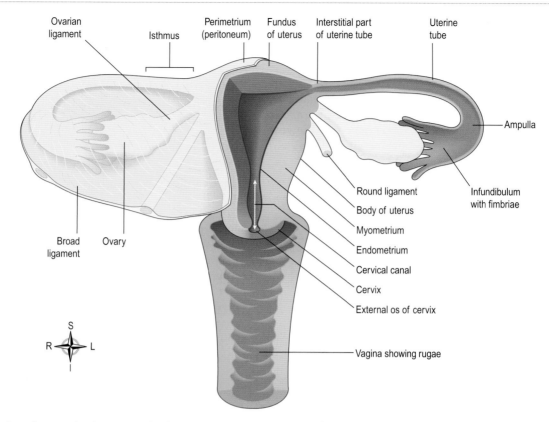

Figure 18.4 The female reproductive organs in the pelvis.

Hymen. The hymen is a thin layer of mucous membrane that partially occludes the opening of the vagina. It is normally incomplete to allow for passage of menstrual flow and is stretched or completely torn away by sexual intercourse, insertion of a tampon or childbirth.

Structure of the vagina

The vaginal wall has three layers: an outer covering of areolar tissue, a middle layer of smooth muscle and an inner lining of stratified squamous epithelium that forms ridges or *rugae*. It has no secretory glands but the surface is kept moist by cervical secretions. Between puberty and the menopause, *Lactobacillus acidophilus*, bacteria that secrete lactic acid, are normally present maintaining the pH between 4.9 and 3.5. The acidity inhibits the growth of most other micro-organisms that may enter the vagina from the perineum or during sexual intercourse.

Blood supply, lymph drainage and nerve supply
Arterial supply. An arterial plexus is formed round the vagina, derived from the uterine and vaginal arteries, which are branches of the internal iliac arteries.

Venous drainage. A venous plexus, situated in the muscular wall, drains into the internal iliac veins.

Lymph drainage. This is through the deep and superficial iliac glands.

Nerve supply. This consists of parasympathetic fibres from the sacral outflow, sympathetic fibres from the lumbar outflow and somatic sensory fibres from the pudendal nerves.

Functions of the vagina

The vagina acts as the receptacle for the penis during sexual intercourse (coitus), and provides an elastic passageway through which the baby passes during childbirth.

Uterus

The uterus is a hollow muscular pear-shaped organ, flattened anteroposteriorly. It lies in the pelvic cavity between the urinary bladder and the rectum (Fig. 18.3).

In most women, it leans forward (*anteversion*), and is bent forward (*anteflexion*) almost at right angles to the vagina, so that its anterior wall rests partly against the bladder below, forming the vesicouterine pouch between the two organs.

When the body is upright, the uterus lies in an almost horizontal position. It is about 7.5 cm long, 5 cm wide and its walls are about 2.5 cm thick. It weighs between 30 and 40 grams. The parts of the uterus are the fundus, body and cervix (Fig. 18.4).

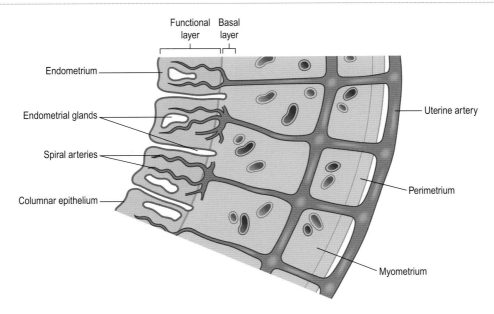

Figure 18.5 Layers of the uterine wall. Green line shows boundary between the functional and basal layers of the endometrium.

Fundus. This is the dome-shaped part of the uterus above the openings of the uterine tubes.

Body. This is the main part. It is narrowest inferiorly at the *internal os* where it is continuous with the cervix.

Cervix ('neck' of the uterus). This protrudes through the anterior wall of the vagina, opening into it at the *external os*.

Structure

The walls of the uterus are composed of three layers of tissue: perimetrium, myometrium and endometrium (Fig. 18.5).

Perimetrium. This is peritoneum, which is distributed differently on the various surfaces of the uterus (Fig. 18.4).

Anteriorly it lies over the fundus and the body where it is folded on to the upper surface of the urinary bladder. This fold of peritoneum forms the *vesicouterine pouch*.

Posteriorly the peritoneum covers the fundus, the body and the cervix, then it folds back on to the rectum to form the *rectouterine pouch* (of Douglas).

Laterally, only the fundus is covered because the peritoneum forms a double fold with the uterine tubes in the upper free border. This double fold is the *broad ligament*, which, at its lateral ends, attaches the uterus to the sides of the pelvis.

Myometrium. This is the thickest layer of tissue in the uterine wall. It is a mass of smooth muscle fibres interlaced with areolar tissue, blood vessels and nerves.

Endometrium. This consists of columnar epithelium covering a layer of connective tissue containing a large number of mucus-secreting tubular glands. It is richly

supplied with blood by *spiral arteries*, branches of the uterine artery. It is divided functionally into two layers:

- The *functional layer* is the upper layer and it thickens and becomes rich in blood vessels in the first half of the menstrual cycle. If the ovum is not fertilised and does not implant, this layer is shed during menstruation.
- The *basal layer* lies next to the myometrium, and is not lost during menstruation. It is the layer from which the fresh functional layer is regenerated during each cycle.

The upper two-thirds of the cervical canal is lined with this mucous membrane. Lower down, however, the mucosa changes, becoming stratified squamous epithelium, which is continuous with the lining of the vagina itself.

Blood supply, lymph drainage and nerve supply

Arterial supply. This is by the uterine arteries, branches of the internal iliac arteries. They pass up the lateral aspects of the uterus between the two layers of the broad ligaments. They supply the uterus and uterine tubes and join with the ovarian arteries to supply the ovaries.

Venous drainage. The veins follow the same route as the arteries and eventually drain into the internal iliac veins.

Lymph drainage. Deep and superficial lymph vessels drain lymph from the uterus and the uterine tubes to the aortic lymph nodes and groups of nodes associated with the iliac blood vessels.

Nerve supply. The nerves supplying the uterus and the uterine tubes consist of parasympathetic fibres from the

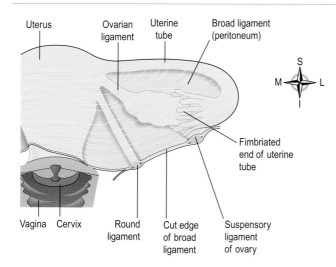

Figure 18.6 The main ligaments supporting the uterus. Left side.

sacral outflow and sympathetic fibres from the lumbar outflow.

Supporting structures

The uterus is supported in the pelvic cavity by surrounding organs, muscles of the pelvic floor and ligaments that suspend it from the walls of the pelvis (Fig. 18.6).

Broad ligaments. These are formed by a double fold of peritoneum, one on each side of the uterus. They hang down from the uterine tubes as though draped over them and at their lateral ends they are attached to the sides of the pelvis. The uterine tubes are enclosed in the upper free border and near the lateral ends they penetrate the posterior wall of the broad ligament and open into the peritoneal cavity. The ovaries are attached to the posterior wall, one on each side. Blood and lymph vessels and nerves pass to the uterus and uterine tubes between the layers of the broad ligaments.

Round ligaments. These are bands of fibrous tissue between the two layers of broad ligament, one on each side of the uterus. They pass to the sides of the pelvis then through the *inguinal canal* to end by fusing with the labia majora.

Uterosacral ligaments. These originate from the posterior walls of the cervix and vagina and extend backwards, one on each side of the rectum, to the sacrum.

Transverse cervical (cardinal) ligaments. These extend one from each side of the cervix and vagina to the side walls of the pelvis.

Pubocervical fascia. This extends forward from the transverse cervical ligaments on each side of the bladder and is attached to the posterior surface of the pubic bones.

Functions of the uterus

After puberty, the endometrium goes through a regular monthly cycle of changes, the *menstrual cycle*, under the control of hypothalamic and anterior pituitary hormones (see Ch. 9). The menstrual cycle prepares the uterus to receive, nourish and protect a fertilised ovum. The cycle is usually regular, lasting between 26 and 30 days. If the ovum is not fertilised, the functional uterine lining is shed, and a new cycle begins with a short period of vaginal bleeding (menstruation).

If the ovum is fertilised the zygote embeds itself in the uterine wall. The uterine muscle grows to accommodate the developing baby, which is called an *embryo* during its first 8 weeks, and a *fetus* for the remainder of the pregnancy. Uterine secretions nourish the ovum before it implants in the endometrium, and after implantation the rapidly expanding ball of cells is nourished by the endometrial cells themselves. This is sufficient for only the first few weeks and the *placenta* takes over thereafter (see Ch. 5). The placenta, which is attached to the fetus by the umbilical cord, is also firmly attached to the wall of the uterus, and provides the route by which the growing baby receives oxygen and nutrients, and gets rid of its wastes. The placenta also has an important endocrine function during pregnancy. It secretes high levels of progesterone, which prevents the muscular uterine walls from contracting in response to the progressive uterine stretching as the fetus grows. At term (the end of pregnancy) the hormone oestrogen, which increases uterine contractility, becomes the predominant sex hormone in the blood. Additionally, oxytocin is released from the posterior pituitary, and also stimulates contraction of the uterine muscle. Control of oxytocin release is by positive feedback (see also Fig. 9.5). During labour, the uterus forcefully expels the baby with powerful rhythmical contractions.

Uterine tubes

The uterine (Fallopian) tubes (Fig. 18.4) are about 10 cm long and extend from the sides of the uterus between the body and the fundus. They lie in the upper free border of the broad ligament and their trumpet-shaped lateral ends penetrate the posterior wall, opening into the peritoneal cavity close to the ovaries. The end of each tube has fingerlike projections called *fimbriae*. The longest of these is the *ovarian fimbria*, which is in close association with the ovary.

Structure

The uterine tubes are covered with peritoneum (broad ligament), have a middle layer of smooth muscle and are lined with ciliated epithelium. Blood and nerve supply and lymphatic drainage are as for the uterus.

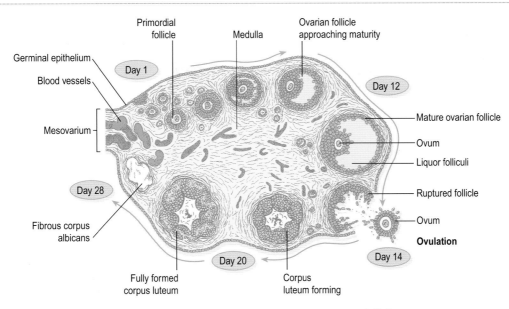

Germinal epithelium

Blood vessels

Mesovarium

Primordial follicle

Medulla

Day 1

Ovarian follicle approaching maturity

Day 12

Mature ovarian follicle

Ovum

Liquor folliculi

Ruptured follicle

Ovum

Ovulation

Day 28

Fibrous corpus albicans

Day 20

Fully formed corpus luteum

Corpus luteum forming

Day 14

Figure 18.7 A section of an ovary showing the stages of development of one ovarian follicle.

Functions

The uterine tubes propel the ovum from the ovary to the uterus by peristalsis and ciliary movement. The secretions of the uterine tube nourish both ovum and spermatozoa. Fertilisation of the ovum usually takes place in the uterine tube, and the zygote is propelled into the uterus for implantation.

Ovaries 18.4

The ovaries (Fig. 18.4) are the female gonads (glands producing sex hormones and the ova), and they lie in a shallow fossa on the lateral walls of the pelvis. They are 2.5–3.5 cm long, 2 cm wide and 1 cm thick. Each is attached to the upper part of the uterus by the ovarian ligament and to the back of the broad ligament by a broad band of tissue, the *mesovarium*. Blood vessels and nerves pass to the ovary through the mesovarium (Fig. 18.7).

Structure

The ovaries have two layers of tissue.

Medulla. This lies in the centre and consists of fibrous tissue, blood vessels and nerves.

Cortex. This surrounds the medulla. It has a framework of connective tissue, or *stroma*, covered by *germinal epithelium*. It contains *ovarian follicles* in various stages of maturity, each of which contains an ovum. Before puberty the ovaries are inactive but the stroma already contains immature (primordial) follicles, which the female has from birth. During the childbearing years, about every 28 days, one or more ovarian follicle (Graafian follicle) matures, ruptures and releases its ovum into the

peritoneal cavity. This is called *ovulation* and it occurs during most menstrual cycles (Figs 18.7 and 18.8). Following ovulation, the ruptured follicle develops into the corpus luteum (meaning 'yellow body'), which in turn will leave a small permanent scar of fibrous tissue called the corpus albicans (meaning 'white body') on the surface of the ovary.

Blood supply, lymph drainage and nerve supply

Arterial supply. This is by the ovarian arteries, which branch from the abdominal aorta just below the renal arteries.

Venous drainage. This is into a plexus of veins behind the uterus from which the ovarian veins arise. The right ovarian vein opens into the inferior vena cava and the left into the left renal vein.

Lymph drainage. This is to the lateral aortic and preaortic lymph nodes. The lymph vessels follow the same route as the arteries.

Nerve supply. The ovaries are supplied by parasympathetic nerves from the sacral outflow and sympathetic nerves from the lumbar outflow.

Functions

The ovary is the organ in which the female gametes are stored and develop prior to ovulation. Their maturation is controlled by the hypothalamus and the anterior pituitary gland, which releases gonadotrophins (follicle stimulating hormone, FSH, and luteinising hormone, LH), both of which act on the ovary. In addition, the ovary has endocrine functions, and releases hormones essential to the physiological changes during the reproductive cycle.

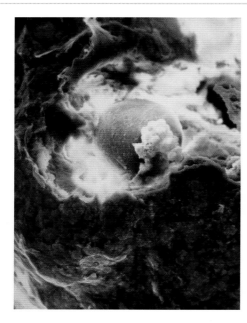

Figure 18.8 The moment of ovulation: scanning electron micrograph of an ovum (pink) emerging through the surface of the ovary (brown).

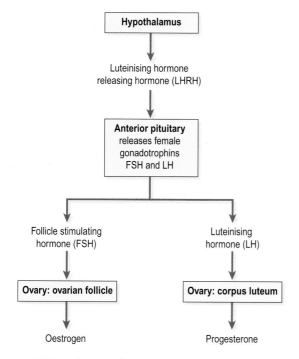

Figure 18.9 Female reproductive hormones and target tissues.

The source of these hormones, oestrogen, progesterone and inhibin, is the follicle itself. During the first half of the cycle, while the ovum is developing within the follicle, the follicle secretes increasing amounts of oestrogen. However, after ovulation, the corpus luteum secretes primarily progesterone, with some oestrogen and inhibin (Fig 18.9). The significance of this is discussed under the menstrual cycle (see below).

Puberty in the female

Puberty is the age at which the internal reproductive organs reach maturity, usually between the ages of 12 and 14. This is called the menarche, and marks the beginning of the childbearing period. The ovaries are stimulated by the gonadotrophins from the anterior pituitary: follicle stimulating hormone and luteinising hormone.

A number of physical and psychological changes take place at puberty:

- the uterus, the uterine tubes and the ovaries reach maturity
- the menstrual cycle and ovulation begin (menarche)
- the breasts develop and enlarge
- pubic and axillary hair begins to grow
- increase in height and widening of the pelvis
- increased fat deposited in the subcutaneous tissue, especially at the hips and breasts.

The reproductive cycle

This is a series of events, occurring regularly in females every 26 to 30 days throughout the childbearing period between menarche and menopause (Fig. 18.10). The cycle consists of a series of changes taking place concurrently in the ovaries and uterine lining, stimulated by changes in blood concentrations of hormones (Fig. 18.10B and D). Hormones secreted during the cycle are regulated by negative feedback mechanisms.

The hypothalamus secretes luteinising hormone releasing hormone (LHRH), which stimulates the anterior pituitary to secrete (see Table 9.1):

- follicle stimulating hormone (FSH), which promotes the maturation of ovarian follicles and the secretion of oestrogen, leading to ovulation. FSH is therefore predominantly active in the first half of the cycle. Its secretion is suppressed once ovulation has taken place, to prevent other follicles maturing during the current cycle
- luteinising hormone (LH), which triggers ovulation, stimulates the development of the corpus luteum and the secretion of progesterone.

The hypothalamus responds to changes in the blood levels of oestrogen and progesterone. It is stimulated by high levels of oestrogen alone (as happens in the first half of the cycle) but suppressed by oestrogen and progesterone together (as happens in the second half of the cycle).

The average length of the cycle is about 28 days. By convention the days of the cycle are numbered from the beginning of the *menstrual phase*, which usually lasts about 4 days. This is followed by the *proliferative phase* (approximately 10 days), then by the *secretory phase* (about 14 days).

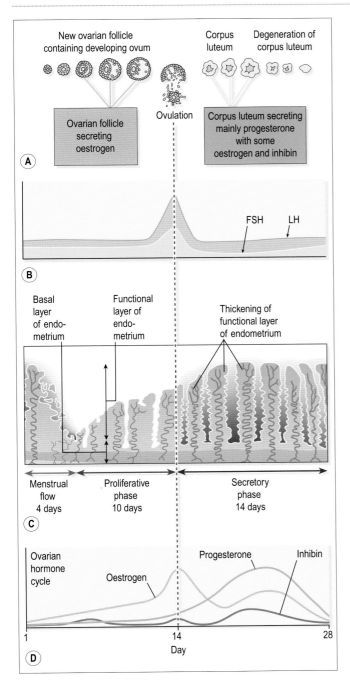

Figure 18.10 Summary of one female reproductive cycle.
A. Ovarian cycle; maturation of follicle and development of corpus luteum. **B.** Anterior pituitary cycle; LH and FSH levels. **C.** Uterine cycle; menstrual, proliferative and secretory phases. **D.** Ovarian hormone cycle; oestrogen, progesterone and inhibin levels.

Menstrual phase

When the ovum is not fertilised, the corpus luteum starts to degenerate. (In the event of pregnancy, the corpus luteum is supported by human chorionic gonadotrophin [hCG] secreted by the developing embryo.) Progesterone and oestrogen levels therefore fall, and the functional layer of the endometrium, which is dependent on high levels of these ovarian hormones, is shed in menstruation (Fig. 18.10C). The menstrual flow consists of the secretions from endometrial glands, endometrial cells, blood from the degenerating capillaries and the unfertilised ovum.

During the menstrual phase, levels of oestrogen and progesterone are very low because the corpus luteum that had been active during the second half of the previous cycle has degenerated. This means the hypothalamus and anterior pituitary can resume their cyclical activity, and levels of FSH begin to rise, initiating a new cycle.

Proliferative phase

At this stage an ovarian follicle, stimulated by FSH, is growing towards maturity and is producing oestrogen, which stimulates proliferation of the functional layer of the endometrium in preparation for the reception of a fertilised ovum. The endometrium thickens, becoming very vascular and rich in mucus-secreting glands. Rising levels of oestrogen are responsible for triggering a surge of LH approximately mid-cycle. This LH surge triggers ovulation, marking the end of the proliferative phase.

Secretory phase

After ovulation, LH from the anterior pituitary stimulates development of the corpus luteum from the ruptured follicle, which produces progesterone, some oestrogen, and inhibin. Under the influence of progesterone, the endometrium becomes oedematous and the secretory glands produce increased amounts of watery mucus. This assists the passage of the spermatozoa through the uterus to the uterine tubes where the ovum is usually fertilised. There is a similar increase in secretion of watery mucus by the glands of the uterine tubes and by cervical glands that lubricate the vagina.

The ovum may survive in a fertilisable form for a very short time after ovulation, probably as little as 8 hours. The spermatozoa, deposited in the vagina during intercourse, may be capable of fertilising the ovum for only about 24 hours although they can survive for several days. This means that the period in each cycle during which fertilisation can occur is relatively short. Observable changes in the woman's body occur around the time of ovulation. Cervical mucus, normally thick and dry, becomes thin, elastic and watery, and body temperature rises by about 1°C immediately following ovulation. Some women experience abdominal discomfort in the middle of the cycle, thought to correspond to rupture of the follicle and release of its contents into the abdominal cavity.

After ovulation, the combination of progesterone, oestrogen and inhibin from the corpus luteum suppresses the hypothalamus and anterior pituitary, so FSH and LH levels fall. Low FSH levels in the second half of the cycle prevent further follicular development in case a pregnancy results from the current cycle. If the ovum is not

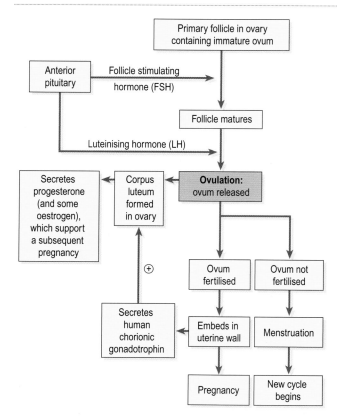

Figure 18.11 Summary of the stages of development of the ovum and the associated hormones.

fertilised, falling LH levels leads to degeneration and death of the corpus luteum, which is dependent on LH for survival. The resultant steady decline in circulating oestrogen, progesterone and inhibin leads to degeneration of the uterine lining and menstruation, with the initiation of a new cycle.

If the ovum is fertilised there is no breakdown of the endometrium and no menstruation. The fertilised ovum (zygote) travels through the uterine tube to the uterus where it becomes embedded in the wall and produces human chorionic gonadotrophin (hCG), which is similar to anterior pituitary luteinising hormone. This hormone keeps the corpus luteum intact, enabling it to continue secreting progesterone and oestrogen for the first 3–4 months of the pregnancy, inhibiting the maturation of further ovarian follicles (Figure 18.11). During that time the placenta develops and produces oestrogen, progesterone and gonadotrophins. ▪ **18.5, 18.6**

This is summarised in Figure 18.11. Box 18.1 summarises the reproductive functions of oestrogen and progesterone.

Menopause

The menopause (climacteric) usually occurs between the ages of 45 and 55 years, marking the end of the childbearing period. It may occur suddenly or over a period of years, sometimes as long as 10 years, and is caused by a progressive reduction in oestrogen levels, as the number of functional follicles in the ovaries declines with age. The ovaries gradually become less responsive to FSH and LH, and ovulation and the menstrual cycle become irregular, eventually ceasing. Several other phenomena may occur at the same time, including:

- short-term unpredictable vasodilation with flushing, sweating and palpitations, causing discomfort and disturbance of the normal sleep pattern
- shrinkage of the breasts
- axillary and pubic hair become sparse
- atrophy of the sex organs
- episodes of uncharacteristic behaviour, e.g. irritability, mood changes
- gradual thinning of the skin
- loss of bone mass predisposing to osteoporosis (p. 431)
- slow increase in blood cholesterol levels that increase the risk of cardiovascular disease in postmenopausal women to that in males of the same age.

Similar changes occur after bilateral irradiation or surgical removal of the ovaries.

Breasts ▪ 18.7

The breasts or *mammary glands* are accessory glands of the female reproductive system. They exist also in the male, but in only a rudimentary form.

Structure

The mammary glands or breasts (Fig 18.12) consist of varying amounts of glandular tissue, responsible for milk

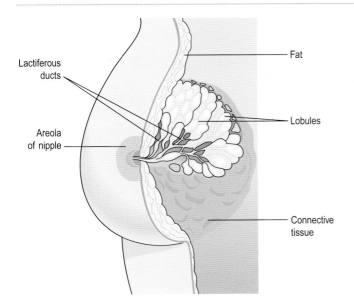

Lactiferous ducts

Fat

Areola of nipple

Lobules

Connective tissue

Figure 18.12 Structure of the breast.

production, supported by fatty tissue and fibrous connective tissue that anchor the breast to the chest wall.

Each breast contains about 20 *lobes*, each of which contains a number of glandular structures called *lobules*, where milk is produced. Lobules open into tiny *lactiferous ducts*, which drain milk towards the nipple. Supporting fatty and connective tissues run through the breast, surrounding the lobules, and the breast itself is covered in subcutaneous fat. In the lactating breast, glandular tissue proliferates (hyperplasia, Fig. 3.41) to support milk production, and recedes again after lactation stops.

The nipple. This is a small conical eminence at the centre of the breast surrounded by a pigmented area, the *areola*. On the surface of the areola are numerous sebaceous glands (Montgomery's tubercles), which lubricate the nipple during lactation.

Blood supply, lymph drainage and nerve supply

Arterial supply. The breasts are supplied with blood from the thoracic branches of the axillary arteries and from the internal mammary and intercostal arteries.

Venous drainage. This is formed by an anastomotic circle round the base of the nipple from which branches carry the venous blood to the circumference, and end in the axillary and mammary veins.

Lymph drainage. (see Fig. 6.1). This is mainly into the superficial axillary lymph vessels and nodes. Lymph may drain through the internal mammary nodes if the superficial route is obstructed.

Nerve supply. The breasts are supplied by branches from the 4th, 5th and 6th thoracic nerves, which contain sympathetic fibres. There are numerous somatic sensory nerve endings in the breast, especially around the nipple.

When these touch receptors are stimulated by sucking, impulses pass to the hypothalamus and secretion of the hormone oxytocin is increased, promoting the release of milk.

Functions

In the female, the breasts are small and immature until puberty. Thereafter they grow and develop under the influence of oestrogen and progesterone. During pregnancy these hormones stimulate further growth. After the baby is born the hormone *prolactin* (p. 219) from the anterior pituitary stimulates the production of milk, and *oxytocin* (p. 220) from the posterior pituitary stimulates the release of milk in response to the stimulation of the nipple by the sucking baby, by a positive feedback mechanism.

Male reproductive system

Learning outcomes

After studying this section, you should be able to:

- describe the structure and function of the testes

- outline the structure and function of the spermatic cords

- describe the secretions that pass into the spermatic fluid

- explain the process of ejaculation

- list the main changes occurring at puberty in the male.

The male reproductive system is shown in Figure 18.13. The functions of the male reproductive organs are:

- production, maturation and storage of spermatozoa
- delivery of spermatozoa in *semen* into the female reproductive tract.

The urethra is also the passageway for urine excretion.

Scrotum

The scrotum is a pouch of pigmented skin, fibrous and connective tissue and smooth muscle. It is divided into two compartments, each of which contains one testis, one epididymis and the testicular end of a spermatic cord. It lies below the symphysis pubis, in front of the upper parts of the thighs and behind the penis.

Testes 18.8

The testes (Fig. 18.14A and B) are the male reproductive glands and are the equivalent of the ovaries in the female.

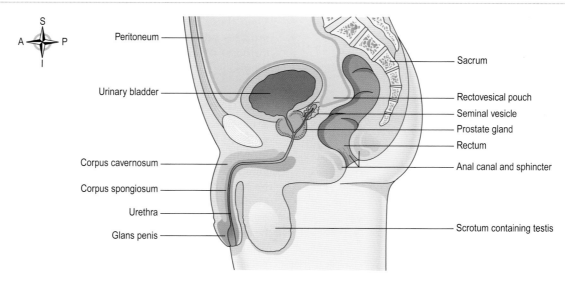

Figure 18.13 The male reproductive organs and their associated structures.

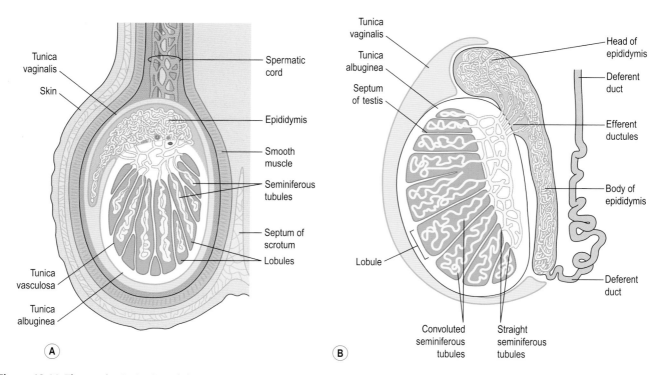

Figure 18.14 The testis. A. Section of the testis and its coverings. **B.** Longitudinal section of a testis and deferent duct.

They are about 4.5 cm long, 2.5 cm wide and 3 cm thick and are suspended in the scrotum by the spermatic cords. They are surrounded by three layers of tissue.

Tunica vaginalis. This is a double membrane, forming the outer covering of the testes, and is a downgrowth of the abdominal and pelvic peritoneum. During early fetal life, the testes develop in the lumbar region of the abdominal cavity just below the kidneys. They then descend into the scrotum, taking with them coverings of peritoneum, blood and lymph vessels, nerves and the deferent duct.

The peritoneum eventually surrounds the testes in the scrotum, and becomes detached from the abdominal peritoneum. Descent of the testes into the scrotum should be complete by the 8th month of fetal life.

Tunica albuginea. This is a fibrous covering beneath the tunica vaginalis. Ingrowths form septa, dividing the glandular structure of the testes into *lobules*.

Tunica vasculosa. This consists of a network of capillaries supported by delicate connective tissue.

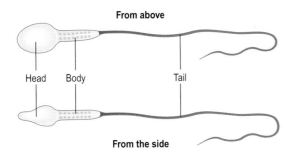

Figure 18.15 A spermatozoon.

From above

Head Body Tail

From the side

Structure

In each testis are 200–300 lobules, and within each lobule are 1–4 convoluted loops of *germinal epithelial cells*, called *seminiferous tubules*. Between the tubules are groups of *interstitial cells (of Leydig)* that secrete the hormone testosterone after puberty. At the upper pole of the testis the tubules combine to form a single tubule. This tubule, about 6 m in its full length, is repeatedly folded and tightly packed into a mass called the epididymis. It leaves the scrotum as the *deferent duct* (vas deferens) in the spermatic cord. Blood and lymph vessels pass to the testes in the *spermatic cords*.

Functions

Spermatozoa (sperm) are produced in the seminiferous tubules of the testes, and mature as they pass through the long and convoluted epididymis, where they are stored. FSH from the anterior pituitary (p. 220) stimulates sperm production. A mature sperm (Fig. 18.15) has a head, a body, and a long whip-like tail used for motility. The head is almost completely filled by the nucleus, containing its DNA. It also contains the enzymes required to penetrate the outer layers of the ovum to reach, and fuse with, its nucleus. The body of the sperm is packed with mitochondria, to fuel the propelling action of the tail that powers the sperm along the female reproductive tract.

Successful spermatogenesis takes place at a temperature about 3°C below normal body temperature. The testes are cooled by their position outside the abdominal cavity, and the thin outer covering of the scrotum has very little insulating fat. ▮ **18.9**

Unlike females, who produce no new gametes after birth, sperm production in males begins at puberty and continues throughout life, often into old age, under the influence of testosterone.

Spermatic cords

The spermatic cords suspend the testes in the scrotum. Each cord contains a testicular artery, testicular veins, lymphatics, a deferent duct and testicular nerves, which come together to form the cord from their various origins in the abdomen. The cord, which is covered in a sheath

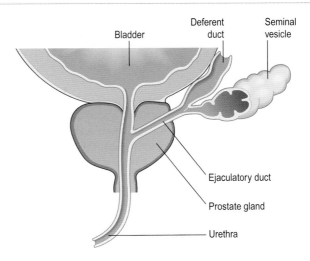

Bladder Deferent duct Seminal vesicle

Ejaculatory duct

Prostate gland

Urethra

Figure 18.16 Section of the prostate gland and associated reproductive structures on one side.

of smooth muscle and connective and fibrous tissues, extends through the inguinal canal (p. 427) and is attached to the testis on the posterior wall.

Blood supply, lymph drainage and nerve supply
Arterial supply. The testicular artery branches from the abdominal aorta, just below the renal arteries.

Venous drainage. The testicular vein passes into the abdominal cavity. The left vein opens into the left renal vein and the right into the inferior vena cava.

Lymph drainage. This is through lymph nodes around the aorta.

Nerve supply. This is provided by branches from the 10th and 11th thoracic nerves.

The deferent duct
This is some 45 cm long. It passes upwards from the testis through the inguinal canal and ascends medially towards the posterior wall of the bladder where it is joined by the duct from the seminal vesicle to form the *ejaculatory duct* (Fig. 18.16).

Seminal vesicles ▮ **18.10**

The seminal vesicles are two small fibromuscular pouches, 5 cm long, lined with columnar epithelium and lying on the posterior aspect of the bladder (Fig. 18.16).

At its lower end each seminal vesicle opens into a short duct, which joins with the corresponding deferent duct to form an ejaculatory duct.

Functions

The seminal vesicles contract and expel their stored contents, seminal fluid, during ejaculation. Seminal fluid, which forms 60% of the volume of semen, is alkaline to protect the sperm in the acidic environment of the vagina, and contains fructose to fuel the sperm during their journey through the female reproductive tract.

Ejaculatory ducts

The ejaculatory ducts are two tubes about 2 cm long, each formed by the union of the duct from a seminal vesicle and a deferent duct. They pass through the prostate gland and join the prostatic urethra, carrying seminal fluid and spermatozoa to the urethra (Fig. 18.16).

The walls of the ejaculatory ducts are composed of the same layers of tissue as the seminal vesicles.

Prostate gland

The prostate gland (Fig. 18.16) lies in the pelvic cavity in front of the rectum and behind the symphysis pubis, completely surrounding the urethra as it emerges from the bladder. It has an outer fibrous covering, enclosing glandular tissue wrapped in smooth muscle. The gland weighs about 8 g in youth, but progressively enlarges (hypertrophies) with age and is likely to weigh about 40 g by the age of 50.

Functions

The prostate gland secretes a thin, milky fluid that makes up about 30% of the volume of semen, and gives it its milky appearance. It contains a clotting enzyme, which thickens the semen in the vagina, increasing the likelihood of semen being retained close to the cervix.

Urethra and penis 📽 18.11

Urethra

The male urethra provides a common pathway for the flow of urine and semen. It is about 19–20 cm long and consists of three parts. The *prostatic urethra* originates at the urethral orifice of the bladder and passes through the prostate gland. The *membranous urethra* is the shortest and narrowest part and extends from the prostate gland to the bulb of the penis, after passing through the perineal membrane. The *spongiose* or *penile urethra* lies within the corpus spongiosum of the penis and terminates at the external urethral orifice in the *glans penis*.

There are two urethral sphincters (Fig. 18.17). The *internal sphincter* is a ring of smooth muscle at the neck of the bladder above the prostate gland. The *external sphincter* is a ring of skeletal muscle surrounding the membranous part.

Penis 📽 18.12

The penis (Fig. 18.17) has a *root* and a *shaft*. The root anchors the penis in the perineum and the shaft (*body*) is

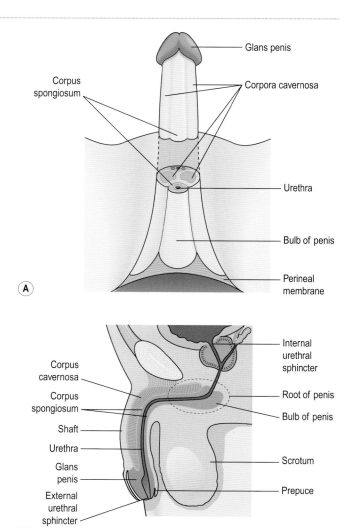

Figure 18.17 The penis. A. Viewed from below. **B.** Viewed from the side.

the externally visible, moveable portion of the organ. It is formed by three cylindrical masses of *erectile tissue* and smooth muscle. The erectile tissue is supported by fibrous tissue and covered with skin and has a rich blood supply.

The two lateral columns are called the *corpora cavernosa* and the column between them, containing the urethra, is the *corpus spongiosum* (Fig. 18.18A). At its tip it is expanded into a triangular structure known as the *glans penis*. Just above the glans the skin is folded upon itself and forms a movable double layer, the *foreskin* or *prepuce*. Arterial blood is supplied by deep, dorsal and bulbar arteries of the penis, which are branches from the internal pudendal arteries. A series of veins drain blood to the internal pudendal and internal iliac veins. The penis is supplied by autonomic and somatic nerves. Parasympathetic stimulation leads to filling of the spongy erectile tissue (Fig. 18.18B) with blood, caused by arteriolar dilation and venoconstriction, which increases blood flow into the penis

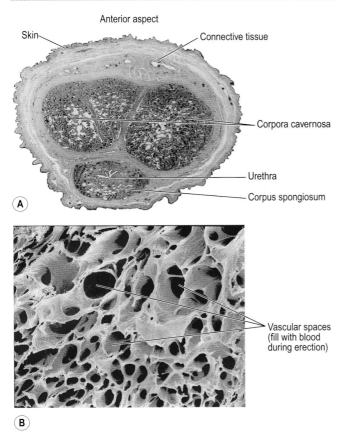

Anterior aspect

Skin

Connective tissue

Corpora cavernosa

Urethra

Corpus spongiosum

Ⓐ

Vascular spaces
(fill with blood
during erection)

Ⓑ

Figure 18.18 The penis. A. Transverse section (light micrograph).
B. Erectile tissue (scanning electron micrograph).

and obstructs outflow. The penis therefore becomes engorged and erect, essential for sexual intercourse.

Ejaculation

During ejaculation, which occurs at male orgasm, spermatozoa are expelled from the epididymis and pass through the deferent duct, the ejaculatory duct and the urethra. The semen is propelled by powerful rhythmical contraction of the smooth muscle in the walls of the deferent duct; the muscular contractions are sympathetically mediated. Muscle in the walls of the seminal vesicles and prostate gland also contracts, adding their contents to the fluid passing through the genital ducts. The force generated by these combined processes leads to emission of the semen through the external urethral sphincter (Fig. 18.19). 18.13

Sperm comprise only 10% of the final ejaculate, the remainder being made up mainly of seminal (50–60%) and prostatic fluids (20–30%), which are added to the sperm during male orgasm, as well as mucus produced in the urethra. Semen is slightly alkaline, to neutralise the acidity of the vagina. Between 2 and 5 mL of semen are produced in a normal ejaculate, and contain between 40

and 100 million spermatozoa per mL. If not ejaculated, sperm gradually lose their fertility after several months and are reabsorbed by the epididymis.

Puberty in the male

This occurs between the ages of 10 and 14. Luteinising hormone from the anterior lobe of the pituitary gland stimulates the interstitial cells of the testes to increase the production of testosterone. Under the influence of testosterone, sexual maturation and other characteristic changes take place, including:

- growth of muscle and bone and a marked increase in height and weight
- enlargement of the larynx and deepening of the voice – it 'breaks'
- growth of hair on the face, axillae, chest, abdomen and pubis
- enlargement of the penis, scrotum and prostate gland
- maturation of the seminiferous tubules and production of spermatozoa
- the skin thickens and becomes oilier.

Human development

Learning outcomes

After studying this section, you should be able to:

- define the terms embryo, fetus, zygote and blastocyst
- outline the main stages of embryonic and fetal development.

Growth of a new human being begins when an ovum is fertilised by a spermatozoon (Fig. 1.19), usually in the uterine tube. The resulting cell is called a *zygote*. Because the ovum and spermatozoon each had 23 chromosomes, it has the full complement of 46 chromosomes. The period between fertilisation and birth (*gestation*) takes about 40 weeks. The first 8 weeks of development is called the *embryonic period* and thereafter the developing individual is called a *fetus*.

Aided by peristalsis of the uterine tube, the zygote travels towards the uterus, a journey that takes about a week, and by 10 days after fertilisation is firmly embedded in the uterine lining. During this time, it undergoes rapid and repeated cell divisions so by the time it implants in the endometrium it has become a *blastocyst*, a hollow ball of 70–100 cells. The blastocyst contains an inner mass of cells, which develops into the fetus and its *amniotic sac*, a bag of membranes enclosing it. The outer layer, the *trophoblast*, becomes an important layer of the *placenta* (p. 115).

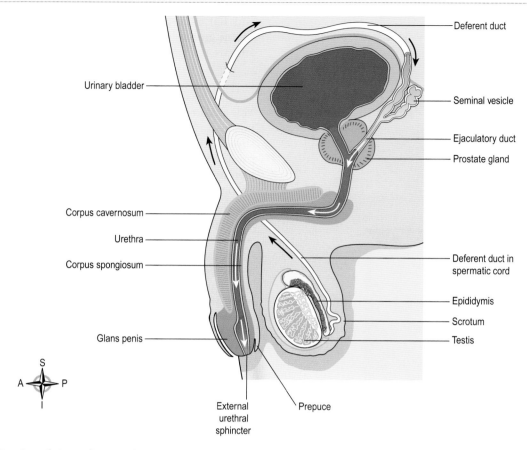

Figure 18.19 Section of the male reproductive organs. Arrows show the route taken by spermatozoa during ejaculation.

Nourishment during intrauterine growth. In the early stages, the embryo is small enough that simple diffusion is adequate to supply the dividing cells but because embryonic growth is so rapid, this quickly becomes unsustainable and between the third and 10th weeks of pregnancy, the placenta (p. 115) develops, attached firmly to the uterine wall. The fetus is attached to the placenta by the *umbilical cord*, and absorbs oxygen and nutrients from the maternal bloodstream as well as excreting its waste products.

The first 3 months
A newborn baby is made up of trillions of cells and many different tissues, all of which have developed from the single-celled zygote formed at fertilisation. Differentiation of cells into specialised tissues, and the organisation of these specialised tissues into the body systems, is largely completed in the first 12 weeks of gestation. A 12-week fetus is very similar to a 40-week fetus, although much smaller.

Later pregnancy
The final 6 months of pregnancy is devoted primarily to the rapid growth of the fetus in preparation for birth and independent life.

Table 18.1 summarises some of the main landmarks in embryonic/fetal development.

Ageing and the reproductive systems

Learning outcomes

After studying this section, you should be able to:

■ describe the effects of ageing on female reproduction

■ describe the effects of ageing on male reproduction.

Ageing and reproduction in the female
Usually between the ages of 45 and 55, the ovarian supply of oocytes runs out and the oestrogen they release therefore declines, at which point the reproductive cycle is disrupted and fertility declines towards zero (menopause, p. 458). At the menopause, although oestrogen levels begin to fall, there is a rapid and sustained rise in gonadotrophin secretion, as the anterior pituitary and

Table 18.1 Some of the main landmarks in embryonic/fetal development

Month	Length	Weight	Main developmental features
1	5 mm	0.02 g	Heart is beating Main respiratory and gastrointestinal organs appearing Neural tube appears (from which the nervous system develops) Limb buds apparent
2	28 mm	2.7 g	Endocrine glands appearing Respiratory tree in place Vascular system laid down Heart development complete Skin, nails and sweat glands present in skin Cartilage models for bones appear Face has human profile
3	78 mm	26 g	Blood cells produced in bone marrow Basic brain and spinal cord structure in place Ossification of bones begins and muscles form Gonads appear (ovaries in females, testes in males)
4	133 mm	150 g	Formation of hair Eyes and ears in place Rapid CNS development Joints formed
9	346 mm	3.2 kg	At birth, many systems immature but otherwise functional. Some important adaptations to independent life required, e.g. in cardiovascular and respiratory function (p. 117)

hypothalamus attempt to maintain activity in the failing ovaries. From middle through to old age, the female reproductive organs, including the breasts, progressively shrink in size. The vulva atrophy and become more fibrous, which may predispose to infection and malignant change. The walls of the vagina become thin and smooth with loss of rugae and glandular secretions.

Ageing and reproduction in the male

There is no equivalent of the female menopause in the older male. Although testosterone secretion tends to decline after age 50, leading to a relative reduction in fertility and sexual desire, it is usually sufficient to maintain sperm production and a man may still be able to father a child until extreme old age.

Sexually transmitted infections

Learning outcomes

After studying this section, you should be able to:

- list the principal causes of sexually transmitted infections

- explain the effects of sexually transmitted infections.

These are common in all cultures and an increasing problem in many countries. Micro-organisms responsible for sexually transmitted infections are unable to survive outside the body for long periods and have no intermediate host.

Chlamydia

The bacterium *Chlamydia trachomatis* causes inflammation of the female cervix. Infection may ascend through the reproductive tract and cause pelvic inflammatory disease (p. 467). In the male, it may cause urethritis, which may also ascend and lead to epididymitis. In both sexes, it is an important cause of subfertility. Chlamydia infection is often present in conjunction with other sexually transmitted diseases. The same organism causes trachoma, an eye infection that is the primary cause of blindness worldwide (p. 211).

Gonorrhoea

This is caused by the bacterium *Neisseria gonorrhoeae*, which infects the mucosa of the reproductive and urinary tracts. In the male, suppurative urethritis occurs and the infection may spread to the prostate gland, epididymis and testes. In the female, the infection may spread from vulvar glands, vagina and cervix to the body of the uterus, uterine tubes, ovaries and peritoneum. Healing by fibrosis in the female may obstruct the uterine tubes, leading to infertility. In the male it may cause urethral stricture.

Non-venereal transmission of gonorrhoea may cause *neonatal ophthalmia* in babies born to infected mothers. The eyes become infected as the baby passes through the birth canal.

Syphilis

This disease is caused by the bacterium *Treponema pallidum*. There are three clearly marked stages. After an incubation period of several weeks, the *primary sore* (chancre) appears at the site of infection, e.g. the vulva, vagina, perineum, penis or round the mouth. In the female the primary sore may be undetected if it is internal. After several weeks the chancre subsides spontaneously. The *secondary stage*, 3–4 months after infection, involves systemic symptoms including lymphadenopathy, skin rashes and mucosal ulceration of the mouth and genital tract. There may then be a latent period of between 3 and 10 years. *Tertiary lesions* (gummas) then develop in many organs, including skin, bone and mucous membranes, and may involve the nervous system, leading to general paralysis and dementia.

Sexual transmission occurs during the primary and secondary stages when discharge from lesions is highly infectious. Congenital transmission from mother to fetus carries a high risk of stillbirth.

Trichomonas vaginalis

These protozoa cause acute vulvovaginitis with irritating, offensive discharge. It is usually sexually transmitted and is commonly present in women with gonorrhoea. Males are often asymptomatic.

Candidiasis

The yeast *Candida albicans* (see also p. 320) is frequently a commensal in the vagina and normally causes no problems. It is normally prevented from flourishing by vaginal acidity, but in certain circumstances it proliferates, causing candidiasis (thrush). Common precipitating factors include:

- antibiotic therapy, which kills the bacteria that keep vaginal pH low
- pregnancy
- reduced immune function
- diabetes mellitus.

In women, persistent itch is the main symptom, with discharge, swelling and erythema of the vulvar area.

Acquired immune deficiency syndrome (AIDS) and hepatitis B infection

These viral conditions may be sexually transmitted, but there are no local signs of infection. For a description of AIDS and HIV see page 386, and for hepatitis B see page 333.

Genital herpes

One form of the herpes virus, Herpes simplex 2 (HSV-2), is associated with genital infections. Initial infection tends to present as clusters of small, painful ulcers on the external genitalia, often with fever and headache. Recurrences of the disease occur because the virus establishes itself within the dorsal root ganglion, from where it can be reactivated from time to time.

Diseases of the female reproductive system

Learning outcomes

After studying this section, you should be able to:

■ describe the causes and consequences of pelvic inflammatory disease

■ define the term imperforate hymen

■ outline the causes and effects of cervical carcinoma

■ discuss the main pathologies of the uterus and uterine tubes

■ describe the causes and effects of ovarian disease

■ describe the causes of female infertility

■ discuss the principal disorders of the female breast.

Pelvic inflammatory disease (PID)

This condition is usually a consequence of sexually transmitted infections. It usually begins as vulvovaginitis and may spread upwards to the cervix, uterus, uterine tubes and ovaries. Upward spread can also occur when infection is present in the vagina before a surgical procedure, childbirth or miscarriage, especially if some of the products of conception are retained. Complications of PID include:

- infertility due to obstruction of uterine tubes
- peritonitis
- intestinal obstruction due to adhesions between the bowel and the uterus and/or uterine tubes
- bacteraemia, which may lead to meningitis, endocarditis or suppurative arthritis.

Disorders of the uterus

Cervical carcinoma

Dysplastic changes, referred to as *cervical intraepithelial neoplasia* (CIN) begin in the deepest layer of cervical epithelium, usually at the junction of the stratified squamous epithelium of the lower third of the cervical canal with the secretory epithelium of the upper two-thirds. Dysplasia may progress to involve the full thickness of epithelium. Not all dysplasias develop into malignant disease, but it is not possible to predict how far development will go, and whether it will remain static or regress. Early detection with a screening programme can allow abnormal tissue to be removed before it becomes malignant. Established malignancy is staged according to how extensive the tumour is. Stage I refers to disease confined to the cervix. Stages II through IV reflect increasing spread, including involvement of the rectum, bladder and structures outwith the pelvis. Early spread is via lymph nodes and local spread is commonly to the uterus, vagina, bladder and rectum. In the late stages spread via the blood to the liver, lungs and bones may occur.

The disease takes 15–20 years to develop and it occurs mostly between 35 and 50 years of age.

The great majority of cases (90% +) are caused by the sexually transmitted human papilloma virus (HPV), which is also believed to cause a large proportion of cancers of the penis and vulva. The risk is therefore greatest in women who are sexually active from an early age with multiple partners and who do not use barrier methods of contraception.

Disorders of the endometrium

The general term for inflammation of the endometrium is *endometritis*, caused by a range of organisms following, for example, childbirth or miscarriage, or by an infected intrauterine contraceptive device. Other more specific conditions include endometriosis, endometrial hyperplasia and endometrial carcinoma.

Endometriosis

This is the growth of endometrial tissue outside the uterus, usually in the ovaries, uterine tubes and other pelvic structures. The ectopic tissue, like the uterine endometrium, responds to fluctuations in sex hormone levels during the menstrual cycle, causing menstrual-type bleeding into the lower abdomen and, in the ovaries, the formation of coloured cysts, 'chocolate cysts'. There is intermittent pain due to swelling, and recurrent haemorrhage causes fibrous tissue formation. Ovarian endometriosis may lead to pelvic inflammation, infertility and extensive pelvic adhesions, involving the ovaries, uterus, uterine ligaments and the bowel.

Endometrial hyperplasia

Hyperplasia of the endometrium is associated with high blood oestrogen levels, e.g. in obesity, oestrogen therapy or an ovarian tumour and may be associated with increased risk of malignant change.

Endometrial carcinoma

This occurs mainly in women who have never been pregnant and is most common between 50 and 60 years of age. The incidence is increased when an oestrogen-secreting tumour is present and in women who are obese, hypertensive or diabetic, because they tend to have high levels of blood oestrogen. As the tumour grows, there is often ulceration and vaginal bleeding. Endometrium has no lymphatics, so lymph spread is delayed until extensive local spread involves other pelvic structures. Distant metastases, spread in blood or lymph, develop later, most commonly in the liver, lungs and bones. Invasion of the ureters leads to hydronephrosis and uraemia, commonly the cause of death.

Disorders of the myometrium

Adenomyosis

This is the growth of endometrium within the myometrium. The ectopic tissue may cause general or localised uterine enlargement. The lesions may cause dysmenorrhoea and irregular excessive bleeding (menorrhagia), usually beginning between 40 and 50 years of age.

Leiomyoma (fibroid, myoma)

These are very common, often multiple, benign tumours of myometrium. They are firm masses of smooth muscle encapsulated in compressed muscle fibres and they vary greatly in size. Large tumours may degenerate if they outgrow their blood supply, leading to necrosis, fibrosis and calcification. They develop during the reproductive period and may be hormone dependent, enlarging during pregnancy and when oral contraceptives are used. They tend to regress after the menopause. Large tumours may cause pelvic discomfort, frequency of micturition, menorrhagia, irregular bleeding, dysmenorrhoea and reduced fertility. Malignant change is rare.

Disorders of the uterine tubes and ovaries

Acute salpingitis

Salpingitis is inflammation of the uterine tubes. It is usually due to infection spreading from the uterus, and only occasionally from the peritoneal cavity. The uterine tubes may be permanently damaged by fibrous scar tissue, which can cause obstruction and infertility. Infection may spread into the peritoneum and involve the ovaries.

Ectopic pregnancy

This is the implantation of a fertilised ovum outside the uterus, usually in a uterine tube. As the fetus grows the tube may rupture and its contents enter the peritoneal cavity, causing acute inflammation (peritonitis) and potentially fatal intraperitoneal haemorrhage.

Ovarian tumours

Most ovarian tumours are benign, usually occurring between 20 and 45 years of age. The rest occur mostly between 45 and 65 years and are divided between borderline malignancy (low-grade cancer) and frank malignancy.

Ovarian cancer is associated with developed societies, higher socioeconomic groups, and, in some families, a genetic susceptibility. Pregnancy and the use of the contraceptive pill have a protective effect. Most malignancies of the ovary arise from epithelium, but some arise from the germ cells of the ovary, or from stromal cells.

Metastatic ovarian tumours

The ovaries are a common site of metastatic spread from primary tumours in other pelvic organs, the breast, stomach, pancreas and biliary tract.

Female infertility

This common condition may be due to:

- blockage of uterine tubes, often the consequence of pelvic inflammatory disease and/or STIs
- anatomical abnormalities, e.g. retroversion (tilting backwards) of the uterus
- endocrine factors; any abnormalities of the glands and hormones governing the menstrual cycle can interfere with fertility
- low body weight, e.g. in anorexia nervosa, or severe malnourishment, and may be associated with low leptin levels (p. 228)
- endometriosis.

Disorders of the breast

Mastitis (inflammation of the breast)

This is usually associated with lactation and breast-feeding, and may or may not involve infection. Usually only one breast is involved. Non-infective mastitis is the result of milk stasis in the breast and causes swelling and pain. Infection (usually by *Staphylococcus aureus*) can occur if the nipple is damaged during suckling, allowing bacteria to enter and spread into the system of milk ducts. Generally the condition responds well to treatment but can progress to more serious complications such as abscess formation.

Tumours of the breast

Benign tumours

Most breast tumours (90%) are benign. Fibroadenomas are the commonest type and occur any time after puberty; incidence peaks in the third decade. Other benign tumours may be cystic or solid and these usually occur in women nearing the menopause. They may originate from secretory cells, fibrous tissue or from ducts.

Malignant tumours

These are usually painless lumps found in the upper outer quadrant of the breast. Fibrosis occurs around the tumour and may cause retraction of the nipple and necrosis and ulceration of the overlying skin.

Early spread beyond the breast is via lymph to the axillary and internal mammary nodes. Local invasion involves the pectoral muscles and the pleura. Blood-spread metastases may occur later in many organs and bones, especially lumbar and thoracic vertebrae. The causes of breast cancer are not known, but risk increases with age and an important predisposing factor appears to be high oestrogen exposure. Women with an early menarche, a late menopause, and no pregnancies have a higher than normal risk because they experience more menstrual cycles in their lifetimes, and each monthly cycle brings with it the oestrogen surge seen during the proliferative phase (p. 457). A genetic component is also likely, with close relatives of breast cancer sufferers having an elevated risk of developing the disease. In about 15% of cases, the disease is linked to the presence of one of two faulty genes, BRCA1 and BRCA2. Women carrying one of these genes have a very high (80–90%) chance of developing the disease, and there is also increased risk of ovarian and bowel cancer. In women carrying these genes, the average age at which the disease appears is significantly lower than in those without the gene. One percent of all breast cancer occurs in men.

Diseases of the male reproductive system

Learning outcomes

After studying this section, you should be able to:

- outline the causes and effects of penile and urethral infections
- describe the main pathologies of the testis
- discuss the principal disorders of the prostate gland
- list the main causes of male infertility.

Infections of the penis

Inflammation of the glans and prepuce may be caused by a specific or non-specific infection. In non-specific infections, or *balanitis*, lack of personal hygiene is an important predisposing factor, especially if *phimosis* is present, i.e. the orifice in the foreskin (prepuce) is too small to allow for its normal retraction. If the infection becomes chronic there may be fibrosis of the foreskin, which increases the phimosis.

Infections of the urethra

Gonococcal urethritis is the most common specific infection. Non-specific infection may be spread from the bladder (cystitis) or be introduced during catheterisation, cystoscopy or surgery. Both types may spread

throughout the system to the prostate, seminal vesicles, epididymis and testes. If infection becomes chronic, fibrosis may cause urethral stricture or obstruction, leading to retention of urine.

Epididymis and testes

Infections

Non-specific epididymitis and orchitis are usually due to spread of infection from the urethra, commonly following prostatectomy. The microbes may spread either through the deferent duct (vas deferens) or via lymph.

Specific epididymitis. This is usually caused by gonorrhoea spread from the urethra.

Orchitis (inflammation of the testis). This is commonly caused by mumps virus, blood-borne from the parotid glands. Acute inflammation with oedema occurs about 1 week after the appearance of parotid swelling. The infection is usually unilateral but, if bilateral, severe damage to germinal epithelium of the seminiferous tubules may result in sterility.

Undescended testis (cryptorchidism)

During embryonic life the testes develop within the abdominal cavity, but descend into the scrotum prior to birth. If they fail to do this and the condition is not corrected, infertility is likely to follow and the risk of testicular cancer is increased.

Hydrocele

This is the most common form of scrotal swelling and is accumulation of serous fluid in the tunica vaginalis. The onset may be acute and painful or chronic. It may be congenital or be secondary to another disorder of the testis or epididymis.

Testicular tumours

Most testicular tumours are malignant, the commonest malignancies in young men. They occur in childhood and early adulthood when the affected testis has not descended or has been late in descending into the scrotum. The tumour tends to remain localised for a considerable time but eventually spreads in lymph to pelvic and abdominal lymph nodes, and more widely in the blood. Occasionally, hormone-secreting tumours develop and may cause precocious development in boys.

Prostate gland

Infections

Acute prostatitis is usually caused by non-specific infection, spread from the urethra or bladder, often following catheterisation, cystoscopy, urethral dilation or prostate surgery. Chronic infection may follow an acute attack. Fibrosis of the gland may occur during healing, causing urethral stricture or obstruction.

Benign prostatic enlargement

Hyperplasia (p. 54) flow of urine, causing urinary retention. Incomplete emptying of the bladder predisposes to infection, which may spread upwards, causing pyelonephritis and other complications. Prostatic enlargement is common in men over 50, affecting up to 70% of men aged over 70. The cause is not clear.

Malignant prostatic tumours

Seven per cent of all cancers in men are prostatic carcinomas. Risk increases with age but the trigger for the malignant change is not known, although there is believed to be a hormonal element. Initially, the growing tumour usually causes symptoms of urinary obstruction, but it spreads quickly and sometimes presents with indications of secondary spread, e.g. back pain from bone metastases, weight loss or anaemia.

Breast

Gynaecomastia

This is proliferation of breast tissue in men. It usually affects only one breast and is benign. It is common in adolescents and older men, and is often associated with:

- endocrine disorders, especially those associated with high oestrogen levels
- cirrhosis of the liver (p. 334)
- malnutrition
- some drugs, e.g. chlorpromazine, spironolactone, digoxin
- Klinefelter syndrome, a genetic disorder with testicular atrophy and absence of spermatogenesis.

Malignant tumours

These develop in a small number of men, usually in the older age groups. One percent of all breast cancers occur in men.

Male infertility

This may be due to endocrine disorders, obstruction of the deferent duct, failure of erection or ejaculation during intercourse, vasectomy, or suppression of spermatogenesis by, e.g. ionising radiation, chemotherapy and other drugs.

For a range of self-assessment exercises on the topics in this chapter, visit Evolve online resources: https://evolve.elsevier .com/Waugh/anatomy/

Glossary

Abduction Movement of a body part away from the midline of the body

Abscess A pus-filled cavity within tissue

Accommodation Focussing adjustment of the eyes to view close objects

Acid Substance that releases hydrogen ions in solution

Acidosis Situation when blood pH falls below the normal pH range

Action potential The electrical current (impulse) conducted along a nerve cell (neurone)

Active transport Movement of substances across a cell membrane, up the concentration gradient, and requiring energy

Acute Of sudden onset

Adaptation Lessening of response by sensory receptors to prolonged stimulation

Adduction Movement of a body part towards the midline of the body

Adenosine triphosphate (ATP) Molecular store of chemical energy for chemical reactions

Adhesions Fusion of two separate tissue layers with fibrous tissue, usually following inflammation

Adipose tissue Fat tissue

Aerobic Requiring oxygen

Aetiology Cause of a disease

Afferent Carrying or travelling towards an organ

Afterload The resistance to blood flow from the heart, determined mainly by the diameter of the arteries

Agranulocyte White blood cell with no granules in its cytoplasm (i.e. lymphocytes and monocytes)

Alkali Substances that accepts hydrogen ions in water or solution

Alkalosis Situation when blood pH rises above the normal pH range

Allele The form of a gene carried on a chromosome

Allergy Targeting and destruction of harmless antigens by the immune system, often with detrimental effects on normal body tissues

Alveolar ventilation The amount of air reaching the alveoli with each breath

Alveolus (pl. alveoli) An air sac in the lungs; also the milk secreting sacs in the mammary glands

Amino acid The building blocks of protein

Anabolism Synthesis of larger molecules from smaller ones

Anaerobic Not requiring oxygen

Anaphase Third phase of mitosis

Anaphylaxis The severest form of allergy, with multiple, potentially fatal, systemic effects

Anastomosis The joining of two tubes, e.g. (i) in blood vessels where there are no capillary beds, (ii) following surgery

Anatomical position Used to maintain consistency of anatomical descriptions – the body is upright, with the head facing forward, the arms at the sides with the palms of the hands facing forward, and the feet together

Aneurysm A weakness in the wall of an artery

Anion A negatively charged ion

Anterior (ventral) Describes a body part nearer the front

Antibody Defensive protein synthesised by B-lymphocytes in response to the presence of antigen

Antigen A protein that stimulates the body's immunological defences

Antimicrobial A substance or mechanism that kills or inhibits growth of micro-organisms

Appendicular skeleton (cf. axial skeleton) The shoulder girdle, upper limbs, pelvic girdle and lower limbs

Arrhythmia An abnormal heart rhythm

Arteriole A small artery

Artery A blood vessel that carries blood away from the heart

Articulation A joint

Atrophy Decrease in cell size resulting in shrinking of an organ or body part

Auditory Related to hearing

Autoimmunity Targeting and sometimes destruction of one's own or 'self' tissues by the immune system

Autoregulation The ability of a tissue to independently control its own blood supply

Autorhythmicity The ability of a tissue to generate its own electrical signals

Autosome Any one of the chromosomes in pairs 1–22 (i.e. all but the sex chromosomes)

Axial skeleton (cf. appendicular skeleton) The skull, vertebral column, sternum (breastbone) and ribs

Bacterium (pl. bacteria) Single-celled micro-organism, common in the external environment, some of which can cause disease

Baroreceptor Sensory receptor sensitive to pressure (stretch)

Basal metabolic rate The energy use of the body when at rest in a warm environment, without having eaten for 12 hours

Benign Non-cancerous or a non-serious condition for which treatment may be required

Blastocyst The hollow ball of cells that, during fetal development, embeds in the uterine wall

Blood–brain barrier The collective term given to the physiological adaptations in the central nervous system that prevents many blood-borne substances from accessing it

Bradycardia Abnormally slow heart rate

Bronchodilation Widening of the larger airways and bronchioles

Buffer A substance that resists a shift in pH of body fluids

Capacitance vessel A vessel that can expand to contain large quantities of blood at low pressure (veins)

Capillary A tiny blood vessel between an arteriole and a venule, which has leaky walls to allow exchange of substances between the blood and tissues

Carbohydrate Group of organic compounds including the sugars and starches

Carcinogen A cancer-causing substance

Carcinoma A tumour arising from epithelial tissue

Cardiac Of the heart

Cardiac output (CO) The amount of blood ejected by one ventricle every minute: CO = heart rate (HR) × stroke volume (SV)

Catabolism Breaking down of larger molecules into smaller ones

Catalyst A substance that speeds up a biochemical reaction without taking part in it

Cation A positively charged ion

Central nervous system The brain and spinal cord

Cerebrospinal fluid (CSF) The fluid bathing the brain and spinal cord

Chemoreceptor A sensory receptor sensitive to chemicals in solution

Chemotaxis The movement of a cell towards a chemical attractant

Chondrocyte Mature cartilage cell

Chromatin The uncoiled state of chromosomes during interphase

Chromosome Sausage-shaped structure consisting of a tightly coiled molecule of DNA visible at the end of interphase

Chronic Long-standing or recurring

Cilia (sing. cilium) Microscopic cell extensions for moving materials through the lumen of a tube

Circadian rhythm The regular, predictable fluctuation of a physiological function over a 24-hour period

Circumduction Movement of a body part to describe a cone shape

Citric acid cycle Important sequence of aerobic metabolic reactions in cellular energy production

Coagulation Blood clotting

Co-dominance The situation when more than one form of a gene is dominant

Coitus The act of sexual intercourse

Commensal A harmless micro-organism that lives in the body or on its surfaces, which may bring advantages to its host, e.g. by producing vitamins, or by preventing the growth of pathogens

Communicable (disease) Transferable from one person to another

Compliance The stretchability of a tissue

Compound A molecule containing more than one element

Concentration gradient Where two areas of, e.g., liquid have different concentrations of a solute

Congenital Inherited

Constriction Narrowing of a tube or vessel due to contraction of circular muscle in its wall

Convergence The turning of the eyes inward to focus on a close object

Cortex The outer layer of a gland or structure

Costal Related to the ribs

Cytoplasm The contents of a cell except the nucleus (i.e. cytosol + organelles)

Deamination Removal of the amine group from an amino acid

Deep A body structure or part that is not close to the body surface

Defaecation Expulsion of faeces from the rectum

Deglutition Swallowing

Dehydration Excessive loss of body water

Deoxyribonucleic acid (DNA) The molecule in which the genetic code is written, and packaged into chromosomes in the nucleus

Diapedesis Movement of an independently motile cell from one place to another

Diaphysis The shaft of a long bone

Diastole Resting period of the heart or its individual chambers

Diastolic blood pressure The pressure recorded in the systemic circulation (often at the arm) when the pressure is at its lowest, corresponding to relaxation of the myocardium; the lower of the two measurements used to denote a blood pressure recording

Differentiation The process of cell specialisation

Diffusion Movement of substances down a concentration gradient, which does not require energy or presence of a membrane

Dilation Widening of a tube or vessel due to relaxation of circular muscle in its wall

Diploid A cell with 46 chromosomes, the whole complement of 23 pairs

Distal Further from the origin of a body part or point of attachment of a limb

Diuresis The passing of urine

Dominant In genetics, the preferential expression of one form of a gene over another

Efferent Carrying or travelling away from an organ

Elasticity The ability of a tissue to stretch and recoil to its original length or shape

Electrolyte An inorganic ion in body fluids, which conducts electricity

Element A chemical whose atoms are all of the same type

Embolus A blood clot or other substance that travels in a blood vessel and may lodge blocking a smaller vessel

Embryo In humans, the first eight weeks of development after fertilisation following which it is referred to as the fetus

Endocrine gland A ductless gland that secretes a hormone which travels to its target organ in the bloodstream

Endogenous Internal, produced by the body

Endothelium Epithelium lining blood vessels

Enzyme A protein substance that speeds up (catalyses) chemical reactions

Epidermis The outermost layer of the skin

Epinephrine Another term for adrenaline

Epiphysis Each end of a long bone

Epithelium Tissue that lines and covers most body organs

Equilibrium The state of physiological balance or equivalence

Erythropoiesis Production of red blood cells

Essential nutrient A nutrient that must be eaten in the diet

Eversion Turning the soles of the feet outwards

Exocrine gland Gland that secretes its product into ducts for transport

Exocytosis Process by which particulate waste is expelled from a cell

Exogenous External; not produced by the body

Expiration (cf. inspiration) The physical process of breathing out

Extension An increase in the angle between two bones, straightening a limb

External respiration Exchange of gases in the lungs

Extracellular Outside a cell

Extrinsic pathway Clotting process triggered by damaged extravascular tissues

Facilitated diffusion A form of diffusion that requires carrier proteins for transfer of substances across cell membranes

Faeces Waste product of digestion excreted through the anus

Fascia Fibrous membrane that supports, covers and separates muscles

Fertilisation The penetration of an ovum by a spermatozoon to form a zygote that can grow into a fetus

Fibre Muscle cell; in nutrition, the indigestible part of the diet also known as non-starch polysaccharide

Fibrinolysis The breakdown of a blood clot

Fibroblast Connective tissue cell that produces collagen fibres

Filtration The movement of small molecules, by hydrostatic pressure, through a selectively permeable membrane

Fistula An abnormal passageway between two organs or an organ and the body surface

Flagella (sing. flagellum) Long cell extensions used for cellular propulsion

Flexion The reducing of the angle between two bones; straightening a limb

Follicle A small secretory gland

Gamete An ovum or spermatozoon (reproductive cell)

Gastric Of the stomach

Gene An area on a chromosome that codes for one particular protein

Genome All the genes in a cell

Genotype The genetic make-up of an individual

Gestation Pregnancy

Glia Nervous tissue that supports neurones

Globulin One class of plasma protein, including antibodies

Glucocorticoids Group of steroid (fat-based) adrenal cortex hormones essential for life

Gluconeogenesis The production of glucose from non-carbohydrate molecules

Glucose Simple sugar used by cells for energy

GLOSSARY

Glycogen Storage, very high molecular weight form of glucose

Glycolysis The anaerobic breakdown of glucose to release some of its stored energy

Granulation tissue Newly formed repair tissue following tissue damage

Granulocyte General term for a white blood cell without cytoplasmic granules

Granulopoiesis The production of white blood cells

Gustation Taste

Haematemesis Vomiting of blood

Haemolysis The breakdown of red blood cells

Haemopoiesis The production of blood cells

Haemorrhage Profuse blood loss

Haemostasis The cessation of blood flow

Haploid A cell with 23 chromosomes (half the total chromosome complement)

Hepatic Of the liver

Heterozygous Genetically, a form of a gene on one chromosome that is different to the form of the same gene on the other chromosome of the pair

High-density lipoprotein A lipid/protein complex in the bloodstream important in transporting cholesterol to the liver for disposal

Hilum Indented area of an organ where blood vessels, nerves and ducts enter and leave

Homeostasis Maintenance of a stable internal environment

Homozygous Genetically, a form of a gene on one chromosome that is the same as the form of the same gene on the other chromosome of the pair

Hormone A substance secreted by an endocrine gland that is transported in the blood and acts on specific target cells elsewhere in the body

Hydrophilic Water loving

Hydrophobic Water hating

Hydrostatic pressure The pressure exerted by a fluid on the walls of its container, e.g. of blood on the walls of blood vessels

Hypersecretion Abnormally high secretion of a body product, e.g. a hormone

Hypersensitivity An abnormal immune response directed either against a harmless antigen (allergy) or a 'self' antigen (autoimmunity)

Hypertension Abnormally high blood pressure

Hypertonic A solution with a solute concentration higher than body fluids

Hypertrophy An increase in cell size resulting in enlargement of an organ or body part

Hyperventilation Abnormally high respiratory effort, associated with loss of excessive amounts of carbon dioxide

Hyposecretion Abnormally low secretion of a body product, e.g. a hormone

Hypotension Abnormally low blood pressure

Hypothermia An abnormally low body temperature (core temperature <35°C)

Hypotonic A solution with a solute concentration lower than body fluids

Hypoventilation An abnormally low respiratory effort, associated with retention of carbon dioxide

Hypoxia Inadequate levels of oxygen in the tissues

Iatrogenic A condition resulting from a healthcare intervention

Idiopathic A condition of unknown cause

Immunity Body defence mechanisms against a specific disease

Incontinence Inability to control the voiding of urine

Infarction Death of a region of tissue due to interruption of its blood supply

Infection The invasion of body tissues by pathogenic organisms

Inferior Structure further from the head

Inflammation Non-specific tissue response to damage

Ingestion Taking in of substances orally, i.e. through the mouth

Insensible water loss Loss of water through the skin and respiratory tract

Insertion (cf. origin) The point where a muscle is attached to the bone in moves

Inspiration (cf. expiration) The physical process of breathing in

Integumentary Of the skin

Internal respiration Exchange of gases in the tissues

Interphase Phase of the cell cycle when there is no division

Interstitial fluid Fluid situated between body cells, also known as tissue fluid

Intracellular Inside a cell

Intrinsic factor A protein secreted by the stomach required for absorption of vitamin B_{12} (the extrinsic factor)

Intrinsic pathway Clotting process triggered by damaged blood vessels

Inversion The turning of the soles of the feet to face each other

Involuntary Not under conscious control

Ion A charged atom (which has either lost or acquired electrons)

Ionising radiation Radiation that generates ions when it passes through atoms; can damage cells by changing the atoms in the molecules that make up living tissue, e.g. X-rays

Ischaemia Impaired blood supply to a body part

Isometric Muscle work where the tension in the muscle rises but the muscle does not shorten, e.g. if trying to lift a weight that is too heavy to move

Isotonic Muscle work where the muscle shortens as the tension rises, allowing, e.g., a load to be lifted by the arm; in chemistry, solutions with a solute concentration the same as body tissues

Isotope A form of an element that has a different number of neutrons from the principal form

Karyotype Photographic presentation of a cell's chromosomes as matched pairs in descending order of size

Lactation Production of breast milk

Lateral Structure further from the midline or at the side of the body

Leukocyte General term for a white blood cell

Leukopenia A low blood white cell count

Ligament Band of connective tissue that binds one bone to another

Lipase Enzyme that breaks down fat

Lipid The general term for any substance that does not dissolve in water but dissolves in non-polar solvents like alcohol

Lipolysis Breakdown of fat

Low-density lipoprotein A lipid/protein complex in the bloodstream associated with deposition of cholesterol in arterial walls

Lumen The central passageway within an internal tube or duct

Lymph Watery fluid drained by the lymphatic system from the tissue spaces

Lysis Destruction of a cell, e.g. haemolysis

Lysozyme An antimicrobial enzyme present in some body fluids

Macrophage A phagocytic cell usually found in connective tissue

Malignant Cancerous

Mastication Chewing

Meatus An opening into a passage

Medial Structure that is nearer to the midline

Median plane An imaginary line that divides the body longitudinally into right and left halves

Mediastinum The region between the lungs, containing the heart, great vessels, trachea and other important structures

Medulla The inner layer of a gland or structure

Meiosis Process of cell division by which gametes are formed

Melaena Blood in the faeces

Menarche The onset of puberty in females, marked by the start of menstruation

Menopause Time of the female life span when reproductive function ceases

Menstruation (menses) Regular shedding of uterine lining, usually monthly, during the reproductive period of the female life span

Metabolic pathway Sequence of metabolic steps in cellular biochemistry

Metabolism All the chemical reaction that take place within the body

Metaphase Second phase of mitosis

Metastasis (pl. metastases) Secondary deposits from a primary malignant tumour

Microbe Micro-organism, e.g. a fungus, bacterium or virus

Micturition Passing urine

Mitosis Cell division giving two identical daughter cells

Mole In chemistry, the quantity of a substance representing its molecular weight in grams

Motor nerve or neurone An efferent nerve that carries impulses from the central nervous system to muscles or glands

Mucosa Lining of body tracts (also mucous membrane)

Mutagen Any substance that causes mutation

Mutation A genetic change that arises during cell division

Myelin A fatty substance that surrounds the axons of myelinated nerves

Myofilaments Intracellular protein threads within muscle cells, made either of actin or myosin, responsible for muscle cell contraction

Necrosis Cell death caused by an injury or a pathological condition

Negative feedback (cf. positive feedback) Any control mechanism that resists and reverses any change from normal in a physiological system

Neoplasm A new growth which may be benign or malignant

Nephron The structure in the kidneys responsible for the formation of urine

Neuromuscular junction The synapse between a motor nerve and a skeletal muscle cell

Neurone Nerve cell

Neurotransmitter Chemical that transmits an impulse between one nerve and the next, or between a nerve and the neuromuscular junction

Non-specific defence The defence mechanisms of the body that are effective against different types of threat, e.g. the skin, inflammation, complement

Norepinephrine Alternative name for noradrenaline

Nucleotide Building block of nucleic acids

Nutrient Any substance that is digested, absorbed and used to promote body function

Oedema Tissue swelling due to collection of fluid in the intercellular spaces

Olfaction Sense of smell

Oncogenic Cancer-causing

Organ Body part, composed of different tissues, that carries out a specific body function

Organelle Intracellular structure that carries out a specific function

Organic A molecule or substance containing carbon

Origin Point of attachment of a muscle to a bone that moves least during muscle contraction

Osteoid The organic constituent of bone tissue

Osteon Structural unit of compact bone

Osteopenia Age-related bone degeneration

Osmoreceptors Specialised sensory receptors sensitive to solute concentration

Osmosis Movement of water down its concentration gradient across a semipermeable membrane

Osmotic pressure The pressure exerted by water in a solution

Ossicles Bones of the middle ear: hammer, anvil and stirrup

Ossification The production of bone tissue

Ovulation The release of a mature ovum from the ovary

Oxidative phosphorylation The aerobic high energy-generating metabolic process of cellular respiration

Oxyhaemoglobin The oxygenated form of haemoglobin

Parasympathetic nervous system Division of the autonomic nervous system that prepares the body for 'rest and repair'

Parietal layer A layer of serous membrane lining a body cavity (cf. visceral layer)

Parturition Childbirth

Passive transport Any form of transport within the body that does not require the use of energy

Pathogen Micro-organism capable of causing disease

Peptidase An enzyme that breaks down protein

Peripheral nervous system Nervous tissue that is not part of the brain or spinal cord

Peripheral resistance The force against which the blood has to push to move through the arterial circulation, determined mainly by the diameter of the arterioles

Peristalsis Rhythmical contraction of smooth muscle in the walls of hollow organs and tubes, e.g. the alimentary canal

pH scale Scale of measurement of acidity or alkalinity

Phagocytosis Defence mechanism by which body cells consume and destroy foreign materials, 'cell eating'

Phenotype The expression of the genes in an individual, e.g. hair colour, height, etc.

Phospholipid Fat-based molecule containing phosphate, essential to the structure of the cell membrane

Pinocytosis Ingestion of small vacuoles into a cell, 'cell drinking'

Plasma Clear, straw coloured liquid portion of the blood

Plasma protein Any one of a group of important proteins synthesised by the liver and carried in the plasma, with diverse physiological functions, e.g. as antibodies or clotting proteins

Platelet (thrombocyte) Small cell fragments involved in blood clotting

Pleural Related to the lungs

Plexus A network formed by a collection of nerves or blood vessels

Polymophonuclear leukocyte A general term for a white blood cell with an irregular nucleus (i.e. basophils, eosinophils and neutrophils)

Polyuria Production of large quantities of urine

Positive feedback (cf. negative feedback) A control mechanism that increases and accelerates any change from normal in a physiological system; much rarer than negative feedback control

Posterior (dorsal) Lying to the back of the body

Preload The amount of blood in the ventricle just prior to ventricular contraction, determined mainly by venous return

Presbycusis Irreversible hearing loss, usually due to ageing, which results from degeneration of the cochlea and begins with an inability to hear high pitched sounds

Presbyopia Stiffening of the lens, usually due to ageing, which impairs the ability of the eye to change focus (accommodate)

Pressure ulcer Damage to superficial tissues caused by prolonged pressure and interrupted blood supply, usually over a bony prominence

Primary wound healing Simple repair of relatively minor tissue damage

Prognosis Likely outcome of a disease

Prophase First phase of mitosis

Pronation The turning of the palms to face backwards

Protein A large polypeptide

Proximal Nearer the origin of a body part or point of attachment of a limb

Puberty The stage of life in males or females where reproductive maturity is achieved

Pulmonary Of the lungs

Pulse The pressure wave generated by the heart, felt along an arterial wall where that artery lies close to the body surface

Pulse pressure Diastolic blood pressure subtracted from the systolic value

Pyrexia Fever

Pyrogen A substance that causes fever

Radiation The transmission of energy in waves

Receptor A molecule, usually on the cell surface, that detects and responds to chemicals in the cell's external environment, e.g. a neurotransmitter. Also, a sensory nerve ending that detects physical changes in the local environment, e.g. a baroreceptor measuring pressure

Recessive Genetically, a form of a gene that can only be expressed if it is present as two identical forms on the chromosome pair

Refraction The bending of light rays as they pass through a lens, e.g. the lens of the eye

Renal Of the kidneys

Resistance vessel A blood vessel, usually an arteriole, with a thick layer of smooth muscle in its tunica media, that constricts or dilates to regulate blood flow and blood pressure

Reticulocyte Immature red blood cell

Retroperitoneal Lying behind the peritoneum

Ribonucleic acid (RNA) Molecule used to transfer genetic instructions from DNA to cytoplasmic ribosomes

Rotation The movement of a body part around its long axis

Rugae Folds in the internal surface of a hollow organ when the organ is relaxed

Sagittal plane An imaginary vertical line dividing the body into right and left halves either down the midline (midsagittal) or on either side of the midline (sagittal)

Salt The product of a reaction between an acid and a base

Saltatory conduction The 'jumping' of a nerve impulse along a myelinated nerve axon, from one node of Ranvier to the next

Scar tissue The nonfunctional tissue that replaces damaged tissue

Secondary wound healing Repair of tissue after extensive damage; a more complex and intense process than primary wound healing

Semipermeability (selective permeability) A property of cell membranes that allows passage of some substances but not others

Senescence Cell ageing and the decline in function that accompanies it

Sensory nerve or neurone An afferent nerve that carries impulses to the central nervous system

Serous fluid The general term for protein-containing fluid secreted by certain membranes, e.g. serous pericardium and visceral pleura

Sex chromosome The X or Y chromosome (pair 23)

Sign An abnormality observed by people other than a patient

Simple propagation The continuous conduction of an impulse along an non-myelinated nerve fibre

Sliding filament theory The accepted mechanism by which actin and myosin filaments within muscle cells slide over one another to permit muscle shortening (contraction)

Specific defence mechanisms Immunity; body's protective mechanisms raised against a specific threat or antigen

Sphincter Circle of muscle surrounding an internal passageway or orifice, used to regulate passage through the opening

Spinal reflex Involuntary, usually protective, action controlled at the level of the spinal cord (i.e. independent of the brain)

Squamous Flattened (epithelial cells)

Stratified Of tissues, having several cell layers

Striated The microscopic appearance of a striped pattern on skeletal and cardiac muscle cells

Stroke volume The volume of blood ejected by the ventricle when it contracts

Superficial Near the body surface

Superior Towards the upper part of the body

Supination Turning the palm to face forwards

Sympathetic nervous system Division of the autonomic nervous system that prepares the body for 'fight or flight'

Symptom An abnormality described by a patient

Synapse The junction between a nerve and the cell it supplies

Syndrome A collection of signs and symptoms that tend to occur together

Systemic circulation The blood supply to all body organs except for the pulmonary arteries and veins

Systole Contraction period of the heart or its individual chambers

Systolic blood pressure The pressure recorded in the systemic circulation (often at the arm) when the pressure is at its highest, immediately following ventricular contraction; the higher of the two measurements used to denote a blood pressure recording

Tachycardia Abnormally fast heart rate

Telophase Fourth (final) phase of mitosis

Telomere Non-coding sections of DNA that cap and protect the ends of each chromosome

Tendon A band of fibrous tissue connecting muscle to bone

Teratogen Any substance or agent known to cause abnormal fetal development

Thrombosis The inappropriate, pathological formation of stationary blood clots within blood vessels

Thrombus (pl. thrombi) Stationary blood clot (clots)

Tissue fluid Fluid between body cells, also known as interstitial fluid

Tolerance The ability of the immune system and its defensive cells and mechanisms to identify, and not attack, 'self' tissues

Tract A bundle of axons in the central nervous system

Transcription Production of mRNA from DNA

Translation Production of protein from mRNA

Transverse plane An imaginary line slicing the body into an upper and a lower part

Trophic hormone Hormone released that causes the release of a second hormone

Trophoblast Outer cell layer of the blastocyst that forms the placenta

Tumour Mass of cells growing outwith the body's normal control mechanisms

Tunica adventitia The outer, supportive lining of blood vessels

Tunica intima The lining of blood vessels (also called endothelium)

Tunica media The middle layer of tissue in larger blood vessels

Urine Liquid waste product made in the kidneys

Vasoconstriction Decrease in diameter (narrowing) of a blood vessel

Vasodilation Increase in diameter (widening) of a blood vessel

Vein A blood vessel that carries blood towards the heart

Venule A small vein

Virus Non-living particle, which may be capable of causing disease

Visceral layer A layer of serous membrane covering a body organ

Voluntary control Conscious control of a body function

Zygote Fertilised egg formed by fusion of an ovum and spermatozoon

Normal values

Note. Some biological measures have been extracted from the text and listed here for easy reference. In some cases slightly different 'normals' may be found in other texts and used by different medical practitioners.

Metric measures, units and SI symbols

Name	SI unit	Symbol
Length	metre	m
Mass	kilogram	kg
Amount of substance	mole	mol
Pressure	pascal	Pa
Energy	joule	J

Decimal multiples and submultiples of the units are formed by the use of standard prefixes.

Multiple	Prefix	Symbol	Submultiple	Prefix	Symbol
10^6	mega	M	10^{-1}	deci	d
10^3	kilo	k	10^{-2}	centi	c
10^2	hecto	h	10^{-3}	milli	m
10^1	deca	da	10^{-6}	micro	μ
			10^{-9}	nano	n
			10^{-12}	pico	p
			10^{-15}	femto	f

Conversion table for kPa/mmHg (for e.g. capillary pressures)
1 mmHg = 0.13 kPa
1 kPa   = 7.5 mmHg
35 mmHg = 4.7 kPa
25 mmHg = 3.3 kPa
15 mmHg = 2.0 kPa
10 mmHg = 1.3 kPa

Hydrogen ion concentration (pH)

Neutral = 7 Acid = 0 to 7 Alkaline = 7 to 14

Normal pH of some body fluids	
Blood	7.35 to 7.45
Saliva	5.8 to 7.4
Gastric juice	1.5 to 3.5
Bile	6.0 to 8.5
Urine	4.5 to 8.0

Some normal plasma levels in adults

Calcium	2.12 to 2.62 mmol/L	(8.5 to 10.5 mg/100 mL)
Chloride	97 to 106 mmol/L	(97 to 106 mEq/L)
Cholesterol	3.6 to 6.7 mmol/L	(140 to 260 mg/100 mL)
Glucose	3.5 to 8 mmol/L	(63 to 144 mg/100 mL)
Fasting glucose	3.6 to 5.8 mmol/L	(65 to 105 mg/100 mL)
Potassium	3.3 to 4.7 mmol/L	(3.3 to 4.7 mEq/L)
Sodium	135 to 143 mmol/L	(135 to 143 mEq/L)
Urea	2.5 to 6.6 mmol/L	(15 to 44 mg/100 mL)

Arterial blood gases

PO_2	12 to 15 kPa	(90 to 110 mmHg)
PCO_2	4.5 to 6 kPa	(34 to 46 mmHg)
Bicarbonate	21 to 27.5 mmol/L	
H^+ ions	36 to 44 nmol/L	(7.35 to 7.45 pH units)

NORMAL VALUES

Blood pressure
Normal adult 120/80 mmHg.
Blood pressure above 140/90 is generally considered high.

Heart rate
At rest	60 to 80/min
Sinus bradycardia	<60/min
Sinus tachycardia	>100/min

Respiration rate
At rest 15 to 18/min
Tidal volume	500 mL
Dead space	150 mL
Alveolar ventilation	15 (500 − 150) = 5.25 L/min

Blood count
Leukocytes	$4 \times 10^9/L$	to	$11 \times 10^9/L$
Neutrophils	$2.5 \times 10^9/L$	to	$7.5 \times 10^9/L$
Eosinophils	$0.04 \times 10^9/L$	to	$0.44 \times 10^9/L$
Basophils	$0.015 \times 10^9/L$	to	$0.1 \times 10^9/L$
Monocytes	$0.2 \times 10^9/L$	to	$0.8 \times 10^9/L$
Lymphocytes	$1.5 \times 10^9/L$	to	$3.5 \times 10^9/L$
Erythrocytes			
female	$3.8 \times 10^{12}/L$	to	$5 \times 10^{12}/L$
male	$4.5 \times 10^{12}/L$	to	$6.5 \times 10^{12}/L$
Thrombocytes	$200 \times 10^9/L$	to	$350 \times 10^9/L$

Diet
1 kilocalorie (kcal) = 4.182 kilojoules (kJ)
1 kilojoule = 0.24 kilocalories

Energy source	Energy released	Recommended proportion in diet
Carbohydrate	1 g = 17 kJ = 4 kcal	55–75%
Protein	1 g = 17 kJ = 4 kcal	10–15%
Fat	1 g = 38 kJ = 9 kcal	15–30%

Daily vitamin requirements for adults

Vitamin	Daily requirement
Fat soluble	
Vitamin A	600–700 mcg
Vitamin D	10 mcg
Vitamin E	Males: 10 mg Females: 8 mg
Vitamin K	1 mcg per kg body weight
Water soluble	
Vitamin B_1	0.8–1 mg
Vitamin B_2	1.1–1.3 mg
Vitamin B_3	12–17 mg
Vitamin B_6	1.2–1.4 mg
Vitamin B_{12}	1.5 mcg
Folic acid	200 mcg
Pantothenic acid	3–7 mg
Biotin	10–20 mcg
Vitamin C	40 mg

Urine
Specific gravity	1.020 to 1.030
Volume excreted	1000 to 1500 mL/day

Glucose is normally absent, but appears in urine when blood glucose levels exceed 9 mmol/L

Body temperatures
Normal	36.8°C: axillary
Hypothermia	≤35°C: core temperature
Death when below	25°C

Cerebrospinal fluid pressure
Lying on the side 60–180 mm H_2O

Intraocular pressure
1.3 to 2.6 kPa (10 to 20 mmHg)

Bibliography

Bain CM, Burton K, McGavigan CJ (2011) *Gynaecology Illustrated* 6th edn Churchill Livingstone

Boron WF, Boulpaep EL (2005) *Medical physiology* Updated edition Saunders: Oxford

Brashers VL (2006) *Clinical applications of pathophysiology: an evidence-based approach* 3rd edn Mosby: St Louis

British Nutrition Foundation. *Nutrition science.* Available online at: http://www.nutrition.org.uk/nutritionscience Available: 8 January 2014

Carroll RG (2006) *Elsevier's integrated physiology* Mosby: Edinburgh

Colledge MR, Walker BR, Ralston SH (2010) *Davidson's principles and practice of medicine* 21st edn Churchill Livingstone: Edinburgh

Cross SS Ed. (2013) *Underwood's Pathology: a Clinical Approach* 6th edn Churchill Livingstone: Edinburgh

Damjanov I (2008) *Pathophysiology* Saunders: Philadelphia

Department of Health (1991) *Dietary reference values of food energy and nutrients for the UK: COMA report* HMSO: London

des Jardins T, Burton GG (2011) *Clinical Manifestations and assessment of respiratory disease* 6th edn Mosby

Folkow B, Svanborg A (1993) *Physiology of Cardiovascular Aging* In Physiological Reviews 73 (4)

Friedman NJ, Kaiser PK (2007) *Essentials of ophthalmology* Saunders: Edinburgh

Gaw A, Murphy MJ, Cowan RA, et al. (2008) *Clinical biochemistry* 4th edn Churchill Livingstone: Edinburgh

Geissler CA, Powers HJ (2011) *Human nutrition* 12th edn Churchill Livingstone: Edinburgh

Guyton AC, Hall JE (2005) *Textbook of medical physiology* 11th edn Saunders: Edinburgh

Huether SE, McCance KL (2012) *Understanding pathophysiology*, 5th edn Mosby: St Louis

Islam N, Strouthidis N, Keegan D, et al. (2009) *Crash course: ophthalmology, dermatology, ENT* Mosby: Edinburgh

Jafek BW, Murrow BW (2005) *ENT secrets* 3rd edn Mosby: London

Kierszenbaum A, Tres LL (2012) *Histology and cell biology: an introduction to pathology* 3rd edn Mosby: Edinburgh

King T (2006) *Elsevier's integrated pathology* Mosby: Edinburgh

Klug WS, Cummings MR, Spencer CA, Palladino MA (2012) *Essentials of Genetics* 8th edn Pearson

Kumar P, Clark M (2012) *Clinical medicine* 8th edn Saunders: Edinburgh

Kumar V, Abbas AK, Aster JC (2013) *Robbins basic pathology* 9th edn Saunders: Edinburgh

Madigan MT, Martinko JM (2006) *Brock Biology of Microorganisms* 11th edn Pearson

Male D, Brostoff J, Roth DB, et al. (2013) *Immunology* 8th edn Mosby: Philadelphia

Martini FH, Nath JL (2012) *Fundamentals of anatomy and physiology* 9th edn Pearson/Benjamin Cummings: San Francisco

Masoro EJ, Austad SN (eds) (2011) *Handbook of the Biology of Aging* 2011 Academic Press

NICE guidelines: *hypertension* http://guidance.nice.org.uk/CG127 Available: 9 January 2014

Patton KT, Thibodeau GA (2013) *Anatomy and physiology* 8th edn Mosby: St Louis

Standring S (2008) *Gray's anatomy: the anatomical basis of clinical practice* 40th edn Churchill Livingstone: Edinburgh

Telser AG, Young JK, Baldwin KM (2007) *Elsevier's integrated histology* Mosby: Edinburgh

Tortora GJ, Derrickson BH (2011) *Principles of Anatomy and Physiology* 13th edn Wiley

Turnpenny P, Ellard S (2012) *Elements of Medical Genetics* 14th edn Elsevier

Vander JF, Gault JA (2007) *Ophthalmology secrets in color* 3rd edn Mosby: St Louis

World Health Organization 2012 *Good health adds life to years. Global brief for World Health Day 2012.* WHO 2012 Geneva. Available online at http://whqlibdoc.who.int/hq/2012/WHO_DCO_WHD_2012.2_eng.pdf (p. 10) Available: 8 January 2014

Young B, Lowe JS, Stevens A, et al. (2006) *Wheater's functional histology: a text and colour atlas* Churchill Livingstone: Edinburgh

Index

Page numbers followed by 'f' indicate figures, 't' indicate tables, and 'b' indicate boxes.